1994
YEAR BOOK OF
ANESTHESIOLOGY AND
PAIN MANAGEMENT®

Statement of Purpose

The YEAR BOOK Service

The YEAR BOOK series was devised in 1901 by practicing health professionals who observed that the literature of medicine and related disciplines had become so voluminous that no one individual could read and place in perspective every potential advance in a major specialty. In the final decade of the 20th century, this recognition is more acutely true than it was in 1901.

More than merely a series of books, YEAR BOOK volumes are the tangible results of a unique service designed to accomplish the following:

- to *survey* a wide range of journals of proven value

- to *select* from those journals papers representing significant advances and statements of important clinical principles

- to provide *abstracts* of those articles that are readable, convenient summaries of their key points

- to provide *commentary* about those articles to place them in perspective.

These publications grow out of a unique process that calls on the talents of outstanding authorities in clinical and fundamental disciplines, trained literature specialists, and professional writers, all supported by the resources of Mosby, the world's preeminent publisher for the health professions.

The Literature Base

Mosby subscribes to nearly 1,000 journals published worldwide, covering the full range of the health professions. On an annual basis, the publisher examines usage patterns and polls its expert authorities to add new journals to the literature base and to delete journals that are no longer useful as potential YEAR BOOK sources.

The Literature Survey

The publisher's team of literature specialists, all of whom are trained and experienced health professionals, examines every original, peer-reviewed article in each journal issue. More than 250,000 articles per year are scanned systematically, including title, text, illustrations, tables, and references. Each scan is compared, article by article, to the search strategies that the publisher has developed in consultation with the 270 outside experts who form the pool of YEAR BOOK editors. A given article may be reviewed by any number of editors, from one to a dozen or more, regardless of the discipline for which the paper was originally published. In turn, each editor who receives the article reviews it to determine whether or not the article should be included in the YEAR BOOK. This decision is based on the article's inherent quality, its probable usefulness to readers of that YEAR BOOK, and the editor's goal to represent a balanced picture of a given field in each volume of the YEAR BOOK. In addition, the editor indicates when to include figures and tables from the article to help the YEAR BOOK reader better understand the information.

Of the quarter million articles scanned each year, only 5% are selected for detailed analysis within the YEAR BOOK series, thereby assuring readers of the high value of every selection.

The Abstract

The publisher's abstracting staff is headed by a physician-writer and includes individuals with training in the life sciences, medicine, and other areas, plus extensive experience in writing for the health professions and related industries. Each selected article is assigned to a specific writer on this abstracting staff. The abstracter, guided in many cases by notations supplied by the expert editor, writes a structured, condensed summary designed so that the reader can rapidly acquire the essential information contained in the article.

The Commentary

The YEAR BOOK editorial boards, sometimes assisted by guest commentators, write comments that place each article in perspective for the reader. This provides the reader with the equivalent of a personal consultation with a leading international authority—an opportunity to better understand the value of the article and to benefit from the authority's thought processes in assessing the article.

Additional Editorial Features

The editorial boards of each YEAR BOOK organize the abstracts and comments to provide a logical and satisfying sequence of information. To enhance the organization, editors also provide introductions to sections or individual chapters, comments linking a number of abstracts, citations to additional literature, and other features.

The published YEAR BOOK contains enhanced bibliographic citations for each selected article, including extended listings of multiple authors and identification of author affiliations. Each YEAR BOOK contains a Table of Contents specific to that year's volume. From year to year, the Table of Contents for a given YEAR BOOK will vary depending on developments within the field.

Every YEAR BOOK contains a list of the journals from which papers have been selected. This list represents a subset of the nearly 1,000 journals surveyed by the publisher and occasionally reflects a particularly pertinent article from a journal that is not surveyed on a routine basis.

Finally, each volume contains a comprehensive subject index and an index to authors of each selected paper.

The 1994 Year Book Series

Year Book of Allergy and Clinical Immunology: Drs. Rosenwasser, Borish, Gelfand, Leung, Nelson, and Szefler

Year Book of Anesthesiology and Pain Management: Drs. Tinker, Abram, Chestnut, Roizen, Rothenberg, and Stoelting

Year Book of Cardiology®: Drs. Schlant, Collins, Engle, Gersh, Kaplan, and Waldo

Year Book of Chiropractic: Dr. Lawrence

Year Book of Critical Care Medicine®: Drs. Rogers and Parrillo

Year Book of Dentistry®: Drs. Meskin, Currier, Kennedy, Leinfelder, Berry, and Roser

Year Book of Dermatologic Surgery: Drs. Swanson, Glogau, and Salasche

Year Book of Dermatology®: Drs. Sober and Fitzpatrick

Year Book of Diagnostic Radiology®: Drs. Federle, Clark, Gross, Madewell, Maynard, Sackett, and Young

Year Book of Digestive Diseases®: Drs. Greenberger and Moody

Year Book of Drug Therapy®: Drs. Lasagna and Weintraub

Year Book of Emergency Medicine®: Drs. Wagner, Burdick, Davidson, McNamara, and Roberts

Year Book of Endocrinology®: Drs. Bagdade, Braverman, Poehlman, Kannan, Landsberg, Molitch, Morley, Odell, Rogol, Ryan, and Nathan

Year Book of Family Practice®: Drs. Berg, Bowman, Davidson, Dietrich, and Scherger

Year Book of Geriatrics and Gerontology®: Drs. Beck, Reuben, Burton, Small, Whitehouse, and Goldstein

Year Book of Hand Surgery®: Drs. Amadio and Hentz

Year Book of Hematology®: Drs. Spivak, Bell, Ness, Quesenberry, and Wiernik

Year Book of Infectious Diseases®: Drs. Keusch, Wolff, Barza, Bennish, Gelfand, Klempner, and Snydman

Year Book of Infertility®: Drs. Mishell, Lobo, and Sokol

Year Book of Medicine®: Drs. Epstein, Greenberger, Cline, Malawista, Utiger, Bone, O'Rourke, and Mandell

Year Book of Neonatal and Perinatal Medicine®: Drs. Klaus and Fanaroff

Year Book of Nephrology®: Drs. Coe, Favus, Henderson, Kashgarian, Luke, Myers, and Curtis

Year Book of Neurology and Neurosurgery®: Drs. Bradley and Crowell

Year Book of Neuroradiology: Drs. Osborn, Eskridge, Grossman, and Harnsberger

Year Book of Nuclear Medicine®: Drs. Hoffer, Gore, Gottschalk, Rattner, Zaret, and Zubal

Year Book of Obstetrics and Gynecology®: Drs. Mishell, Kirschbaum, and Morrow

Year Book of Occupational and Environmental Medicine: Drs. Emmett, Frank, Gochfeld, and Hessl

Year Book of Oncology®: Drs. Simone, Longo, Ozols, Steele, Glatstein, and Bosl

Year Book of Ophthalmology®: Drs. Laibson, Adams, Augsburger, Benson, Cohen, Eagle, Flanagan, Nelson, Rapuano, Reinecke, Sergott, and Wilson

Year Book of Orthopedics®: Drs. Sledge, Poss, Cofield, Frymoyer, Griffin, Hansen, Johnson, Simmons, and Springfield

Year Book of Otolaryngology–Head and Neck Surgery®: Drs. Paparella and Holt

Year Book of Pain: Drs. Gebhart, Haddox, Jacox, Payne, Rudy, and Shapiro

Year Book of Pathology and Clinical Pathology®: Drs. Gardner, Bennett, Cousar, Garvin, and Worsham

Year Book of Pediatrics®: Dr. Stockman

Year Book of Plastic, Reconstructive, and Aesthetic Surgery: Drs. Miller, Cohen, McKinney, Robson, Ruberg, and Whitaker

Year Book of Podiatric Medicine and Surgery®: Dr. Kominsky

Year Book of Psychiatry and Applied Mental Health®: Drs. Talbott, Frances, Breier, Meltzer, Perry, Schowalter, and Yudofsky

Year Book of Pulmonary Disease®: Drs. Bone and Petty

Year Book of Rheumatology: Drs. Sergent, LeRoy, Meenan, Panush, and Reichlin

Year Book of Sports Medicine®: Drs. Shephard, Drinkwater, Eichner, Sutton, Torg, Col. Anderson, and Mr. George

Year Book of Surgery®: Drs. Copeland, Deitch, Eberlein, Howard, Luce, Ritchie, Seeger, Souba, and Sugarbaker

Year Book of Thoracic and Cardiovascular Surgery: Drs. Ginsberg, Lofland, and Wechsler

Year Book of Transplantation: Drs. Ascher, Hansen, and Strom

Year Book of Ultrasound: Drs. Merritt, Babcock, Carroll, Goldstein, and Mittelstaedt

Year Book of Urology®: Drs. Gillenwater and Howards

Year Book of Vascular Surgery®: Dr. Porter

1994

The Year Book of ANESTHESIOLOGY AND PAIN MANAGEMENT®

Editor-in-Chief

John H. Tinker, M.D.
Professor and Head, Department of Anesthesia, University of Iowa, College of Medicine, Iowa City, Iowa

Editors

Stephen E. Abram, M.D.
Professor and Vice Chairman, Department of Anesthesiology, Pain Management Center, Medical College of Wisconsin, Milwaukee,, Wisconsin

David H. Chestnut, M.D.
Professor of Anesthesia and Obstetrics and Gynecology, Vice Chairman for Administration, Department of Anesthesia, University of Iowa College of Medicine, Iowa City, Iowa

Michael F. Roizen, M.D.
Professor and Chairman, Department of Anesthesia and Critical Care; Professor of Medicine, University of Chicago, Chicago, Illinois

David M. Rothenberg, M.D.
Associate Professor, Director, Division of Critical Care, Department of Anesthesiology, Rush-Presbyterian/St. Luke's Medical Center, Chicago, Illinois

Robert K. Stoelting, M.D.
Professor and Chair, Department of Anesthesia, Indiana University School of Medicine, Indianapolis, Indiana

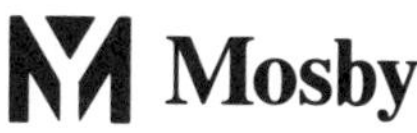

St. Louis Baltimore Boston Chicago London Madrid Philadelphia Sydney Toronto

Vice President and Publisher, Continuity Publishing: Kenneth H. Killion
Sponsoring Editor: Bernadette Buchholz
Illustrations and Permissions Coordinator: Bernadette R. Bauer
Manager, Literature Services: Edith M. Podrazik, R.N.
Senior Information Specialist: Terri Santo, R.N.
Information Specialist: Nancy Dunne, R.N.
Senior Medical Writer: David A. Cramer, M.D.
Senior Project Manager: Max F. Perez
Project Supervisor: Tamara L. Smith
Senior Production Editor: Wendi Schnaufer
Production Coordinator: Sandra Rogers
Editorial Coordinator: Rebecca Nordbrock
Proofroom Manager: Barbara M. Kelly

Printed in the United States of America
Composition by International Computaprint Corporation
Printing/binding by Maple-Vail

Mosby–Year Book, Inc.
11830 Westline Industrial Drive
St. Louis, MO 63146

Editorial Office:
Mosby–Year Book, Inc.
200 North LaSalle St.
Chicago, IL 60601

International Standard Serial Number: 1073-5437
International Standard Book Number: 0-8151-5986-2

Table of Contents

Mosby Document Express

Copies of the full text of the original source documents of articles abstracted or referenced in this publication are available by calling Mosby Document Express, toll-free, at **1 (800) 55-MOSBY.**

With Mosby Document Express, you have convenient, 24-hour-a-day access to literally every article on which this publication is based. In fact, through Mosby Document Express, virtually any medical or scientific article can be located and delivered by FAX, overnight delivery service, international airmail, electronic transmission of bitmapped images (via Internet), or regular mail. The average cost of a complete, delivered copy of an article, including up to $4 in copyright clearance charges and first-class mail delivery, is $12.

For inquiries and pricing information, please call the toll-free number shown above. To expedite your order for material appearing in this publication, please be prepared with the code shown next to the bibliographic citation for each abstract.

Journals Represented

Mosby subscribes to and surveys nearly 1,000 U.S. and foreign medical and allied health journals. From these journals, the Editors select the articles to be abstracted. Journals represented in this YEAR BOOK are listed below.

AORN: Journal of the American Operating Room Nurses Association
Acta Anaesthesiologica Scandinavica
American Journal of Cardiology
American Journal of Medicine
American Journal of Obstetrics and Gynecology
American Journal of Roentgenology
American Surgeon
Anaesthesia
Anaesthesia and Intensive Care
Anesthesia and Analgesia
Anesthesiology
Annals of Emergency Medicine
Annals of Internal Medicine
Annals of Thoracic Surgery
Archives of Internal Medicine
Archives of Pathology and Laboratory Medicine
Archives of Physical Medicine and Rehabilitation
Arthritis and Rheumatism
Arthroscopy
British Journal of Anaesthesia
British Journal of Surgery
British Medical Journal
Canadian Journal of Anaesthesia
Cancer
Chest
Circulation
Clinical Science
Critical Care Medicine
European Heart Journal
European Journal of Vascular Surgery
European Respiratory Journal
Gastrointestinal Endoscopy
Hepatology
International Journal of Obstetric Anesthesia
International Journal of Pediatric Otorhinolaryngology
Journal of Applied Physiology: Respiratory, Environmental and Exercise Physiology
Journal of Clinical Anesthesia
Journal of Consulting and Clinical Psychology
Journal of General Internal Medicine
Journal of Laryngology and Otology
Journal of Pediatric Surgery
Journal of Pediatrics
Journal of Reproductive Medicine
Journal of Thoracic and Cardiovascular Surgery
Journal of Trauma
Journal of Vascular Surgery
Journal of the American College of Cardiology
Journal of the American Medical Association
Journal of the Royal Society of Medicine

Lancet
Laryngoscope
Medical Journal of Australia
Neurosurgery
New England Journal of Medicine
New Zealand Medical Journal
Obstetrics and Gynecology
Orthopedics
Pain
Regional Anesthesia
S.A.M.J./S.A.M.T.-South African Medical Journal
Scandinavian Journal of Thoracic and Cardiovascular Surgery
Scandinavian Journal of Work, Environment and Health
Spine
Stroke
Surgery
Surgical Neurology
Transfusion
Western Journal of Medicine

Standard Abbreviations

The following terms are abbreviated in this edition: acquired immunodeficiency syndrome (AIDS), central nervous system (CNS), cerebrospinal fluid (CSF), computed tomography (CT), electrocardiography (ECG), human immunodeficiency virus (HIV), and magnetic resonance (MR) imaging (MRI).

Publisher's Preface

We are delighted to welcome John H. Tinker, M.D., and his associates, David M. Rothenberg, M.D., and David H. Chestnut, M.D., and to welcome back Michael F. Roizen, M.D., Robert K. Stoelting, M.D., and Stephen E. Abram, M.D., as editors of the 1994 YEAR BOOK OF ANESTHESIOLOGY AND PAIN MANAGEMENT.

This team is carrying on the tradition of distinguished editorial direction for the YEAR BOOK OF ANESTHESIOLOGY AND PAIN MANAGEMENT. We congratulate them and extend our appreciation for their superb work with the YEAR BOOK series.

Dr. Stoelting has been involved with the series since 1982. This is his final volume; we are truly grateful for the enormous amount of time and effort he has dedicated to this publication.

For the 1995 edition and beyond, Dr. Tinker and the editorial board will be joined by Margaret Wood, M.D., to carry on the tradition of excellence.

Introduction

Accepting a new challenge always involves a "learning curve." I hope the readers of the YEAR BOOK OF ANESTHESIOLOGY AND PAIN MANAGEMENT will grant me leeway as I try to fill the shoes of Dr. Ronald D. Miller who so ably served as Editor-in-Chief of this publication during the years 1982 through 1993. This publication has a long and distinguished history and is in a way returning "home," because its founding Editor-in-Chief, Dr. Stuart C. Cullen, was the academic founder of the Department of Anesthesia here at the University of Iowa. Another big set of shoes to fill.

This past year, most "hallway discussion" and much discussion at "scientific meetings" was all-too-often centered on economic issues, "health-care reform," outcomes, provider-specific outcome-related data releases, mergers, alliances, and the like. Legitimate science as it relates to improvement in drugs, techniques, monitors, and actual care of our patients tended to receive short shrift. Indeed, perhaps because so many have focused on "health-care reform" this past year, and because so much of what has been written recently about health-care reform is either unmitigated drivel, hopelessly out of date the day it was published, or both, it is reasonable for the clinical anesthesiologist to refocus on what we do so well, namely *care for our patients*. Despite the hue and cry mentioned above, considerable legitimate science has shown promise and progress this past year. Accordingly, my fellow editors and I have chosen these articles for your consideration. I ask the reader to digest the abstracts for their science, and not just the comments for their entertainment (and hopefully educational) values. I will list some important developments below.

With respect to mechanisms of anesthesia, new information indicated that genetic manipulations can alter sensitivity to anesthetic agents. This may unleash the power of molecular genetics in the study of specific mechanisms of anesthetic actions. In a fascinating paper, removal of the cerebral cortex does not change the minimum alveolar concentration! . . . at least in the rat. I wonder what *that* means.

In this YEAR BOOK OF ANESTHESIOLOGY AND PAIN MANAGEMENT, several controversies about N-methyl D-aspartate (NMDA) receptor antagonists, especially whether they may be cerebral protectants and whether they potentiate anesthetics, are addressed. So also is the issue of whether nitric oxide alters anesthetic potency. Nitric oxide itself is one of the hottest topics, with numerous studies of its effects on various vascular beds and other interesting areas, including clinical trials in neonates and adults with severe pulmonary/vascular dysfunction.

We have needed an "awareness monitor" for many years. This issue of the YEAR BOOK OF ANESTHESIOLOGY AND PAIN MANAGEMENT contains articles about new studies of auditory evoked potentials that may get us closer to that Holy Grail, in addition to several other studies of awareness and its ramifications during anesthesia.

This edition contains considerable examples of modern health services research, with numerous studies of outcome-related and cost-efficacy topics. The "regional vs. general" anesthesia battle is revisited. We have included a report of more than 45,000 ambulatory anesthetics and their outcomes.

The new anesthetic desflurane is of considerable interest, especially with respect to its acceptability compared with propofol and other agents in the important arena of postoperative nausea and vomiting.

The ongoing American Society of Anesthesiologists Closed Claims Study weighed in this year with an elegant report on mortality and morbidity related to anesthesia in pediatric patients. There are numerous other pediatric anesthesia studies of interest, with perhaps the hottest topic being postanesthetic apnea.

In the cardiovascular arena, hemodilution, coronary physiology, coronary pharmacology, and sympathetic responses to anesthesia were of considerable interest, as was the vasodilator adenosine. As often happens when I select papers about cardiovascular topics, several papers are selected to complain about them, often because 1 dose of 1 drug was used to compare with 1 dose of another drug instead of designing legitimate pharmacologic dose-response studies. Also as usual, numerous papers attempted to predict the incidence of myocardial ischemia and/or its consequences. I do not think success has crowned those efforts. The slogan "steal-prone anatomy" is nearly dead now, thanks to further studies reported in this edition. Anticoagulants are of interest in the cardiovascular arena as usual, and we are still struggling with the development of better monitors. Neurologic dysfunction after bypass remains problematic.

We included a number of articles about nerve injury and other peripheral postoperative neurologic deficits.

With respect to new drugs, studies of the opioid remifentanyl, the volatile anesthetics sevoflurane and desflurane, the new local anesthetic articaine, and numerous others are included. We still do not have perfect diagnostic abilities in the arena of malignant hyperthermia, and several papers are included to bring the reader up to date on that subject.

This year, the old problem of whether anesthetics affect postoperative infection resistance has been revisited.

One of the most novel ideas of the year is to use the police ethanol "breathalyzer" with a low concentration of intravenous ethanol during transurethral prostatectomy as a monitor for water intoxication! Halothane hepatotoxicity is probably best explained by trifluoroacetylated liver proteins that can then act as haptens. We now seem to have a pretty good handle on the mechanism of that old bugaboo, despite the fact that some internists call any postoperative jaundice "halothane hepatitis," whether or not halothane was given to the patient.

Obstetric anesthesia continues to be of great interest in our clinical science. Morbidly obese parturients are reported on in this edition. Spinal needles are undergoing interesting changes in their design. Cognitive deficits in women after childbirth were studied. It may now be possible to do better monitoring than just fetal heart rates by using intrapartum petal pulse oximetry (it is about time somebody did something better than simply heart rate). Intraspinal/epidural opiates come in for their fair share of attention (or more). Aspiration of gastric contents and prevention of same are still legitimate subjects for study in obstetric anesthesia (and elsewhere).

Neuromuscular blocker research has continued with emphasis on histamine and the possibility that the histamine releasers may lead to bronchospasm.

This edition carries a report about the possibility that prolonged propofol anesthesia may lead to seizures during awakening.

In critical care medicine, in keeping with our traditional practices, most articles chosen were predominantly published in nonanesthesiology journals. This chapter contains articles on monitoring equipment, cardiovascular resuscitation, respiratory failure, acute lung injury, mechanical ventilation and airway management, renal and acid base physiology, sepsis and infection, ethics, economics, and containment in the intensive care unit. Care that appears futile in the intensive care unit and in the emergency room is receiving considerable attention both in the lay and medical press.

In the area of critical care medicine again, inhalational nitric oxide is one of the hottest topics. We present an article on liquid perflurocarbons to improve oxygenation as well as other articles that deal with various new modes of pressure support ventilation. Articles also address risk variables for developing ventilator-associated pneumonia.

There might be some (slight) cause for hope that "newer cardiopulmonary resuscitation (CPR)" might work a little better than our standard CPR.

Numerous issues regarding postoperative and chronic pain management continue to receive literature attention. The use of intra-articular opioids vs. local anesthetics is still controversial. One study demonstrated benefit with morphine but not bupivacaine; one showed better analgesia with morphine plus bupivacaine than with either drug alone; and one study showed an analgesic effect from bupivacaine but not morphine. One could not be faulted for abandoning this technique until a more definitive answer is found.

Studies of the effect of systemic analgesics on postoperative pain cover a variety of issues, including possible preemptive effects of nonsteroidal anti-inflammatory drugs and systemic opioids (i.e., preoperative vs. postoperative administration), analgesic effect of dopaminergic and serotoninergic agonists, and intranasal and oral transmucosal opioid administration.

A popular issue regarding epidural analgesia for postoperative pain is the controversy regarding the spinal effects of epidural infusions of fentanyl and sufentanil. Most recent studies suggest that epidural infusions of lipid-soluble drugs work almost entirely by a systemic mechanism. Similarly, epidural clonidine has been shown to be only slightly more effective than systemic clonidine for postoperative pain. In another study, epidural clonidine, somewhat surprisingly, appeared to be associated with respiratory depression.

Epidural anesthesia was associated with superior analgesia and better pulmonary function than general in one study, but it failed to provide fewer pulmonary complications. Another study showed that epidural anesthesia was associated with less pain and nausea and earlier discharge time among outpatients.

In the area of cancer pain, a well-conducted, controlled study demonstrated that patients treated with neurolytic celiac plexus blocks achieved good analgesia with lower opioid doses and fewer side effects than patients treated with analgesics alone. A surprising study reported on a number of cancer patients receiving high-dose morphine who were able to achieve good analgesia and minimal side effects with relatively much lower doses of methadone. Tumor spread in an animal model was reversed by morphine analgesia. The possible implications among cancer patients undergoing surgery are obvious.

The chronic pain treatment literature includes a clinical trial of an intrathecal NMDA antagonist, stellate ganglion morphine injections, a description of the natural history of lumbar radiculopathy, low-level laser therapy, and investigations on the pathophysiology of fibromyalgia and herpes zoster.

A tremendous variety of pharmacologic studies in animals has led to new insights into pain mechanisms and to some interesting possibilities for future clinical interventions. There is little agreement on how quickly and under what circumstances animal data should be brought into clinical trials.

Returning to my original theme that despite the "gloom and doom" of health-care reform and despite President and Mrs. Clinton telling us that the profession in which we all have been toiling for so may years, so many hours each day and night, is somehow sick or broken, the truth is that we do administer more than 25 million anesthetics yearly in the United States alone with a remarkable track record of safety and efficacy. The truth is that our science is alive and well and progressing along many fronts. The truth is that our trainees are as bright and eager as ever (or better). As the HMOs, PPOs, IPAs, gatekeepers, DRGs, RBRVSs, ODSs, etc., attempt to regulate our behavior, take their financial cuts, and do whatever else they choose to do, there are still sick patients, plenty of them, seemingly getting younger, smaller, older, and bigger, not to mention sicker, every year. In 500 B.C., Heraclitus allegedly said, "Doctors cut, burn and torture the sick and then demand an undeserved fee for such service."

Medicine always was and will be political. Our advantage over quackery is our scientific base and our reliance on the scientific method whenever possible. Much of medicine is still experiential, not experimental, but readers of this edition of the YEAR BOOK OF ANESTHESIOLOGY AND PAIN MANAGEMENT will, I think, come away believing that scientific inquiry is alive and well in our specialty. I gratefully acknowledge the superb contributions of our colleagues in the specialty and my fellow editors of the YEAR BOOK OF ANESTHESIOLOGY AND PAIN MANAGEMENT.

John H. Tinker, M.D.

1 Preoperative Evaluation

Preadmission Clinics

Preadmission Anaesthesia Consultation Clinic
Conway JB, Goldberg J, Chung F (Univ of Toronto)
Can J Anaesth 39:1051–1057, 1992   101-94-1-1

Objective.—More and more ambulatory surgical patients are arriving for surgery without a formal preoperative anesthesiology assessment. As a result, many surgical procedures must be delayed or canceled. There is little information in the literature on one possible solution to this problem: the preadmission anesthesia consultation clinic. An initial experience in a newly established preadmission anesthesia consultation clinic was evaluated.

Clinic Description.—The clinic was established at a Canadian tertiary care hospital. Staff surgeons were asked to refer their high-risk surgical patients who might need special preoperative evaluation or preparation. All patients referred were seen by an attending staff anesthetist. For each patient, the anesthetist was asked to note whether the consultation was appropriate, i.e., did the patient require further preoperative evaluation or preparation or was the anesthetist able to obtain clear patient information affecting anesthetic management. Surgery was done 1 or 2 weeks later to allow the institution of any necessary preoperative measures.

Initial Results.—The investigators performed a prospective study of the first 400 patients referred to the clinic. Sixty percent of the patients had cardiovascular disease; 27% had coronary artery disease. Eighty-one percent of the referrals were appropriate, and many of the inappropriate referrals were from 1 surgeon who consistently referred healthy patients. Thirty-five percent of the patients had additional tests and 9% needed further consultation. The rate of surgical delay was 5% and the incidence of cancellations was 3%; these figures could have been reduced to .75% and 1.5%, respectively, with optimal functioning of the clinic. Ninety-two percent of the patients thought that the anesthetic consultation had improved their care and made them better informed.

Conclusion.—A preadmission anesthesia consultation clinic has the potential to reduce hospital costs while improving operating room efficiency. Most of the delays and cancellations noted in this study could have been eliminated if preadmission laboratory tests were better orga-

nized and if surgeons waited for the test results before scheduling surgery.

▶ This article reviewed the use of the preadmission anesthesia consultation clinic in this Canadian hospital to reduce delays before surgery and to reduce cancellations on the day of surgery. The authors found that from the hospital's standpoint, this setting up of a preadmission testing center appeared to be very cost-benefit effective, as they reduced delays from something around 17% to 5% and cancellations on the morning of surgery from 5% to around 1.5%. It looked like that type of reduction and improvement in care would result in less unoccupied operating rooms. Of interest, the consultations were all done by an attending staff anesthetist, and "in no case was there a delay or cancellation because of disagreement between the consultant anaesthetist and the anaesthetist providing perioperative care." I think this represents a key point and one that we have used in our preoperative clinic for the 7 years it has been in operation. That is, the people in the preoperative area have to ensure that they do a comprehensive enough history and physical examination so that unnecessary delays do not occur, and they have to see the patients far enough in advance to ensure that laboratory data and consultations are done and are pursued diligently and in such a fashion as to expedite surgery. In the 7 years, we have had almost 21,000 patients and we have had only 4 delays because of disagreement between the consultant anesthesiologist in the clinic and the one providing care on the day of surgery that were not caused by changes in patient history between the 2 time periods.

This article is useful to review some of the processes of setting up the clinic and some of the benefits of it. One item that makes me think there are still benefits from exchanging information is that all patients in Canada get a urinalysis whether or not they need it, apparently because the public hospital act of Ontario requires it. Much regulation in the United States, like much other government regulation, increases cost. It is too bad we cannot figure out a system that allows for the best information and care to be instantly translated to medical practice. It seems to me that much of the regulations that are promulgated often have unintended negative effects of either driving up the cost of care or rendering it impossible for the physician to do what is best for the patient. This article, although showing how an excellent group has tried to improve the quality of care, also reveals how government regulation impedes some of those changes.—M.F. Roizen, M.D.

Preoperative Potassium

Health Status and the Preoperative Change in Serum Potassium Concentration
Hahn RG, Löfgren A, Nordin AM (Huddinge Univ Hosp, Sweden)
Acta Anaesthesiol Scand 37:329–333, 1993
101-94-1–2

Background.—Anesthetists testing for preanesthetic abnormal serum potassium (S-K) levels often rely on blood tests performed on hospital admission, 1 or more days before surgery. However, the S-K level often changes between hospital admission and anesthesia induction. The effects of health status and medication on the preoperative change in S-K levels were studied in a group of unselected elderly men scheduled for urologic surgery.

Methods.—One hundred fifty men aged 45–88 years participated in the study. No oral medication was taken on the day of surgery.

Findings.—One third of the men had a change of .4 mmol/L or more. Increases were as common as decreases. Patients receiving calcium channel blocker or diuretic treatment had an increase in the S-K concentration preoperatively. Patients taking oral antidiabetics had a reduction. Beta-adrenoceptor antagonist use did not significantly predict changes in S-K concentrations.

Conclusion.—Changes in S-K were common before surgery in the patients studied. However, only a small proportion of the variance could be explained by health status and medication.

▶ This article again shows that S-K measurements seem to be much ado about nothing. They vary, have no relationship to morbidity or mortality, and undoubtedly cause more harm from their pursuit than benefit from their treatment. Maybe we should even stop writing about them or commenting on them. I look forward to the day when I can say, "Serum potassium measurements, in relatively healthy people—may they rest in peace."—M.F. Roizen, M.D.

Cardiac Risk Evaluation and Screening

Cardiac Risk Screening of Peripheral Arterial Surgical Patients by the Use of Combined Simple Clinical and Non-Invasive Cardiodynamic Parameters
Jivegård L, Haljamäe H, Holm J, Johansson SR (Sahlgrenska Hosp, Göteborg, Sweden)
Eur J Vasc Surg 7:180–187, 1993   101-94-1–3

Introduction.—Peripheral arterial surgical procedures are associated with a considerable risk of cardiac complications and death. Patients undergoing such procedures have a high incidence of coronary atherosclerosis impairing left ventricular function, but these risk factors may not be identified preoperatively. It was hypothesized that the predictive value of clinical cardiac risk indices would be improved by evaluation of hemoglobin concentration and cardiodynamic function.

Methods.—The prospective study included 195 patients undergoing 195 arterial surgical procedures during a 24-month period. Forty patients had diabetes and 88 had hypertension. A nurse examined all patients preoperatively using the Detsky multifactorial clinical cardiac risk index

(DRI), hemoglobin concentration, and resting computerized bioimpedance cardiodynamic measurements. The most common procedures were elective operations for lower-limb ischemia; standard arterial surgical techniques were used. Events recorded were cardiac death (CD) and potentially lethal cardiac complications (PLCs). Cardiac death was defined as death within 30 days after surgery from arrhythmia or progressive low cardiac output; PLCs were defined as nonfatal acute myocardial infarction, alveolar pulmonary edema, or life-threatening arrhythmia within 30 days after surgery.

Results.—There were 6 CDs and 11 PLCs within 30 days after surgery for an overall rate of serious cardiac complications of 8.7%. At a mean follow-up of 20 months, 148 patients (75.9%) were still alive. Cardiac death was best predicted by combining cardiodynamic measurements and DRI; PLC was best predicted by combining DRI and the hemoglobin concentration of the blood. The combination of DRI $\leq$ 10 and hemoglobin > 120 g/L identified a low-risk group with no CD or PLC.

Conclusion.—The sensitivity of clinical cardiac risk indices is low when applied to patients scheduled for peripheral arterial surgical procedures. The preoperative noninvasive cardiodynamic measurements used in this study, when combined with the hemoglobin concentration and the DRI, offer an inexpensive way of identifying low-risk patients. The more extensive and costly cardiac tests can thus be reserved for a more limited group of high-risk patients.

▶ It should be noted that most findings in this article resulted from a Detsky score differential of 10 or less and a hemoglobin concentration of greater than 120. Detsky's score, to remind ourselves, uses myocardial infarction, angina class, unstable angina within 3 months, ECG rhythm other than sinus or more than 5 premature ventricular contractions/min documented, suspected severe aortic valvular disease, age older than 70 years, emergency operation, poor general medical status, and pulmonary edema as its classifications. Thus, you can basically have only 1 of those conditions and still be at a low DRI that was correlated with good outcome in this study.

I believe that more and more we are going to see a swing away from technology and back toward the wise old clinician trying to walk the patient up 2 flights of stairs or using a hand bicycle ergometer for those who are arteropaths to see whether they can keep their pulse rate above 99 for 2 minutes while exercising as predictors of low cardiac morbidity.—M.F. Roizen, M.D.

Prognostic Value of Noninvasive Cardiac Tests in the Assessment of Patients With Peripheral Vascular Disease

Rose EL, Liu XJ, Henley M, Lewis JD, Raftery EB, Lahiri A (Northwick Park

Hosp and Clinical Research Centre, Harrow, Middlesex, England)
Am J Cardiol 71:40–44, 1993   101-94-1-4

Introduction.—Death from coronary artery disease is frequent in patients with peripheral vascular disease (PVD); thus, a prospective study was done of 145 patients with intermittent claudication who were seen in the vascular clinic of a district general hospital. Another 91 patients scheduled for elective surgery for abdominal aortic aneurysm, occlusive PVD, or carotid artery disease were also evaluated.

Methods.—A resting ECG was a routine part of the evaluation. Noninvasive cardiac studies including exercise ECG recording, Holter monitoring, nuclide ventriculography, and dipyridamole-thallium imaging were done for 168 of the 236 patients, including all those scheduled for surgery.

Results.—Cardiac events, including 4 deaths from congestive failure, 2 sudden cardiac deaths, and 1 death from myocardial infarction, occurred in 21 patients in all and in 18 of the 168 patients who had noninvasive cardiac studies. Clinical evidence of coronary artery disease was the best predictor of cardiac events. The heart-lung thallium-201 ratio and the left ventricular ejection fraction (LVEF) significantly improved the prediction of cardiac events.

Conclusion.—Although clinically evident coronary artery disease is the chief risk indicator in patients with PVD, useful information may be obtained by determining the LVEF or by analyzing the pulmonary uptake of radiothallium during dipyridamole stress.

▶ Clinical evidence of cardiovascular disease was the best predictor of adverse events after peripheral vascular surgery. The clinical evidence included a history of myocardial infarction; a history of angina or congestive heart failure; and left ventricular hypertrophy by echocardiography criteria. How the study participants actually questioned patients for angina or prior myocardial infarction was not revealed in the study. Thus, important improvements that can be made on this study involve revealing the method of questioning for cardiovascular disease, as well as what exercise tolerance and heart rate tolerance patients have to minor exercise tests.—M.F. Roizen, M.D.

Extent of Jeopardized Viable Myocardium Determined by Myocardial Perfusion Imaging Best Predicts Perioperative Cardiac Events in Patients Undergoing Noncardiac Surgery
Brown KA, Rowen M (Univ of Vermont, Burlington)
J Am Coll Cardiol 21:325–330, 1993   101-94-1-5

Introduction.—Recommendations for perioperative care in patients scheduled for noncardiac surgery who have transient radiothallium defects may be based in part on the extent of the perfusion abnormality, but it is not clear that this is a valid approach. Such defects are thought to represent jeopardized but viable myocardium. The risk of perioperative cardiac events (cardiac death, nonfatal myocardial infarction, and unstable angina) was related to the presence of transient defects on dipyridamole thallium-201 imaging in 231 consecutive patients undergoing noncardiac operations. Most had vascular reconstructive or bypass procedures.

Methods.—Each of 3 planar projections of the thallium perfusion scintigram was divided into 3 segments, and each of these segments was interpreted as being normal or exhibiting a transient or fixed defect. The ability of clinical factors and the imaging findings to predict perioperative cardiac events was estimated by stepwise multivariate logistic regression analysis.

Results.—Five patients died of cardiac causes, and 7 each had nonfatal myocardial infarction and unstable angina. The only significant predictors of cardiac death or nonfatal infarction were the number of myocardial segments wtih transient thallium defects and a history of diabetes. Use of a calcium channel blocker was an additional predictive factor when all cardiac events were considered.

Recommendation.—Because the risk of cardiac events after noncardiac surgery is most closely related to the extent of myocardium at risk, the extent of transient radiothallium defects should be routinely quantified in preoperative perfusion imaging.

▶ This study showed that people with transient myocardial defects on perfusion imaging have approximately a threefold increased incidence of cardiac events in the perioperative period compared with those without transient defects. This ratio is about half of that found in well-done studies in the literature (1). However, an even better predictor would be wall motion abnormalities on stress echo, or perhaps we are going back to exercise tolerance or ability to exercise with either hands or legs to get the heart rate greater than 99 beats/min for 2 minutes. Neither of these variables was tested in this study. Will we ever find the right preoperative test or preoperative assessment mode? That is, will people ever use the routine ones such as exercise tolerance or history to supplement these expensive tests?—M.F. Roizen, M.D.

Reference

1. Mantha S, et al: *Anesth Analg* 78:5266, 1994.

Effects of Surgical Stress and Volatile Anesthetics on Left Ventricular Global and Regional Function in Patients With Coronary Artery Disease: Evaluation by Computer-Assisted Two-Dimensional Quantitative Transesophageal Echocardiography

Houltz E, Gustavsson T, Caidahl K, Kirnö K, Lamm C, Milocco I, Ricksten S-E (Univ of Gothenburg, Sweden; Chalmers Univ of Technology, Gothenburg, Sweden)
Anesth Analg 75:679–687, 1992   101-94-1-6

Background.—Little is known about the effects of halothane, enflurane, and isoflurane on central hemodynamics and left ventricular global and regional function in patients with coronary artery disease. The effects of these agents when used to control intraoperative hypertension were examined in a prospective, randomized study.

Methods and Findings.—Thirty-nine patients with coronary artery disease composed the study population. Increased arterial blood pressure during sternotomy resulted from an increase in vascular resistance accompanied by increases in heart rate and filling pressures, but the global area ejection fraction (GAEF) declined. There were no changes in the segmental area ejection fraction (SAEF)–GAEF ratio during sternotomy. Inhaled anesthetics restored arterial blood pressure through a comparable reduction in vascular resistance. Isoflurane produced an increase in the cardiac index that was not seen with halothane or enflurane. Halothane reduced the GAEF, but isoflurane and enflurane had no effect. Isoflurane reduced the SAEF-GAEF ratios of 2 segments corresponding to the inferolateral wall of the left ventricle that was, in 1 segment, significantly more marked than with halothane and enflurane. Neither halothane nor enflurane changed regional wall motion.

Conclusion.—In patients wtih coronary artery disease, isoflurane is more likely to cause regional wall motion changes than halothane or enflurane. Regional wall motion changes induced by isoflurane appeared to be more pronounced in patients with other types of coronary anatomy than steal-prone coronary anatomy.

▶ In these patients, isoflurane tended to be associated with a more hyperdynamic circulation than either halothane or enflurane, when the volatile anesthetic was deliberately used to drop arterial pressure back to control levels after sternotomy. If isoflurane is not as much of a myocardial depressant, but more of a peripheral vasodilator than the other 2, then this hyperdynamism is explainable by that fact. If that in turn is true, then it is possible that the regional myocardial wall motion abnormalities observed by the authors to be more likely with isoflurane could be related to that hyperdynamism.

How clinically relevant is this study? Do we deliberately push the volatile anesthetic very hard after sternotomy to get the pressure back down to pre-sternotomy levels? I do not know the answer to that question, but I do know that only 15 μg of fentanyl per kg was "on board" when these measurements were made. Many cardiac anesthetists would opine that higher doses of fentanyl might have greatly smoothed these differences between the volatile agents. On the other hand, as we move toward earlier and earlier extubation, with less and less fentanyl as a "baseline," these differences might become important.—J.H. Tinker, M.D.

Assessment of Gastrointestinal Bleeding

Haemoglobin in Gut Lavage Fluid as a Measure of Gastrointestinal Blood Loss

Brydon WG, Ferguson A (Univ of Edinburgh, Scotland)
Lancet 340:1381–1382, 1992
101-94-1–7

Introduction.—A number of factors may interfere with currently available methods of detecting and measuring gastrointestinal bleeding, such as dilution by fecal bulk, inability to detect upper gastrointestinal bleeding, or the need to collect feces for several days. The clinical usefulness of measuring hemoglobin in whole-gut lavage fluid for the detection of gastrointestinal bleeding was examined.

Methods and Results.—The investigators performed whole-gut lavage in healthy subjects as well as in patients with various gastrointestinal diseases. They used the HemoQuant method for measurement of hemoglobin in the clear lavage fluid. Eleven healthy subjects had lavage fluid hemoglobin concentrations of .5 to 5.1 mg/L, which corresponded to a daily blood loss of .1 to 1.1 mL. In contrast, hemoglobin concentrations were significantly higher in 7 of 16 patients with active inflammatory bowel disease and normal or borderline in patients with inactive disease. Hemoglobin concentrations were normal in 4 patients with recent acute bleeding from gastric lesions and in 6 of 7 patients with benign colonic polyps. Higher concentrations—corresponding to estimated blood losses of 2.6 to 24.5 mL/day—were found in patients with colorectal cancer, severe diverticular disease, rectal varices, and iron-deficiency anemia thought to be caused by gastrointestinal bleeding.

Conclusion.—Gastrointestinal bleeding can be assessed by measurement of hemoglobin in whole-gut lavage fluid. The technique is a safe and easy one with many advantages over fecal collections. In many cases, lavage fluid can be obtained with no additional cost or patient discomfort.

▶ Whole-gut lavage, for those who are not familiar with it, as I was not familiar with it, in this case, is a measurement of blood in the first sample of clear fluid passed per rectum after oral Golytely administration. After the initial administration of Golytely, you get rid of solid feces and then gradually clear, and the first volume of completely clear fluid is what was collected and measured. As unappetizing as this may sound, it does seem like a low-cost method to measure gastrointestinal blood loss. Will we be seeing it routinely in patients, and should we be aware of its meaning? I do not know if we will be seeing it routinely, but, if we do, this article does help us by defining normal values.—M.F. Roizen, M.D.

Water With Premedication

Effects of Giving Water 20–450 ML With Oral Diazepam Premedication 1–2 H Before Operation

Søreide E, Holst-Larsen H, Reite K, Mikkelsen H, Søreide JA, Steen PA (Rogaland Central Hosp, Stavanger, Norway; Ullevaal Univ Hosp, Oslo, Norway)
Br J Anaesth 71:503–506, 1993   101-94-1–8

Introduction.—Recent studies have suggested that it is safe to avoid clear fluids for only 2–3 hours before surgery. The amount of water taken with tablets may influence the clinical effects of oral premedication, but little is known of the effects of giving variable amounts of water within 2 hours before induction of anesthesia, the time when most patients receive oral premedication.

Study Design.—Seventy-five patients scheduled for elective gynecologic laparoscopy were studied in an attempt to determine the proper volume of water that should accompany 10 mg of oral diazepam given 1–2 hours before induction of anesthesia. Groups of 25 patients were given 20, 150, or 300–450 mL of water. In all cases, anesthesia was induced with atropine, midazolam, and fentanyl and was maintained with enflurane and 67% nitrous oxide in oxygen.

Results.—Thirst and oral dryness were significantly reduced in all groups, but the effect was limited in patients given only 20 mL of water. Sedative effects were comparable in all groups. Only the patients given 150 mL of water reported significantly less anxiety. After surgery, there were no differences in thirst, sore throat, nausea, or gastric fluid volume and pH.

Conclusion.—Diazepam tablets given 1–2 hours before anesthesia should be taken with 150 mL of cold water.

2 Anesthetic Technique, Procedures, and Equipment

Preoxygenation

End-Tidal Oxygen Measurement Compared With Patient Factor Assessment for Determining Preoxygenation Time

Machlin HA, Myles PS, Berry CB, Butler PJ, Story DA, Heath BJ (Alfred Hosp, Melbourne, Australia)

Anaesth Intensive Care 21:409–413, 1993   101-94-2-1

Introduction.—The benefits of preoxygenation are widely accepted, but the time needed to sufficiently oxygenate the lungs has not been definitively established. A large series of patients undergoing elective surgery was studied to determine the time required for adequate preoxygenation.

Methods.—Two hundred patients were included in the study in which end-tidal oxygen concentration was measured. A variety of patient fac-

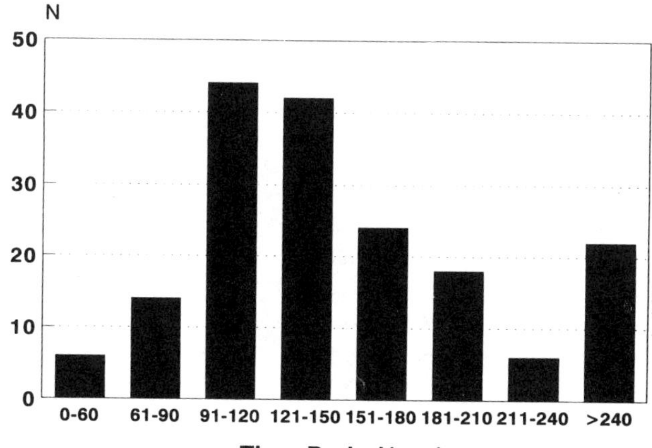

Fig 2–1.—Frequency distribution of time periods required to achieve an end-tidal oxygen concentration of 90% (*n* = 177). (Courtesy of Machlin HA, Myles PS, Berry CB, et al: *Anaesth Intensive Care* 21:409–413, 1993.)

tors was analyzed to determine whether any of them predicted the time needed to preoxygenate a patient.

Findings.—Twenty-three patients (11.5%) could not be preoxygenated adequately, usually because of a poor mask fit. The mean preoxygenation time was 154 seconds. Twenty-three percent of the patients who could be adequately preoxygenated needed more than 3 minutes. A clinically useful predictive equation could not be established (Fig 2–1).

Conclusion.—The time required for adequate preoxygenation cannot be accurately predicted. A routine 3 minutes may not be sufficient for many patients. However, measuring end-tidal oxygen concentration is useful for determining the end point for preoxygenation.

▶ Preoxygenation is more accurately described as denitrogenation. Body habitus and/or co-existing lung disease may influence the effectiveness of various preoxygenation regimens. In healthy, awake patients, the increase in arterial hemoglobin oxygen saturation achieved with 4 vital capacity breaths of 100% oxygen over 30 seconds is similar to that achieved during breathing 100% oxygen for 3 to 5 minutes at normal tidal volumes.—R.K. Stoelting, M.D.

Preoxygenation Techniques: The Value of Nitrous Oxide

Khoo ST, Woo M, Kumar A (Natl Univ of Singapore)
Acta Anaesthesiol Scand 37:23–25, 1993   101-94-2–2

Introduction.—Using the pulse oximeter, the maximum safe level of inspired nitrous oxide that can be given during preoxygenation was determined. This noninvasive method detects hypoxemia long before it is clinically apparent.

Patients and Methods.—Seventy-five healthy patients scheduled for elective surgery took part in the study. They were divided into 3 equal groups for preoxygenation, receiving 100% oxygen (group I), a mixture of 50% oxygen and 50% nitrous oxide (group II), or a mixture of 30% oxygen and 70% nitrous oxide (group III). All patients were then induced with thiopentone, paralyzed with suxamethonium, and intubated orally. The 3 groups were compared for changes in the arterial oxygen saturation, recorded every 5 seconds after the start of thiopentone injection.

Results.—Control saturation values, obtained after application of the finger probe of the pulse oximeter, were comparable in the 3 groups; the median control saturation of the patients was 98%. All 3 groups showed significant increases in the arterial oxygen saturation relative to control values. Further increases occurred after thiopentone induction. Although patients in all 3 groups desaturated below their preinduction values during intubation, none desaturated significantly below their respective control values (Fig 2–2). No patient showed clinical signs of hypoxemia.

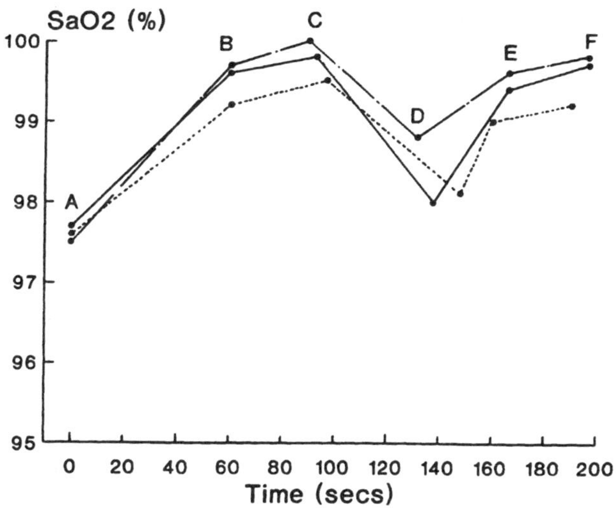

Fig 2–2.—Changes in arterial oxygen saturation (Sao_2) during preoxygenation, induction of anesthesia, and intubation. A is the control; B is the preinduction, Sao_2 after 1 minute of preoxygenation, start of thiopentone injection; C is the start of suxamethonium injection; D is the lowest Sao_2 recorded during suxamethonium-induced apnea; E is Sao_2 immediately postintubation; F is 30 seconds after intubation and manual ventilation with 100% oxygen. Group I (*solid line*), group II (*dash-dot-dash line*), group III (*dashed line*). (Courtesy of Khoo ST, Woo M, Kumar A: *Acta Anaesthesiol Scand* 37:23–25, 1993.)

Conclusion.—A mixture of oxygen and nitrous oxide for preoxygenation will accelerate the buildup of alveolar nitrous oxide concentration and facilitate induction. In this study, preoxygenation for 1 minute with either 100% oxygen or mixtures of 30% or 50% oxygen in nitrous oxide were equally effective in preventing arterial desaturation. Patients with cardiopulmonary disease or other medical problems may require longer periods of preoxygenation.

▶ I cannot endorse the logic of including nitrous oxide in the preoxygenation period based on a more rapid "build-up of alveolar nitrous oxide concentration" and to "facilitate induction" with thiopental.—R.K. Stoelting, M.D.

Laryngoscopy and Intubation

Mandibulohyoid Distance in Difficult Laryngoscopy

Chou H-C, Wu T-L (Kaiser Permanente Med Ctr, Hayward, Calif)
Br J Anaesth 71:335–339, 1993   101-94-2–3

Introduction.—Difficult laryngoscopy has been attributed to a variety of factors. To define a predictive indicator of difficult intubation, the lateral cervical x-ray scans were reviewed for 11 patients in whom conventional rigid laryngoscopy by experienced anesthetists failed.

Methods.—Radiographs of the 11 patients were compared with those of 100 controls and 1 patient with a severely receding jaw and protruding upper incisors in whom intubation was performed without difficulty. Measurements were taken of the vertical distance between the mandible and the hyoid bone (mandibulohyoid distance), and the positions of the mandibular angle and hyoid bone were determined in relation to the cervical vertebrae. Data were analyzed separately by gender.

Results.—Significant differences were noted in the mean mandibulohyoid distances of both male study and control subjects (33.8 mm vs. 21.4 mm) and female study and control subjects (26.4 mm vs. 15.4 mm). Patients in whom the trachea was difficult to intubate tended to have a relatively long mandibulohyoid distance. In both men and women patients with a long mandibulohyoid distance, the mandibular angle tended to be situated more rostrally; among women patients, the hyoid bone tended to be situated more caudally.

Conclusion.—The interaction of many anatomical factors can result in difficult laryngoscopy. A relatively short mandibular ramus or a relatively caudal larynx may contribute to problems with intubation. Of the 11 patients, 5 had a receding jaw, but this characteristic did not prevent intubation in a patient with a relatively normal mandibulohyoid distance. The mandible and hyoid bones are easily identified anatomical landmarks; they may provide a preoperative indication of a difficult intubation.

▶ It is unlikely that any single anatomical finding will always predict the ease or difficulty of tracheal intubation using direct laryngoscopy. Nevertheless, the ability to visualize the uvula with the patient sitting and facing the examiner during a preoperative evaluation (Mallampati class I) is reassuring and, in my experience, 100% predictive of successful tracheal intubation.—R.K. Stoelting, M.D.

Orotracheal Intubation in Patients With Potential Cervical Spine Injuries: An Indication for the Gum Elastic Bougie
Nolan JP, Wilson ME (Royal United Hosp, Bath, England)
Anaesthesia 48:630–633, 1993   101-94-2–4

Background.—Patients with injuries to the cervical spine may require urgent tracheal intubation without causing further damage, but the best method of achieving intubation remains controversial. One school of thought suggests immobilization of the neck in a neutral position using manual in-line stabilization and application of cricoid pressure. However, because the position of the head differs from that ideal for intubation, it may be more difficult to view the larynx.

Methods.—In 157 patients undergoing elective surgery, the conditions for emergency tracheal intubation of patients with cervical spine injury

Grades of View at Laryngoscopy

	Grade			
	1	2	3	Total
Optimum position	129 (82.2)	26 (16.5)	2 (1.3)	157 (100)
Neutral, manual in-line stabilisation position	75 (47.8)	48 (30.6)	34 (21.6)	157 (100)

Note: Values in parentheses are percentages.
(Courtesy of Nolan JP, Wilson ME: *Anaesthesia* 48:630–633, 1993.)

were simulated during induction of anesthesia. The view of the larynx during laryngoscopy with the head in the optimum intubating position was compared with that obtained when manual in-line stabilization of the cervical spine and cricoid pressure were used. The amount of larynx exposed was classified as grade 1 when at least some of the glottis was seen, grade 2 when only the arytenoids were exposed, grade 3 when the glottis could not be viewed, and grade 4 when neither the glottis nor the epiglottis was seen. With the head maintained in a neutral position with manual in-line stabilization and application of cricoid pressure, the time taken to achieve intubation with the aid of a gum elastic bougie was compared with the time needed with direct visual intubation.

Results.—During laryngoscopy with cervical stabilization, the view of the larynx was reduced by at least 1 grade in about 45% of patients, and the epiglottis could not be seen in 22% (table). Although the visual technique was quicker (median time, 20 seconds), intubation took longer than 45 seconds in 6 patients. Furthermore, 5 patients could not be directly intubated. With the use of the gum elastic bougie, all patients were successfully intubated within 45 seconds (median, 25 seconds), including all 5 failed visual intubations.

Conclusion.—The use of a gum elastic bougie is recommended for intubating the acute trauma patient with suspected cervical spine injury, particularly when the glottis is not immediately visible.

Urgent Paralysis and Intubation of Trauma Patients: Is It Safe?
Rotondo MF, McGonigal MD, Schwab CW, Kauder DR, Hanson CW (Hosp of the Univ of Pennsylvania, Philadelphia)
J Trauma 34:242–246, 1993
101-94-2–5

Background.—There has been reluctance to apply urgent paralysis and orotracheal intubation in the management of trauma patients, because of fear of an increase in the incidence of intubation mishaps and pulmonary complications. Since 1987, this technique has been applied in patients with complex injury or combative behavior. To evaluate the corre-

Intubation Mishaps, Pulmonary Complications, and Injury Severity
Scores by Location of Procedure

	Operating Room	Trauma Admitting Area and Radiology Suite
Number of intubation mishaps		
Multiple attempts	11	3
Aspiration	0	7
Esophageal intubations	1	2
Totals	12	12
Number of pulmonary complications	4	11*
Number of intubation mishaps and pulmonary complications	1	1
ISS	13.6 ± 7.9	20.6 ± 15.8†

Note: Injury Severity Scores (ISS) reported as mean ± 1 SD.
* $P < .001$, Student's t-test.
† $P < .012$, Fisher's exact test.
(Courtesy of Rotondo MF, McGonigal MD, Schwab CW, et al: *J Trauma* 34:242–246, 1993.)

lations between the use of paralysis and intubation and intubation mishaps and pulmonary complications, a retrospective study was conducted.

Setting.—Between January and December of 1989, 851 patients meeting major trauma triage guidelines were evaluated. Of those, 231 (27%) underwent urgent paralysis and orotracheal intubation within 8 hours of admission. Intubation was performed by the anesthesia resident (postgraduate year 2–4). All procedures used the rapid-sequence induction technique.

Outcome.—A total of 204 patients had assessable medical records. Indications for urgent paralysis and intubation were emergency surgery in 131, airway control in 30, combativeness in 24, and hyperventilation in 19. The procedure was performed in the operating room in 121 cases (59%), in the trauma admitting center in 82 cases, and in another location in 1 case.

There were 24 (12%) intubation mishaps, including 14 multiple attempts, 7 aspirations, and 3 esophageal intubations. Although patients intubated in the trauma admitting area were more severely injured and had more pulmonary complications, the occurrence of intubation mishaps was not related to the procedure location (table). Among the 194 patients who survived at least 24 hours, 15 (8%) had pulmonary complications, including pneumonia in 8, persistent infiltrates in 5, and severe atelectasis in 2. No deaths were related to intubation mishaps or pulmonary complications. There was no statistical relationship between the occurrence of intubation mishaps and subsequent pulmonary complications, although patients with pulmonary complications had significantly higher scores on the Abbreviated Injury Scale and Injury Severity Score.

Conclusion.—Urgent paralysis and orotracheal intubation in patients who have sustained trauma is a safe and efficient means to gain rapid airway and control combative behavior.

▶ Both of these studies (Abstracts 101-94-2-4 and 101-94-2-5) suggest that emergency intubation of trauma patients can be safely facilitated by the use of general anesthesia and muscle relaxants, in association with cricoid pressure and manual in-line cervical stabilization. This practice is opposed by those who insist that awake fiberoptic intubation, awake blind nasal intubation, or cricothyroidotomy are the optimal methods of securing the airway of a patient with a suspected cervical spine injury. Results of the gum elastic bougie being used in actual trauma patients still need to be evaluated, as this first study was only simulated. Relative to the overall safety of urgent paralysis, it is interesting to note that in the latter study, all aspirations occurred outside of the operating room, the conclusion being that the safest method of emergency intubation in the trauma or cervical spine injury patient is the one that uses the most experienced hands.—D.M. Rothenberg, M.D.

Tracheal Tube Cuff Inflation As an Aid to Blind Nasotracheal Intubation

Van Elstraete AC, Pennant JH, Gajraj NM, Victory RA (Univ of Texas, Dallas)
Br J Anaesth 70:691–693, 1993   101-94-2-6

Background.—Inflation of the tracheal tube cuff has been described in a case report as a way to avoid malpositioning in blind nasotracheal intubation. However, the efficacy of this maneuver has not been tested formally.

Methods.—The efficacy of tracheal tube cuff inflation in the oropharynx as an aid to blind nasotracheal intubation was studied in a prospective, randomized trial. Twenty patients, American Society of Anesthesiologists class I and II, undergoing elective oral surgery were included. The trachea was intubated once using the tube cuff inflation technique and once with the tracheal tube cuff deflated (Fig 2–3).

Findings.—Intubation was successful in 45% of patients while the cuff was deflated. In 40%, it was successful on the first attempt. With the tracheal tube cuff inflated, intubation was successful in 95% of the patients. Seventy-five percent of those were successful on the first attempt. The difference in the success rates was significant. Intubation times did not differ significantly.

Conclusion.—In normal patients, inflation of the tracheal tube cuff in the oropharynx increases the success rate of blind nasotracheal intubation. It has not yet been established whether this technique would im-

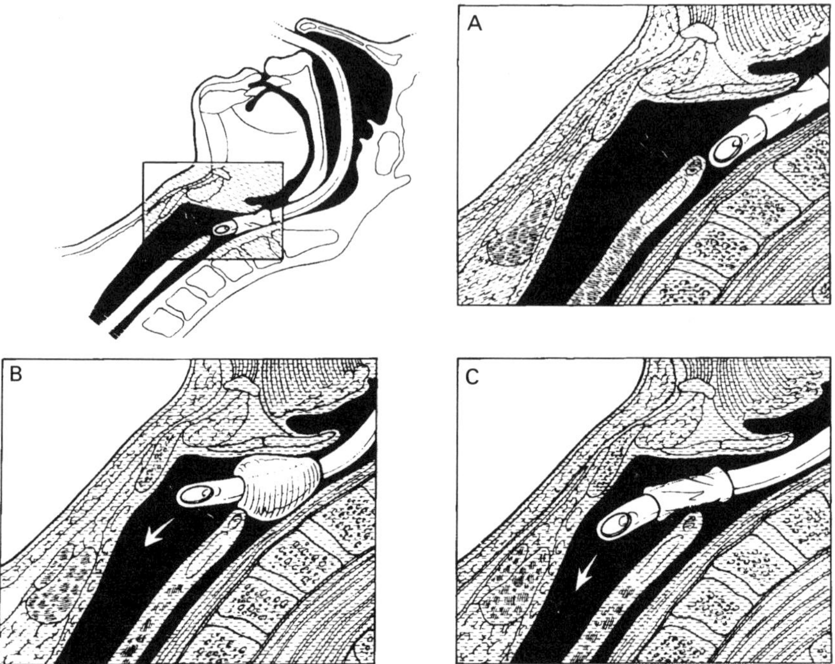

Fig 2–3.—Technique of tracheal tube (*TT*) cuff inflation in the oropharynx for blind nasotracheal intubation. **A,** the tip of the TT is positioned in the oropharynx; *B,* the cuff is inflated using 15 mL of air and the TT is advanced until the cuff contacts the vocal cords; **C,** the cuff is deflated and the TT is advanced into the trachea. (Courtesy of Van Elstraete AC, Pennant JH, Gajraj NM, et al: *Br J Anaesth* 70:691–693, 1993.)

prove the success rate of blind nasotracheal intubation in patients who are difficult to intubate.

▶ Fiberoptic laryngoscopy is threatening to make blind nasotracheal intubation an historic technique. Nevertheless, the potential value of an inflated tracheal tube cuff while the tube is in the pharynx is intriguing and worth trying the next time you attempt this technique. Remember, however, to deflate the cuff before advancing the tube through the glottis.—R.K. Stoelting, M.D.

Tracheal Intubation Without the Use of Muscle Relaxants: A Technique Using Propofol and Varying Doses of Alfentanil

Scheller MS, Zornow MH, Saidman LJ (Univ of California, San Diego)
Anesth Analg 75:788–793, 1992   101-94-2-7

Background.—For some patients receiving propofol and alfentanil for induction of anesthesia, the trachea can be intubated with no need for concomitant neuromuscular blockade. The airway management, tracheal intubation, and hemodynamic responses in patients receiving alfentanil

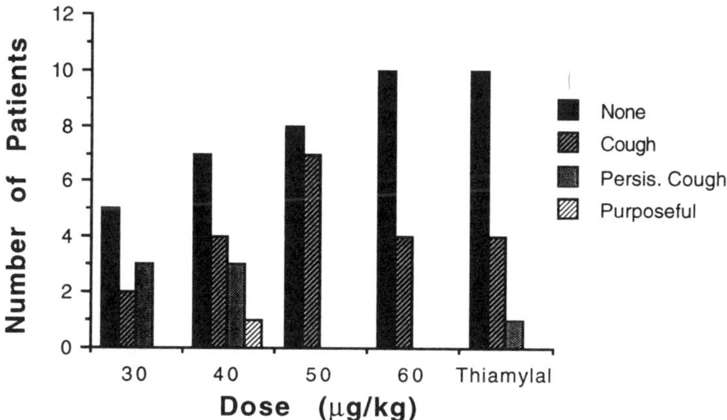

Fig 2–4.—Response to tracheal intubation. *None* denotes no coughing or movement. *Cough* denotes 1 or 2 coughs after insertion of tracheal tube. *Persis. Cough* denotes 3 or more coughs. *Purposeful* denotes purposeful movement during or after tracheal intubation. (Courtesy of Scheller MS, Zornow MH, Saidman LJ: *Anesth Analg* 75:788–793, 1992.)

and propofol vs. a standard thiamylal/succinylcholine induction sequence were studied.

Methods.—The subjects were 75 outpatients scheduled for various surgical procedures. All were in American Society of Anesthesiologists physical status I or II with Mallampati class I airways. Premedication with midazolam, 1 mg intravenously, was given to all patients before induction. They were then randomized into 5 groups: 1 received *d*-tubocurarine, 3 mg; thiamylal, 4 mg/kg; and succinylcholine, 1 mg/kg intravenously; the other 4 received alfentanil at 30, 40, 50, or 60 µg/kg. The last 4 groups received no muscle relaxants. One blinded investigator was responsible for airway management.

Results.—All patients were easily ventilated by mask and all had adequate jaw relaxation. One third of the patients receiving the lowest dose of alfentanil could not be intubated because of poor cord exposure or closed vocal cords. The cord position was more often better in the other 3 alfentanil groups (Fig 2-4). After induction, all alfentanil groups had a decreased heart rate and arterial blood pressure, with no differences between groups. The thiamylal/succinylcholine patients had a significantly increased heart rate after induction. They also had a significantly increased mean arterial pressure after laryngoscopy and tracheal intubation.

Conclusion.—With premedication, healthy outpatients with good airway anatomy can undergo tracheal intubation with the combination of alfentanil, 40 µg/kg, and propofol, 2 mg/kg. Acceptable jaw mobility, mask ventilation, vocal cord exposure or position, or movement in response to ventilation may not require muscle relaxants. This technique may avoid the adverse effects of muscle relaxants for selected patients.

▶ A nondepolarizing muscle relaxant replacement for succinylcholine will neutralize many of the reasons for considering tracheal intubation without the aid of skeletal muscle relaxation. In this regard, mivacurium has an attractive duration of action whereas rocuronium has the more desirable onset of action. Perhaps someone will find a way to combine the attractive features of both.—R.K. Stoelting, M.D.

Estimation of the Correct Length of Tracheal Tubes in Adults

Patel N, Mahajan RP, Ellis FR (St James's Univ Hosp, Leeds, England; Pinderfields Gen Hosp, Wakefield, England)
Anaesthesia 48:74–75, 1993   101-94-2–8

Background.—Determining the correct length of a tracheal tube is very important. Such tubes should be tailored for each individual patient. Existing formulas and tables for estimating tube length are not completely satisfactory. A simple method was developed.

Methods and Findings.—Predicted tube lengths were established before induction of anesthesia for each of 108 patients needing tracheal intubation. The upper end of the cuff was aligned externally with the cricoid cartilage, leaving the more proximal part of the tube lying alongside the neck toward the angle of the mandible. The tube was then curved forward, toward the upper incisor teeth, and the length at the teeth or gums was noted. The anesthetist intubated the trachea without knowing the predicted length of the tube. The tube length was standardized in relation to the vocal cords, and the actual length of the inserted tube was documented. The estimated length was then compared with the actual

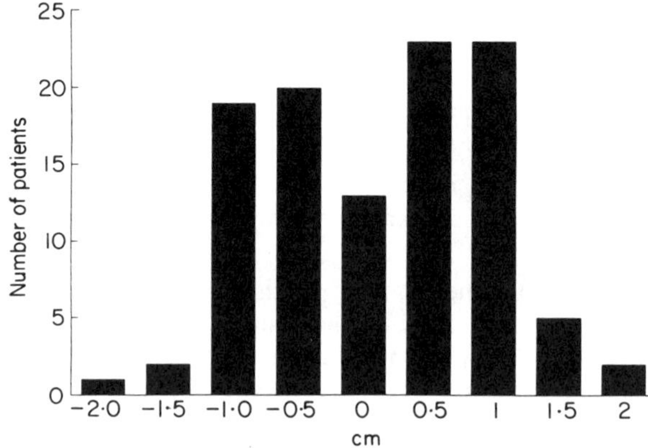

Fig 2–5.—Differences between estimated and actual lengths of tracheal tubes. (Courtesy of Patel N, Mahajan RP, Ellis FR: *Anaesthesia* 48:74–75, 1993.)

length. Estimated lengths were within 1 and 1.5 cm of the actual length in 91% and 97% of the patients, respectively (Fig 2–5).

Conclusion.—The presented method for estimating the required length of tracheal tubes is simple, quick, noninvasive, and reliable. In all patients studied, the clinical signs indicated correct placement of the tracheal tube. Careful clinical checks are still needed, however, and difficult cases of tube placement require radiographic or endoscopic confirmation.

▶ Confirmation of tracheal placement of the tube is best determined by capnography, not radiographic or endoscopic examinations.—R.K. Stoelting, M.D.

The Laryngeal Mask Airway

The Laryngeal Mask Airway Facilitates Intubation at Cesarean Section: A Case Report of Difficult Intubation
Hasham FM, Andrews PJD, Juneja MM, Ackerman WE III (Univ of Louisville, Ky; Norton Hosp, Louisville, Ky)
Int J Obstet Anesth 2:181–182, 1993   101-94-2–9

Introduction.—The laryngeal mask airway (LMA) has been successfully used in the United Kingdom in cases of failed or difficult intubation. In the present case, the LMA was used after failed intubation for emergency cesarean section, and subsequently to facilitate endotracheal intubation.

Case Report.—Woman, 33, was admitted in established labor at the end of her fifth pregnancy. Variable and late fetal heart rate decelerations prompted a decision to perform operative delivery under spinal anesthesia. Fetal bradycardia of 60 beats per minute developed when the patient was positioned for spinal block, indicating the need for immediate section delivery. The glottic structures could not be visualized using various blades, but a size 3 LMA was readily passed, allowing manual ventilation with 100% oxygen. Subsequently anesthesia was maintained with 2.5% and then 1% isoflurane in 50% nitrous oxide–oxygen. After delivery, the LMA was exchanged for a size 8 tracheal tube using a medium-size exchanger. Cricoid pressure was maintained throughout. Oxygen saturation never decreased to less than 93%.

Discussion.—Use of a LMA was an effective emergency procedure in this patient. Endotracheal intubation was elected to protect the airway should aspiration occur. A small endotracheal tube may be passed directly through the LMA.

▶ The LMA may serve 2 roles in the management of failed intubation at cesarean section. First, the LMA may be used as an alternative to mask ventilation. Second, the LMA may be used to facilitate endotracheal intubation, as was done in this case. It seems prudent to learn to use the LMA in *elective* cases, so that one does not use it for the first time in a case of failed intubation.—D.H. Chestnut, M.D.

Cricoid Pressure May Prevent Insertion of the Laryngeal Mask Airway

Ansermino JM, Blogg CE (Churchill Hosp, Oxford, England; Radcliffe Infirmary, Oxford, England)
Br J Anaesth 69:465–467, 1992   101-94-2-10

Background.—The laryngeal mask airway (LMA) is an effective alternative for achieving a clear airway when tracheal intubation is difficult or impossible. Maintaining cricoid pressure during LMA insertion after failed intubation has been recommended, although there have been no data to support this practice. The effect of applying cricoid pressure on the ability to insert the LMA correctly was studied.

Methods.—Forty-two women aged 18–40 years who were undergoing elective surgery were randomly assigned to 2 groups. After induction of anesthesia, the LMA was inserted with cricoid pressure in 1 group and without it in the other.

Findings.—Insertion was successful after the first or second attempt in 19 of the 22 patients in the noncricoid pressure group and in only 3 of 20 patients in the cricoid pressure group. After removal of cricoid pressure, the LMA was inserted successfully in all 17 patients (Fig 2–6).

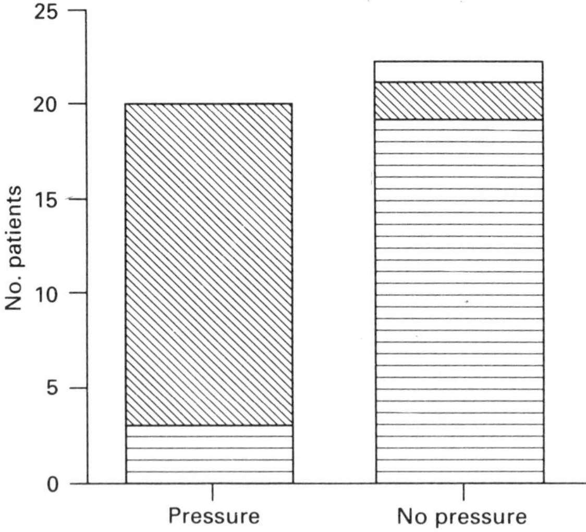

Fig 2–6.—Success and failure of insertion of LMA in patients with and without cricoid pressure. *Open space* indicates failure; *diagonal lines,* achieved after removal of screen; *horizontal lines,* achieved at first or second attempt. (Courtesy of Ansermino JM, Blogg CE: *Br J Anaesth* 69:465–467, 1992.)

Conclusion.—After failed intubation in patients with a significant risk of regurgitation and for whom ventilation can be maintained with a face mask while cricoid pressure is applied, it appears safer to continue with face mask anesthesia than to try to insert a LMA. When a clear airway cannot be maintained, inserting a LMA may be an alternative to cricothyroid puncture.

▶ A LMA is unquestionably no substitute for a cuffed tracheal tube if the greatest perceived risk to the patient is regurgitation and aspiration. Nevertheless, to abandon the LMA in favor of mask ventilation with cricoid pressure on the assumption that the latter is the best protection against aspiration seems unreasonable. In this situation, I would opt for a patent upper airway provided by the LMA and give up cricoid pressure.—R.K. Stoelting, M.D.

Comparison of the Anesthetic Requirement for Tolerance of Laryngeal Mask Airway and Endotracheal Tube
Wilkins CJ, Cramp PGW, Staples J, Stevens WC (Oregon Health Sciences Univ, Portland)
Anesth Analg 75:794–797, 1992   101-94-2-11

Introduction.—One way to avoid some of the problems in ensuring a patent airway and adequate ventilation during anesthesia may be the use of the laryngeal mask airway (LMA). This device can provide a clear airway for patients in whom conventional mask anesthesia is difficult or impossible and in whom tracheal intubation is difficult or undesirable. The LMA was tolerated at much lighter levels of anesthesia than was an endotracheal tube (ET) in one investigation.

Methods.—Twenty unpremedicated, nonsmoking patients, 18 to 40 years of age, were randomized to receive either an ET or LMA. All patients were of American Society of Anesthesiologists physical status I or II and had an operation lasting longer than 1 hour. The airway was inserted after induction of anesthesia with intravenous propofol.

Patients with an ET received vecuronium, .015 mg/kg intravenously, followed by succinylcholine, 1.5 mg/kg. Isoflurane and nitrous oxide, approximately 66% in oxygen, were the only means of anesthetic maintenance. Gas concentrations were measured by a spectrometer sampling from the breathing circuit end of the airway. As the procedure was coming to a close, the end-tidal nitrous oxide concentration was decreased to less than 3 vol% and the isoflurane concentration to .8 vol%. The end-trial isoflurane concentration was then decreased in .1% increments, and the patients were observed for any reaction to their LMA or ET.

Results.—The 2 groups were similar in terms of age, gender distribution, duration of nitrous oxide exposure, propofol dosage, time to achieving final end-tidal isoflurane concentration, and time to rejecting the airway. The mean end-tidal isoflurane concentration was .55% for reaction to the ET vs. .35% for reaction to the LMA. Signs of airway rejection included swallowing, coughing, or biting, sometimes with head movements.

Conclusion.—The clinical impression that the LMA is tolerated at lighter levels of isoflurane anesthesia than is the ET was confirmed. This may result in less cardiovascular depression and quicker recovery times, as well as fewer episodes of coughing, breath holding, and bronchospasm during emergence from anesthesia.

▶ The LMA should mimic an oropharyngeal airway with regard to upper airway stimulation. I agree that this might require less depressant anesthesia than that needed to obtund tracheal stimulation. Regardless of the airway in place, it is useful to avoid sudden movements of the patient's head, which could elicit a response characterized as "coughing."—R.K. Stoelting, M.D.

Portable Suction Devices

Evaluation of Three Portable Suction Devices
Simon EJ, Davidson JAH, Boom SJ (Western Infirmary, Glasgow, Scotland)
Anaesthesia 48:807–809, 1993   101-94-2–12

Introduction.—Portable suction equipment must sometimes be used to clear the pharynx of secretions and vomitus in emergency resuscitation. A number of types of portable units are available.

Methods and Results.—Three types of portable suction units—the hand-held Res-Q-Vac, the Dräger Sujector 2000, and the Laerdal battery-powered unit—were evaluated and compared with a wall-mounted Ohmeda suction unit connected to a central vacuum supply. The 4 types of suction were tested for their ability to aspirate 140 mL of mock gastric contents. The mean aspiration times were 7.39 seconds for the Res-Q-Vac, 8.6 seconds for the Dräger unit, 11.4 seconds for the Laerdal unit, and 7.27 seconds for the Ohmeda unit.

Discussion.—The portable suction units tested compare favorably with the wall-mounted equipment. Equipment design may dictate which unit is most appropriate for a particular situation given differences in size, power supply, and portability. The Res-Q-Vac is the most portable and least costly unit, and because it is manually powered, it does not require batteries or compressed gas.

▶ For those of you involved in administration of cardiopulmonary resuscitation services or purchasing portable suction devices, this is an important article. I would guess that very few of us use the Res-Q-Vac, which was the least expensive and most effective device in this evaluation. I think we will evaluate it and may well choose which device we routinely use.—M.F. Roizen, M.D.

Rapid Induction

Vital Capacity Rapid Inhalation Induction Technique: Comparison of Sevoflurane and Halothane

Yurino M, Kimura H (Asahikawa Med College, Hokkaido, Japan)
Can J Anaesth 40:440–443, 1993   101-94-2–13

Background.—Previous studies have demonstrated the safety and acceptability of using the vital capacity rapid inhalation induction (VCRII) technique to induce anesthesia with halothane and oxygen. Advantages of this VCRII technique include prompt induction without triggering an excitatory phase, and a lack of anesthesia "hangover." Halothane and sevoflurane were compared using the VCRII technique.

Patients and Methods.—Thirty-two adult, demographically similar volunteers, who had never experienced anesthesia, were included in the study. Fifteen volunteers were randomly assigned to the 2% halothane group and 17 to the 4.5% sevoflurane group. No participant received premedication and all breathed air before induction. Each volunteer was asked to take a vital capacity breath after which anesthesia induction was initiated and maintained for 5 minutes. The participants then breathed oxygen until they recovered consciousness. An objective observer, blinded to the agents used, asked the volunteers questions as they regained consciousness concerning how many commands had been heard during induction, how they would characterize the smell of the anesthetic, and whether they would object to undergoing VCRII again.

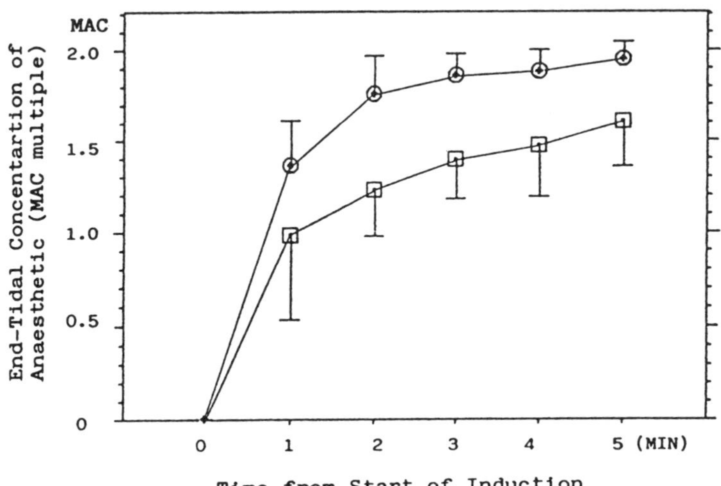

Fig 2–7.—End-tidal concentration (ex)/rend as minimum alveolar concentration (MAC) multiple of sevoflurane (*circles*) increased more rapidly with VCRII than halothane (*squares*). (Courtesy of Yurino M, Kimura H: *Can J Anaesth* 40:440–443, 1993.)

<table>
<tr><td colspan="3" align="center">Incidence of Complications During Induction
of Anesthesia</td></tr>
<tr><td></td><td>Sevoflurane
(n = 17)</td><td>Halothane
(n = 15)</td></tr>
<tr><td>Induction</td><td></td><td></td></tr>
<tr><td>– Complicated</td><td>3/17 (17.6%)*</td><td>5/15 (33.3%)</td></tr>
<tr><td>– Uncomplicated</td><td>14/17 (82.4%)</td><td>10/15 (66.7%)</td></tr>
<tr><td>1 Coughing</td><td>–</td><td>3/15 (20.0%)</td></tr>
<tr><td>2 Laryngospasm</td><td>–</td><td>–</td></tr>
<tr><td>3 Breath holding</td><td>–</td><td>–</td></tr>
<tr><td>4 Movement</td><td>3/17 (17.6%)</td><td>2/15 (13.3%)</td></tr>
<tr><td>5 Secretion</td><td>–</td><td>–</td></tr>
</table>

*P < .05 vs. halothane.
(Courtesy of Yurino M, Kimura H: *Can J Anaesth* 40:440–443, 1993.)

Results.—Anesthesia induction was successful among both groups. However, the mean induction for halothane was slower at 153 seconds when compared with the 81-second time for sevoflurane. In addition, end-tidal halothane concentrations increased more slowly than those of sevoflurane (Fig 2–7). Measurements such as heart rate, blood pressure, and arterial oxygen saturation did not differ among the participant groups. Overall, the participants in the sevoflurane group had fewer complications than did those in the halothane group. No serious complications, such as severe coughing, laryngospasm, breath holding, or excess secretions, were noted in any patients. Only 3 of 17 sevoflurane participants experienced complicated induction compared with 5 of the 15 halothane participants (table). All volunteers stated that they would be willing to undergo the VCRII procedure again. In addition, the smell of sevoflurane at 65% acceptance level was perceived as more pleasant than that of halothane with only a 13% acceptance level.

Conclusion.—All subjects found VCRII acceptable, but the slower induction time for halothane was frustrating for the anesthetist mainly because of the chance for pronounced excitatory phenomena. Because sevoflurane causes less airway irritation, has a more pleasant odor, and has a shorter induction time, it is favored over halothane when using the VCRII technique.

▶ In the movies, the villain pours an unknown liquid on a handkerchief and covers the victim's face. The victim falls to the ground in just 2–3 seconds or less. The last agent we had that could in fact produce near-single breath induction was cyclopropane, which was often given for "rapid sequence" inductions, having the patient take 3 or 4 maximal breaths. With desflurane and sevoflurane, with blood gas solubility coefficients of .41 and .6, respectively, rapid inhalation induction is a distinct possibility. Unfortunately, with desflurane, pungency probably precludes this kind of induction, but with sevoflurane, near-single breath induction is possible as is shown by this paper. Whether it is desirable or not, in any given set of modern clinical circumstances, I do not know. Whether the criminal element will attach themselves to this phenomenon, I cannot even begin to speculate about.—J.H. Tinker, M.D.

Computer-Assisted Anesthesia

Pilot Study of an Expert System Adviser for Controlling General Anaesthesia
Greenhow SG, Linkens DA, Asbury AJ (Univ of Sheffield, England; Western Infirmary, Glasgow, Scotland)
Br J Anaesth 71:359–365, 1993   101-94-2–14

Objective.—An attempt was made to develop an expert system using on-line clinical data to estimate the adequacy of anesthesia, and to automatically provide on-line advice about the delivery of anesthetic agents. The result was the real-time expert system for advice and control (RESAC).

The System.—Clinical data and on-line measurements are merged in RESAC using the technique of Bayesian inference and "fuzzy" logic. Data entry is designed to be rapid and intuitive, minimizing keyboard use. The system requires a knowledge of when surgical stimulation begins, data on patient characteristics such as body size and the state of health, and information on the reasonable physiologic ranges for each patient. A test commentary on the perceived adequacy of anesthesia is provided at 1-minute intervals.

Validation.—The performance of RESAC was evaluated in 7 patients using a variety of anesthetic techniques including neuromuscular blockade, 2 analgesics, and positive-pressure ventilation. Questionnaire responses were analyzed as a gauge of system performance. In most instances, the anesthetists were confident enough to follow the dosage advice given by RESAC.

Conclusion.—Initial experience with RESAC suggests that it provides reasonable advice in most instances. Although many problems remain, the use of an on-line expert system clearly has merit.

▶ This fascinating study described the first use of an expert system that I have seen that uses both Bayesian inference and fuzzy "logic." The anesthesiologist then administered what the machine suggested and looked at the outcome. The attempt here, obviously, is to model the human mind and expert systems in a machine so that more efficient anesthesia can be given without as-skilled humans involved. If this system is to work, more refinement is necessary, but the system showed promise. I guess that is bad for those of us who believe that we are needed, and I cannot help believing that human judgment is needed for giving anesthesia. The go-to-sleep and wake-up is not very difficult, but the judgments one has to make in critically ill patients and in serious operations, I believe, are too great to be programmed at this time. One clear error in this system is the lack of duplication of essential data; that is, blood pressure was obtained from only 1 monitor, heart rate from only 1 monitor, etc. I think that duplicative systems are needed if we are going to have a system such as this be a benefit at all, or even for that matter to be tested.—M.F. Roizen, M.D.

Anesthetics and Bowel Function

Anaesthetic Technique Does Not Influence Postoperative Bowel Function: A Comparison of Propofol, Nitrous Oxide and Isoflurane
Jensen AG, Kalman SH, Nyström P-O, Eintrei C (Univ Hosp Linköping, Sweden)
Can J Anaesth 39:938–943, 1992   101-94-2–15

Introduction.—Anesthetics have the potential for contributing to postopertive morbidity by altering gastrointestinal physiology, either by impairing intestinal motor activity or by an action on the cardiovascular system. Propofol and isoflurane, which are thought to have minimal effects on postoperative bowel function, were compared with nitrous oxide, an agent that demonstrably impairs bowel function.

Design.—Sixty patients aged 18–85 years who were scheduled for surgery on the colon and rectum were randomly assigned to anesthesia with isoflurane and nitrous oxide, propofol in air, or propofol with nitrous oxide. Fentanyl and vecuronium were used in all 3 groups. All operations were done by the same anesthetic and surgical teams. The postoperative status was inferred from the acute physiology score (APS) based on the Acute Physiology and Chronic Health Evaluation II classification, the passage of gas, the tolerance of enteral feeding, the hospital stay, and complications within 30 days of surgery.

Results.—The time needed to achieve a normal APS was similar in all groups, as were the times to passage of flatus and tolerance of oral intakes. The postoperative hospital stay was comparable in all groups, and complications were equally frequent.

Conclusion.—The anesthetic agents used had minimal influence on the postoperative course of colorectal surgery in these patients.

▶ I am singularly unimpressed with the criteria we seem to have for assessing postoperative bowel function, namely passage of gas, tolerance of enteral feeding, hospital stay, and complications up to 30 days after surgery. You would think that as important an organ as the bowel would have attracted more scientific interest in assessing its function.—J.H. Tinker, M.D.

3 Complications Related to Anesthesia and Critical Care

Regional Anesthesia Complications

Dural Puncture

Dural Taps Revisited: A 20-Year Survey From Birmingham Maternity Hospital

Stride PC, Cooper GM (Birmingham Maternity Hosp, England)
Anaesthesia 48:247–255, 1993   101-94-3-1

Introduction.—An investigation of the problem of dural tap and subsequent postdural puncture headache (PDPH) drew on the records of the Birmingham Maternity Hospital. Data were collected on 34,819 epidurals performed from 1969 through 1988.

Methods.—Epidural blockade was introduced in 1969 to prevent maternal bearing down in the second stage of labor. Bupivacaine (.5%) was used to maintain blockade, and forceps were used electively for delivery; this policy was relaxed in the mid-1980s. Epidural drips were introduced in 1970. Beginning in 1974, blood patches were offered to all patients with significant PDPH. During the study period, 460 dural taps were recorded. The full notes of these patients were examined.

Results—The overall incidence of dural tap was 1.3% for the 20-year study period. Three regimens were used from 1969 through 1973 for the management of PDPH. Thirty-five patients received no specific measures to prevent headaches; 32 patients were discouraged from bearing down in the second stage of labor to minimize leakage of CSF. A third group of 68 patients received an epidural drip of compound sodium lactate solution after delivery. None of these measures significantly reduced the incidence of PDPH, although those who received an epidural drip had a lower proportion of severe headaches when compared with the no-treatment group. The onset of headache was delayed by epidural drip. From 1974 on, epidural drip was an established measure for patients with dural tap. Whether bearing down was discouraged or not, and despite the provision of a drip, nearly 50% had severe headache. Of the 135 blood patches completed in the 1974–1988 period, 86 patients had complete and permanent relief of PDPH from a single patch.

Conclusion.—The onset of PDPH may be as late as 6 days after the precipitating event. In general, a late onset means a shorter duration. Location of epidural space by the loss of resistance to injection of saline was associated with a lower incidence of dural tap (.6%) than either the Macintosh balloon or loss of resistance to injection of air. Discouragement of maternal bearing down after dural tap appears to be ineffective prophylaxis against PDPH. Prophylactic patching is not used at the study institution. Caffeine offers no relief, but bedrest may be helpful in those who have headache. Although blood patching is a safe and established therapy, 14% of these patients continued to have severe symptoms. An alternative is epidural patching with Dextran 40, a technique that might be applicable to certain patients (e.g., Jehovah's Witnesses).

▶ I do not perform a prophylactic blood patch for several reasons. First, not every patient who is subjected to unintentional dural puncture experiences a PDPH. Second, when performing a blood patch, it is preferable to inject the blood as close as possible to the site of the dural puncture. Unfortunately, one is never certain of the location of the catheter tip. Third, I am reluctant to inject blood through a catheter that may not remain sterile. On the other hand, I offer a therapeutic blood patch at the first sign of a PDPH in patients who have suffered an unintentional dural puncture with an 18-gauge epidural needle. I disagree with the authors' conclusion that caffeine is ineffective. In my practice, intravenous caffeine offers substantial (albeit often temporary) relief in a significant number of women with PDPH. Unfortunately, caffeine rarely provides permanent relief in patients who have had an unintentional dural puncture with a large epidural needle.—D.H. Chestnut, M.D.

Acute Deterioration of Mental Status Following Epidural Blood Patch
Beers RA, Cambareri JJ, Rodziewicz GS (State Univ of New York, Syracuse)
Anesth Analg 76:1147–1149, 1993   101-94-3–2

Introduction.—Epidural blood patch (EBP) has been well documented as a safe and effective treatment for postlumbar puncture headache. Acute mental deterioration beginning shortly after an EBP treatment for postlumbar puncture headache was examined.

Case Report.—Man, 70, was seen for an elective transurethral prostatectomy. On the third postoperative day, he complained of a severe postural headache and nausea, which persisted after conservative management. Therefore, EBP was performed and relief was obtained. However, the next day, problems with balance and lethargy were noted. By the next day, headache had returned and confusion was noted. Within 4 hours, the patient responded to vigorous nonnoxious stimuli. Computed tomography of the head showed a right parasagitta cerebellar lesion with obstructive hydrocephalus. External ventriculostomy was performed with a dramatic improvement in mental status. No infection was detected. Several days later, a posterior fossa craniotomy was performed for total resection of a benign meningioma.

Discussion.—The CSF leak, which was responsible for the initial headache, may have triggered hemorrhage and edema within the tumor, yet permitted drainage to relieve this pressure. Sealing off this leak with EBP may then have brought on the obstructive hydrocephalus. Atypical neurologic symptoms after spinal anesthesia or EBP should be thoroughly evaluated before deciding they are simply complications of the procedures performed.

▶ This is a classic example of the admonition that proof of cause and effect based only on temporal association with another event is the weakest form of scientific evidence.—R.K. Stoelting, M.D.

PERIPHERAL NERVE INJURY

Peripheral Nerve Injury Caused by Injection Needles Used in Regional Anaesthesia: Influence of Bevel Configuration, Studied in a Rat Model
Rice ASC, McMahon SB (St Thomas' Hosp, London)
Br J Anaesth 69:433–438, 1992   101-94-3–3

Background.—Nerve injury during the delivery of regional anesthesia can result from direct trauma caused by the injection needle. Bevel design and needle size are probably important factors in this mechanism of injury. The immediate and long-term effects of sciatic nerve impalement by short and long bevelled needles were studied in a rat model.

Methods.—Three methods were used to assess neural trauma and its consequences. Stained longitudinal nerve sections were evaluated by light microscopy and scored for injury. Extravasation of Evan's Blue dye after antidromic electric nerve stimulation was also used to test unmyelinated fiber function. Finally, the flexion withdrawal times from a noxious stimulus were measured.

Findings.—Lesions induced by short bevelled needle impaling a nerve fascicle were more severe, more common, and took longer to heal than lesions induced by long bevelled needles. Injury from short bevelled needle impalement was associated with persisting signs of damage for 28 days.

Conclusion.—The recommendation that short bevelled needles be used to prevent nerve injury during induction of regional anesthesia should be reexamined. The use of long bevelled needles may be better, especially if the bevel is aligned parallel to the nerve fibers.

▶ As a confirmed iconoclast, I loved this paper. I have long been dead set against deliberately impaling nerves with any needle, short beveled or long beveled. When you poke a nerve, I just do not see how damage could help but result, whether temporary or permanent. I realize that the idea behind the short beveled needle was that the injectate would go where you wanted instead of out the back side of the "sheath." There may even be evidence that this is so, but I have not seen it. I think the main point this paper has to make is that deliberately inserting needles in nerves will result in nerve damage.—J.H. Tinker, M.D.

Common Peroneal Nerve Palsy Associated With Epidural Analgesia

Cohen DE, Van Duker B, Siegel S, Keon TP (Univ of Pennsylvania, Philadelphia)

Anesth Analg 76:429–431, 1993   101-94-3–4

Background.—A foot drop after surgery in the lithotomy position or after major pelvic explorations often indicates peroneal nerve damage. A common peroneal nerve palsy associated with a continuous epidural infusion for postoperative analgesia was described.

Case Report.—Girl, 14 years, had an exploratory laparotomy for bowel obstruction with general anesthesia. During an exploratory laparotomy 2 months earlier, an unresectable ovarian tumor with diffuse peritoneal metastases was discovered, and a colostomy was created. After the second procedure, the patient was placed in a right lateral decubitus position, and an 18-gauge Hustead needle was placed in the epidural space at the L3–4 interspace. The loss-of-resistance technique was used. A 20-gauge nonstyletted epidural catheter was then threaded 2 cm past the end of the needle after injection of a test dose of .25% bupivacaine with 1 part per 200,000 epinephrine. Another dose of the solution was given before the girl was awakened. The patient was taken uneventfully to the postanesthesia care unit, where she complained of severe abdominal pain. An additional bolus of 5 mL of .25% bupivacaine with 1 part per 200,000 epinephrine was given. At this time, an epidural infusion of .05% bupivacaine and preservative-free morphine, .05 mg/mL diluted in 5% dextrose in water at 5 mL per hour was given. The patient still reported abdominal pain. A sensory and incomplete motor block of her left leg was noted 20 minutes after the additional bolus. Another bolus of 5 mL was given, and the infusion was increased to 8.5 mL per hour. Half an hour later, she still had abdominal pain. Examination revealed a complete motor and sensory block of her left leg. There were sensory deficits in the right leg. Another bolus was administered, and her infusion was again increased. After this, a T8 sensory level was noted on the left side, with an incomplete sensory block to T8 on the right. After 60 mg of intravenous ketrolac, the patient no longer reported pain.

The next morning, the patient was sedated and comfortable but had a L1–2 sensory level on the left. The bupivacaine concentration in the epidural infusion was decreased by half, and her leg numbness resolved. However, numbness in her left foot persisted. It was weak, with an inability to dorsiflex. Bupivacaine was discontinued, but the foot symptoms continued. The epidural catheter was removed the next day. Closer assessment revealed a persistent foot drop, inability to evert and invert the foot, and numbness on the dorsum of the foot and lateral part of the calf. Physical therapy was begun. By 7 days after the surgery, some sensation to the dorsum of the foot had returned. Improvement continued, and by discharge 2 weeks after injury, the patient had almost complete return of sensation and function.

Conclusion.—It is recommended to check for the presence or absence of sensory blockade intermittently and have standing orders on the adequacy of ventilation and level of consciousness monitoring of patients with continuous epidural infusions. If any sensation loss occurs, nurses should check pressure points and change the position of the patient frequently. The concentration of the local anesthetic is also reduced until paresthesias of the legs are gone.

▶ How do you get an injury to the common peroneal nerve without the lithotomy position, without leg casts, without metal braces for the legs or knee supports, etc? The authors incriminate the postoperative period in this case. I have long believed that many nerve injuries are the result of "routine" care for 24–48 hours postoperatively that often involves the patient lying quietly supine, or even restrained in that position with forearms supinated and the elbows extended. I am convinced that we get blamed for some postoperative nerve injuries as if they had occurred in the operating room, when they may well have occurred postoperatively. I am sure that that is what happened here (beyond a "reasonable degree of medical certainty"—for those of you who do not know medical legal jargon, that is 51% or more, but it does not have to be 99%).—J.H. Tinker, M.D.

Complications of Spinal/Epidural Anesthesia or Analgesia

The Effect of Epidural Anaesthesia and Size of Spinal Needle on Post-Operative Hearing Loss
Öncel S, Hasegeli L, Uğuz MZ, Savaci S, Önal K, Oyman S (State Hosp, Yeşilyurt, Izmir, Turkey)
J Laryngol Otol 106:783–787, 1992   101-94-3–5

Introduction.—Vestibulocochlear nerve lesions after spinal anesthesia are reported to occur in 2–3.7 per thousand cases. Pure tone audiometry was used to examine the effects of epidural and spinal anesthesia on vestibulocochlear dysfunction.

Patients and Methods.—Study subjects were 45 patients scheduled to undergo elective urologic operations. All were in good general health and had no severe hearing loss. The patients were randomized to receive epidural anesthesia, spinal anesthesia with 25-gauge needles, or spinal anesthesia with 22-gauge needles. Both spinal and epidural anesthesia were performed via L3-L4, using 2% lignocaine. Patients were evaluated for headache and function at cranial nerves III, IV, VI, VII, and VIII. Pure tone audiograms were performed preoperatively and on the third and fourth postoperative days. Hearing in both ears was evaluated at frequencies of 125 to 8,000 Hz.

Results.—None of the patients experienced postoperative headache or had cranial nerve lesions. Patients in the epidural group showed no statistically significant hearing loss in the postoperative period compared with the preoperative period. The greatest loss was observed in 22-gauge spinal anesthesia group. On average, there was a 10-dB hearing loss in both ears at 125 Hz, 250 Hz, and 500 Hz. When the 22-gauge and 25-gauge groups were compared, a statistically significant difference was observed at 125 Hz, 250 Hz, 4 KHz, and 6 KHz.

Conclusion.—Spinal anesthesia results in a transient hearing impairment. In the patients who received spinal anesthesia with a 22-gauge needle, the hearing loss was mainly in the low frequencies and was not accompanied by headache. Significant hearing loss, however, is associated with headache. Pure tone audiometry is a more sensitive indicator of CSF loss, and resulting hearing loss in the low frequencies, than postoperative headache.

▶ Hearing loss in low frequencies with or without a postspinal headache is not likely to be appreciated by the physician in the absence of a specific complaint by the patient. The clinical significance, if any, of this observation remains to be determined.—R.K. Stoelting, M.D.

Comparison of an Ephedrine Infusion With Crystalloid Administration for Prevention of Hypotension During Spinal Anesthesia

Gajraj NM, Victory RA, Pace NA, Van Elstraete AC, Wallace DH (Univ of Texas, Dallas)
Anesth Analg 76:1023–1026, 1993   101-94-3–6

Introduction.—An infusion of ephedrine may be more effective than preblock crystalloid administration in reducing the incidence of hypotension during spinal anesthesia. Previous studies have added ephedrine to crystalloid treatment; this study evaluated the efficacy of ephedrine infusion alone in patients scheduled for postpartum tubal ligations with spinal anesthesia.

Methods.—The 54 patients were randomly allocated to receive either 15 mL of crystalloid per kg or an ephedrine infusion. Spinal anesthesia was performed in the sitting position using 70–90 mg of hyperbaric 5% lidocaine. Patients in the ephedrine group immediately received an infusion at a rate of 5 mg/min for 2 minutes, then 1 mg/min for the next 18 minutes. The infusion rate was increased or decreased if hypotension or hypertension occurred. Patients in both groups received a 10-mg bolus of ephedrine intravenously if hypotension developed.

Results.—The mean total dose of ephedrine was 15.2 mg in the crystalloid group and 37.4 mg in the ephedrine infusion group, a significant

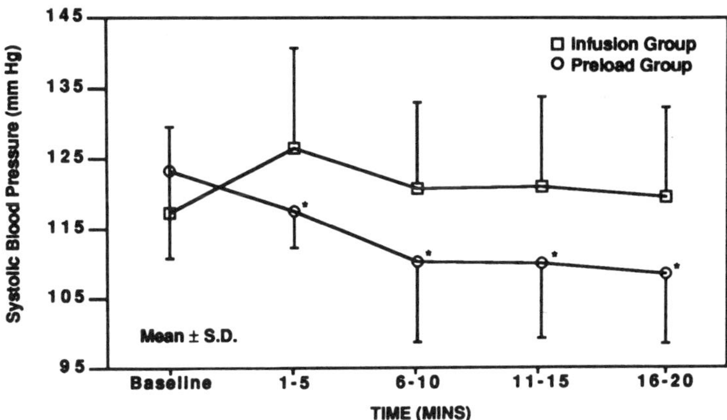

Fig 3–1.—Mean systolic blood pressures for the ephedrine infusion (*squares*) and crystalloid groups (*circles*) during the 20 minutes after spinal anesthesia. *Significant difference between groups ($P < .05$). (Courtesy of Gajraj NM, Victory RA, Pace NA, et al: *Anesth Analg* 76:1023–1026, 1993.)

difference. The crystalloid group received a mean of 1.4 boluses of ephedrine, compared with a mean of .4 boluses in the infusion group. The incidence of hypotension was significantly higher in the crystalloid group (55%) than in the ephedrine infusion group (22%) (Fig 3–1). Nausea and vomiting occurred at similar rates in the 2 groups. No patient had hypertension develop, and the maximum heart rate was similar in both groups.

Conclusion.—An ephedrine infusion without preblock crystalloid administration was more effective than crystalloid administration in reducing the incidence of hypotension during spinal anesthesia. The effectiveness of crystalloid administration is questionable, and the procedure may be undesirable in certain patients, such as those with congestive cardiac failure or renal impairment.

▶ Treatment of hypotension after development of sympathetic nervous system blockade owing to spinal anesthesia is based on the relative risk of the blood pressure decrease to the patient. I would be reluctant to advocate a prophylactic continuous infusion of ephedrine in a patient population characterized as young and without cardiovascular disease (postpartum tubal ligations). Conversely, intravenous fluid administration is not likely to provide the desired response when a prompt increase in blood pressure is needed. In these instances, I reach for a "vasopressor."—R.K. Stoelting, M.D.

Failure of Anaesthesia After Accidental Subdural Catheter Placement

van der Maaten JMAA, van Kleef JW (Leiden Univ Hosp, The Netherlands)
Acta Anaesthesiol Scand 36:707–709, 1992   101-94-3-7

Background.—Failure to achieve subarachnoid block, a well-documented complication, usually results from deposition of the local anesthetic outside the subarachnoid space. Subdural catheter placement after an attempted continuous subarachnoid anesthetic and analgesia failure was proved radiologically.

Case Report.—Woman, 37, had internal osteosynthesis of a right ankle fracture. The patient was otherwise healthy and had not had any previous lumbar puncture. The anesthesiologist planned a continuous epidural technique. The patient was placed in the right lateral position and a 1.3-mm Tuohy needle was inserted at L3–4. Immediately after loss of resistance, CSF flowed from the needle. Continuous subarachnoid anesthesia was then begun. A 1.1-mm single endhole radiopaque Teflon catheter was inserted easily cephalad, 3 cm beyond the needle tip. After aspiration of clear CSF, bupivacaine was injected slowly. After 20 minutes, there were no signs of sympathetic or sensory blockade. After further aspiration, lignocaine was injected. Ten minutes later, there was still no change in sensory perception or skin temperature. The catheter was withdrawn 1 cm, and CSF again flowed. More lignocaine was injected, and after 5 minutes, there was a poor, diffuse sensory blockade in L1–2 and some vasodilation in the leg. Repeated aspiration resulted in free flow of CSF. Finally, a higher dose of 5% heavy lignocaine was injected. There was no further change in sympathetic or sensory blockade. Surgery was performed with the use of general anesthesia, without complications. Two hours after the first injection of local anesthetic, no sensory or sympathetic blockade was detected. A radiologic assessment demonstrated spread of contrast medium in the subdural space from the tip of the catheter, at the L3 level, in a caphalad direction. The patient's postoperative recovery was uneventful.

Conclusion.—In this patient, an epidural anesthetic was complicated by dural puncture. Attempted conversion to a continuous subarachnoid infusion technique then resulted in failure of the anesthesia. Accidental subdural catheter placement was confirmed by radiologic study.

▶ In the past, failed spinal anesthesia after injection of tetracaine was attributed to "inactive thermolabile drug." I suspect the explanation described in this case report was also responsible for many failed spinal anesthetics previously attributed to the drug.—R.K. Stoelting, M.D.

Cauda Equina Syndrome: A Consequence of Lumbar Disk Protrusion or Continuous Subarachnoid Analgesia?

Ackerman WE III, Andrews PJD, Juneja MM, Rigor BM (Univ of Louisville,

Ky; Norton Hosp, Louisville, Ky)
Anesth Analg 76:898–901, 1993   101-94-3–8

Introduction.—Epidural analgesia during labor has been shown to be both safe and effective. Cauda equina syndrome in a patient with lumbar disk disease discovered post partum was studied. During the first stage of labor in this patient, the epidural catheter had migrated to a subarachnoid position.

Case Report.—Parturient, 29, gravida 2, para 1, was admitted in labor at 2:32 A.M. At 7:30 P.M., the cervix was dilated 6 cm and epidural anesthesia was initiated. A 17-gauge Tuohy epidural needle was inserted at the L3–4 interspace, with the patient in the sitting position. An 18-gauge epidural catheter was inserted without paresthesias. Blood was detected and the catheter was replaced at the L4–5 interspace, without blood, CSF, or paresthesias. About 95 minutes later, the patient complained of difficulty in moving both legs. Aspiration of the catheter revealed free-flowing clear fluid that was glucose-positive. A diagnosis of subarachnoid migration of the epidural catheter was presumed. It was decided to use the catheter for intermittent subarachnoid analgesia. Post partum, the patient complained of pain in the sciatic nerve distribution of the left lower extremity and left buttocks and was unable to void or defecate. There were no symptoms of epidural abscess or hematoma. She was discharged on the fourth postpartum day with instructions for self-catheterization of the bladder. The patient was referred to a neurologist. At 4 weeks' post partum, electromyography was performed and was compatible with a L5 to S1 radiculopathy and myelopathy. Magnetic resonance imaging demonstrated posterior disk protrusion. One year after the delivery, the patient has only minimal improvement.

Discussion.—The etiology of this case is not known but was probably multifactorial and may not be related to the anesthetic. The etiology of cauda equina syndrome is difficult to diagnose when regional anesthesia has been administered, especially in the case of inadvertent dural puncture. The use of an epidural catheter for continuous spinal anesthesia once it has punctured the dura should be investigated by prospective laboratory studies with an appropriate model.

▶ See the comment for Abstract 101-94-3–2.—R.K. Stoelting, M.D.

The Effect of Head-Down Tilt on Arterial Blood Pressure After Spinal Anesthesia

Miyabe M, Namiki A (Kushiro City Gen Hosp, Japan; Sapporo Med College, Japan)
Anesth Analg 76:549–552, 1993   101-94-3–9

Introduction.—The head-down tilt has been used for hemodynamic improvement in a number of hypotensive states, although the procedure

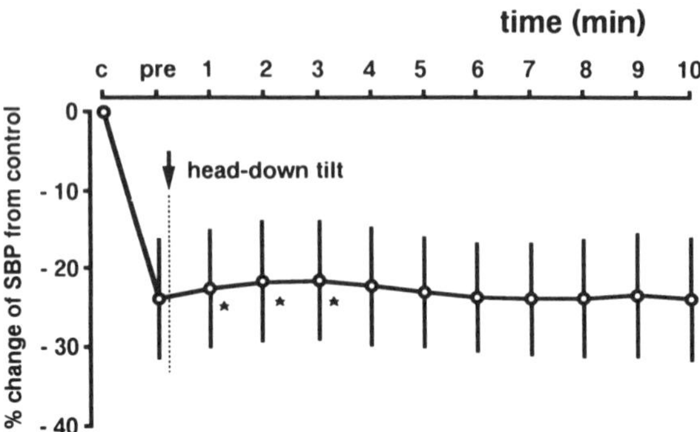

Fig 3–2.—*Abbreviations: c,* SBP before spinal block; *pre,* SBP just before head-down tilt was performed. The effect of head-down tilt on hypotension after spinal block. Data are mean ± standard deviation (*n* = 40). **P* < .05 compared with pre. (Courtesy of Miyabe M, Namiki A: *Anesth Analg* 76:549–552, 1993.)

remains controversial. Whether the head-down tilt position is effective in treating or preventing hypotension in patients who have undergone spinal block was determined.

Methods.—Ninety women scheduled for major elective gynecologic surgery were evaluated. None were receiving medications that could affect arterial blood pressure or heart rate. The 10-degree head-down tilt was used after arterial blood pressure had decreased in 40 patients, and a prophylactic tilt was used in 50 patients. In the latter group, 24 patients were tilted for 20 minutes immediately after injection of local anesthetic (head-down group), and 26 were maintained in the horizontal position (horizontal group). The systolic blood pressure (SBP) was measured before the patient was positioned for lumbar puncture and at 1-minute intervals after injection of the anesthetic with an automated device.

Results.—After spinal block, the average SBP decreased 24%. After head-down tilt, the SBP increased up to a 21% to 22% depression level from the control for 3 minutes, then decreased to a 22% to 24% depression level (Fig 3–2). The patients were divided into 3 groups based on the degree of decrease of the SBP after spinal block. Group I decreased 10%, group II decreased 20%, and group III decreased 30% from the control. In group I, the SBP remained lower than the level just before the head-down tilt was applied. In group II, the SPB did not differ from the pre–head-down tilt value after 4 minutes. And in group III, the SBP decreased 35% from the control, increased for the first 3 minutes, then remained at that level. The cephalad spread of analgesia at 20 minutes after spinal block was higher in the head-down tilt group than in the horizontal group.

Conclusion.—The head-down tilt increased the SBP only in severe hypotension (30% decrease from control). In 2 such cases, however, the SBP did not increase after the head-down tilt. Also indicated is that prophylactic performance of the tilt could not prevent the decrease in the SBP after the spinal block. The effect of the head-down tilt to increase blood pressure appears to be counteracted by the higher cephalad spread of analgesia.

▶ Hypotension owing to spinal anesthesia is presumed to reflect primarily decreased venous return with a resulting decrease in cardiac output. If the head-down position improves venous return more than it facilitates cephalad spread of the anesthesia, it would seem, along with other therapies (fluids, sympathomimetics), to be indicated. Under no circumstances is the head-up tilt indicated in a misguided attempt to limit cephalad spread of the spinal anesthetic.—R.K. Stoelting, M.D.

Continuous Spinal Anesthesia: Where Do Spinal Catheters Go?
Van Gessel EF, Forster A, Gamulin Z (Hôpital Cantonal Universitaire, Geneva)
Anesth Analg 76:1004–1007, 1993   101-94-3–10

Objective.—The incidence of technical problems related to continuous spinal anesthesia (CSA) was determined. This procedure, like epidural anesthesia, requires insertion of a catheter. The influence of catheter tip position on block height after injection of a hypobaric spinal anesthetic in CSA was also investigated.

Methods.—Study subjects were 29 consecutive elderly patients undergoing CSA for traumatic hip surgery. Lumbar puncture was performed with an 18-gauge Tuohy needle at the L3–4 (or L2–3) interspace. An attempt was made to uniformly thread all catheters in a cephalad direction. Threading was defined as difficult if cephalad insertion was impossible on the first try. All patients received 7.5 mg of either tetracaine or bupivacaine as hypobaric solutions in the lateral decubitus position. The catheters were injected with radiographic dye after the surgical procedure and radiographically examined for verification of position.

Results.—One case was excluded from analysis. Of the 28 remaining catheters, 24 were threaded easily in the subarachnoid space and 4 required the maneuver used for difficult threading. In 59% of the cases, determination of the level of lumbar puncture was falsely judged, and the puncture was performed 1 or 2 spaces higher than assumed. Twenty catheters were successfully placed cephalad, 6 remained coiled in a horizontal position, and 2 took a caudal direction. Anesthesia was adequate in all cases. There was no correlation between the position of the tip of the catheter and the sensory levels achieved with the same dose of local anesthetic.

Conclusion.—Technical problems were encountered in 14% of the patients undergoing CSA. In 2 of these 4 patients, catheters were not threaded in the desired cephalad direction. Most lumbar punctures were performed higher than assumed, probably because of bony abnormalities of the lower vertebrae or skeletal deformities in these elderly patients. The direction taken by the intrathecal catheter could not be predicted, yet the final position of the tip did not influence the distribution of hypobaric local anesthetics in the subarachnoid space. Nevertheless, CSA carried a potential risk of damage to the spinal cord.

▶ Continuous spinal anesthesia has many attractive features. The dilemma is balancing the benefits of this technique against potential risks, ranging from pooling and neurotoxicity of local anesthetics to direct trauma from a more cephalad position of the catheter than realized.—R.K. Stoelting, M.D.

Auditory Function After Spinal Anesthesia
Wang LP, Magnusson M, Lundberg J, Törnebrandt K (Lund Univ Hosp, Sweden)
Reg Anesth 18:162–165, 1993   101-94-3–11

Background.—Recent reports mention transient hearing loss as a side effect of spinal anesthesia in patients having transurethral resection of the prostate (TURP). In theory, such hearing loss could result from dural puncture, plasma hypo-osmolarity secondary to absorption of irrigation fluid, the local anesthetic itself, or cerebral ischemia resulting from arterial hypotension.

Study Design.—Hearing function was assessed using refined audiometric techniques in 18 men undergoing TURP or other transurethral procedures. Six patients were operated on with the use of epidural anesthesia; 12 had spinal anesthesia induced using a 26-gauge spinal needle and bupivacaine in a glucose solution. Audiometry was repeated on the second postoperative day.

Results.—Serum osmolarity declined significantly only in the epidural group. One patient in the spinal group had severe postdural puncture headache, nausea, and vomiting and also described vertigo and deafness. The auditory symptoms lasted 5 days. With this exception, audiometry showed no changes in hearing level at any frequency. Regional anesthesia did not affect the mean hearing level or speech discrimination in any group.

Conclusion.—Minor hearing loss is not a problem when spinal anesthesia is induced with a 26-gauge needle. An occasional patient may have severe but transient low-frequency hearing loss regardless of how small a needle is used for dural puncture.

▶ See the comment for Abstract 101-94-3–5.—R.K. Stoelting, M.D.

Postoperative Pulmonary Complications: Epidural Analgesia Using Bupivacaine and Opioids Versus Parenteral Opioids

Jayr C, Thomas H, Rey A, Farhat F, Lasser P, Bourgain J-L (Institut Gustave-Roussy, Villejuif, France)
Anesthesiology 78:666–676, 1993　　　　　　　　　　　101-94-3–12

Background.—Epidural analgesia may enhance respiratory mechanics postoperatively compared with parenteral opioid analgesia.

Objective.—Pulmonary complications and the duration of hospitalization were compared in patients requiring major abdominal surgery for cancer who received morphine either by continuous subcutaneous infusion or epidurally in a prospective, double-blind, 14-month study.

Methods.—A total of 153 patients was randomized in the study. Either general anesthesia with intravenous fentanyl was followed by postoperative analgesia using continuous subcutaneous morphine, or general anesthesia combined with epidural bupivacaine was followed by the epidural administration of bupivacaine and morphine. Analgesia was estimated using a visual analogue pain scale.

Results.—Epidural analgesia provided significantly better analgesia in the first 2 postoperative days, at rest or with a cough. Vital capacity was better preserved in epidurally treated patients, and arterial oxygen tension immediately after surgery was higher in this group. Clinical pulmonary complications and radiographic chest abnormalities were comparably frequent in the 2 groups. Intestinal function recovered more rapidly in the epidural group, but significantly more patients in this group had systolic hypotension on the first postoperative day. Hospital times were similar.

Conclusion.—Postoperative epidural analgesia using an opioid and a local anesthetic provided adequate pain relief in this trial but did not reduce respiratory morbidity or shorten the hospital stay compared with subcutaneous morphine.

▶ This randomized, prospectively stratified study demonstrated benefits from epidural analgesia in terms of postoperative pain, vital capacity, and intestinal motility, but it failed to demonstrate a reduction in pulmonary complications. As competition for shrinking health-care dollars increases, will we be able to justify added expense for analgesic interventions if patient comfort is the only added benefit?—S.E. Abram, M.D.

Intravascular Migration of an Epidural Catheter During Postoperative Patient-Controlled Epidural Analgesia

Bush DJ, Kramer DP (Univ of Michigan, Ann Arbor)
Anesth Analg 76:1150–1151, 1993　　　　　　　　　　　101-94-3–13

Introduction.—A case of symptomatic intravenous migration of an epidural catheter as a complication of a previously effective patient-controlled epidural analgesia (PCEA) was examined.

Case Report.—Woman, 38, underwent hysterectomy under combined epidural and general anesthesia. A multiorifice epidural catheter was used. After surgery, PCEA was commenced with .25% bupivacaine containing 5 μg/mL of fentanyl infused at a background rate of 6 mL/hr with patient-initiated boluses of 5 mL every 20 minutes. In the general ward, the patient had 6 successful demands from the epidural pump with satisfactory analgesia. Fourteen hours after surgery, she had increased wound pain. Absence of blood on aspiration of the catheter and use of a test dose of 1% lidocaine with epinephrine did not suggest catheter misplacement. The pain recurred and aspiration of the epidural catheter produced blood-stained fluid. The catheter was removed and PCEA was discontinued.

Discussion.—Symptomatic intravascular migration of an epidural catheter can occur during satisfactory PCEA. In this patient, perhaps 1 of the distal holes of the multiorifice epidural catheter was initially in an epidural blood vessel but temporarily occluded until some later event cleared the obstruction. When PCEA is used with relatively low levels of monitoring on the general floor, small bolus doses of the drugs should be used, and patients should be encouraged to report strange or new symptoms.

▶ This case report emphasizes the controversy that still exists regarding the optimal level of monitoring for postoperative epidural analgesia.—S.E. Abram, M.D.

Extradural Air As a Cause of Paraplegia Following Lumbar Analgesia
Nay PG, Milaszkiewicz R, Jothilingam S (St Mary's Hosp, London; Hammersmith Hosp, London; Lister Hosp, Stevenage, England)
Anaesthesia 48:402–404, 1993   101-94-3–14

Background.—One way to locate the extradural space is the "loss of resistance to air" technique. This technique was complicated by paraplegia caused by nerve root displacement by extradural air in 1 patient.

Case Report.—Woman, 52, was seen at a pain clinic for a 10-year history of intermittent low back pain. She was obese with extensive fat over the lumbar spine. The patient requested general anesthesia for the performance of lumbar extradural anesthesia because of the severity of her back pain. After induction of general anesthesia, the extradural space was located using a 16-gauge Tuohy needle and the loss of resistance to air technique. Four attempts and about 40 mL of air were needed before a satisfactory position could be found. The epidural catheter was placed, and bupivacaine and methylprednisolone were injected. No immediate complications were apparent.

Eight hours later, the patient had persistent weakness and numbness of the left leg. She had a left-sided sensory deficit in the dermatomal distribution of L2–L4 with decreased hip, knee, and ankle power. On CT, performed for suspected extradural hematoma causing cord compression, large amounts of air were observed in the extradural space, apparently displacing the cauda equina. Intravenous dexamethasone was given, and the patient was free of motor and sensory deficits by the next morning. On follow-up CT 3 days later, the epidural air had largely resorbed.

Discussion.—This is the first report of prolonged paresthesia and paresis of the left leg after use of the loss-of-resistance-to-air technique for locating the epidural space. Symptoms resulted from nerve root compression. When using this technique, the anesthesiologist should avoid large volumes of air and take special care in patients with "difficult" backs.

▶ This paper is an example of "hype." The air did not cause paraplegia if you believe that the term paraplegia generally refers to a permanent injury. Another problem with this paper is to understand exactly why so much air got into this patient. The authors stated that "the procedure was difficult due to excessive subcutaneous fat." As a fat person myself, I would argue that perhaps the authors should have stated that *they* had trouble doing the procedure. This is like your kid saying, "Mommy, the vase fell off the shelf," or my resident stating, "Dr. Tinker, the arterial cannula wouldn't thread." In both these instances, and in this case report, human failure is excused by the presence of some inanimate obstruction. I believe we would be a lot better off if we were to say, "I knocked the vase off the shelf," or "I could not thread the arterial line," or "I injected a lot of air during multiple attempts at epidural placement in this patient."—J.H. Tinker, M.D.

RETROBULBAR BLOCK

Retrobulbar Hemorrhage After 12,500 Retrobulbar Blocks

Edge KR, Nicoll JMV (King Khaled Eye Specialist Hosp, Riyadh, Saudi Arabia)
Anesth Analg 76:1019–1022, 1993   101-94-3–15

Introduction.—Retrobulbar hemorrhage is a common complication of retrobulbar anesthesia. The prevalence of retrobulbar hemorrhage, the predisposing risk factors, and the risk of visual impairment after hemorrhage were investigated in a case-control study.

Study Design.—During a 5-year period from 1984 to 1989, 12,500 retrobulbar anesthetics were administered at the King Khaled Eye Specialist Hospital by 13 anesthesiologists. For each patient who had a hemorrhage, the next patient in the series was used as a comparative control.

Results.—Of 12,500 cases, 55 had retrobulbar hemorrhages, for an overall prevalence of .44%. The presence of vascular complications significantly increased the prevalence of hemorrhage. No relationship was detected between the amount of experience the surgeon had and the frequency of hemorrhage. There was no difference in visual outcome between patients with hemorrhage and those without.

Conclusion.—The incidence of retrobulbar hemorrhage after retrobulbar anesthesia in this large series was .44%. If managed properly, the hemorrhage is not likely to cause permanent visual impairment. As acquired vascular disease is a risk factor for retrobulbar hemorrhage, an alternative technique should be considered for such patients.

▶ Because many patients undergoing surgery that could benefit from a retrobulbar block are elderly, the presence of the significant risk factor (acquired vascular disease) identified in this study would most likely be a common problem.—R.K. Stoelting, M.D.

CELIAC PLEXUS BLOCK

Celiac Plexus Block: Efficacy and Safety of the Anterior Approach
Romanelli DF, Beckmann CF, Heiss FW (Lahey Clinic Med Ctr, Burlington, Mass)
AJR 160:497–500, 1993   101-94-3–16

Introduction.—For patients with chronic abdominal pain of celiac ganglion origin, especially that caused by pancreatic carcinoma, celiac plexus block with percutaneous injection is a widely used treatment. The anterior approach to celiac block offers several advantages over the posterior approach; including a quicker procedure, less discomfort, and lower risk of neurologic complications. The anterior approach to celiac plexus block was evaluated in 17 consecutive patients.

Methods.—All patients were referred with chronic abdominal pain believed to be of celiac ganglion origin. All had celiac plexus block by an anterior approach under CT control. Pain relief was assessed retrospectively from medical and nursing records and graded from 1+ to 4+ corresponding to no change and complete relief, respectively. In-hospital analgesic usage was also evaluated.

Results.—Thirteen of 14 patients with pancreatic carcinoma and 2 of 3 with other causes of pain had successful ethanol injection. Of the pancreatic carcinoma group, 79% had at least 2+ relief of pain, and most of these had 3+ or greater relief. In this group, the mean daily analgesic usage declined a mean of 58% after the procedure. The 3 patients with other diagnoses had little or no significant benefit from the procedure. Overall, only 3 of the 17 patients had complications, and all were relatively mild.

Conclusion.—This experience demonstrates the safety and efficacy of the anterior approach to celiac plexus block in patients with pain from pancreatic carcinoma. The reduced amount of neurolytic agent injected yields a lower rate of neurologic complications. This treatment should be considered whenever pancreatic cancer pain does not respond to medications.

▶ The efficacy of this technique is difficult to assess given the retrospective design and vague criteria for success. What is particularly interesting about this and other studies of the anterior approach is the lack of complications related to peritoneal soiling. Apparently the passage of a needle through the bowel, which is bound to occur in many of these patients, is of little consequence.—S.E. Abram, M.D.

Complications Associated With General Anesthesia

Acute Respiratory Failure Neuropathy: A Variant of Critical Illness Polyneuropathy

Gorson KC, Ropper AH (Tufts Univ, Boston)
Crit Care Med 21:267–271, 1993   101-94-3-17

Introduction.—Bolton et al. described "critical illness neuropathy" in patients who were weaned with difficulty from the ventilator or had generalized weakness resulting from an axonal neuropathy after sepsis and multiple-organ failure. Five critically ill patients had an acute respiratory failure preceding a severe axonal polyneuropathy. The sequence of successfully treated acute respiratory failure, followed by continued ventilator dependence with generalized weakness, caused diagnostic difficulty.

Patients.—Mechanical ventilation was initially required for severe bronchospasm or acute respiratory distress syndrome (table). Four patients received neuromuscular blocking agents and 4 received brief high doses of corticosteroids. Four patients had multiple-organ failure and 3 had sepsis.

Findings.—All patients had life-threatening respiratory failure followed by acute areflexic quadriplegia with relative preservation of sensory function. Unexplained respiratory failure and weakness were recognized when neuromuscular blockade was withdrawn, but weakness was evident earlier in 2 patients including 1 who had not received the drugs. The spinal fluid protein concentrations were normal. Electrophysiologic studies showed severe, acute axonal motor neuropathy in 4 patients; 1 patient had initial normal studies but later showed denervation. Two quadriparetic patients died at 2.5 months, 1 remained weak and ventilator-dependent, and 2 recovered to walk in 4–6 months.

Discussion.—Severe axonal motor neuropathy after acute respiratory failure in patients treated with glucocorticoids and neuromuscular blockade probably represents a variant of "critical illness polyneuropathy" that can be recognized from the temporal course of a conversion from primarily pulmonary to a pattern of neuromuscular ventilatory failure. Acute generalized paralysis after respiratory failure has also been attrib-

Features of Patients With Neuropathy After Respiratory Failure

Pt.	Age (yr)/Sex	Respiratory Failure	Interval *	Steroid †	NM Blockade †	Sepsis	Outcome
1	63/M	COPD exacerbated	25 days	14 days	19 days	—	Died
2	72/F	Asthma	13 days	10 days	8 days	— ‡	Ventilated
3	76/F	ARDS	45 days	28 days	24 days	+ ‡	Died
4	74/M	COPD exacerbated	57 days	3 months	None	+	Walked in 6 months
5	35/M	ARDS	33 days	None	30 days	+	Walked in 4 months

Abbreviations: NM, neuromuscular; *COPD*, chronic obstructive pulmonary disease; *ARDS*, adult respiratory distress syndrome.
* From onset of respiratory failure to apparent neuropathy.
† Duration of usage.
‡ Myocardial infarction.
(Courtesy of Gorson KC, Ropper AH: *Crit Care Med* 21:267–271, 1993.)

uted to acute steroid myopathy, acute catabolic myopathy from sepsis, a poorly defined structural myopathy, or neuromuscular change resulting from prolonged neuromuscular blockade. There have also been reports of residual neuromuscular blockade attributable to impaired excretion or accumulation of metabolites, particularly in patients with renal or liver failure.

▶ This syndrome remains difficult to attribute to a single etiology. Most recent concern centers around the toxicity of prolonged vecuronium infusions (1); however, only 1 of the 5 patients in this study received this drug (4 of 5 received pancuronium, which has also been implicated in causing prolonged muscle weakness). Whether many of the previously reported cases of neuromuscular blockade–induced muscle weakness were really polyneuropathy of critical illness is still open to speculation.—D.M. Rothenberg, M.D.

Reference

1.   Segredo V, et al: N *Engl J Med* 327:524, 1992.

Intraoperative Exacerbation of Parkinson's Disease
Reed AP, Han DG (Mount Sinai School of Medicine, New York)
Anesth Analg 75:850–853, 1992   101-94-3–18

Background.—Parkinson's disease affects about 1% of the population older than age 50 years. A patient with advanced Parkinson's disease had an intraoperative exacerbation during regional anesthesia.

Case Report.—Man, 73, was undergoing repair of a large recurrent left inguinal hernia. His Parkinson's disease medications included carbidopa, levodopa, amantadine, and selegiline. Missing or delaying a dose of levodopa resulted in severe generalized body tremors and rigidity. This patient also took lanoxin and isordil for congestive heart failure. He had a permanent pacemaker for sick sinus syndrome. Spinal anesthesia was planned for the current surgery. Hyperbaric bupivacaine, 12 mg, and fentanyl, 10 μg, were injected into the CSF at the L4–5 interspace, and a T-9 level was achieved within 10 minutes. Vital signs were unchanged. One hour after anesthesia was initiated, about 45 minutes into the surgery, the ECG showed a prominent artifact resembling coarse ventricular fibrillation. It had been about 5 hours since he took his levodopa. Assessment of the chest and upper extremities revealed fine tremors progressing to more gross tremors over 10 minutes. The patient, who was still awake and alert, reported feelings of discomfort. His signs and symptoms were similar to manifestations of Parkinson's disease. Levodopa and carbidopa were given orally while surgery continued, and his symptoms resolved about 20 minutes later. After surgery, the patient admitted that he sometimes took an extra dose of levodopa.

Conclusion.—Patients with advanced Parkinson's disease are at risk for perioperative exacerbations. Levodopa should be given orally about 20 minutes before anesthesia is induced in many patients. Levodopa may be given again during and after surgery. Regional anesthesia may be preferable to allow for communication of the patient's subjective feelings.

▶ Equally important to maintaining levodopa during the perioperative period is the avoidance of drugs (phenothiazines and butyrophenones) that are dopamine antagonists at the basal ganglia. The significant observation in this case report was the development of symptoms with only about 5 hours elapsing since the last dose of levodopa. It is usually taught that interruptions for more than 6 to 12 hours can result in abrupt loss of therapeutic benefit derived from the drug.—R.K. Stoelting, M.D.

Risk Factors Associated With Vasovagal Reactions During Colonoscopy
Herman LL, Kurtz RC, McKee KJ, Sun M, Thaler HT, Winawer SJ (Mem Sloan-Kettering Cancer Ctr, New York; Cornell Univ, New York)
Gastrointest Endosc 39:388–391, 1993   101-94-3–19

Purpose.—As the use of colonoscopy increases, so does experience with its complications. Although the serious complications of perforation and hemorrhage are well described, other complications, such as vasovagal reaction, have been less studied. The syndrome of colonoscopy-associated vasovagal reaction was studied, and an attempt was made to identify risk factors for it.

Methods.—During 60 days, 223 consecutive patients underwent colonoscopy at a gastrointestinal endoscopy unit. They were observed for signs of vasovagal reaction, defined as diaphoresis, sustained bradycardia of less than 60 beats/min or a 10% decrease in heart rate, and/or hypotension. The definition of hypotension was blood pressure less than 90/60 mm Hg or a reduction of more than 10% below a baseline measurement taken after sedation but before beginning the procedure. Thirty-seven patients (16.5%) met these criteria for vasovagal reaction. They were compared with a randomly selected group of 100 of the other patients.

Findings.—The 2 groups had similar demographic characteristics, cardiopulmonary disease, cardiac medications, procedural success or difficulty, endoscopist, procedure tolerance, or colonic preparation. The mean midazolam dose was 4.6 mg in the vasovagal group, compared with 3.9 mg in the control group. Forty-three percent of the patients in the vasovagal group had severe diverticulosis, compared with 16% of the controls. Some medical intervention was required in 35% of the vasovagal patients (6% of the overall series).

Conclusion.—Careful monitoring during colonoscopy will reveal a high incidence of vasovagal reactions. It is less common, however, for a patient to require intervention for such a reaction. Even when intervention is needed, these vasovagal reactions do not appear to carry any significant sequelae.

▶ Diagnosis of colonoscopy-associated vasovagal reaction based on a heart rate less than 60 beats/min or a 10% decrease in heart rate in the presence of midazolam sedation seems very imprecise. It is not surprising that the incidence of vasovagal reactions was high and the need for intervention rare.—R.K. Stoelting, M.D.

Is Uvular Edema a Complication of Endotracheal Intubation?

Diaz JH (Tulane Univ, New Orleans, La)
Anesth Analg 76:1139–1141, 1993

101-94-3-20

Background.—Postanesthetic uvular edema is a rare complication of endotracheal intubation reported in children and adults. A patient with

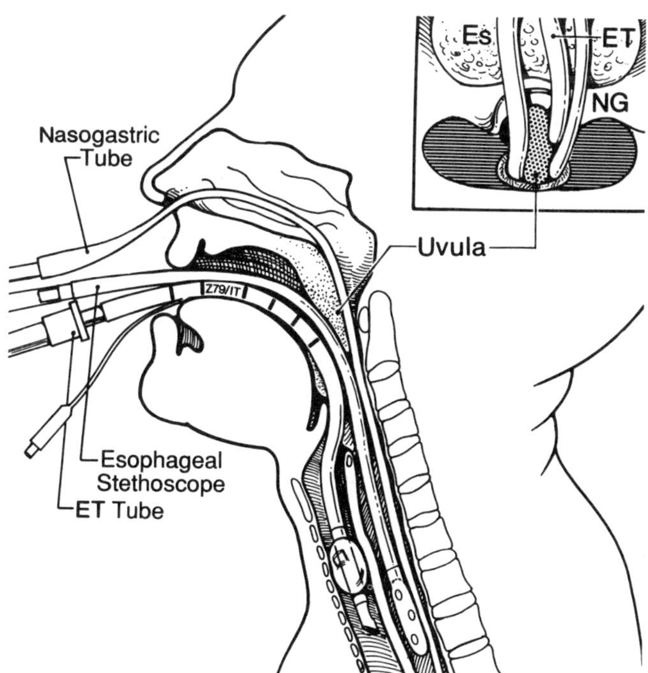

Fig 3–3.—Sagittal section of an adult's upper airway shows a possible mechanism of postanesthetic uvular edema. Entrapment of the uvula between pharyngeal tubes may lead to venous and lymphatic engorgement of the uvula, especially during prolonged anesthesia in the supine position. (Courtesy of Diaz JH: *Anesth Analg* 76:1139–1141, 1993.)

this complication after atraumatic endotracheal intubation with a sterile single-use endotracheal tube was seen.

Case Report.—Man, 66, was undergoing transabdominal exploration of the lumbosacral plexus bilaterally for isolation and removal of plexiform neurofibromas. He had neurofibromatosis. The trachea was intubated without trauma, and the endotracheal tube cuff was inflated. A 14-French Salem sump was passed into the stomach through the right nostril, and an esophageal stethoscope was inserted into the esophagus through the mouth on the side opposite the oral endotracheal tube. No other airways were used. Anesthesia was maintained with isoflurane and fentanyl. On the patient's admission to the postanesthetic care unit, about 6 hours after initial intubation, the trachea was extubated. During extubation, the patient's uvula was prolapsed between the endotracheal and nasogastric tubes. The uvula appeared longer than usual but not swollen or distorted. Twenty hours after surgery, the patient complained of a sore throat and a feeling of something hanging down the middle of his throat that made him gag when he sat upright. Examination showed a uniformly swollen, grossly edematous, cherry-red uvula with a thick white exudate along the left side and distal tip. Dexamethasone, 12 mg, was given intravenously, and humidified oxygen by face mask was continued. A regimen of oral mouth rinses was prescribed. The patient was encouraged to remain supine. Within 48 hours after surgery, he became asymptomatic. His uvula returned to near-normal size, and he was discharged home 6 days after his operation.

Conclusion.—The patient's long uvula was entrapped between the nasogastric and endotracheal tube. The uvula may have been enmeshed among the endotracheal tube, the nasogastric tube, and the esophageal stethoscope during the 6-hour operation with the patient in the supine position (Fig 3–3). The pinched uvula then became progressively engorged with venous blood and lymph, causing gagging from a foreign-body sensation when the patient sat upright.

▶ This is a surprisingly rare complication considering the potential for trauma to this structure that accompanies nearly every general anesthetic that includes tracheal intubation.—R.K. Stoelting, M.D.

Intraoperative Somatosensory Evoked Potential Monitoring Predicts Peripheral Nerve Injury During Cardiac Surgery
Hickey C, Gugino LD, Aglio LS, Mark JB, Son SL, Maddi R (Brigham and Women's Hosp, Boston)
Anesthesiology 78:29–35, 1993   101-94-3–21

Introduction.—The incidence of brachial plexus injury after open heart surgery is reported in some studies to be as high as 18%. Somatosensory evoked potentials (SEPs) were monitored during cardiac surgery to determine whether such peripheral nerve injury can be predicted intraoperatively. The use of SEP monitoring has been shown to minimize the risk of sciatic nerve injury during hip surgery.

Methods.—Thirty consecutive, neurologically normal patients scheduled for elective coronary artery bypass surgery agreed to undergo monitoring of SEPs from bilateral median and ulnar nerves. The SEPs were analyzed for changes during central venous cannulation and during use of the Favoloro and Canadian self-retaining sternal retractors, events implicated in brachial plexus injury. Neurologic examinations were performed within 24 hours of completion of surgery by a researcher unaware of the results of SEP monitoring.

Results.—Four patients showed transient changes in SEPs at the time of central venous cannulation. These changes completely resolved within 5 minutes and were not associated with postoperative neurologic deficits. Significant changes in SEPs were seen in 21 patients during use of the Canadian and Favoloro retractors. Waveforms returned to baseline levels intraoperatively in 16 patients and were not associated with postoperative neurologic deficits. Five patients, however, had evidence of nerve deficits that persisted to the end of surgery. Neurologic injury was associated with the Favoloro retractor in 3 cases and with the Canadian retractor in 2 cases.

Conclusion.—Brachial plexus injury is common after cardiac surgery. When SEP waveforms are normal or improving at the end of the operation, peripheral nerve dysfunction is minor and transient. The continued presence or progression of a significant change toward a flat line trace indicates a level of dysfunction that will be clinically evident postoperatively. Only 6% of patients in this series retained their deficits 1 week after surgery. Examination of SEP changes may lead to the development of operative techniques and instruments designed to minimize nerve injury.

▶ Of the 30 patients involved in this study, 5 developed arm neurologic deficits postoperatively. This seems like an enormously high incidence to me, although the authors cited corroborative evidence from other studies. Although intraoperative SEP monitoring seems to have been predictive of postoperative injury, the next step is to figure out how to make the whole thing go away, i.e., not cause injury in the first place. Some have suggested that tucking his/her arms down at the sides of the patient, combined with the retractors mentioned by the authors, may be the problem. Perhaps we should be hanging the arms from suspension devices, such as those used during obesity surgery. Some cardiac anesthesiologists even place the arms above the patient's head (a practice with which I cannot agree). Clearly, if peripheral nerve injury is this common, however transient, then we need to rethink our positioning of patients for this kind of surgery.—J.H. Tinker, M.D.

Anaesthetic Practice and Postoperative Pulmonary Complications

Pedersen T, Viby-Mogensen J, Ringsted C (Univ of Copenhagen)
Acta Anaesthesiol Scand 36:812–818, 1992   101-94-3–22

Introduction.—Although the type and site of surgery are known risk factors for postoperative pulmonary complications, the contributions of anesthetic technique are less well recognized. The important risk factors for development of such complications, including anesthetic technique.

Methods.—Data were collected prospectively on 7,306 patients undergoing abdominal, urologic, gynecologic, or orthopedic surgery. Based on a previous study, risk factors analyzed were age, presence or absence of chronic obstructive lung disease, type of surgery and whether it was emergency or elective, and type and duration of anesthesia.

Findings.—At least 1 postoperative pulmonary complication occurred in 4.1% of patients. In the more than 6,000 patients receiving general anesthesia, the pulmonary complication rate was 4.5%. The complication rate neared 13% for patients receiving pancuronium, compared with just more than 5% for those receiving atracurium. Although this difference disappeared after stratification for the type of surgery and duration of anesthesia, logistic regression analysis found an increased risk of postoperative pulmonary complications in lengthy procedures in which pancuronium was used.

The pulmonary complication rate was less than 2% for patients receiving regional anesthesia. For patients having major orthopedic surgery, the complication rate was 11.5% for those receiving regional anesthesia compared with 3.6% for those receiving general anesthesia. Logistic regression identified 6 significant predictors of pulmonary complications. In order, they were advanced age, major abdominal surgery, emergency surgery, history of chronic obstructive lung disease, pancuronium anesthesia lasting longer than 1.5 hours, and pancuronium anesthesia.

Conclusion.—Some significant predictors of postoperative pulmonary complications were identified. Pancuronium anesthesia, especially when given for long operations, is a significant predictor. General anesthesia entails a higher risk than regional anesthesia for patients undergoing major orthopedic operations.

▶ This paper is the latest salvo in the "regional vs. general" battle that has been controversial for all of my career in anesthesia and before that. The only subgroup of the approximately 7,000 patients who were included in this study that showed a significant difference in pulmonary morbidity between regional vs. general anesthesia included those undergoing major orthopedic surgery. The question not addressed by the authors, however, is the validity of retrospectively dividing this large group into smaller subgroups. A number of studies show that if you take any large group of patients, study them for anything, and then *retrospectively* divide them into smaller cohorts, on any criteria, you will find significant differences appearing between subgroups. It is logical to think that if you had 100 such subgroup cohorts, then if you accepted statistical significance at the $P < .05$ level, you would find signficant differences in 5 groups, between "treatment A vs. treatment B." In fact, the mathematicians tell us that this is not so. They tell us that if you divided a large group into such cohorts and applied fictitious "treatment A vs. treatment B" to these cohorts in a random fashion, *approximately 40% of the cohorts will develop statistical significance.* All this really tells us is that it is invalid to divide large groups into smaller cohorts. I very strongly question the validity of the findings of this paper.—J.H. Tinker, M.D.

Forearm Amputation After Radial Artery Cannulation

Upper Limb Amputation Following Radial Artery Cannulation

Bright E, Baines DB, French BG, Cartmill TB (Children's Hosp, Camperdown, New South Wales, Australia)
Anaesth Intensive Care 21:351–353, 1993   101-94-3–23

Introduction.—Arterial cannulation for arterial blood pressure and blood gas monitoring has become a routine procedure with few reported major complications. A patient had hand and forearm ischemia requiring above-elbow amputation after "uncomplicated" radial artery cannulation.

Case Report.—Girl, 14 years, was operated on for acyanotic tetralogy of Fallot by a visiting cardiac surgical team in Fiji. Before the operation, an 18-gauge cannula was placed in a right forearm vein and a 22-gauge cannula in the left radial artery on the first attempt. After induction, a 5.5-French gauge triple-lumen catheter was placed in the right atrium via the right internal jugular vein. The patient had a complicated form of tetralogy of Fallot, requiring patching of a large ventricular septal defect and transannular patch augmentation of the right ventricular outflow tract. Low-dose dopamine and adrenaline were needed to wean the patient from bypass. She was kept on ventilation in the intensive care unit postoperatively.

Overnight, her left hand became pale, with poor capillary return and a damped arterial waveform. No blood could be aspirated, and the cannula was removed. After extubation, she complained of pain in the arm. By 24 hours, the hand was obviously nonviable. The patient was returned to the operation room for removal of thrombi from the radial and ulnar arteries and extensive fasciotomy and carpal tunnel release. The patient was given heparin infusion. Rethrombosis developed within 6 hours in both arteries; thrombectomy was repeated and the heparin dose was increased. The hand appeared viable during the next 24 hours, and the visiting surgical team left. The next day, however, the radial pulse disappeared and the forearm became nonviable. This required reexploration and above-elbow amputation. The patient had a good cardiac result.

Discussion.—This case serves as a reminder of the possibility of complications from the routine procedure of radial artery cannulation. Although the cause of the thrombosis in this case is unknown, the surgical setting and lack of continuing care certainly played a role in the patient's disastrous outcome.

▶ The authors have presented this case to remind us that this devastating complication still lurks after radial artery cannulation. We impale the radial artery with impunity, sometimes piercing it many more times than just once during our attempts to cannulate it. After we puncture it, we jam our Teflon catheters into it, sometimes wrinkling them, stating "the catheter wouldn't thread." We prefer not to think of the damage we might be doing. In my years as a cardiac anesthetist, I have seen this complication 1 other time in a previously healthy patient. It was just as devastating then as it was in this case.—J.H. Tinker, M.D.

Delayed Ischaemia of the Hand Necessitating Amputation After Radial Artery Cannulation

Mangar D, Laborde RS, Vu DN (Univ of South Florida, Tampa)
Can J Anaesth 40:247–250, 1993   101-94-3–24

Introduction.—A rare case of ischemic injury to the hand occurred after placement of a left radial artery catheter. The patient subsequently underwent amputation of the left hand and right leg.

Case Report.—Man, 35, was scheduled for right femoral-tibial bypass. The patient had a 25-year history of insulin-dependent diabetes mellitus, end-stage renal disease, coronary artery disease, peripheral vascular disease, and hypertension. He had had a silent myocardial infarction and a left hemispheric cerebrovascular accident and had undergone a number of surgical procedures related to his medical problems. The patient also had a 20-year history of smoking 2–3 packs of cigarettes per day. A left radial artery catheter, which had been placed atraumatically before surgery under general anesthesia, was accidently pulled out the following morning by the patient. His left hand had no evidence of ischemia or hematoma. Ten days later, however, the patient complained of pain, coldness, and discoloration. Two weeks after the surgery, the patient underwent right below-knee amputation. A right above-knee and left hand amputation were performed 1 week later.

Discussion.—Gross pathologic examination revealed that both the ulnar and radial arteries were calcified, with as much as 95% occlusion. Severe, obliterative atherosclerotic peripheral vascular disease with extensive calcification and focal organizing thrombosis was apparent at microscopic examination. The patient had cigarette burns to his left hand that he had never felt, indicating vascular compromise. A previously treated, occluded left forearm arteriovenous fistula may have further compromised flow. Other sites of arterial access, such as the superficial temporal or axillary artery, should be used in patients with severe peripheral vascular disease.

▶ Overall, the safety of radial artery cannulation is impressive and, in my opinion, provides useful information far in excess to remote risks. Nevertheless, like any medical intervention, this invasive monitor should be selected on an individual patient basis. Patients with severe peripheral vascular disease may be at increased risk for vascular compromise after radial artery cannulation. Likewise, they may also greatly benefit from the continuous information derived from an intra-arterial catheter during major operative procedures.—R.K. Stoelting, M.D.

Aspiration of Gastric Contents
(see also Anesthesia for Obstetrics and Gynecology)

Preoperative Drinking Does Not Affect Gastric Contents
Phillips S, Hutchinson S, Davidson T (Kingston Hosp, Surrey, England)
Br J Anaesth 70:6–9, 1993   101-94-3-25

Background.—Several researchers have questioned the need for preoperative fasting. Whether allowing unrestricted clear fluids until 2 hours before anesthesia would change gastric volume and pH, affect anesthetic complications such as regurgitation or aspiration, and increase patient comfort was investigated.

Methods.—One hundred adults undergoing elective surgery were enrolled in the prospective, randomized trial. Patients were assigned to an experimental group, in which intake of free clear fluids was allowed up to the time of premedication, or to a control group, in which fasting for 6 hours before surgery was required. The residual volume and pH of gastric contents after anesthesia induction were measured.

Findings.—The experimental group consumed a mean 388 mL of fluids in the 6 hours preceding surgery. Drinking liquids before surgery did not affect the mean residual gastric volume of pH (table). The experimental group had less thirst preoperatively. There were no problems with aspiration or regurgitation.

Conclusion.—Allowing patients to drink clear fluids until 2 hours before anesthesia is induced for elective surgery may improve their comfort without compromising their safety. Ingesting unrestricted clear fluids until oral premedication did not affect gastric volume or gastric contents pH in the current series.

▶ These data are consistent with numerous other studies that confirm that ingestion of clear liquids up until 2 hours before the induction of anesthesia in the absence of known risk factors (emergency surgery, anticipated difficult upper airway management, obesity, diabetes mellitus) does not increase gastric fluid volume. The best protection against vomiting and regurgitation in the vast majority of patients is the skillful anesthesiologist who maintains a patent upper airway.—R.K. Stoelting, M.D.

| | Residual Gastric Volume (RGV) and pH | | | |
	Study group	Control group	CI	P
RGV (ml)	21 (0–80)	19 (0–63)	−5 to +9	0.58
pH	2.64 (1.07–6.82)	2.26 (1.25–7.03)	−2.5 to +0.8	0.07
Percent of patients with				
RGV > 0.4 ml kg^{-1}	26	22	−13 to +21	0.64
pH < 2.5	76	87	−24 to +6	0.25
Both	20	20	−16 to +17	0.96

Abbreviation: CI, confidence interval for difference.
Note: Values for RGV and pH are means with range in parentheses.
(Courtesy of Phillips S, Hutchinson S, Davidson T: *Br J Anaesth* 70:6-9, 1993.)

4 Physiology and Pathophysiology Related to Anesthesia

Cardiovascular

Effects of Acute Isovolemic Hemodilution and Anesthesia on Regional Function in Left Ventricular Myocardium With Compromised Coronary Blood Flow

Spahn DR, Smith LR, McRae RL, Leone BJ (Duke Univ, Durham, NC)
Acta Anaesthesiol Scand 36:628–636, 1992   101-94-4–1

Introduction.—Isovolemic hemodilution has been proposed as an alternative to transfusion therapy, but it reduces the oxygen-carrying capacity of arterial blood and therefore may lead to regional myocardial dysfunction in patients with coronary artery disease.

Objective and Methods.—The threshold of hemodilution-induced regional myocardial dysfunction was determined in a canine model of critical left anterior descending (LAD) coronary artery stenosis. Isovolemic hemodilution was produced with dextran 70 to hematocrit levels of 35%, 25%, and 15%. Halothane was administered at end-tidal concentrations of .7%, .9%, 1.1%, and 1.3% at each level of hemodilution. Regional left ventricular contractility was quantified by sonomicrometry in the flow-compromised LAD territory and in noncompromised regions of the left ventricular myocardium.

Results.—Both arterial and coronary perfusion pressures declined during hemodilution, as did left ventricular contractility. There was a slight increase in left ventricular end-diastolic pressure. Systolic shortening in the LAD region was significantly compromised at maximal hemodilution. Postsystolic shortening was not increased in the compromised area of myocardium. The effects of hemodilution on global cardiovascular function and regional myocardial function were not altered by exposure to halothane (Fig 4–1).

Conclusion.—In this canine model, moderate hemodilution is relatively well tolerated in myocardial areas where coronary blood flow is

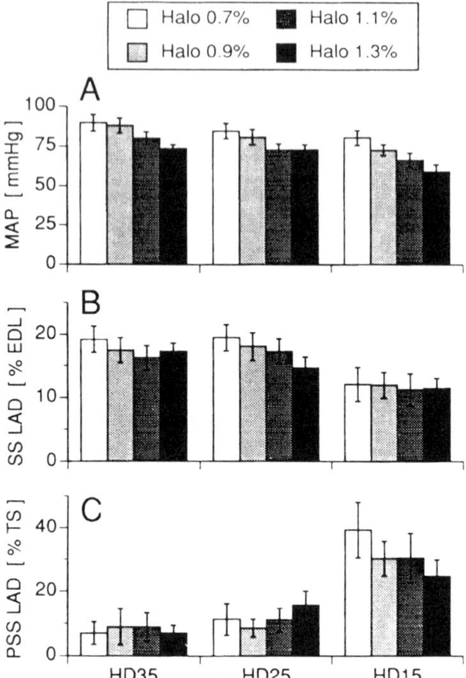

Fig 4–1.—Responses of **(A)** mean arterial pressure (*MAP*), **(B)** systolic shortening in the coronary flow compromised LAD territory (*SS LAD*), and **(C)** postsystolic shortening in the LAD territory (*PSS LAD*) to different (.7% to 1.3%) end-tidal halothane concentrations at 3 hemodilutional stages. *HD 35* signifies hematocrit of 35%; *HD25*, hematocrit of 25%; *HD15*, hematocrit of 15%. (Courtesy of Spahn DR, Smith LR, McRae RL, et al: *Acta Anaesthesiol Scand* 36:628–636, 1992.)

compromised. The critical level of isovolemic hemodilution in dogs lies between hematocrit levels of 15% and 25%.

▶ This group has tackled, systematically, the important task of figuring out how low we might be able to go in hemoglobin levels, during blood conservation practices, in order to avoid placing patients who have coronary artery disease at risk of myocardial ischemia or worse. This work is in dogs, of course, with their much better developed ventricular myocardial collateral systems. Nonetheless, this paper and others from this group show clearly that even in the presence of a severely stenosed coronary, levels of hemodilution that would have been unheard of just 10 years ago are clearly tolerated. I also think the elegant model they have developed will prove very useful as we begin to use plain-old "isovolemic hemodilution" by adding recombinant or other types of stroma-free hemoglobin.—J.H. Tinker, M.D.

Sympathetic Hyperactivity During Desflurane Anesthesia in Healthy Volunteers: A Comparison With Isoflurane
Ebert TJ, Muzi M (Med College of Wisconsin, Milwaukee)
Anesthesiology 79:444–453, 1993   101-94-4-2

Background.—On anesthesia induction, desflurane is associated with more tachycardia and hypertension than isoflurane. Microneurography was used to determine whether these cardiovascular effects were related to sympathetic outflow.

Methods.—Fourteen healthy volunteers aged 20–31 years were studied. Arterial pressure was measured from the radial artery, forearm blood flow as determined by strain gauge plethysmography, and sympathetic nerve activity (SNA) directed to skeletal muscle blood vessels was noted using a tungsten needle placed percutaneously into the peroneal nerve. Thiopental, 5 mg/kg, and vecuronium, .2 mg/kg, were administered, and 2 minutes later, desflurane or isoflurane was titrated gradually to the inspired gas over minutes to 1.5 minimum alveolar concentration (MAC).

Findings.—Desflurane anesthesia initiation produced significant changes, including a 2.5-fold increase in SNA, hypertension, tachycardia, facial flushing, and tearing. Moderate upper airway obstruction developed in 3 volunteers about 4 minutes after desflurane was initiated, despite neuromuscular blockade. No volunteers given isoflurane had those responses. Both agents were associated with a progressive decline in blood pressure and forearm vascular resistance. Muscle SNA increased gradually. The heart rate was unchanged in individuals receiving desflurane until 1.5 MAC was reached, at which time tachycardia occurred. A transition from 1 to 1.5 MAC desflurane produced significant increases in the heart rate, hypertension, and a doubling of SNA persisting for several minutes. No subject given isoflurane had these responses.

Conclusion.—Titrating desflurane after thiopental induction and increasing desflurane concentration from 1 to 1.5 MAC produce sympatho-excitation, hypertension, and tachycardia in healthy, young volunteers. Desflurane should be used with great caution in patients who may be placed at risk by such changes.

▶ The sympathetic responses documented here during rapid increases in desflurane concentration are likely largely due to pungency-related airway irritation. It is important to remember that desflurane's potency is considerably lower than that of isoflurane. Thus, larger increments in inspired concentration must be used if one is going to change the blood level in comparison with isoflurane, to the same percentages of MAC. I think most people agree now that this phenomenon observed and recorded by these authors is more mundane than they may have thought, namely it is probably due to airway irritation and pungency. I selected this paper partly to discuss the desflurane sympathetic response phenomenon, but also to showcase a truly elegant technique of recording human peripheral sympathetic responses.—J.H. Tinker, M.D.

Pulmonary

Respiratory Response to CO_2 in Patients With Chronic Obstructive Pulmonary Disease in Acute Respiratory Failure

Tardif C, Bonmarchand G, Gibon J-F, Hellot M-F, Leroy J, Pasquis P, Milic-Emili J, Derenne J-P (Hôpital Charles Nicolle, Rouen, France; Hôpital de la Pitié-Salpêtrière, Paris)
Eur Respir J 6:619–624, 1993   101-94-4-3

Background.—In patients with acute respiratory failure (ARF) resulting from chronic obstructive pulmonary disease (COPD), oxygen administration results in increased arterial carbon dioxide tension ($PaCO_2$),

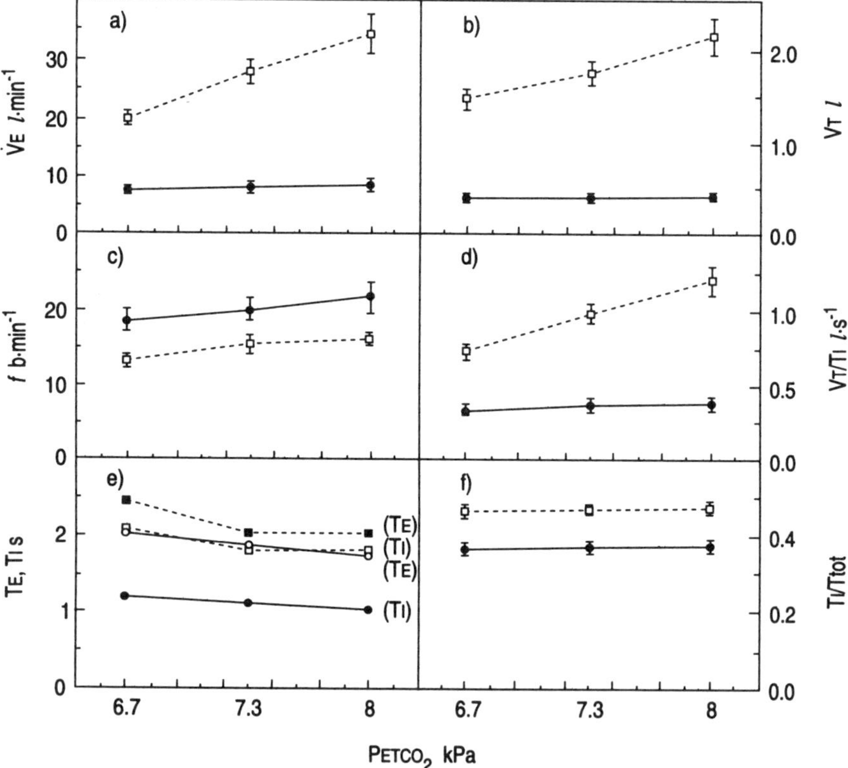

Fig 4–2.—*Abbreviation: P_{ETCO_2},* end-tidal carbon dioxide tension. Ventilatory responses to CO_2 in patients with COPD (*solid lines*) and in normal subjects (*dashed lines*). **a,** minute ventilation (V̇E); **b,** tidal volume (VT); **c,** respiratory frequency (*f*); **d,** mean inspiratory flow (VT/TI); **e,** inspiratory time (TI), expiratory time (TE); **f,** duty cycle (TI/Ttot). (Courtesy of Tardif C, Bonmarchand G, Fibon J-F, et al: *Eur Respir J* 6:619–624, 1993.)

leading to the hypothesis that sensitivity to hypercapnia is blunted. It is now known that hypoxia is not a primary chemoreceptor drive, but the blunted sensitivity to CO_2 remains unexplored.

Study Design.—Twenty-five patients with COPD with ARF and 26 normal subjects were studied to determine the respiratory response to CO_2. All patients were mechanically ventilated to bring their arterial oxygen tension, $PaCO_2$, pH, and bicarbonate levels to near-normal values to allow assessment of the chemoreceptor-respiratory center response under normal standard acid-base conditions. Carbon dioxide rebreathing tests were performed in the spontaneously breathing, intubated patients after arterial blood gases were near normal levels. Ventilatory and mouth occlusion pressure $(P_{.1})$ responses to CO_2 were determined. Similar respiratory responses were recorded in normal subjects (excluding arterial blood gases).

Results.—The slopes of ventilatory responses to CO_2 were significantly lower in patients with COPD, compared with normal controls (Fig 4–2). However, the drive from CO_2 receptor stimulation still accounted for an important part of ventilation. Increasing $PaCO_2$ from 5.3 kPa to 8 kPa (40 to 60 mm Hg) increased minute ventilation from 6.3 L/min to 9.6 L/min. The CO_2 drive was responsible for this 34% increase in ventilation. The slopes of the $P_{.1}$ responses were significantly lower in patients than in normal controls. However, in half of the patients, the $P_{.1}$ responses to CO_2 were in the normal range. In addition, at an end-tidal carbon dioxide tension of 7.3 kPa, the $P_{.1}$ values did not differ significantly between patients and controls. Therefore, the overall neural drive to breathe was probably well above normal.

Conclusion.—Contrary to previous reports of a severely blunted chemoreceptor response to CO_2, the CO_2 drive appears to be a major determinant of respiratory stimulation in many patients with ARF resulting from COPD.

The Pathophysiologic Changes Following Bile Aspiration in a Porcine Lung Model
Porembka DT, Kier A, Sehlhorst S, Boyce S, Orlowski JP, Davis K Jr (Univ of Cincinnati, Ohio; Cleveland Clinic Found, Ohio)
Chest 104:919–924, 1993   101-94-4-4

Purpose.—To date, bile aspiration remains an underappreciated aspiration syndrome. A porcine lung model was used to evaluate the physiologic response and the histopathology of lung tissue after the administration of sublethal doses of bile.

Methods.—Twenty-one domestic swine, weighing 11–19 kg, were included in the study. Of those, 15 were placed into 1 of 3 equal groups. Control group swine received physiologic saline (pH 7.45), study group 1 was given strained gastric contents (pH 2.24), and study group 2 received strained bile (pH 7.19). Intratracheal installation at .5 mL/kg was used for all solutions. The lungs of 6 additional animals, including 2 gastric, 2 bile, and 2 physiologic saline, were evaluated after aspiration by scanning electron microscopy (SEM). An additional untreated animal served as the SEM control. The physiologic findings were analyzed via analysis of variance (ANOVA) for repeated measures; SEM and histopathologic results were scored by an observer blinded to the groups and were assessed via ANOVA and Scheffe tests.

Results.—Significant deterioration of the partial pressure of oxygen in arterial blood (PaO$_2$), shunt fraction, static compliance, and the alveolar-arterial gradient were noted in the bile aspiration group. In addition, the bile-exposed lungs revealed greater pathologic changes compared with the gastric- or saline-exposed lungs, as determined by light histopathologic and SEM results.

Conclusion.—Bile aspiration can lead to significant lung injury and physiologic deterioration of PaO$_2$. After gastric aspiration, the development of noncardiac pulmonary edema should alert the clinician to possible bile aspiration. The benefits of surfactant instillation in this clinical setting need to be elucidated.

▶ A low pH and/or the presence of particulate matter are accepted risk factors for development of aspiration pneumonitis. The likelihood of aspiration of bile with near-neutral pH seems remote but, on the basis of these data, deserving of consideration as a risk factor.—R.K. Stoelting, M.D.

Metabolic

The Independent Metabolic Effects of Halothane and Isoflurane Anaesthesia

Carli F, Ronzoni G, Webster J, Khan K, Elia M (Northwick Park Hosp, Harrow, England; MRC Dunn Nutrition Unit, Cambridge, England)
Acta Anaesthesiol Scand 37:672–678, 1993   101-94-4–5

Objective.—The metabolic effects of anesthetic agents are not well known. Whether halothane and isoflurane alone cause changes in circulating concentrations of hormones, various metabolites and amino acids, and the flux of some substrates across the forearm was examined.

Patients and Methods.—Twelve women scheduled for elective abdominal hysterectomy agreed to participate in the study. Six were randomized to isoflurane and 6 to halothane. Anesthesia was administered for 2 hours before surgery and during the hour-long operation. Four patients in each group took part in arteriovenous catheterization to assess the exchange of metabolites across the forearm. Blood samples were obtained from all patients during anesthesia and recovery to measure concentrations of various hormones, metabolites, selected amino acids, and albumin. Measurements of carbon dioxide production, oxygen consumption,

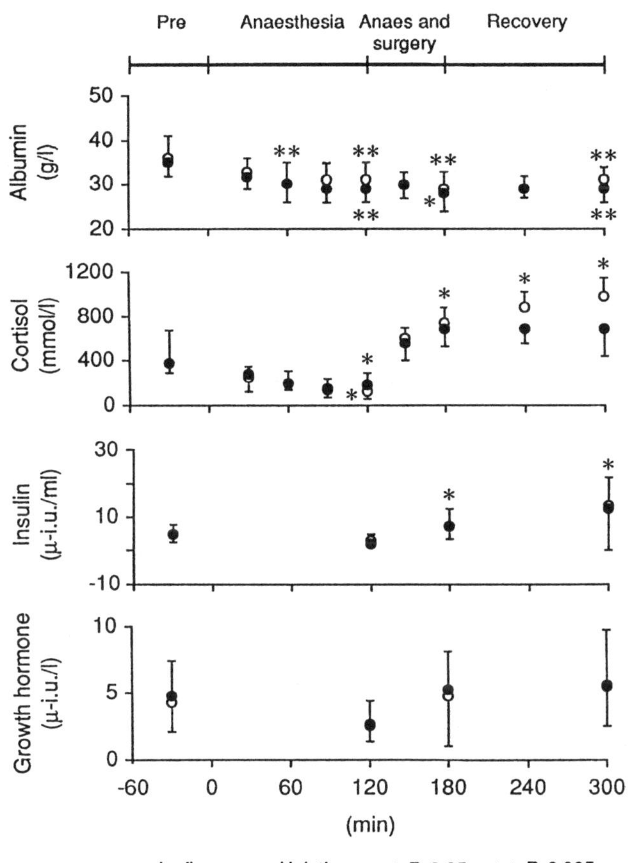

Fig 4–3.—Plasma concentrations of albumin and hormones in the 2 groups studied during the 4 periods. Data are presented as mean and SD. *P* values vs. preanesthesia levels. (Courtesy of Carli F, Ronzoni G, Webster J, et al: *Acta Anaesthesiol Scand* 37:672–678, 1993.)

and the respiratory exchange ratio were taken before anesthesia, before and at the end of surgery, and during the recovery period.

Results.—Whole body oxygen consumption decreased significantly by more than 20% during anesthesia, both with and without surgery. The circulating concentration of most amino acids exhibited little or no change during the period of anesthesia alone. However, there was a tendency for the flux of most metabolites to decrease, a tendency that persisted during surgery. The albumin concentration decreased during anesthesia alone, and plasma cortisol concentration demonstrated a twofold reduction. The onset of surgery brought about a rapid increase in plasma cortisol concentration and a significant increase in circulating concentrations of glucose and lactate. Hypoalbuminemia persisted, however, after the initiation of surgery. In both the halothane and isoflurane groups, heart rate increased during anesthesia, and systolic and diastolic blood pressures decreased significantly. Forearm blood flow increased during isoflurane anesthesia alone, but this change was not observed in the halothane group (Fig 4-3).

Conclusion.—The metabolic effects of surgical trauma have been extensively investigated, yet little research has dealt with the effects of anesthesia alone. Halothane and isoflurane alone appear to have a minimal effect on the circulating concentration of various metabolites. Both agents had an important effect on the concentration of cortisol and albumin, however. An unexpected finding was the significant decrease in plasma cortisol during anesthesia alone.

▶ I included this paper because for years we have paid lip service to the effects of anesthetics on endocrine function (other than the direct cardiovascular endocrine hormones). Anesthesia-related postoperative complications such as perioperative myocardial infarction may be related to the so-called stress injury of anesthesia and/or surgery. Activation of complement, hypercoagulability, alterations in renal function, and other stress indicators clearly do have effects, but we often have little or no idea what they might be. This elegant paper gets us back into that kind of study again by looking at effects of anesthetics on plasma cortisol and other hormonal concentrations. On the other hand, watching plasma concentrations fluctuate and trying to understand what is causing those fluctuations, plus what those fluctuations are doing to the overall stress response is, as one wag put it, "like trying to understand the ocean by watching bottles bounce up and down in New York and Hong Kong harbors."—J.H. Tinker, M.D.

5 Pharmacology of Anesthetics, Relaxants, and Adjuvants

Mechanisms of Anesthetic Action

Is There a Cutoff in Anesthetic Potency for the Normal Alkanes?

Liu J, Laster MJ, Taheri S, Eger EI II, Koblin DD, Halsey MJ (Univ of California, San Francisco)
Anesth Analg 77:12–18, 1993   101-94-5-1

Background.—The anesthetic potencies of normal alkanes from methanes to octane reportedly increase as the chain length increases. The apparent inability of n-alkanes, which have greater chain lengths, to provide anesthesia is called the cutoff phenomenon. Because the cutoff phenomenon is theoretically important, the anesthetizing partial pressures of n-alkanes from methane to decane were studied.

Methods and Results.—Vapor pressures and anesthetizing partial pressure were measured in 10 consecutive normal alkanes. All produced anesthesia in rats, defined by the lack of movement in response to tail-clamp or electric tail stimulation. The anesthetizing partial pressure was determined as the mean between the concentrations just permitting and preventing movement. Nonane and decane did not produce anesthesia given alone at saturated vapor pressures, but their anesthetic properties were shown by their ability to reduce the anesthetic requirement for isoflurane. Anesthetic potency increased and vapor pressure declined with increasing chain length. The reduction in vapor pressure far exceeded the potency increase. The ratio of the partial pressure needed for anesthesia to the saturated vapor pressure was .48 for nonane and .19 for decane.

Conclusion.—There appears to be no cutoff phenomenon from n-methane to n-decane. However, larger alkanes apparently have vapor pressures too low to permit their potency to be evident when given alone.

▶ Past literature has contended that the long-chain alkanes nonane and decane exhibit the so-called cutoff phenomenon, i.e., for some reason they do not produce anesthesia. These authors have shown that no cutoff phenome-

"

non really exists, but rather that the vapor pressures are such that older studies were unable to deliver anesthetizing partial pressures. What does all this mean? Basically, it means that the Meyer-Overton lipid-solubility association with general anesthesia, however imperfect, still works, although it may need to be modified, because it does not predict the potency of these 2 alkanes very well. Is any of this relevant to clinical practice? I have always been fascinated by the observation that most clinical anesthesiologists do not appear to give a "tinker's damn" (sorry about the pun) about why anesthetics work. Is this kind of knowledge arcane? I think the answer to that question might be yes if we had perfect anesthetics today. We do not, and therefore my answer to these authors and others of their ilk is "keep working." We need these kinds of studies.—J.H. Tinker, M.D.

Volatile Anesthetic Requirements Differ in Mice Selectively Bred for Sensitivity or Resistance to Diazepam: Implications for the Site of Anesthesia

McCrae AF, Gallaher EJ, Winter PM, Firestone LL (Univ of Pittsburgh, Pa; VA Med Ctr, Portland, Ore; Oregon Health Sciences Univ, Portland)
Anesth Analg 76:1313–1317, 1993   101-94-5-2

Background.—One approach to determining the general anesthetic target involves genetic selection procedures. In this approach, animals are bred for sensitivity or resistance to general anesthetics, and correlations with specific neuronal structural or functional defects are sought. For instance, murine strains have been developed to be sensitive or resistant to the obtunding effects of diazepam, defined by their ability to maintain balance on a rotating rod. In the current study, halothane and enflurane requirements were tested to determine whether diazepam-sensitive (DS) and diazepam-resistant (DR) mice might be similarly divergent in the obtunding response to general anesthetics.

Methods and Findings.—Loss-of-righting reflex was defined as the end point using a carousel in a chamber. For both anesthetics, the DS animals had a lower median effective dose than the DR animals. The decrease paralleled diazepam susceptibility. With halothane, the median effective dose was .72 and .87 in the DS and DR groups, respectively. The results obtained with enflurane were comparable.

Conclusion.—There was an association between an inbred difference in response to diazepam and an altered volatile anesthetic requirement. This relationship suggests that a common underlying mechanism mediates these 2 phenotypes.

▶ The very fact that scientists can genetically alter mice toward resistance or sensitivity to diazepam is fascinating in itself. This new study showed that these differing phenotypes of mice also seem to differ, in the same direction, in their sensitivities to halothane and enflurane, at least. This in turn implies common underlying mechanisms for general anesthesia between intravenous drugs such as diazepam and inhalation anesthetics. If this is so, it is very newsworthy, because we have always rigidly separated these 2 types of agents, i.e., those that apparently work on conventional receptors, e.g., the intravenous drugs, and those that appear to work in "physical solution," e.g., the inhalation agents. That some elements of sensitivity or resistance to both these kinds of anesthetics might be genetically determined could be a major breakthrough because it could allow us, through gene identification, to understand the nature of the expression of that gene. That knowledge, in turn, could allow us to understand what the expression of that gene has to do with anesthesia. In short, I think molecular genetics may be able to help us make significant strides in understanding the molecular mechanisms that underlie general anesthesia.—J.H. Tinker, M.D.

Neuroprotective Doses of *N*-Methyl-D-Aspartate Receptor Antagonists Profoundly Reduce the Minimum Alveolar Anesthetic Concentration (MAC) for Isoflurane in Rats

Kuroda Y, Strebel S, Rafferty C, Bullock R (Wellcome Surgical Inst, Glasgow, Scotland; Univ of Glasgow, Scotland)
Anesth Analg 77:795–800, 1993   101-94-5–3

Background.—In animal studies of focal cerebral ischemia, N-methyl-D-aspartate (NMDA) receptor antagonists, which block a glutamate receptor, have been associated with cerebral protection. The effect of neuroprotective doses of dizocilpine, a noncompetitive NMDA antagonist, and of D-CPP-ene and CGS 19755, 2 competitive NMDA antagonists, on the minimum alveolar anesthetic concentration (MAC) of isoflurane was studied in rats.

Methods and Results.—A single bolus injection of any of the antagonists significantly reduced the MAC of isoflurane. This reduction was sustained. At a dose of .15 mg/kg, dizocilpine reduced MAC by 33% to 38%; at .5 mg/kg, it reduced MAC by 48% to 54%. D-CPP-ene in doses of 1.5 and 4.5 mg/kg reduced MAC by 32% to 37% and 39% to 45%, respectively. In doses of 3 and 10 mg/kg, CGS 19755 decreased MAC by 19% to 24% and 49% to 58%, respectively. Dizocilpine resulted in a small, transient reduction in the mean arterial blood pressure, whereas the competitive antagonists did not.

Conclusion.—Neuroprotective doses of NMDA antagonists consistently decrease the MAC of isoflurane. These data are consistent with the notion that glutaminergic receptor activity is involved in determining the anesthetic state. Competitive NMDA antagonists may be clinically useful because of their minimal effects on systemic physiology.

▶ The new NMDA receptor antagonists may or may not be cerebral protectants, but this study clearly showed that they do have anesthetic potency. It is likely, as much recent literature has shown, that glutaminergic receptor activity, when inhibited, plays a role in general anesthesia. If general anesthesia is cerebral protective (and some kinds are, some might not be), and if the "excitotoxic" theory of CNS damage during and after ischemia holds true, then inhibition of the excitatory amino acid effects on the brain might not only be protective but also anesthetic. Again, as I have said in several other comments throughout this year's Year Book of Anesthesiology and Pain Management, we seem to be getting pretty close to understanding basic mechanisms of general anesthesia.—J.H. Tinker, M.D.

Measuring Recovery From General Anaesthesia Using Critical Flicker Frequency: A Comparison of Two Methods

Salib Y, Plourde G, Alloul K, Provost A, Moore A (McGill Univ, Montreal)
Can J Anaesth 39:1045–1050, 1992   101-94-5-4

Background.—The critical flicker frequency (CFF)—the frequency at which a flickering light source is perceived as continuous—is considered one of the best ways of evaluating recovery of mental function postoperatively. Most often the method of limits is used, whereby the flicker frequency is slowly changed until the subject reports the onset or loss of flicker. With this method, the CFF depends on the perceptual threshold and also on response bias, a confounding factor. The effects of response bias and response delay may be avoided by using a forced-choice method in which the subject observes the light for 2 brief periods with the light flickering in only 1 of them and then must state during which period the light flickers.

Study Design.—These 2 methods were compared in 20 healthy patients, aged 20–65 years, who received either midazolam or thiopentone for induction. The patients were not premedicated. Fentanyl was given 2 minutes before induction, and, after tracheal intubation, anesthesia was maintained with nitrous oxide and isoflurane in oxygen. The CFF was estimated before induction and 1, 2, and 3 hours after arrival in the recovery area.

Findings.—The CFF values were higher using the forced-choice technique than with the limit method. Values for midazolam were lower than those for thiopentone using both methods. The 2 methods correlated at a level of .6 at 1 hour, and at .8 at 2 hours; no correlation was evident for measurements made 3 hours postoperatively.

Conclusion.—The forced-choice method of estimating CFF is preferred when evaluating recovery from anesthesia. In addition, it may help to take changes in pupillary diameter into account.

▶ This group has attained leadership in the race to develop reliable methods to assess the depth of general anesthesia. Now they have come up with a quantifiable method of understanding the degree of recovery from anesthesia. I think this is excellent science.—J.H. Tinker, M.D.

Anesthetic Potency (MAC) Is Independent of Forebrain Structures in the Rat

Rampil IJ, Mason P, Singh H (Univ of California, San Francisco)
Anesthesiology 78:707–712, 1993   101-94-5–5

Background.—The mechanisms by which general anesthetics produce unresponsiveness to surgical incision and other noxious stimuli remain unknown. Anesthetics may achieve this effect by depressing a site or sites in the cerebral cortex and thalamus. Alternatively, noxious-evoked movement may be suppressed through actions in the hindbrain or spinal cord. The neural structures that subtend the somatomotor response associated with anesthesia were further investigated.

Methods.—Fourteen rats were anesthetized with isoflurane in oxygen, and bilateral parietal-temporal craniotomies were performed. The minimum alveolar concentration (MAC), the concentration that blocks movement evoked by a noxious stimulus, was tested repeatedly in each rat by using tail-clamping and Dixon's up-down concentration method. Baseline MACs were established. Seven rats were then subjected to aspiration decerebration, and MAC was tested repeatedly again.

Results.—In the 7 rats in the control group the mean MAC remained constant at 1.3% for more than 6 hours. The baseline MAC in the rats undergoing aspiration decerebration was 1.26%. These rats showed no change in the MAC compared with control rats as long as 11 hours after decerebration. The nocifensive movements occurring in all animals consisted of alternating proximal flexion and extension, resembling ambulation in 2 or more extremities simultaneously.

Conclusion.—In this rat model, anesthetic potency, relative to movement elicited by noxious stimulation, did not change in acutely decerebrated animals. Therefore, the anesthetic-induced unresponsiveness to noxious stimuli as measured by MAC testing apparently does not depend on cortical or forebrain structures in the rat.

▶ I do not normally subject readers of the YEAR BOOK OF ANESTHESIOLOGY AND PAIN MANAGEMENT to rat studies, but this one is at least provocative if not a landmark. The authors destroyed the entire cerebral cortex of these rats and did not find that anesthetic potency, at least as measured by MAC, was changed at all! This is a remarkable finding, to say the least. This means that decerebrate rats were able to move in response to supramaximal tail-clamp stimulation at concentrations below MAC and were not able to move in concentrations above MAC. Furthermore, this study showed that the MAC for the decerebrated rats was the same as the MAC for the same rats intact. What to make of all this? Clearly, movement in response to noxious stimulus does not require the cortex, and equally clearly, the important site of anesthetic action here in these decerebrated rats was not the cerebrum!

We will be buzzing about this paper for a long time. It just might turn out to be a landmark in our understanding of how and where anesthetics act in vivo.—J.H. Tinker, M.D.

Studies of Nitric Oxide

Nitric Oxide Synthase Inhibitor Dose-Dependently and Reversibly Reduces the Threshold for Halothane Anesthesia: A Role for Nitric Oxide in Mediating Consciousness?
Johns RA, Moscicki JC, DiFazio CA (Univ of Virginia, Charlottesville)
Anesthesiology 77:779–784, 1992   101-94-5-6

Background.—Nitric oxide (NO) is now recognized as a cell messenger for the activation of soluble guanylate cyclase. It is produced from L-arginine by NO synthase in a wide range of tissues, including the vascular endothelium and the brain. Inhalational anesthetics inhibit NO production by vascular endothelium and also lower the resting cyclic guanosine monophosphate content in some areas of the brain. Halothane reduces neurotransmission by amino acid neurotransmitters including L-glutamate, which increases the content of cyclic guanosine monophosphate through stimulating NO production.

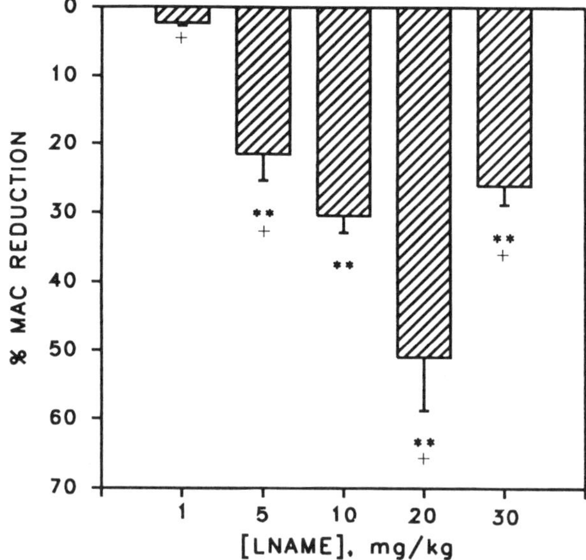

Fig 5–1.—Halothane MAC reduction by increasing concentrations of nitro^G-L-arginine-methyl-ester (LNAME). Data are presented as mean ± SEM; n = 9 (1 mg/kg), 6 (5 mg/kg), 18 (10 mg/kg), 7 (20 mg/kg), and 3 (30 mg/kg). **Significantly different from control (P < .01); *plus sign* indicates significantly different from previous concentration (P < .01). (Courtesy of Johns RA, Moscicki JC, DiFazio CA: *Anesthesiology* 77:779–784, 1992.)

Objective.—To clarify the role of the L-arginine-to-NO pathway in anesthesia, the effects of the specific NO synthase inhibitor nitro^G-L-arginine methyl ester on the minimum alveolar concentration (MAC) for halothane anesthesia were examined in rats.

Results.—Bolus injections of inhibitor in doses up to 30 mg/kg led to a dose-dependent reduction in the MAC for halothane (Fig 5–1). The reduction in MAC was immediately and totally reversed by infusing L-arginine, but not D-arginine. The reduction in MAC for halothane was associated with increased blood pressure and a small reduction in heart rate.

Interpretation.—Inhibiting the NO pathway seems to reduce the level of consciousness and augment anesthesia. However, the NO synthase inhibitor might act on specific arginine transporters on the cell membrane or on other metabolic paths involved in arginine metabolism.

▶ I could not resist including this outstanding example of basic science directly related to mechanisms of anesthesia. Dr. Johns and his colleagues at Virginia are directing their enormous basic science talents at anesthetics and their mechanisms of action. At the same time, they are potentially opening wide vistas for understanding neurologic mechanisms of general anesthesia.—J.H. Tinker, M.D.

Inhaled Nitric Oxide for the Adult Respiratory Distress Syndrome
Rossaint R, Falke KJ, López F, Slama K, Pison U, Zapol WM (Freie Universität Berlin; Harvard Med School, Boston)
N Engl J Med 328:399–405, 1993   101-94-5–7

Background.—Patients with adult respiratory distress syndrome experience pulmonary hypertension and right-to-left shunting of venous blood. Vasodilators can reduce the abnormally elevated pulmonary vascular resistance but may lead to systemic arterial hypotension, right ventricular ischemia, and heart failure. The hypothesis that inhaled nitric acid would selectively improve perfusion of ventilated lung regions, thus improving gas exchange and reducing pulmonary hypertension, was tested.

Methods.—Ten consecutive patients with severe adult respiratory distress syndrome entered the study. Patients ranged in age from 17 to 46 years; none had a history of lung disease. Nitric oxide was inhaled in 2 concentrations for 40 minutes at a time. During the inhalation period, hemodynamic variables, gas exchange, and ventilation-perfusion distributions were measured by multiple inert-gas–elimination techniques. Results were compared with those obtained with an intravenous infusion of prostacyclin at a rate of 4 ng/kg of body weight/min. Seven patients were treated with continuous inhalation of nitric oxide in a concentration of 5 to 20 ppm for 3 to 53 days.

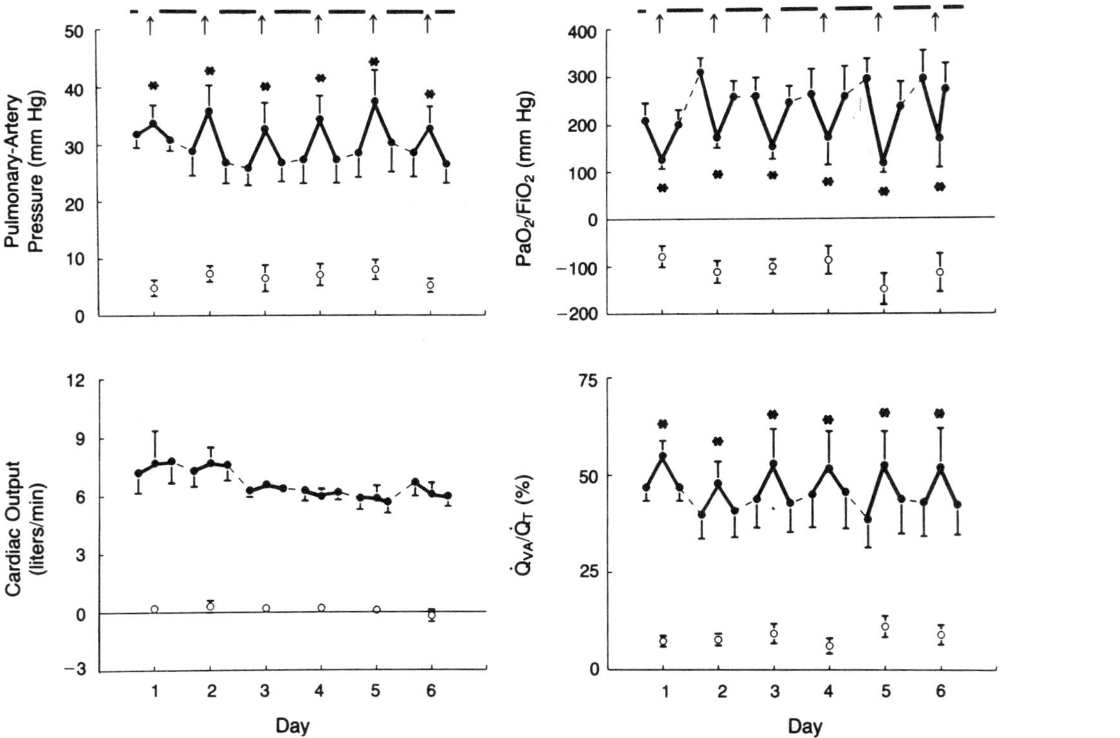

Fig 5–2.—Hemodynamic function and gas exchange before, during, and after brief interruptions (*arrows*) of nitric oxide inhalation (*bars*) during the first 6 days of treatment. Values are means ± SE (*solid symbols*). Also shown (*open symbols*) are the means ± SE of the individual differences between the values for the effect of treatment and the means of the values determined before and after interruption of nitric oxide therapy. The standard errors for the treatment effects were small, indicating that the effects of nitric oxide were clear and precisely estimated. Each *asterisk* denotes a significant difference from the means of the values determined before and after interruption of nitric oxide therapy. (Courtesy of Rossaint R, Falke KJ, López F, et al: *N Engl J Med* 328:399–405, 1993.)

Results.—Nitric oxide inhalation usually resulted in a prompt reduction in the pulmonary artery pressure (PAP) and a concomitant increase in the arterial oxygenation efficiency. During inhalation of nitric acid at 18 ppm, the PAP decreased by 6 mm Hg from baseline; no significant difference was noted between 18 and 36 ppm. Intrapulmonary shunting decreased from 36% to 31% at a concentration of 18 ppm. The mean arterial pressure and cardiac output remained unchanged during nitric oxide administration. The intravenous infusion of prostacyclin reduced PAP, arterial oxygenation efficiency, and systemic arterial pressure but increased intrapulmonary shunting. Continuous nitric oxide inhalation consistently lowered PAP and augmented the arterial oxygenation efficiency. During daily brief interruptions of continuous nitric oxide therapy, PAP consistently increased and arterial oxygenation efficiency was consistently decreased (Fig 5–2).

Conclusion.—Inhalation of nitric acid for 3 to 53 days remained effective in reducing PAP and improving oxygen exchange, without causing tachyphylaxis. The impact of inhaled nitric acid on outcome in adult respiratory distress syndrome remains to be determined.

▶ The ability to provide pulmonary vasodilation while sparing systemic involvement appears to make inhalational nitric oxide an ideal agent in patients with primary or secondary pulmonary hypertension. Clinical studies to date represent about 100 adult patients who have received this therapy with the results being similar to those presented in this article. Nitric oxide has also been used with success in the pediatric population, i.e., newborns with pulmonary hypertension. The toxicity of nitric oxide inhaled for longer periods needs to be determined. Hopefully, complications from this therapy will be minimal, and finally, after many years of serving up ineffective systemic vasodilators to treat pulmonary hypertension, this target-specific therapy will prove to be a truly "free lunch."—D.M. Rothenberg, M.D.

Inhalation of Nitric Oxide Reduced Pulmonary Hypertension After Cardiac Surgery in a 3.2-kg Infant

Selldén H, Winberg P, Gustafsson LE, Lundell B, Böök K, Frostell CG (St Göran Hosp, Stockholm; Karolinska Inst, Stockholm; Karolinska Hosp, Stockholm)

Anesthesiology 78:577–580, 1993   101-94-5–8

Introduction.—Pulmonary vasospasm and severe pulmonary hypertension are frequently seen after surgery for congenital heart disease, and they create a difficult management problem. Nitric oxide (NO) is an endothelium-derived relaxing factor that in low dosage has produced selective pulmonary vasodilation in awake sheep and also in healthy humans who have inhaled a hypoxic gas mixture.

Case Report.—Female infant, born at 31 weeks' gestation, had respiratory insufficiency shortly after birth and also had esophageal atresia, an annular pancreas, and a ventricular septal defect. The gastrointestinal malformations were corrected surgically, but severe tracheomalacia necessitated endotracheal intubation. An increasing left-to-right shunt and heart failure prompted closure of the septal defect at age 3 months. Pulmonary vasospasm developed immediately after surgery and responded to intravenously administered dobutamine and nitroglycerin. Subsequently, oxygenation declined as the pulmonary artery pressure increased to near-systemic levels, and alveolar infiltrates were found in both lungs. Periods of manual hyperventilation and loop diuretics were ineffective, but inhalation of 30 ppm of NO, followed by 10 ppm for 30 minutes, was followed by a marked decrease in pulmonary artery pressure and improved oxygenation. The effects persisted after NO was discontinued. The patient was disconnected from the ventilator after 1 week.

Discussion.—Inhalation of a low concentration of NO for a limited time permanently improved gas exchange and relieved acute pulmonary hypertension in this infant. However, there are potential risks from administering NO in the clinical setting, including methemoglobinemia and the spontaneous formation of NO_2.

▶ Nitric oxide, as most of you know, is sweeping the world right now. It may be very useful for treatment of pulmonary hypertension that develops in premature and other infants during the battle those infants must wage with respiratory distress syndrome. The key to understanding the use of this treatment is to understand that dosage is critical and that the toxic therapeutic ratio is very low. Furthermore, these infants can be rapidly made methemoglobinemic, which will be counterproductive to say the least. This paper, however exciting, does not mean that every neonatology unit should go out and buy some sort of gadget to administer NO.

The other interesting part about NO is whether or not we can figure out ways to get this fascinating gas delivered to the other side of the circulation so as to benefit clinical situations in which arteriolar vasodilation is needed. So far, the half-life of NO is so short that it does not get past the lungs, but I predict that we will be seeing new drugs that are essentially vehicles for carrying NO across the lungs. The only one of these kinds of substances we currently have is sodium nitroprusside, which has stood a long test of time despite its warts. It would be nice to have a drug that would deliver NO to systemic arterioles without releasing cyanide.—J.H. Tinker, M.D.

Inhaled Nitric Oxide Selectively Reverses Human Hypoxic Pulmonary Vasoconstriction Without Causing Systemic Vasodilation
Frostell CG, Blomqvist H, Hedenstierna G, Lundberg J, Zapol WM (Danderyd Hosp, Sweden; Uppsala Univ, Sweden; Karolinska Inst, Stockholm; et al)
Anesthesiology 78:427–435, 1993   101-94-5–9

Objective.—Nitric oxide (NO) is an important endothelium-derived relaxing factor that acts as a local vasodilator. Such clinical vasodilators as sodium nitroprusside and nitroglycerin work by releasing NO intracellularly. The pulmonary and systemic circulatory effects of NO in humans were assessed.

Methods.—The subjects were 9 healthy adult volunteers. All were studied while awake and breathing air, 12% oxygen in nitrogen, and the same oxygen-nitrogen mixture plus 40 ppm of NO, with the fraction of inspired oxygen maintained at .12. Measurements of pulmonary artery and radial artery pressures began 6 minutes after inhalation of each new gas mixture and continued for 4 minutes.

Findings.—Partial pressure of oxygen in the alveoli decreased from 106 mm Hg on air to 47 mm Hg on 12% oxygen. At the same time, pulmonary artery pressure increased from 15 to 20 mm Hg and cardiac output from 6 to 8 L/min. When NO was added, the pulmonary artery pressure decreased to the air-breathing level, whereas the partial pressure of oxygen in the alveoli and the arterial blood partial pressure of carbon dioxide remained unchanged. Nitrous oxide–induced pulmonary vessel dilation brought no changes in systemic vascular resistance or mean arterial pressure. In a further experiment, none of the measured parameters changed significantly when the subjects breathed 40 ppm NO in 21% oxygen. Hypoxia, with or without NO inhalation, was not associated with any change in plasma endothelin–like immunoreactivity concentrations.

Conclusion.—Full antagonism of severe hypoxia by NO inhalation in humans was documented. The vasodilator effect of NO is completely confined to the pulmonary circulation. Careful studies of the potential vasodilator effects of NO in various lung diseases are needed.

▶ This landmark human volunteer study will soon be followed by case reports of the use of this exciting "new" substance, formerly thought to be simply a deadly poisonous gas, in patients with various kinds of pulmonary vasoconstrictive problems, including newborn infants with respiratory distress syndrome. When you think about it, this is not the first (nor will it be the last) substance formerly thought to be a poison that is now being tried as therapy. On the other hand, it is not easy to administer and it does cause methemoglobinemia.—J.H. Tinker, M.D.

Evaluation of a New System for Ventilatory Administration of Nitric Oxide

Stenqvist O, Kjelltoft B, Lundin S (Sahlgren Hosp, Göteborg, Sweden)
Acta Anaesthesiol Scand 37:687–691, 1993   101-94-5–10

Introduction.—Nitric oxide could play an important role in the treatment of ventilation-perfusion mismatch by selectively decreasing pulmo-

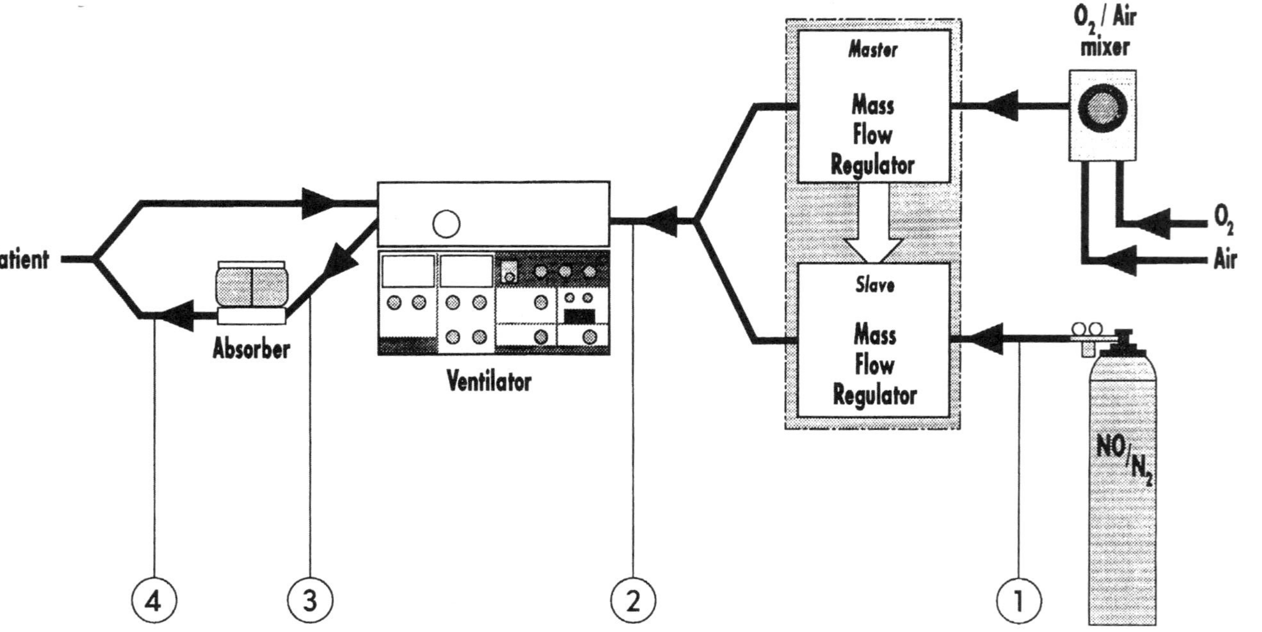

Fig 5–3.—Schematic graph of the nitric oxide (NO) administration system. *Digits* in graph indicate sampling sites for NO and nitrogen dioxide analysis. *1*, pressure regulator outlet; 2, ventilator gas inlet; 3, after passage of ventilator, before absorber in inspiratory limb; *4*, after absorber. (Courtesy of Stenqvist O, Kjelltoft B, Lundin S: *Acta Anaesthesiol Scand* 37:687–691, 1993.)

nary vascular resistance and improving right ventricular function. However, delivery is a problem because nitric oxide is toxic at high concentrations. A newly developed system of delivery of nitric oxide to inspiratory gas was examined and evaluated.

Methods.—The system consisted of 2 mass flow regulators and a soda-lime absorber for scavenging of nitrogen dioxide (Fig 5–3). Three different techniques of nitric oxide analysis were used for system analysis: infrared, chemiluminescence, and the electrochemical fuel cell, the latter being suitable for routine clinical use. Ultraviolet methods were used to analyze nitrogen dioxide. The highest recommended level of nitrogen dioxide for occupational health and safety is 5 ppm.

Results.—Nitrogen dioxide levels were highest before the absorber in the inspiratory limb of the breathing system—5 ppm at 100% oxygen and 100 ppm nitric oxide using "infant" respiratory settings. For "adult" settings, the corresponding value was 3.2 ppm. With use of the absorber, nitrogen dioxide levels were reduced to well below 1 ppm. When 20 ppm of nitric oxide was used—a clinically relevant level—no nitrogen dioxide was found beyond the absorber, regardless of oxygen concentration. Gas cylinders containing nitric oxide mixed in nitrogen had an initially high nitrogen dioxide concentration of about 12 ppm and had to be flushed before use.

Conclusion.—Delivery of toxic levels of nitric oxide can be avoided by limiting concentration in the gas cylinder to 500 ppm. Concentration of higher oxides can be controlled by use of a soda-lime absorber in the inspiratory limb of the breathing system. At clinically relevant doses of nitric oxide in 100% oxygen, nitrogen dioxide levels are undetectable as long as an absorber is used.

▶ Anyone thinking of casually walking down to the neonatal intensive care unit, or the adult ICU for that matter, with a cylinder of nitric oxide and turning it on in order to effect some nice pulmonary vasodilation should read this paper. Nitric oxide is deadly. Overdose can rapidly result in overwhelming methemoglobinemia. This paper clearly showed that one does not administer nitric oxide without thinking carefully about the pharmacy as well as the pharmacology.—J.H. Tinker, M.D.

Studies of Ketorolac

Ketorolac, Nasal Polyposis, and Bronchial Asthma: A Cause for Concern
Haddow GR, Riley E, Isaacs R, McSharry R (Stanford Univ, Calif)
Anesth Analg 76:420–422, 1993   101-94-5-11

Background.—The use of ketorolac alone or in combination with narcotic analgesics has been recommended for the management of postoperative pain. However, ketorolac may interfere with platelet function and increase blood loss. Ketorolac was used in one case when a life-threatening complication occurred.

Case Report.—Man, 84, with metastatic melanoma underwent a right modified radical neck dissection, excision of nasal polyps, antrostomy, and sphenoethmoidectomy for chronic sinusitis. Two years earlier he had been hospitalized for asthma and emphysema, at which time corticosteroid treatment was sustained. Medications included triamcinolone, albuterol, beclomethasone, prednisone, theophylline, and ipvatropium. He took his usual medications before the present surgery. Anesthesia was induced with thiopental, fentanyl, and vecuronium and maintained with isoflurane ventilation. He received atropine during surgery. After surgery, 60 mg of ketorolac was administered intravenously for pain relief. Within 15 minutes, the patient reported difficulty in breathing. Albuterol nebulization was begun, but at 30 minutes there was no improvement. Oxygen saturation decreased to 85%. Another bolus of 100 mg of hydrocortisone was administered, and nebulization with albuterol and triamcinolone was again given. Oxygen saturation increased to 96%. However, respiratory effort decreased. Oxygen saturation again declined to 85%, and no breath sounds could be heard by auscultation of the chest. Arterial blood gas analysis 45 minutes after administration of ketorolac showed a pH_a of 7.15, a partial pressure of carbon dioxide ($PaCO_2$) of 86 mm Hg, and a partial pressure of oxygen (PaO_2) of 56 mm Hg. One hundred mg of ketamine and 100 mg of succinylcholine was administered, and the trachea was intubated. His pH_a was 7.27, the $PaCO_2$ was 54 mm Hg, and the PaO_2 was 466 mm Hg with a fractional concentration of oxygen in inspired gas of 1. He was taken to the intensive care unit, where he improved overnight after treatment with hydrocortisone and nebulized β-adrenergic agonists. The next morning, tracheal extubation was successful.

Conclusion.—The development of acute bronchial asthma in this case illustrates some potential problems with the use of ketorolac. Nasal polyposis and asthma, both easily recognized before surgery, should alert anesthesiologists to the possibility of sensitivity to the nonsteroidal anti-inflammatory drugs.

▶ The potential exacerbation of bronchial asthma in patients with nasal polyps who receive aspirin is a well-known, although rare complication. Ketorolac, like aspirin, is a nonsteroidal anti-inflammatory drug, although the clinician is more inclined to equate this drug's analgesic effects with morphine rather than aspirin. This report reminds us that ketorolac may have side effects traditionally recognized to be part of therapy with nonsteroidal anti-inflammatory drugs.—R.K. Stoelting, M.D.

Ketorolac-Induced Bronchospasm
Zikowski D, Hord AH, Haddox JD, Glascock J (Emory Univ, Atlanta, Ga)
Anesth Analg 76:417–419, 1993   101-94-5–12

Introduction.—The nonsteroidal anti-inflammatory drug (NSAID) ketorolac tromethamine is gaining in popularity because it does not carry many of the side effects associated with the opioid analgesics. It does, however, have its own list of adverse reactions, similar to those reported for other drugs of its class. A patient with ketorolac-induced bronchospasm was reported.

Case Report.—Man, 61, was hospitalized for repair of a hiatal hernia associated with esophageal stricture. He had a lifelong history of asthma, for which he took theophylline, albuterol, and ipratropium. He reported an allergy to aspirin, which caused swelling of the extremities and face. His postoperative course was unremarkable, until he complained of left shoulder pain. This pain, believed to be referred pain caused by the presence of tubes on the left side of his chest, was treated with ketorolac, 60 mg by intramuscular injection.

The patient began complaining of dyspnea on arrival in the intensive care unit and soon become tachypneic, cyanotic, and lethargic, with audible wheezing. He was immediately intubated and placed under controlled ventilation, with rapid improvement in his mental status. Treatment was begun with β_2-adrenergic agonist aerosols and aminophylline by continuous intravenous infusion. Later, the patient's family reported that he had experienced similar asthmatic incidents, requiring emergency intubation, after taking aspirin. Bronchospasm resolved, and the patient was extubated within 36 hours. Later, the patient revealed that he had previously undergone several nasal polypectomies. The patient was discharged with instructions to avoid NSAID. He was given a written description of his reaction because of his inability to give an accurate history.

Conclusion.—Although bronchospasms resulting from NSAIDs have been reported before, they have not been associated with ketorolac. When a patient reports a history of adverse reactions to aspirin and other NSAIDs, this must be taken seriously. It is easy to become complacent about ketorolac because of its excellent effectiveness and relatively low incidence of adverse reactions.

▶ See the comment for Abstract 101-94-5–11.—R.K. Stoelting, M.D.

Studies of Dexmedetomidine

Intramuscular Dexmedetomidine as Premedication for General Anesthesia: A Comparative Multicenter Study

Scheinin H, Jaakola M-L, Sjövall S, Ali-Melkkilä T, Kaukinen S, Turunen J, Kanto J (Turku Univ Central Hosp, Finland; Regional Hosp of Rauma, Finland; Tampere Univ Hosp, Finland; et al)
Anesthesiology 78:1065–1075, 1993   101-94-5–13

Introduction.—The alpha-2-agonists offer several beneficial effects in anesthesia. The potent new selective alpha-2-agonist dexmedetomidine shows promise as a preanesthetic agent; in 1 study, it decreased thiopental requirements by as much as 50% in patients undergoing dilation and curettage. The efficacy and safety of intramuscular dexmedetomidine as premedication in surgical patients receiving standard anesthetic management were determined in a double-blind, randomized, multicenter study.

Methods.—The 192 patients, all in American Society of Anesthesiologists physical status I or II were scheduled to undergo elective abdominal hysterectomy, cholecystectomy, or intraocular surgery. Sixty-four patients received dexmedetomidine, 2.5 μg/kg intramuscularly 60 minutes before induction, and saline placebo 2 minutes before induction (DEXPLA group). Another 64 patients received a combination of midazolam, .08 mg/kg intramuscularly 60 minutes before induction, and fentanyl, 1.5 μg/kg intravenously 2 minutes before induction (MIDFENT group). The remaining 64 patients received a combination of intramuscular dexmedetomidine and intravenous fentanyl (DEXFENT). Anesthesia was induced with thiopental and maintained with 70% nitrous oxide in oxygen, with fentanyl given according to clinical and cardiovascular criteria. Enflurane was also given in patients undergoing cholecystectomy.

Results.—Preoperative sedation and anxiolysis were similar with dexmedetomidine and midazolam. The intubation-induced blood pressure was about 25 mm Hg higher and the heart rate 15 beats/min greater in the DEXPLA and MIDFENT groups than in the DEXFENT group. The DEXFENT group needed 56% less intraoperative fentanyl and the DEXPLA group 31% less than the MIDFENT group. Patients in the 2 dexmedetomidine groups needed significantly more intraoperative fluids or vasopressors for hypotension and glycopyrrolate for bradycardia. Although there were no significant differences in oxygen saturation or analgesic or antiemetic requirements, the dexmedetomidine groups continued to show reductions in blood pressure and heart rate at the end of the 3-hour follow-up. Thirty-three percent of the DEXFENT group and 20% of the DEXPLA group had bradycardia, compared with just 8% of the MIDFENT group.

Conclusion.—In patients undergoing surgery, premedication with dexmedetomidine, 2.5 μg/kg intramuscularly, is effective in achieving preoperative sedation and anxiolysis, attenuating the response to intubation, and reducing intraoperative opioid requirements. However, it is associated with a high incidence of intraoperative hypotension and bradycardia and must therefore be used cautiously.

▶ The clinician will ultimately determine the cost-benefit ratio that is appropriate for dexmedetomidine. It seems likely that healthy patients undergoing short operations will represent a group where dexmedetomidine-induced bradycardia and hypotension will be an unacceptable cost for decreasing the dose of fentanyl or other short-acting drugs such as propofol and desflurane.—R.K. Stoelting, M.D.

Direct Coronary and Cerebral Vascular Responses to Dexmedetomidine: Significance of Endogenous Nitric Oxide Synthesis

Coughlan MG, Lee JG, Bosnjak ZJ, Schmeling WT, Kampine JP, Warltier DC (Med College of Wisconsin, Milwaukee; Zablocki VA Med Ctr, Milwaukee, Wis)

Anesthesiology 77:998–1006, 1992   101-94-5-14

Introduction.—Dexmedetomidine alters coronary and cerebral blood flow and arterial pressure via stimulation of vascular smooth muscle α_2 receptors. Endothelium-derived relaxing factor, believed to be nitric oxide, may oppose the direct vasoconstrictor effects of α_2-adrenergic agonists. A functional endothelium in the coronary collateral vessels of dogs was identified.

Methods.—This study examined the direct effects of dexmedetomidine on isolated canine proximal and distal coronary arteries, coronary collateral vessels, and middle cerebral arteries. Specimens of each vessel were suspended in tissue baths, and responses were measured in the presence of indomethacin, 10^{-5} M, and in the presence and absence of the nitric oxide synthesis inhibitor N^{G}nitro-l-arginine methyl ester (L-NAME).

Results.—In doses of 3×10^{-8} to $3 \times 10^{-3.9}$ M, dexmedetomidine caused significant constriction—as much as 73% of potassium chloride–induced contraction for the middle cerebral artery. For vessels other than the cerebral arteries, L-NAME enhanced this constriction. In the middle cerebral artery, proximal coronary arteries, and coronary collateral vessels, the selective α_2-adrenergic antagonist atipamezole eliminated the response to low concentrations of dexmedetomidine, but not to high concentrations. In the distal coronary arteries, atipamezole also abolished the response to high concentrations.

Conclusion.—Dexmedetomidine appears to have direct vasoconstrictive effects in a number of isolated canine vessels. Vascular nitric oxide synthesis modulates these actions in the coronary arteries and coronary collateral vessels, but not in the middle cerebral arteries. The cerebral blood flow effects of dexmedetomidine in humans remain unknown.

▶ The effect of dexmedetomidine in causing cerebral and coronary vasoconstriction is disappointing. It seemed to have such potential as an agent to decrease perioperative morbidity. Maybe I am throwing the baby out with the bath water, but I wonder whether all alpha-2 agents will cause coronary vasoconstrictive effects when administered intravenously.—M.F. Roizen, M.D.

Studies of Propofol

Propofol Attenuates the Myogenic Response of Vascular Smooth Muscle

MacPherson RD, Rasiah RL, McLeod LJ (Univ of Tasmania, Hobart, Australia)
Anesth Analg 76:822–829, 1993   101-94-5–15

Introduction.—Vascular smooth muscle normally dilates and then constricts in response to stretching secondary to an increased internal pressure. This myogenic response is most evident in small arteries and arterioles. Propofol is an intravenous anesthetic that reduces arterial pressure and cardiac output for reasons that are not clear. One possibility is that the decline in peripheral resistance reflects a direct effect of propofol on arterial beds.

Methods.—The effects of propofol on the myogenic response of isolated, pressurized arteries of the rabbit ear were examined in segments preconstricted with either norepinephrine or 5-hydroxytryptamine. The vessels were illuminated, and intraluminal perfusion pressure was recorded with a pressure transducer. A pressure increase of 60 to 100 mm Hg was induced either in jumps over 500 ms or in ramps over 2 minutes. Propofol was added in concentrations of 1.6 and 4.2×10^{-4} and 1.6×10^{-3} M.

Results.—In control experiments, preconstricted arterial vessels dilated and then rapidly regained their initial diameter. Slow dilation took place during pressure ramps, but the vessels essentially retained their resting diameter. Exposure to propofol resulted in dilation of the preconstricted vessels. Dilation was most pronounced with pressure ramps. After a pressure jump, the vessels were less able to recover their initial diameter.

Conclusion.—Propofol attenuates the myogenic response to increasing intraluminal pressure in arteries of the rabbit ear. This effect is distinct from the vasodilator action of the drug.

▶ This article instructs us that peripheral cardiovascular control is more complex than simply vasodilation; propofol may cause cardiovascular changes by both primary vasodilation and by blocking normal myogenic responses to vasodilation. This article may be one of the most innovative and important of the year.—M.F. Roizen, M.D.

Delayed Seizures Following Sedation With Propofol

Finley GA, MacManus B, Sampson SE, Fernandez CV, Retallick R (Izaak Walton Killam Children's Hosp, Halifax, NS, Canada; Dalhousie Univ, Halifax, NS, Canada)
Can J Anaesth 40:863–865, 1993   101-94-5–16

Background.—Since propofol became available for clinical use, it has been welcomed by patients and anesthetists alike. The rapid recovery and lack of postoperative nausea makes this drug a valuable tool in emergency and outpatient surgery. However, unusual muscular movements have been seen in children during propofol induction. Seizures and other withdrawal symptoms have followed its use for prolonged sedation of children.

Case 1—Girl, 13 years, with progressive glomerulonephritis resulting in chronic renal failure required bone marrow aspiration and biopsy. She was sedated with fentanyl followed by freshly opened propofol, 1 mg/kg, intravenously and lidocaine without epinephrine by infiltration at the biopsy site. The patient was responsive throughout, alert within minutes, and fully awake with normal head control and ambulation 2 hours later. After about 6 hours, she was given nifedipine sublingually twice for blood pressures of 165/102 mm Hg, which subsequently decreased to 140/86 mm Hg. She became sweaty and dizzy 10 minutes later (which had never happened before after nifedipine) and then experienced a generalized tonic-clonic seizure for 90 seconds. Her blood pressure was 149/72 mm Hg, and she had 2 more seizures lasting a minute each. She finally made a complete neurologic recovery with no subsequent seizures.

Case 2—Boy, 11 years, previously healthy, was admitted with a sore throat, anorexia, weight loss, and fever. Propofol, 5.2 mg/kg, was administered intravenously in small bolus doses for sedation, and lidocaine, 15 mg without epinephrine, was used for anesthesia for bone marrow biopsy, aspiration, and lumbar puncture. The boy awoke within 25 minutes. Four hours later, he had a generalized tonic seizure lasting 20 seconds.

Discussion.—Seizure, opisthotonus, or unusual muscle activity have been reported after administration of propofol to adults and adolescents. It has been suggested that the seizures may be subcortical in origin. Drug-induced decerebrate rigidity or glycine antagonism may be possible causes. Some have implied that there may be dose-related effects on both inhibitory and excitatory neurons. The popular use of propofol in outpatient and emergency surgery therefore raises some concern. Many patients travel home on the day of surgery. Seizures such as those described could be frightening and potentially dangerous. Although other factors may have contributed to the seizures in these 2 patients, the apparent association with propofol sedation should stimulate further research to determine the relevant risk factors.

▶ Propofol has emerged as a valuable addition to management of outpatients. Nevertheless, even a rare incidence of delayed seizures caused by this drug is a cause for concern. As the authors concluded, more data are needed to put this issue in perspective. Until then, I will not alter my use of propofol, although a history of a preexisting seizure disorder should probably be a reason to more carefully consider the risk-benefits of this drug.—R.K. Stoelting, M.D.

Change of Ectopic Supraventricular Tachycardia to Sinus Rhythm During Administration of Propofol

Hermann R, Vettermann J (Johann Wolfgang Goethe-Univ Clinic, Frankfurt, Germany)
Anesth Analg 75:1030–1032, 1992   101-94-5-17

Introduction.—Paroxysmal supraventricular tachycardia in children may result from altered normal automaticity of the sinus node or abnormal automaticity of atrial cell compounds other than those taking part in normal pacemaker function. Because persistent tachycardia may result in congestive heart failure, perioperative provocation of such paroxysms should be avoided. The use of propofol to convert ectopic supraventricular tachycardia to sinus rhythm during a surgical procedure in a child was reported.

Case Report.—Boy, 3.5 years, was to undergo adenoidectomy and tympanic membrane incision for recurrent otitis media. He had a history of supraventricular tachycardia based on chronic ectopic atrial tachycardia. He had daily paroxysmal tachycardiac episodes lasting 1 to 2 hours and a prevailing "normal" beat of 140 to 175 beats/min with brief periods at 75 beats/min and was under home ECG monitoring.

The day of surgery, he received premedication with midazolam and his regular morning doses of verapamil and methyl-digoxin. The ECG showed a heart rate of 165 beats/min; anesthesia was achieved with injections of propofol, 2.7 mg/kg, and nalbuphine, .35 mg/kg. The trachea was successfully intubated, then another 20 mg of propofol was given. At this point, the heart rate converted to a normal sinus rhythm at 75 beats/min. Maintenance anesthesia was effected with repeated doses of propofol, 10 to 20 mg every 10 minutes, while ventilation continued with an inspired oxygen fraction of .3 and an inspired fraction of nitrous oxide of .7. Throughout the operation, the child remained in sinus rhythm, varying between 75 and 110 beats min with an apparently normal P wave. Approximately a half-hour after extubation, his heart rate increased suddenly to 215 beats/min and did not return to normal sinus rhythm. His heart rate decreased to 160 beats/min in the recovery room, where the ECG was the same as preoperatively. The patient was discharged in good condition.

Discussion.—With repeated doses of propofol, prevalent supraventricular tachycardia was successfully converted to normal sinus rhythm in a child undergoing surgery. Even for patients who do not have such a response to other volatile anesthetics, propofol may be an appropriate drug for patients with supraventricular tachycardia.

▶ It is not reasonable to accept a cause-and-effect relationship between propofol and conversion of supraventricular tachycardia to normal sinus rhythm based on a single case report. Nevertheless, propofol has been reported to produce bradycardia and even heart block in occasional patients (1).—R.K. Stoelting, M.D.

Reference

1. James MF, et al: *Br J Anaesth* 62:213, 1989.

Anaphylactoid Reaction to Propofol

McHale SP, Konieczko K (Northwick Park Hosp, Harrow, England)
Anaesthesia 47:864–865, 1992   101-94-5–18

Introduction.—A case of anaphylactoid reaction after the induction of anesthesia was reported. Intradermal testing performed after the incident showed that the patient had a positive reaction to propofol.

Case Report.—West Indian man, 46, was admitted for polygastrectomy. Preoperative investigations were normal, and the patient was not noted to be atopic. Anesthesia was induced by propofol (170 mg), to which lignocaine (20 mg) had been added. Suxamethonium (100 mg) was given to facilitate tracheal intubation. The patient was administered a propofol infusion, starting at a rate of 10 mg/kg^{-1}/hr^{-1}. The tracheal tube was withdrawn slightly when air entry to the left lung appeared to be decreased. The patient's lungs were manually ventilated with some difficulty, and atracurium (35 mg) was administered. His heart rate at this time was 156 beats/min^{-1}, systolic arterial blood pressure was 40 mm Hg, peripheral oxygen saturation was 84%, and end-expiratory carbon dioxide tension was 5.8%. A rash was observed on the patient's arms and abdomen. The propofol infusion was stopped, and the patient was treated immediately with Haemaccel (500 mL) and intravenous ephedrine (30 mg). The patient showed rapid improvement, and the operation proceeded after hydrocortisone (100 mg) was given intravenously. The patient recovered with no further problems after the incident of anaphylaxis during anesthesia.

Discussion.—A blood sample taken 24 hours after the operation showed a high level of IgE. Six weeks later, the patient was tested for reactions to a variety of anesthetic agents. The reaction to propofol was positive. The estimated frequency of anaphylaxis during general anesthesia is estimated at between 1:4,500 and 1:20,000. Propofol has been implicated in relatively few cases. The positive results obtained by intradermal tests in this patient could have been caused by either 2,6 di-isopropylphenol or the intralipid solution in which it is solubilized.

▶ Allergic reactions involving antigen-antibody interactions in patients receiving propofol for the first time imply a prior unrecognized sensitization owing to a chemically similar substance. It is speculated that the phenyl nucleus and/or the isopropyl group of propofol may serve as antigenic sites common to other drugs and materials (soaps, cosmetics) as well. It has been suggested that patients with known drug allergies, especially to muscle relaxants, are at increased risk for experiencing an allergic reaction after administration of propofol.—R.K. Stoelting, M.D.

Studies of Opiates (see also Pain Management)

Nalbuphine Is Better Than Naloxone for Treatment of Side Effects After Epidural Morphine

Cohen SE, Ratner EF, Kreitzman TR, Archer JH, Mignano LR (Stanford Univ, Calif)
Anesth Analg 75:747–752, 1992   101-94-5-19

Introduction.—Epidural morphine provides excellent analgesia to postoperative patients but carries a high risk of side effects including pruritus, nausea, and vomiting. Accordingly, a comparison was made between nalbuphine and naloxone when given to cesarean section patients experiencing side effects caused by epidural morphine.

Methods.—Patients who requested treatment for pruritus or nausea after administration of 5 mg of epidural morphine received as many as 3 intravenous doses of .2 mg of naloxone or 5 mg of nalbuphine in a double-blind study. Pain, sedation, nausea/vomiting, and pruritus were evaluated before and 30 minutes after each dose.

Results.—The initial dose of nalbuphine reduced the frequency of vomiting and the severity of both nausea and pruritus, whereas naloxone had no such effects. Sedation scores increased after nalbuphine but were unchanged after naloxone. Pain scores increased only after naloxone administration. More naloxone-treated patients required a second or third dose.

Conclusion.—Nalbuphine appears to be superior to naloxone in the initial treatment of pruritus and nausea caused by epidural morphine in women undergoing cesarean section. Apart from being ineffective, naloxone partially reverses analgesia.

▶ For several years, we have successfully administered nalbuphine, 5 mg intravenously, for treatment of pruritus or nausea in patients who received epidural or intrathecal morphine for postcesarean analgesia. Nalbuphine effectively treats these side effects while preserving analgesia. One potential disadvantage of nalbuphine is that it results in mild sedation. In theory, this might potentiate the respiratory depression that results from epidural or intrathecal morphine administration. However, some studies have noted that nalbuphine reverses the respiratory depression that results from intraspinal morphine, despite causing an increased level of sedation.—D.H. Chestnut, M.D.

Effects of Epidural Morphine and Intramuscular Diclofenac Combination in Postcesarean Analgesia: A Dose-Range Study

Sun H-L, Wu C-C, Lin M-S, Chang C-F (Cathay Gen Hosp, Taipei, Taiwan, Republic of China)
Anesth Analg 76:284–288, 1993   101-94-5–20

Introduction.—Although 3–5 mg, epidural morphine, is widely used for analgesia after cesarean section, it provides good to excellent pain relief in only 70% to 85% of women. The efficacy of combinations of epidural morphine and intramuscular diclofenac in postcesarean analgesia was investigated in a double-blind, randomized study.

Methods.—One hundred twenty parturients were assigned to 1 of 6 groups. Women in groups A, B, C, D, and E received .5, 1, 2, 3, and 4 mg of epidural morphine, respectively, in 10 mL of normal saline solution and 75 mg of diclofenac intramuscularly. Women in group F were given 4 mg of epidural morphine in 10 mL of normal saline solution and 3 mL of normal saline solution intramuscularly. Epidural injections were given after the placenta was delivered, and intramuscular injections were given after the women arrived in the recovery room. Verbal analogue pain scores and pruritus scores were obtained periodically after the epidural injection. Subjective assessments of overall pain were elicited at 24 hours.

Findings.—Women in group A had the highest pain scores and needed more supplemental meperidine than women in groups C, D, E, and F. None of the women in groups D or E asked for supplemental pain relief. Wound pain scores among groups B, C, D, E, and F did not differ. Compared with women in group F, those in groups D and E had better relief of uterine contraction pain from 4 to 12 hours. Overall pain relief among the 6 groups did not differ. Also comparable was the incidence of nausea and/or vomiting, pruritus, and bleeding. Pruritus severity did not appear to be associated with morphine doses. No bradypnea was observed.

Conclusion.—When combined with 75 mg of intramuscular diclofenac, 3 and 4 mg of epidural morphine appears to be better than 4 mg of epidural morphine alone for relieving pain after cesarean section. The best combination for such pain relief seems to be 3 mg of epidural morphine and 75 mg of intramuscular diclofenac. Compared with epidural morphine alone, this combination produces better analgesia, particularly for relieving uterine cramps, without raising the incidence of adverse effects.

▶ Some physicians have expressed concern that postcesarean administration of a nonsteroidal anti-inflammatory drug (NSAID) might increase the likelihood of postpartum hemorrhage. To my knowledge, no study has confirmed that administration of a single dose of a NSAID increases the risk of postpartum bleeding. Both laboratory and clinical studies suggest that concurrent administration of an intraspinal opioid and a NSAID results in at least an additive, and perhaps a synergistic effect. It may be advantageous to give smaller doses of 2 drugs to minimize the side effects of a larger dose of either drug alone.—D.H. Chestnut, M.D.

Acute Toxic Delirium in a Patient Using Transdermal Fentanyl
Steinberg RB, Gilman DE, Johnson F III (Baystate Med Ctr, Springfield, Mass; Tufts Univ, Boston)
Anesth Analg 75:1014–1016, 1992   101-94-5–21

Introduction.—Transdermal drug delivery systems are now used for a variety of indications. Transdermal fentanyl can be very useful for patients with chronic pain, providing effective analgesia and few complications. A patient who had acute toxic delirium after using transdermal fentanyl was studied.

Case Report.—Woman, 71, who had undergone hemimandibulectomy and maximal radiation therapy for squamous cell carcinoma, was seen with increasing jaw pain. She was given Duragesic patches and told to increase her dose by 25 μg/hr once daily until pain control was achieved. Pain persisted despite a dose of 125 μg/hr, and her family reported the patient was having delusions. Confusion, agitation, and paranoia persisted for 9 days of hospitalization despite treatment with morphine sulfate, as much as 120 mg/day orally; lorazepam; and haloperidol, as much as 9 mg/day. Psychiatric consultation revealed a confused, disoriented, combative woman with flat affect and in no obvious pain. Toxic delirium was diagnosed, and the transdermal fentanyl patches were removed. The patient was started with intravenous morphine at 4 mg/hr. The patient's combativeness resolved, and she denied feeling pain; sitters and antipsychotic medications were discontinued. Intravenous morphine was continued at doses of 4 to 5 mg/hr, and the patient remained on supportive care only until her discharge to an extended care facility on day 28.

Discussion.—This patient had acute toxic delirium associated with the use of transdermal fentanyl for cancer pain. Narcotic resistance and delirium probably resulted from accumulated norfentanyl in her system. Blood gas measurement could have ruled out the possibility of opiate overdose with respiratory depression.

▶ Norfentanyl is a recognized and presumed nontoxic metabolite of fentanyl. In the absence of impaired biliary or urinary clearance, its accumulation would seem unlikely. Nevertheless, this patient's symptoms resolved when the transdermal fentanyl was discontinued, and, clinically, this is the important observation.—R.K. Stoelting, M.D.

Morphine Does Not Affect the Awakening Concentration of Sevoflurane

Katoh T, Suguro Y, Kimura T, Ikeda K (Hamamatsu Univ, Japan)
Can J Anaesth 40:825–828, 1993   101-94-5–22

Introduction.—Patients rapidly waken from sevoflurane anesthesia and may experience pain as a result. Intraoperative use of analgesics may delay rapid recovery, thereby countering that advantage of sevoflurane.

Methods.—The effect of intraoperative morphine on the end tidal sevoflurane concentration associated with eye opening on verbal command was investigated. Twenty-four healthy, American Society of Anesthesiologists physical status I patients scheduled for elective extremity or surface procedures were included in the study. Either .1 mg of morphine per kg^{-1} or placebo was given intravenously about 1 hour before the end of surgery, at which time the end-tidal sevoflurane concentration was lowered at a rate of less than .01% per minute.

Results.—The end-tidal sevoflurane concentration at the time the patient could respond to verbal command was .58% for placebo recipients and .57% in patients given morphine. In both groups, this concentration declined with advancing age, and adjusting for age did not alter the findings.

Conclusion.—Intraoperative morphine administration does not alter the awakening concentration of sevoflurane during recovery from anesthesia.

▶ This paper is interesting for several reasons. First, it is a compilation of experience in Japan with the interesting anesthetic sevoflurane. Second, it shows that once again, the ratio of minimum alveolar concentration (MAC) awake to MAC is about .3. Previous studies with other anesthetics have shown that this ratio ranges between .3 and .4 or so. The fact that this range is so constant implies a physical mechanism of action rather than a "chemical" one that involves bonding to receptors or other kinds of covalent bonding. I am less interested in the fact that morphine did not affect it very much, because this would be expected with an agent as fast acting as sevoflurane.—J.H. Tinker, M.D.

Effects of Remifentanil, a New Short-Acting Opioid, on Cerebral Blood Flow, Brain Electrical Activity, and Intracranial Pressure in Dogs Anesthetized With Isoflurane and Nitrous Oxide

Hoffman WE, Cunningham F, James MK, Baughman VL, Albrecht RF (Univ of Illinois, Chicago; Glaxo, Inc Research Inst, Research Triangle Park, NC)
Anesthesiology 79:107–113, 1993   101-94-5–23

Objective.—Remifentanil is a new short-acting opioid that is metabolized by blood and tissue esterase activity. Its analgesic and cardiovascular effects are similar to, but of shorter duration than, those of alfentanil. An animal study examined the time to onset of response and recovery and the magnitude of electroencephalographic (EEG) and regional cerebral blood flow (rCBF) response with equipotent doses of remifentanil and alfentanil.

Methods.—After baseline measurements during maintenance of anesthesia with 1% end-tidal isoflurane and 50% nitrous oxide, 25 dogs were given approximately equipotent high and low doses of remifentanil, .5 and 1 μg/kg/min, and alfentanil, 1.6 and 3.2 μg/kg/min. Each dose was infused for 30 minutes, followed by a 30-minute recovery period. Blood pressure, heart rate, and intracranial pressure were monitored continuously; EEG measurements were made by aperiodic analyses, and rCBF was evaluated using radioactive microspheres.

Results.—Both opioids brought 25% to 30% reductions in blood pressure and heart rate, whereas cortex, hippocampus, and caudate blood flow decreased 40% to 50% during infusion. Flow changes in the lower blood regions were modest at most. The EEG picture shifted from low-amplitude, high-frequency at baseline to high-amplitude, low-frequency during infusion. Dogs receiving remifentanil showed a return to baseline of heart rate, EEG, and rCBF during the 30-minute recovery period, but those receiving alfentanil did not. After decreasing during infusion, blood pressure and intracranial pressure increased above baseline during the recovery period in dogs receiving remifentanil.

Conclusion.—The short-acting opioids remifentanil and alfentanil have similar cardiovascular and cerebral effects. However, recovery is faster after remifentanil. The increasing arterial and intracranial pressures during recovery in dogs receiving remifentanil warrant further study.

▶ I think we will be hearing a lot about this new ultrashort-acting synthetic opioid. As with any new drug, I urge our readers to be aware of enthusiastic early reports, but there is no reason to believe that this drug is anything other than an opioid in a much shorter-acting form.—J.H. Tinker, M.D.

Studies of Thiopental, Etomidate

Effects of Etomidate on the Adrenocortical and Metabolic Adaptation of the Neonate
Crozier TA, Flamm C, Speer CP, Rath W, Wuttke W, Kuhn W, Kettler D (Univ of Göttingen, Germany)
Br J Anaesth 70:47–53, 1993   101-94-5–24

Background.—The condition of the neonate immediately after cesarean delivery is influenced by the anesthetic induction agent. The effects of etomidate and methohexitone on plasma cortisol and blood glucose levels in the neonate were compared.

Methods.—Twenty-two neonates delivered by elective cesarean and 18 delivered by emergency cesarean section were included. Apgar scores, blood sugar, and plasma levels of cortisol and etomidate were documented at birth and 2 and 6 hours later.

Findings.—No differences in Apgar scores were attributable to the induction agent. Median levels of cortisol in cord blood were minimal. Cortisol levels increased in the infants of mothers given methohexitone and declined in the infants of mothers given etomidate. This effect was most apparent 2 hours after delivery. No differences were recorded at 6 hours after birth. Concentration changes associated with the induction agent differed significantly during the trial. Blood glucose levels were minimal in all infants and did not differ between groups. Seventeen neonates had moderate to severe hypoglycemia, 9 in the etomidate group and 8 in the methohexitone group. The ratio of the mean fetal to maternal etomidate concentration was .48, with an umbilical arterial etomidate concentration of 83 ng/mL^{-1}. The mean etomidate concentration was 9.3 ng/mL^{-1} and 6 ng/mL^{-1} at 2 and 6 hours, respectively.

Conclusion.—No evidence was found to preclude the use of etomidate for inducing anesthesia for cesarean section. To avoid hypoglycemia, all infants delivered by cesarean section should be fed early, regardless of the anesthetic given.

▶ Etomidate appears to be a satisfactory induction agent for those patients who require general anesthesia for cesarean section. I reserve etomidate for use in those patients for whom thiopental and ketamine are undesirable.—D.H. Chestnut, M.D.

Determinants of Thiopental Induction Dose Requirements
Avram MJ, Sanghvi R, Henthorn TK, Krejcie TC, Shanks CA, Fragen RJ, Howard KA, Kaczynski DA (Northwestern Univ, Chicago)
Anesth Analg 76:10–17, 1993   101-94-5–25

Objective.—Women and older patients of both sexes need less thiopental for anesthetic induction. However, these differences may be caused by differences in cardiac output and lean body mass rather than by age and sex per se. This hypothesis was studied in 60 elective surgical patients.

Methods.—The patients were 30 men and 30 women, 10 from each of 3 age groups: 18 to 45 years, 46 to 65 years, and older than 65 years. Anesthesia was induced in all patients with thiopental in a 150-mg/min infusion. The investigators compared the groups for thiopental dose needed to reach a clinical end point (dropping a syringe barrel) and an electroencephalogram (EEG) end point (burst suppression).

Results.—Univariate analysis identified outliers in the relationships of age, weight, lean body mass, and cardiac output to thiopental dose. Differential weighting of data points allowed the construction of a robust multiple linear regression model. The model for thiopental dose at the clinical end point selecting the regressor variables of age, weight, and sex was comparable to that for age, lean body mass, and sex. With the EEG end point, the dose was better defined by models using the variables of age, weight, and cardiac output or age, lean body mass, and cardiac output. Despite age-related variations in cardiac output, age was always a selected variable. Sex-related differences in weight and lean body mass minimized the importance of sex as a selected variable.

Conclusion.—Age and body weight or lean body mass are the most important predictors of the thiopental dose required for induction. Gender and cardiac output are relatively minor determinants. The use of thiopental infusion rather than the bolus administrated may have minimized the importance of cardiac output while maximizing that of weight or lean body mass.

▶ During residency I was taught that age and lean body mass are the most important determinants of thiopental dose requirements. I guess those classic, wise, old wives tales that the old clinicians passed along to us are now validated scientifically.—M.F. Roizen, M.D.

Metoclopramide Decreases Thiopental Hypnotic Requirements

Mehta D, Bradley EL Jr, Kissin I (Univ of Alabama, Birmingham)
Anesth Analg 77:784–787, 1993   101-94-5–26

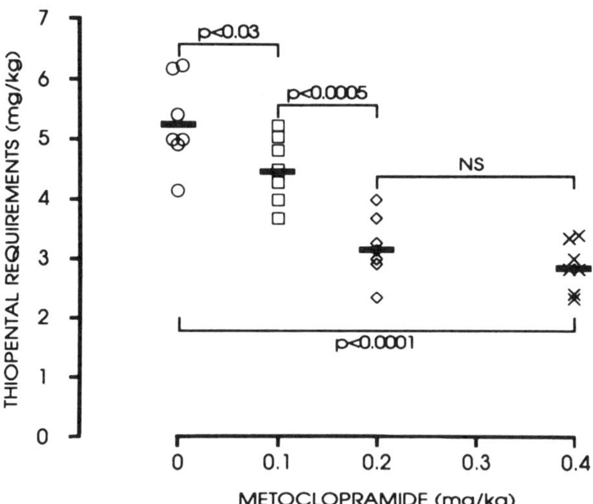

Fig 5–4.—Thiopental requirements for induction of anesthesia in patients receiving different doses of MCA. Each *symbol* (*times sign, diamond, square,* and *circle*) represents an individual induction dose, and the *horizontal bar* represents the mean value in a group of 7 patients. (Courtesy of Mehta D, Bradley EL Jr, Kissin I: *Anesth Analg* 77:784–787, 1993.)

Background.—Metoclopramide (MCA), a dopamine receptor antagonist, prevents nausea and vomiting and has a potential to facilitate hypnosis. The role of dopamine receptors in the anesthetic effects of general anesthetics is controversial, however. A randomized, double-blind study investigated whether MCA decreases thiopental requirements for induction of anesthesia and compared the effects of MCA with those of droperidol (DPD).

Methods.—Study participants were 96 unpremedicated female patients between the ages of 18 and 60 years. The effect of MCA on thiopental hypnotic requirements was determined by 2 methods, thiopental titrations (A series) and bolus injections of predetermined doses (B series) of thiopental. The former method was used for evaluating the reference drug, DPD (C series). Loss of the ability to open eyes on verbal command was used as a hynotic end point. Twenty-eight patients were used in both series A and C, and 40 patients were used in series B. Each series had saline control groups.

Results.—The mean thiopental requirements in series A were 5.3 mg/kg in controls and 4.5, 3.2, and 2.9 mg/kg, respectively, in the MCA .1-, .2-, and .4-mg/kg groups (Fig 5–4). In series B of the experiments, MCA in a dose of .2 mg/kg shifted the thiopental dose-response curve to the left along the dose axis. Thus, the median effective dose value of thiopental decreased from 2.7 mg/kg to 1.5 mg/kg, a reduction of 44%. Series C demonstrated that DPD reduced the thiopental hypnotic requirements almost to the same degree as MCA. The ceiling effect was observed at doses of .01 and .02 mg/kg.

Conclusion.—Metoclopramide decreases thiopental requirements. This decrease appears to be dose-dependent, its maximum reaching 45% at an MCA dose of .2 mg/kg. A ceiling effect was observed above this dose. The titration method provides the same results as the method based on bolus injections of predetermined doses of thiopental. The similarity between the thiopental-sparing effects of MCA and DPD, drugs with quite different pharmacokinetic characteristics, suggests that the blockade of D_2 receptors might be the main mechanism underlying this effect.

▶ The occasional recommendation that metoclopramide be administered intravenously before induction of anesthesia in patients considered at risk for an increased gastric volume should also consider this drug interaction. The potential clinical significance, however, of decreased thiopental hypnotic requirements is unresolved.—R.K. Stoelting, M.D.

Studies of Volatile Anesthetics

Effects of Isoflurane and Enflurane on Intracellular Ca^{2+} Mobilization in Isolated Cardiac Myocytes

Wilde DW, Davidson BA, Smith MD, Knight PR (Univ of Michigan, Ann Arbor; State Univ of New York at Buffalo)
Anesthesiology 79:73–82, 1993

101-94-5–27

Background.—Isoflurane and, particularly, enflurane have depressant effects on the myocardium, presumably through an action on the excitation-contraction pathway. It has been hypothesized that the negative inotropic action of these drugs entails both a limit on membrane calcium entry and a change in intracellular calcium ion release.

Methods.—Intracellular calcium ion transients were recorded in myocytes of the rat ventricle, loaded with fura-2, by fluorescence microscopy. Transients were stimulated by membrane depolarization produced with a suction electrode or by elevating the potassium ion concentration. In other experiments, 15 mM of caffeine was used to induce the release of calcium ion from the sarcoplasmic reticulum. The transients were analyzed for net amplitude, maximal rate of increase, average rate of decline in the intracellular calcium ion concentration, and duration.

Results.—Both enflurane and isoflurane reduced electrically stimulated calcium ion transients in a dose-dependent manner. Transient amplitude was reduced more by enflurane than by isoflurane, and enflurane also had more marked effects on the maximal rate of increase of intracellular calcium ion. Both agents lowered the steady-state increase in intracellular calcium induced by potassium ion. Both agents, particularly enflurane, inhibited the caffeine-sensitive release of calcium from the sarcoplasmic reticulum.

Conclusion.—The negative inotropic actions of enflurane and isoflurane entail depressed calcium ion influx during membrane excitation and also reduce calcium ion release from the sarcoplasmic reticulum.

▶ Many anesthesiologists are fond of saying things such as "We don't know how anesthetics actually work," or "We don't know how anesthetics actually depress the myocardium." I would argue that our basic science-oriented colleagues know a great deal about how anesthetics work and how they depress various organs including myocardium. I included this elegant paper in this year's Year Book of Anesthesiology and Pain Management because I think clinical anesthesiologists should understand that in recent years, with newer techniques, much has been learned. Clearly alterations in regulation of calcium input and in regulation of sarcoplasmic reticulum are contributory to the depressant effects of volatile anesthetics on cardiac function.—J.H. Tinker, M.D.

Influence of Age on Awakening Concentrations of Sevoflurane and Isoflurane

Katoh T, Suguro Y, Ikeda T, Kazama T, Ikeda K (Hamamatsu Univ, Japan)
Anesth Analg 76:348–352, 1993   101-94-5–28

Background.—Age is one of the most important factors influencing the minimum alveolar concentration (MAC). However, there have been no reports on the relationship between age and end-tidal concentration on awakening. The effects of age, duration of anesthesia, gender, and type of surgery on end-tidal concentrations on awakening from anesthesia with sevoflurane and isoflurane were evaluated.

Methods.—Thirty-nine healthy patients, American Society of Anesthesiologists physical status I, were included. The end-tidal anesthetic level was maintained at a constant concentration for at least 15 minutes after surgery. The end-tidal concentration was reduced if patients did not open their eyes on request, and it was maintained again at a constant level for 15 minutes. The anesthetic concentration halfway between the value allowing response and the value just preventing response was noted.

Findings.—The end-tidal concentrations on awakening were .62% for sevoflurane and .41% for isoflurane. These concentrations were significantly correlated with age but not with anesthesia duration, gender, or surgery type.

Conclusion.—Awakening concentration declines at a rate similar to the decrease in MAC with increasing age. Thus, the ratios to MAC are fairly constant at .34 for isoflurane and sevoflurane.

▶ The authors concluded here, logically, that as MAC decreases with age, so does the anesthetic concentration at which the patient will awaken. This would somehow imply that older people are more "sensitive" to anesthetics. Although this seems to be an accepted fact, I have not come across any neurophysiologic or subcellular reason why this should be so. Older people, in fact, tend to need *less* sleep at night. I do not think we understand this business of the effect of age on anesthetic sensitivity very well at all.—J.H. Tinker, M.D.

Minimum Alveolar Concentration of Sevoflurane in Elderly Patients

Nakajima R, Nakajima Y, Ikeda K (Hamamatsu Univ, Japan)
Br J Anaesth 70:273–275, 1993   101-94-5–29

Background.—The minimum alveolar concentration (MAC) of sevoflurane in children and adults has been reported. The MAC of sevoflurane in elderly persons was investigated, and the magnitude of the change with age was quantified.

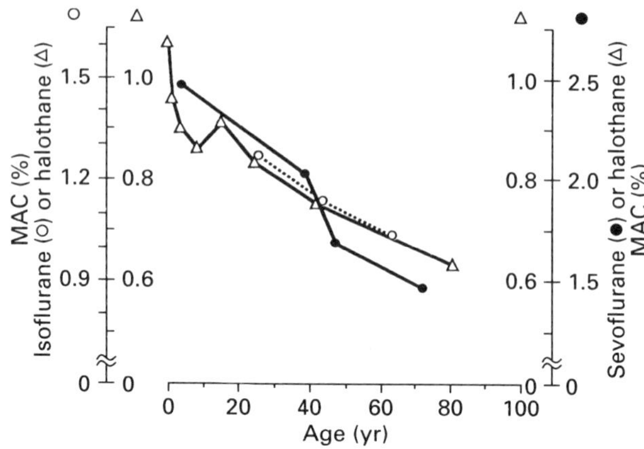

Fig 5–5.—Halothane (*triangle*), isoflurane (*open circle*), and sevoflurane (*filled circle*) MAC at various ages. Halothane data were determined by Gregory, Eger, and Munson; isoflurane data were determined by Stevens and colleagues; and sevoflurane data were determined at younger ages by Katoh and Ikeda and Scheller, Saidman, and Partridge. The ratio of the Y-axis is 1.5 for isoflurane-halothane and 2.5 for sevoflurane-halothane. (Courtesy of Nakajima R, Nakajima Y, Ikeda K: *Br J Anaesth* 70:273–275, 1993.)

Methods and Findings.—Twenty patients, aged 63–82 years, with American Society of Anesthesiologists status I–II, were studied. The MAC of sevoflurane was 1.48%, a value smaller than values previously reported for children and other adults. The magnitude of the change in MAC with age was comparable to that associated with halothane and isoflurane. The calculated anesthetic ED_{95}, the dose that prevented 95% of the patients from moving, was 1.98% (Fig 5–5).

Conclusion.—Many researchers have found that the anesthetic requirements for elderly patients are lower than those of children and younger adults. The current findings are consistent with these previous findings, indicating that elderly persons need a smaller MAC for sevoflurane anesthesia than younger adults and children.

▶ These authors have found an appropriate MAC reduction for age with sevoflurane, similar to that which has been seen in the past for other volatile anesthetics. This consistency is not what you would expect if anesthetics worked on traditional receptors, but it is what you would expect if, as we believe, anesthetics were working in various cellular and subcellular membrane structures to disrupt functions by physical means.—J.H. Tinker, M.D.

Treatment of Intra-Operative Hypertension With Enflurane, Nicardipine, or Human Atrial Natriuretic Peptide: Haemodynamic and Renal Effects

Goto F, Kato S, Sudo I (Kitasato Univ, Kanagawa, Japan; Saiseikai Utsuno-miya Hosp, Japan)
Can J Anaesth 39:932–937, 1992   101-94-5–30

Objective.—Various treatments for intraoperative hypertension were evaluated in 32 patients, 20 men and 12 women aged 30 to 69 years, who underwent gastrectomy for gastric cancer. Hypertension was defined as an intraoperative systolic pressure exceeding 160 mm Hg.

Management.—In 11 patients, intraoperative hypertension was treated by increasing the inspired enflurane concentration. In 11 others, the blood pressure was kept within the range of 110 to 150 mm Hg by infusing nicardipine at rates of .5–2 μg per kg per minute. In the remaining 10 patients, the blood pressure was controlled by infusing human atrial natriuretic peptide (hANP) at rates of .05–.2 μg per kg per minute.

Results.—All treatments effectively controlled the arterial pressure. Urine flow and the urinary excretion of sodium and phosphate increased after nicardipine and hANP administration. The fractional distal reabsorption of sodium was suppressed by hANP only. Creatinine clearance increased in the patients receiving hANP but did not change in nicardipine-treated patients.

Conclusion.—Either nicardipine or hANP may safely be used to treat intraoperative hypertension.

▶ These 2 compounds, namely nicardipine and ANP, are fascinating in different ways. Nicardipine has been extensively tested as a more or less pure vasodilating calcium channel blocker. It has not been introduced in the United States. During its testing, it seemed to me that nicardipine would be the kind of drug that might conceivably replace nitroprusside, although it is too long acting to really be given as a continuous infusion. The hANP is an exciting peptide and may well have a place in our armamentarium for treatment of intra- and postoperative hypertension. It is also not (yet) available in the United States. I think it is interesting that we often read about these fascinating new compounds in the literature from outside the United States and the compounds often go on into general usage in those countries and not in the United States. Financial considerations play an enormous role in these decisions. I wonder whether somewhere reposing in the economic trash bin of drugs not deemed economically worthy of going through the enormous time and expenditure required for Food and Drug Administration introduction there might rest the next penicillin or halothane. The other criticism that I have heard from Europeans and Asians alike is that they are being closely watched by the United States and are serving a bit of a "guinea pig" role while we simply wait and watch the results of the actions of these new drugs on their own populations. How about that for a radical thought? Be that as it may, in the case of these 2 newer substances, I have no idea whether they will prove clinically useful, but they are exciting compounds.—J.H. Tinker, M.D.

Depression of Neuromuscular Function in a Patient During Desflurane Anesthesia

Kelly RE, Lien CA, Savarese JJ, Belmont MR, Hartman GS, Russo JR, Hollmann C (Cornell Univ, New York)
Anesth Analg 76:868–871, 1993   101-94-5-31

Introduction.—Desflurane is a potent, volatile anesthetic; its minimal alveolar anesthetic concentration (MAC) has been established as 7.25%. The first surgical patient in whom neuromuscular depression resulted from desflurane anesthesia was described.

Case Report.—Man, 32, scheduled for bilateral varicocele repair, had neuromuscular function monitored while receiving an infusion of atracurium while under desflurane anesthesia. After premedication with midazolam and fentanyl, thiopental was administered and ventilation was controlled with desflurane in oxygen at inspired concentrations from 3% to 13%. The train-of-four (TOF) ratio faded after 10 minutes of desflurane, and the T1 amplitude declined shortly afterward. The TOF ratio was maximally depressed by 70%, and the T1 amplitude by 76%. Neuromuscular function recovered almost totally within 6 minutes of discontinuance of desflurane. The end-tidal level decreased to 1% within 4 minutes. Recovery was complete within 11 minutes. The changes were reproduced by reintroducing desflurane. Function was normal when the end-tidal concentration reached .5 MAC (3.5%).

Interpretation.—Desflurane may have distinct prejunctional and postjunctional neuromuscular effects, resulting in neuromuscular depression at higher concentrations than previously reported. The substantial lag between the end-tidal desflurane concentration and the onset and end of neuromuscular blockade may result in a difference between blood-gas and blood-muscle partition coefficients.

▶ All the volatile anesthetics have some effect on neuromuscular function, starting with the old observation that diethyl ether depressed spinal synaptic transmission, thus leading to abdominal relaxation. This fascinating case led to a contention by the authors that there is a differential pattern of recovery due to regional solubility characteristics of this new agent. Those differences resulted in substantial lag periods between the obvious reduction in end-tidal desflurane concentration and recovery of the patient's neuromuscular junction clinically. Some have contended that clinical end-tidal measurement of desflurane was not necessary because of its insoluble nature, i.e., the inspired concentration came pretty close to giving the anesthetist the information he/she needed about end-tidal and, therefore, presumably arterial/brain/ neuromuscular junction concentrations. This case report makes me concerned that even if we do insist on end-tidal desflurane measurement (as I have done in our department), we may still not understand what is going on at the neuromuscular junction.—J.H. Tinker, M.D.

Airway Irritation Produced by Volatile Anaesthetics During Brief Inhalation: Comparison of Halothane, Enflurane, Isoflurane and Sevoflurane

Doi M, Ikeda K (Hamamatsu Univ, Japan)
Can J Anaesth 40:122–126, 1993

101-94-5–32

Introduction.—Airway irritation is an important feature of the volatile anesthetics, particularly when they are used for induction. Sevoflurane appears to cause little airway irritation. The airway irritation produced by 4 volatile anesthetics—halothane, enflurane, isoflurane, and sevoflurane—was compared.

Methods.—The subjects were 11 healthy male volunteers. Each agent was tested at 2 concentrations, equivalent to 1 and 2 minimum alveolar concentration. Respiratory inductive plethysmography was used to measure tidal volume, respiratory frequency, and changes in functional residual capacity after 15 seconds of inhalation of each anesthetic. Cough reflex was also assessed, as were the patient's subjective ratings of airway irritation.

Findings.—With inhalation of each anesthetic came a decrease in tidal volume and functional residual capacity and an increase in respiratory frequency. Isoflurane caused significant changes in those parameters most often, followed by enflurane, halothane, and sevoflurane. The patient's subjective ratings placed the 4 agents in the same order. Sevoflurane administration did not induce a cough reflex.

Conclusion.—The clinical impression that sevoflurane is associated with less airway irritation than the other, newer volatile anesthetics was confirmed. This may be a considerable advantage, at least for anesthesia in children. Sevoflurane is also preferred to halothane because of its lower arrhythmogenicity.

▶ This paper represents a competent attempt to quantitate pungency. I think it contains methodology that future authors will find useful in studying airway irritation produced by anesthetics. It also reinforces my belief that the lack of pungency, coupled with the rapid uptake of sevoflurane, may sound the death knell for halothane in pediatric anesthesia.—J.H. Tinker, M.D.

Quantification of the Degradation Products of Sevoflurane in Two CO_2 Absorbants During Low-Flow Anesthesia in Surgical Patients

Frink EJ Jr, Malan TP, Morgan SE, Brown EA, Malcomson M, Brown BR Jr (Univ of Arizona, Tucson)
Anesthesiology 77:1064–1069, 1992

101-94-5–33

Background.—Sevoflurane is a new inhalational agent that produces degradation products on interaction with carbon dioxide (CO_2) absorbants. Quantification of these products during low-flow or closed-circuit

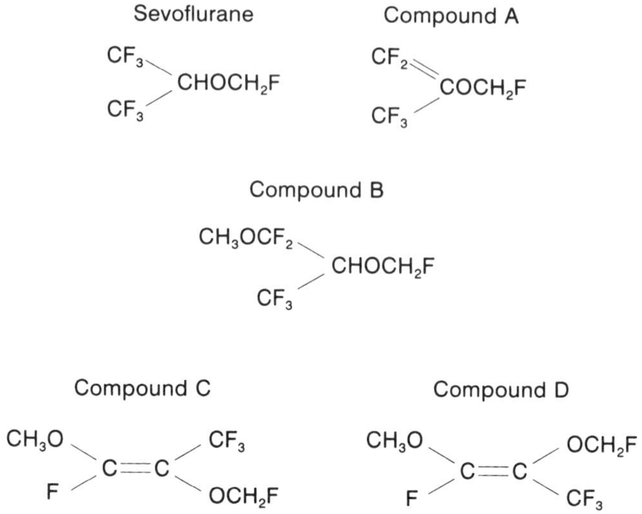

Fig 5–6.—Diagram of sevoflurane and 4 degradation products evaluated in study. Sevoflurane = fluoromethyl 2,2,2-trifluoro-1-(trifluoromethyl) ethyl ether; compound A = fluoromethyl-2,2-difluoro-1-(trifluoromethyl) vinyl ether; compound B = fluoromethyl-2-methoxy-2,2 difluoro-1-(trifluoromethyl) ethyl ether; compound C = D(isomers)-fluoromethyl-2-methoxy-2 fluoro-1-(trifluoromethyl) vinyl ether. (Courtesy of Frick EJ Jr, Malan TP, Morgan SE, et al: *Anesthesiology* 77:1064–1069, 1992.)

anesthesia has not been well evaluated. A low-flow anesthetic technique was used to assess degradation products in patients receiving sevoflurane anesthesia for more than 3 hours. These products have been labeled compounds A, B, C, and D and are shown in Figure 5–6.

Methods.—Sevoflurane anesthesia was administered to 16 patients by using a circle absorption system with oxygen (O_2) flow of 500 mL/min and an average nitrous oxide (N_2O) flow of 273 mL/min. For the first 8 patients, soda lime was the CO_2 absorbant, and for the second 8, baralyme was the CO_2 absorbant.

Findings.—The only degradation product detectable in the low-flow anesthetic circuit was fluoromethyl-2, 2-difluoro-1-(trifluoromethyl) vinyl ether (compound A). Compound A concentrations increased in the first 4 hours of anesthesia with soda lime and baralyme and decreased between 4 and 5 hours when baralyme was used. The mean maximum inhalation level of compound A using baralyme was 20.3 ppm, compared with a mean of 8.16 ppm with soda lime. This difference was not statistically significant. One patient had a maximal concentration of 60.8 ppm during low-flow anesthesia with baralyme. Exhalation concentrations of compound A were less than inhalation concentrations, which suggested patient uptake. Baralyme was associated with higher peak CO_2 absorbant temperatures than soda lime. There were no detectable abnormal changes in hepatic or renal function as many as 48 hours after anesthesia.

Conclusion.—Sevoflurane delivered in a low-flow circuit for 3–5 hours generally produced low levels of a single degradation product. The concentrations of compound A noted in this study were well below the levels reported to cause toxicity in animals. However, further research is needed to assess the potential variability in production of compound A.

▶ Sevoflurane has 2 major drawbacks for clinical use, the first of which is the attack on the fluoromethoxy carbon by hepatic mixed function oxidase (cytochrome P450 and isozymes). The second potential drawback to sevoflurane use is its breakdown by soda lime into "compound A," which is volatile and probably toxic. This study is likely to be of considerable interest because sevoflurane has anesthetic properties that are of considerable interest. This study shows that 16 patients can be anesthetized with sevoflurane in the presence of soda lime without injury. It does not show that millions of patients, with all kinds of preexisting medical conditions, exposed to all sorts of flows, all sorts of concentrations, under all sorts of clinical conditions, with usual American anesthesia circuits including soda lime, will necessarily be as safe.—J.H. Tinker, M.D.

Comparison of the Direct Effects of Sevoflurane, Isoflurane and Halothane on Isolated Canine Coronary Arteries

Nakamura K, Toda H, Hatano Y, Mori K (Kyoto Univ, Japan; Wakayama Med College, Japan)
Can J Anaesth 40:257–261, 1993   101-94-5-34

Background.—Studies on canine epicardial arteries have shown that isoflurane, like adenosine, preferentially dilates the small coronary arteries. Halothane, like nitroglycerin, dilates the larger arteries. The effects of sevoflurane on coronary blood flow remain uncertain.

Objective and Methods.—A study was designed to compare the direct effects of sevoflurane with those of the other agents on both proximal large canine coronary arteries 2.5–3.2 mm in outer diameter, and distal small vessels measuring .6–.9 mm. The vessels were cut into vascular rings and precontracted with potassium chloride so as to compare their relaxant responses to the anesthetics with the maximum response to papaverine.

Results.—Sevoflurane, halothane, and isoflurane all produced dose-dependent relaxation of both large and small coronary arteries. Halothane had a greater relaxing effect on large arteries, whereas isoflurane had a more marked effect on small arteries. Sevoflurane, in concentrations of 1.7% to 5.1%, had equivalent relaxant effects on large and small arteries.

Conclusion.—Sevoflurane seems less likely than isoflurane to produce coronary steal in patients with coronary artery disease.

▶ I included this paper in the YEAR BOOK OF ANESTHESIOLOGY AND PAIN MANAGEMENT this year despite the fact that it is a dog study because it makes several important points. First, although we compare anesthetics with respect to their "anesthetic" potency by using the minimum alveolar concentration (MAC), this does not at all imply that we can rely on the MAC to make comparisons between anesthetics with respect to many other effects, especially those on the heart and its coronary arteries. This paper is a classic example of that.

The second reason I chose this paper is because it is definitive evidence that, unlike isoflurane, sevoflurane is not much of a dilator of small coronary arteries. This implies but does not prove that sevoflurane will not be accused of "coronary steal." At least this is a promising start. I hope we will not have to go through years of suspicion and controversy, as we did with isoflurane, before overwhelming evidence of clinical usage denied the original speculations that isoflurane might produce coronary steal.—J.H. Tinker, M.D.

Halothane Hepatitis Patients Have Serum Antibodies That React With Protein Disulfide Isomerase

Martin JL, Kenna JG, Martin BM, Thomassen D, Reed GF, Pohl LR (Natl Heart, Lung and Blood Inst, Bethesda, Md; Johns Hopkins Med Insts, Bethesda, Md; Natl Inst of Mental Health, Bethesda, Md; et al)
Hepatology 18:858–863, 1993   101-94-5–35

Introduction.—For more than 3 decades, halothane has been the most widely used anesthetic agent in the world. Postoperative hepatotoxicity, which can occur in susceptible individuals, is usually mild and self-limited. A rarer, more severe complication is halothane hepatitis. This syndrome occurs in approximately 1 in 10,000 anesthetized patients and results in death in 40% to 50% of cases. The role of trifluoroacetylated (TFA)-modified liver microsomial proteins in the pathogenesis of halothane hepatitis was examined. The vast majority of affected patients have serum antibodies that react with 1 or more specific liver microsomial proteins covalently altered by the trifluoroacetyl chloride metabolite of halothane.

Methods.—A 57-kD TFA liver microsomial neoantigen associated with halothane hepatitis and native 57-kD protein were purified from liver microsomes of halothane-treated and untreated rats, respectively. The purified TFA and native 57-kD proteins were used as test antigens in an enzyme-linked immunosorbent assay. Sera were obtained from 40 patients with a clinical diagnosis of halothane hepatitis and from various control participants. Five controls had multiple halothane exposures and no evidence of liver dysfunction, 5 had neither halothane exposure nor liver dysfunction, and 5 were medical personnel with exposure to subclinical doses of halothane. Additional controls were 5 patients with a diagnosis of primary biliary cirrhosis, 5 with acute fulminant liver disease, 5 with chronic active liver disease, and 2 with viral hepatitis who had been exposed to halothane.

Results.—Serum antibodies from halothane hepatitis patients reacted with both TFA and native 57-kD proteins to a significantly greater extent than did serum antibodies from the 32 control patients. The 57-kD protein has been identified as rat liver protein disulfide isomerase, and the antibodies raised against it also reacted with a protein of approximately 58 kD in human liver microsomes.

Conclusion.—The TFA protein disulfide isomerase is 1 of the immunogens associated with halothane hepatitis. The antibody response seen in patients with the syndrome implies that the TFA-modified forms of the proteins somehow become exposed to the immune system.

▶ Today, there are still anesthesiologists who cling to the notion that there is no such thing as "halothane hepatotoxicity." It does exist. There is no doubt of that. Furthermore, although we went off on a bit of a wild goose chase about halothane's reductive metabolism for a few years, we now seem to be back on track in directions that make sense. Halothane's reductive metabolism, although it occurs, probably never made much sense as a possible cause of halothane hepatotoxicity, because of its miniscule percentage of the total metabolism of halothane. On the other hand, a mechanism that involves the intermediate of trifluoroacetic acid or its ion, which is of course the major metabolite of halothane, and which is produced from approximately 17% of an inhaled dose during a halothane anesthetic, makes sense as being related to the mechanism of halothane hepatotoxicity. These authors have shown that trifluoroacetic acid can produce "trifluoroacetylated" liver microsomal proteins. These trifluoroacetylated proteins then can become "neoantigens" and can elicit antibody formation. These authors have shown that there is a reasonable mechanism by which we can, in essence, become allergic to halothane! I think this paper is 1 of the better basic science explanations of a clinical phenomenon related to anesthesia that has come along in many years. It is entirely likely that these folks are "on track" toward the explanation of at least much of what we have called "halothane hepatitis."—J.H. Tinker, M.D.

Surfactant in Aspiration

Prevention of Respiratory Failure After Hydrochloric Acid Aspiration by Intratracheal Surfactant Instillation in Rats
Eijking EP, Gommers D, So KL, de Maat MPM, Mouton JW, Lachmann B (Erasmus Univ, Rotterdam, The Netherlands)
Anesth Analg 76:472–477, 1993 101-94-5–36

Background.—The surfactant system is very likely involved in the pathophysiology of respiratory failure brought on by hydrochloric acid (HCl)

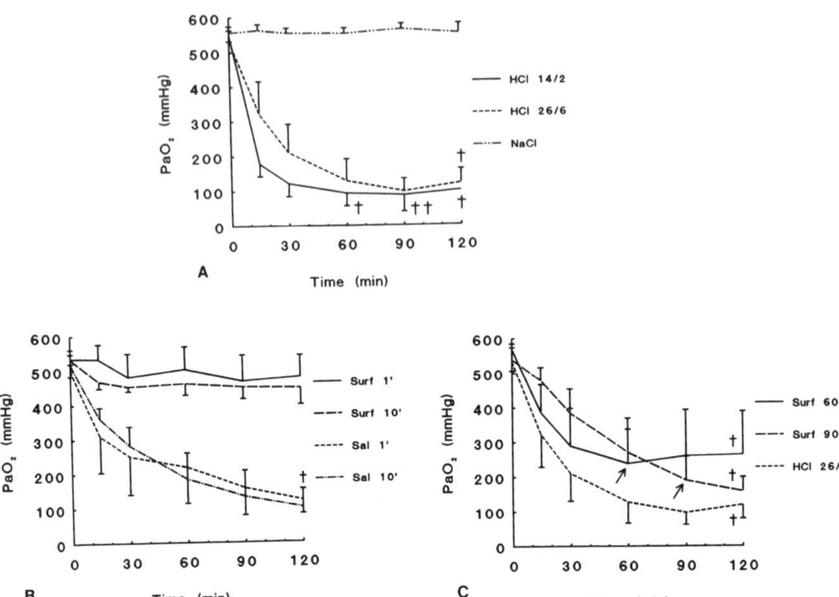

Fig 5–7.—Partial pressure of oxygen in arterial blood (Pao_2) values (mean $\pm$ 1 SD) of the different groups. **A,** rats ventilated at $P_{peak} = 14$/positive end-expiratory pressure (PEEP) = 2 cm H_2O or $P_{peak} = 26$/PEEP = 6 cm H_2O after HCl aspiration (HCl 14/2 and HCl 26/6, respectively) and rats receiving saline (NaCl) instead of HCl; **B,** rats receiving surfactant or saline, 1 or 10 minutes after HCl aspiration (Surf 1′, Surf 10′, Sal 1′, and Sal 10′, respectively); **C,** rats receiving surfactant 60 or 90 minutes after HCl aspiration (Surf 60′and Surf 90′, respectively), and, again, rats ventilated at $P_{peak} = 26$/PEEP = 6 cm H_2O (HCl 26/6). †, 1 rat died: ↑, surfactant instillation. (Courtesy of Eijking EP, Gommers D, So KL, et al: Anesth Analg 76:472–477, 1993.)

aspiration. The effects of various ventilation strategies and intratracheal surfactant instillation at different time intervals on the course of pulmonary gas exchange in rats were investigated.

Methods.—Forty-nine rats were anesthetized and mechanically ventilated via a tracheostomy. Intratracheal .1 N HCl was next instilled at 3 mL/kg to induce respiratory failure. Animals were then placed in 1 of 9 groups. The peak airway pressure/positive end-expiratory pressure of 14/2 and 26/2 were used to ventilate groups 1 and 2 through 9, respectively. Surfactant (200 mg/kg) was given intratracheally to group 3 and 4 animals at 1 and 10 minutes after HCl aspiration. Saline was given to group 5 and 6 animals at 1 and 10 minutes after HCl aspiration. Groups 7 and 8 were given surfactant at 60 and 90 minutes after HCl aspiration, and group 9 was given saline instead of HCl.

Results.—Gas exchange deterioration was noted in groups 1, 2, 5, 6, 7, and 8. However, respiratory failure was prevented in groups 3 and 4. Surfactant treatment prevented further reduction of the partial pressure of oxygen in arterial blood values in group 7 after gas exchange deterioration, although no effect on gas exchange was noted for group 8 animals. In group 9, intratracheal saline instillation had no effect on gas exchange (Fig 5–7).

Conclusion.—Surfactant should be given as quickly as possible after aspiration of gastric contents to deflect development of respiratory failure.

▶ It would be premature based on these animal data to advocate this therapy "to deflect development of respiratory failure." Nevertheless, when known acid aspiration is promptly followed by arterial hypoxemia, the clinician deserves availability of all possibly beneficial therapies. In these rare instances, intratracheal surfactant instillation, along with other more traditional treatments, may become a consideration.—R.K. Stoelting, M.D.

H_2-Receptor Blockers

Interaction of H_2-Receptor Antagonists and Benzodiazepine Sedation: A Double-Blind Placebo-Controlled Investigation of the Effects of Cimetidine and Ranitidine on Recovery After Intravenous Midazolam
Sanders LD, Whitehead C, Gildersleve CD, Rosen M, Robinson JO (Univ of Wales, Cardiff)
Anaesthesia 48:286–292, 1993

101-94-5-37

Background.—Cimetidine and ranitidine are H_2-receptor antagonists used in the treatment of peptic ulcers. In addition, cimetidine, and to a lesser extent, ranitidine, inhibit cytochrome P450. Many patients being treated with these drugs routinely undergo endoscopy and receive benzodiazepines for sedation. Theoretically, patients receiving cimetidine should metabolize benzodiazepines more slowly, because of the inhibition of cytochrome P450. Early studies investigating this effect have produced inconclusive results. The effect of cimetidine on recovery from intravenous benzodiazepine administration in healthy volunteers was investigated in a randomized, double-blind study.

Patients and Methods.—Ten participants were randomly assigned to receive a placebo, 10 to receive cimetidine, and 8 to receive ranitidine. Midazolam was administered intravenously in a dose of .07 mg/kg on day 1 of testing. Participants began placebo, 400 mg daily of cimetidine, or 150 mg/day of ranitidine on the second day and continued medication for 6 days. On day 9, participants once again received midazolam intravenously. The participants were trained as necessary to achieve steady-state levels in 10 tests measuring memory, cognition, and psychomotor ability. Testing was then performed before and after the first midazolam administration, and after the second period of sedation on day 9.

Results.—Individual variance notwithstanding, there was a clearly measurable degree of impairment on all psychomotor tests performed after the first administration of midazolam. A similar, overall level of impairment was also observed after sedation on day 9. However, the group taking cimetidine had an overall impairment score significantly higher than either of the other groups 2.5 hours after sedation. These differences were not reflected in either memory test or subjective assessments.

Conclusion.—Recent studies have shown that most patients leave the hospital within 2 hours of receiving benzodiazepine for gastroscopy. These results suggest that patients treated with cimetidine may still be impaired at this point.

▶ This is a potentially important drug interaction that has been previously described for diazepam and cimetidine. Midazolam metabolism is reported to be unchanged by H_2-receptor antagonists (1). Therefore, it is unexpected that midazolam-treated patients would experience enhanced sedation when treated with H_2-antagonists as reported here.—R.K. Stoelting, M.D.

Reference

1. Greenblatt DJ, et al: *Anesth Analg* 65:176, 1986.

Metoclopramide-Enhanced Analgesia for Prostaglandin-Induced Termination of Pregnancy

Rosenblatt WH, Cioffi AM, Sinatra R, Silverman DG (Yale Univ, New Haven, Conn)
Anesth Analg 75:760–763, 1992   101-94-5–38

Introduction.—A single dose of metoclopramide previously was found to significantly decrease the patient-controlled analgesia (PCA) morphine requirement of women having prostaglandin-induced termination of pregnancy. Repeated doses of metoclopramide were evaluated to determine whether the drug would further reduce pain and accelerate expulsion of the fetus.

Methods.—Thirty-seven women, American Society of Anesthesiologists physical status II, were undergoing elective abortions in the second trimester. After intra-amnionic injection of prostaglandin, the women were randomly assigned to receive 10 mg of intravenous metoclopramide or saline concurrent with PCA initiation. Four hours later, a second identical dose was administered.

Findings.—Patients given metoclopramide had significantly earlier fetal and placental passage, associated with a 66% reduction in PCA morphine by the time of fetal delivery. Patients given metoclopramide were also discharged from the hospital significantly earlier and had fewer second-day hospital stays. Visual analogue scale scores obtained 45 minutes after each infusion were reduced from baseline only in patients given metoclopramide. There were no significant between-group differences in pain or interval morphine usage.

Conclusion.—Repeated doses of metoclopramide significantly reduced the duration of induced labor and, therefore, total PCA morphine needs. This resulted in an earlier discharge from the hospital for women undergoing prostaglandin-induced labor. The analgesic-potentiating effect of metoclopramide was demonstrated within 45 minutes of its administration.

▶ In an earlier study, Vella et al. (1) observed that women in labor who received both meperidine and metoclopramide had lower pain scores than women who received both meperidine and promethazine. In the present study, the authors confirmed their earlier study (2) that suggested that metoclopramide enhanced patient-controlled intravenous opioid analgesia. It is curious that women in the metoclopramide group had a faster labor than women in the control group. It would be interesting to determine whether metoclopramide hastens labor at term.—D.H. Chestnut, M.D.

References

1. Vella L, et al: *Br Med J* 290:1173, 1985.
2. Rosenblatt WH, et al: *Anesth Analg* 73:553, 1991.

Does Ranitidine Provide Protection Against Acid Gastroesophageal Reflux?

Verbessem D, Camu F, Van de Velde A (Flemish Free Univ, Brussels, Belgium)
Can J Anaesth 40:4–9, 1993   101-94-5-39

Introduction.—Pulmonary aspiration of gastric contents is a serious problem in surgical patients. The prevalence of troublesome gastroesophageal acid reflux (GOR) in adults is reported to be 5% to 8%. Ranitidine inhibits basal and nocturnal gastric acid secretion, but the drug's effect on the incidence and characteristics of GOR has not been studied in detail. The effects of ranitidine and placebo on GOR were compared in patients without a history of the condition.

Methods.—Sixty healthy adult patients took part in the study. All required general anesthesia with tracheal intubation for elective nongastrointestinal-abdominal or gynecologic procedures. Excluded were patients with a history of hiatus hernia, dyspepsia, peptic ulcer, or gastrointestinal diseases. Randomization was to a single dose of ranitidine, 50 mg, either intravenously or intramuscularly (IM), or to placebo administered intravenously 90 minutes before surgery. Gastroesophageal pH was monitored continuously for 6 hours in the lower esophagus using a flexible calibrated glass electrode. The occurrence of acid GOR was defined as a pH of less than 4 for 30 seconds.

Results.—Both ranitidine treatments reduced the number of total acid reflux episodes and the reflux index. The total duration of the reflux episodes with a pH of less than 4 was shorter in both ranitidine groups than in the placebo group. Ranitidine, relative to placebo, reduced the number of patients with acid reflux episodes longer than 5 minutes, and it reduced the number of very acid refluxes (pH < 2.5). During reflux episodes, the mean pH value remained higher in both ranitidine groups.

Conclusion.—Both IM and intravenous administration of a single dose of ranitidine reduced, but did not eliminate, episodes of GOR in surgical patients. Overall, the number of reflux episodes with a pH of less than 4 was 76 in the placebo group, 15 in the IM ranitidine group, and 18 in the intravenous ranitidine group. The mean duration of such episodes was shorter in the IM group than in the intravenous or placebo groups.

▶ The incidence of GOR as evidenced by a decrease in esophageal pH during induction of anesthesia in healthy adults is near zero (1). Evidence of reflux is most likely to accompany difficult upper airway management or reaction to the presence of a tracheal tube at the conclusion of anesthesia (2). It is unlikely that any drug, including ranitidine, will decrease the incidence of reflux owing to these mechanisms.—R.K. Stoelting, M.D.

References

1. Hardy JF, et al: *Can J Anaesth* 37:502, 1990.
2. Warner MA, et al: *Anesthesiology* 78:56, 1993.

Increased Volume of Gastric Contents in Diabetic Patients Undergoing Renal Transplantation: Lack of Effect With Cisapride
Reissell E, Taskinen M-R, Orko R, Lindgren L (Helsinki Univ Central Hosp)
Acta Anaesthesiol Scand 36:736–740, 1992   101-94-5-40

Introduction.—Diabetic gastroparesis is characterized by a delay in gastric emptying without gastric outlet obstruction. The resulting increase in gastric contents increases the risk of acid inspiration during anesthesia induction. Cisapride is a new gastrointestinal prokinetic agent that might alleviate this problem. The effect of oral cisapride on gastric volume in 24 patients with diabetes and 24 uremic patients without diabetes receiving a renal transplant under general anesthesia was examined.

Methods.—Patients received either 10 mg of cisapride or placebo in a randomized, double-blind fashion about 100 minutes before anesthesia and 3 times daily for 2 days postoperatively. After anesthesia induction, gastric contents were aspirated and pH and volume were measured. Stomach emptiness was verified by gastroscopy.

Results.—High gastric volumes were detected in half of the patients with diabetes and in 4 of the patients without diabetes. The pH did not differ between the 2 groups. There was also no difference in postoperative constipation.

Conclusion.—Cisapride had no effect on preoperative gastric emptying or on short-term postoperative bowel function in surgical patients with diabetes.

▶ There may be an important distinction between liquids and solids when evaluating the efficacy of drugs on gastric emptying in diabetic patients with gastroparesis. Indeed metoclopramide and, presumably, cisapride, are more effective for speeding gastric emptying of solids than liquids (1).—R.K. Stoelting, M.D.

Reference

1. Wright RA, et al: *Am J Med Sci* 289:240, 1985.

Ondansetron

Comparison of Ondansetron Versus Placebo to Prevent Postoperative Nausea and Vomiting in Women Undergoing Ambulatory Gynecologic Surgery

McKenzie R, Kovac A, O'Connor T, Duncalf D, Angel J, Gratz I, Tolpin E, McLeskey C, Joslyn A (Magee-Womens Hosp, Pittsburgh, Pa; Univ of Kansas, Kansas City; Kenmore Mercy Hosp, NY; et al)

Anesthesiology 78:21–28, 1993   101-94-5–41

Background.—Nausea and emesis after surgery remain a problem, especially in ambulatory surgical patients. The incidence of nausea and emesis during the 24-hour postoperative period in patients given ondansetron was compared with that in patients given placebo.

Methods.—Five hundred eighty women aged 18–70 years were enrolled in the randomized, prospective, double-blind trial. All were having gynecologic procedures with general opioid anesthesia on an outpatient basis. Ondansetron (1, 4, or 8 mg) or placebo was given before induction of anesthesia.

Findings.—Data on 544 women were analyzed. All doses tested were significantly more effective than placebo in decreasing the incidence of emesis after surgery (Fig 5–8). All doses were more effective in patients with no history of emesis after surgery. The 4- and 8-mg doses were more effective than placebo in patients with a history of emesis after surgery. The doses tested were generally well tolerated. In 5 patients, the serum level of aspartate transaminase (AST) was increased. Subsequently, the level of AST decreased to preoperative levels in all 3 patients tested.

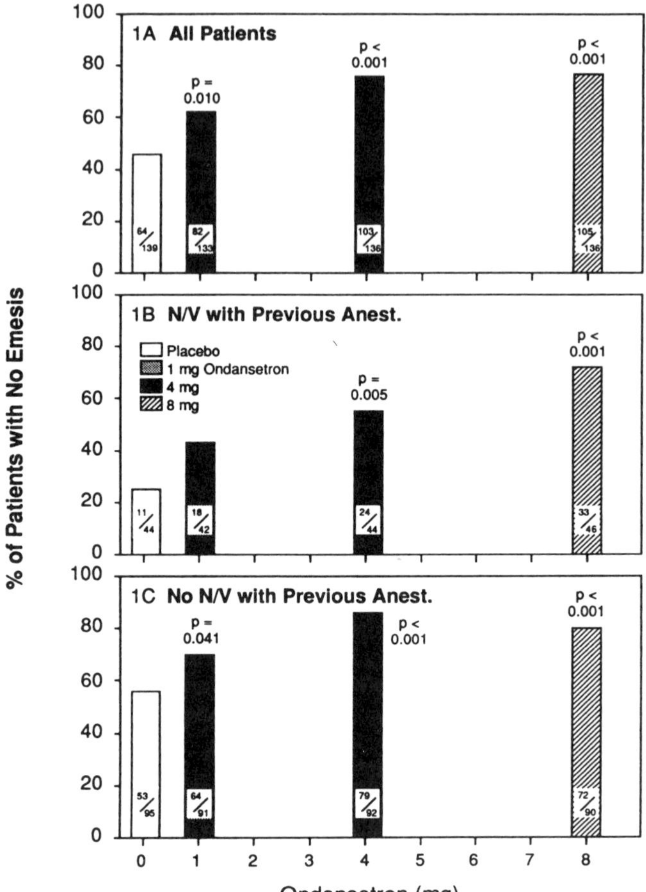

Fig 5–8.—*Abbreviations: N/V,* nausea and vomiting; *Anest.,* anesthesia. Percentage of patients in each study group who had no emesis during the 24-hour study. (Courtesy of McKenzie R, Kovac A, O'Connor T, et al: *Anesthesiology* 78:21–28, 1993.)

Conclusion.—Ondansetron given intravenously in 4- and 8-mg doses was highly effective in preventing postoperative nausea and emesis in this patient population. There were no significant adverse effects.

▶ There is no question that ondansetron is an effective antiemetic. Unanswered are the more compelling questions related to prophylactic use and, if so, what patients, cost vs. benefit, and efficacy compared with less expensive alternatives (droperidol). It is of interest that many postoperative patients are willing to be more sedated and even experience more pain if they could be spared the psychological and physical distress of nausea and vomiting (1). This suggests that patient's priorities might be different from the presumptions of caregivers (2).—R.K. Stoelting, M.D.

References

1. Orkin FK: *Anesth Analg* 74:225, 1992.
2. Kapur PA: *Anesth Analg* 78:5, 1994.

Local Anesthetics (see also Pain Management)

Onset and Duration of Hypoalgesia of Lidocaine Spray Applied to Oral Mucosa—A Dose Response Study

Schønemann NK, van der Burght M, Arendt-Nielsen L, Bjerring P (Univ Hosp, Aarhus, Denmark; Univ of Aalborg, Denmark)
Acta Anaesthesiol Scand 36:733–735, 1992   101-94-5–42

Background.—Lidocaine spray is recommended as a topical analgesic before painful procedures in the mouth and upper airways. Precise information is not available, however, regarding the onset, efficacy, and duration of analgesia after lidocaine spray is applied to the oral mucosa. The laser stimulation method was used to determine just when procedures should be performed and whether a repeated application of lidocaine would be beneficial.

Methods.—Twenty-four healthy adults volunteered for the study. Lidocaine was applied to the inside of the lower lip of each subject; 12 were exposed to 30 mg of lidocaine and 12 were exposed to 60 mg of lidocaine. The second group received 2 applications of 30 mg of lidocaine administered 1 minute apart. Pain thresholds induced by argon-laser stimulation were measured to determine the optimal period of analgesia.

Results.—After 1 or 2 minutes, both groups registered a significant increase in pain thresholds. In the 30-mg group, the pain threshold reached a maximum at a mean of 4.7 minutes after lidocaine application and returned to a normal value in a mean of 10.8 minutes. The 60-mg group reached the maximum pain threshold at a mean of 5.68 minutes and returned to the normal range in a mean 13.2 minutes. The difference in maximal effect on pain thresholds did not differ significantly between the 2 groups.

Conclusion.—Lidocaine is an effective topical analgesia, although local oral application does not produce total analgesia. Doses higher than 15 mg of lidocaine per cm^2 do not increase the pain threshold. For patients undergoing painful procedures in the oral cavity and upper airways, the procedures should be performed within 3 to 8 minutes after application of a single 30-mg dose of lidocaine spray.

▶ My only experience with this is the application of viscous lidocaine to the oral mucosa, which in the 1 subject evaluated (R.K.S.) resulted in prompt numbness. I also think that laryngotracheal lidocaine produces prompt anesthesia to the local presence of a tracheal tube. This is why I recommend a direct laryngoscopy consisting of tracheal lidocaine followed immediately by tracheal intubation.—R.K. Stoelting, M.D.

Cardiac Electrophysiologic Effects of Articaine Compared With Bupivacaine and Lidocaine

Moller RA, Covino BG (Brigham and Women's Hosp, Boston)
Anesth Analg 76:1266–1273, 1993   101-94-5–43

Background.—Articaine, a local anesthetic, differs from lidocaine and bupivacaine structurally in that it contains a thiophene ring. The cardiodepressant effects of articaine were compared with those of lidocaine and bupivacaine.

Methods.—An isolated rabbit heart model was used in the randomized, blinded study. Hearts were removed, and the right septal wall was placed in a warm, aerated, Tyrode's solution-perfused chamber. The effects of the 3 anesthetics on action potentials from the Purkinje fiber and ventricular muscle tissues were then assessed.

Findings.—Action potential overshoot, amplitude, and maximal rate of depolarization (V_{max}) were depressed to a similar degree by bupivacaine and articaine. The effects of bupivacaine persisted significantly longer than those of articaine and lidocaine. With all 3 anesthetics, rate-dependent reductions in steady-state (SS) V_{max} were obtained. At their highest levels, bupivacaine and lidocaine reduced SS V_{max} from the first V_{max} response. However, articaine decreased SS V_{max} at 3 Hz only; at 1 and 2 Hz, articaine increased it. During bolus concentration superfusion of the local anesthetics, bupivacaine blocked Purkinje fiber–ventricular muscle conduction significantly longer than articaine or lidocaine.

Conclusion.—Articaine was generally no more potent than lidocaine in depressing cardiac electrophysiologic variables. In addition, both articaine and lidocaine were far less potent than bupivacaine in this respect.

▶ This paper is representative of a search for a suitable replacement for bupivacaine. Bupivacaine is a superb local anesthetic, but its cardiotoxicity has been problematic. Articaine might fit that need.

Frankly, in addition to its excellence, the other reason I included this paper in this year's YEAR BOOK OF ANESTHESIOLOGY AND PAIN MANAGEMENT is to pay tribute to my good friend, the late Benjamin G. Covino. Ben will long be remembered as a major contributor to our specialty. I do not know whether this will be the last original paper published with his name on it, but he certainly will live on in the knowledge he has created, plus his living legacy of outstanding trainees. Ben, I know I speak for all of anesthesiology when I say, "We salute you."—J.H. Tinker, M.D.

Magnesium Sulfate

High-Dose Magnesium Sulfate Attenuates Pulmonary Oxygen Toxicity

Flink EB, Dedhia HV, Dinsmore J, Doshi HM, Banks D, Hshieh P (West Virginia Univ, Morgantown)
Crit Care Med 20:1692–1698, 1992   101-94-5–44

Introduction.—Oxygen toxicity results in pathologic changes in the lung that resemble the histologic findings of the adult respiratory distress syndrome (ARDS). Rats exposed to 100% oxygen die in a few days and show the severe histologic damage in the lung characteristic of ARDS. The effects of magnesium sulfate therapy in a rat model of acute oxygen toxicity were evaluated. A number of experimental studies suggest that magnesium significantly affects lung structure and mediator reactions. An in vitro study was also conducted in which varying concentrations of magnesium sulfate were mixed with arachidonate.

Methods.—Thirty-four Sprague-Dawley rats in which an arterial catheter had been inserted for the collection of blood samples were exposed to 100% oxygen for 96 hours or until death. Eighteen animals served as controls and received no magnesium therapy, 8 received a low dosage of magnesium sulfate (1.6 to 3.6 mEq/day), and 8 received a high dosage (7.2 to 9.6 mEq/day). The lungs were excised within an hour after death and examined for damage on a scale of 1 to 4, based on the degree of alveolar congestion, hemorrhage and edema, degree of alveolar epithelial injury, and extent of hyaline membrane formation.

Results.—In the low-dose group, the mean peak level of plasma magnesium concentration was in the desired range, but the mean trough level decreased far below this range. Animals in this group did not have a statistically significant difference in lung damage from controls. Rats receiving higher doses of magnesium sulfate maintained a serum magnesium concentration recognized as therapeutic in eclampsia (4 to 6 mEqL, 2 to 3 mmol/L). The score for the high-dose magnesium group was statistically different from that of the control group, indicating better preservation of lung parenchyma. When sodium arachidonate at 1 mmol/L was mixed with varying concentrations of magnesium sulfate, an opaque solution was formed with 2 mmol/L and a clear solution was formed with .5 mmol/L.

Conclusion.—High-dose magnesium sulfate therapy reduced lung injury caused by acute toxicity in rats. A preliminary experiment and a review of the literature suggest that magnesium in body fluids can bind to and alter the metabolism of arachidonic acid. The removal of arachidonate may lead to decreased levels of its metabolites capable of causing lung injury.

▶ The list of potential benefits of intravenous magnesium continues to grow. No longer only used to treat preeclampsia and eclampsia, clinical and experimental data suggest that magnesium is beneficial to limit myocardial infarct size, to prevent and treat a multitude of dysrhythmias, as a bronchodilator, as a CNS protectant, and as an analgesic.—D.M. Rothenberg, M.D.

Vancomycin

Hypoxia Following Perioperative Administration of Vancomycin
Gopalan K, Dhandha SK (Children's Hosp of Michigan, Detroit)
Anesth Analg 76:200–201, 1993   101-94-5–45

Background.—The glycopeptide antibiotic, which acts against staphylococci, streptococci, and other gram-positive organisms, has been associated with a number of reactions resulting from histamine release. Several nonhistamine reactions have also been reported, probably mediated by IgG and complement. Two children with decreased oxygen saturation (SpO_2) and increased alveolar-arterial gradient resulting from perioperative vancomycin use were studied.

Case Report.—Infant, 4 months, was undergoing elective suboccipital decompression for Arnold-Chiari malformation. The patient had undergone repair of a lumbar myelomeningocele at birth and had no respiratory signs or symptoms other than a mild coryza. Anesthesia was induced with halothane and nitrous oxide in oxygen, and intravenous pancuronium was given to assist in intubation. An infusion of vancomycin was given, 20 mg/kg/hr; however, 10 minutes into this infusion, SpO_2 began to decline, with no response to increasing forced inspiratory oxygen (FIO_2). Mild hypotension responded to a bolus of 5% albumin. Although the lungs were easily ventilated with 100% oxygen, SpO_2 persisted at 90%. At a FIO_2 of .9, the PaO_2 was 89 mm Hg and the $PaCO_2$ 36 mm Hg. There were no signs of increased airway pressure, bronchospasm, or bronchial intubation, and endotracheal tube suctioning produced no secretions. Vancomycin was stopped and the patient was given diphenhydramine, 2.5 mg intravenously. The SpO_2 improved during the next 10 minutes and was maintained at 100% with a FIO_2 of .5 in air. The remainder of the operation and the postoperative course were unremarkable.

Conclusion.—Adverse reaction to perioperative vancomycin in children may present with a decrease in SpO_2. The large intrapulmonary shunt observed in these patients may result from the opposition of hypoxic pulmonary vasoconstriction by mast cells.

▶ The histamine-releasing potential of vancomycin ("red-man syndrome"), especially when the drug is infused rapidly intravenously, is well known. The diversity of the possible effects of histamine is emphasized by this report suggesting that decreases in SpO_2 in the absence of other signs and symptoms may reflect drug-induced release of this chemical mediator.—R.K. Stoelting, M.D.

Glycopyrrolate

Glycopyrrolate vs. Atropine During Anaesthesia for Laryngoscopy and Bronchoscopy

Grønnebech H, Johansson G, Smedebøl M, Valentin N (Univ of Copenhagen, Hellerup, Denmark)
Acta Anaesthesiol Scand 37:454–457, 1993   101-94-5-46

Background.—Glycopyrrolate has been reported to be better than atropine in reducing salivation, maintaining a stable cardiac rate and rhythm, and patient recovery. These traits would make glycopyrrolate an attractive alternative to atropine in patients having laryngoscopy or bronchoscopy. The 2 drugs were compared in 90 patients.

Methods.—Forty-five patients undergoing direct laryngoscopy and 45 undergoing bronchoscopy were studied. In most cases, the procedures

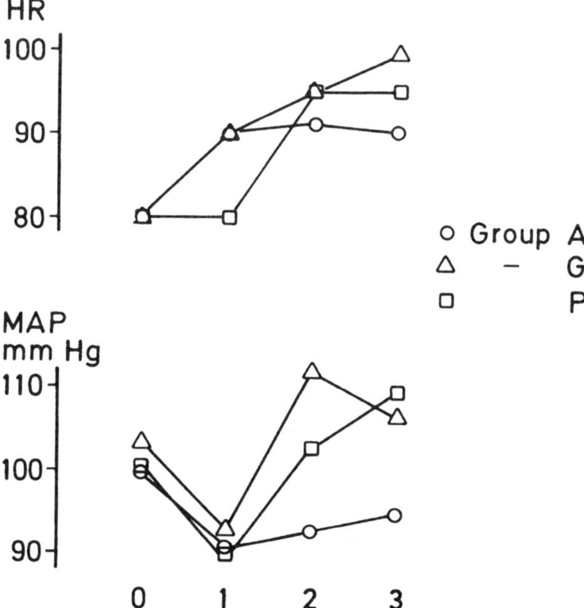

Fig 5–9.—Median values of heart rate (*HR*), **top panel,** and of mean arterial pressure (*MAP*), **bottom panel,** before premedication, 0; before induction, 1; 5 minutes, 2, and 10 minutes, 3, after the induction of anesthesia. (Courtesy of Grønnebech H, Johansson G, Smedebøl M, et al: *Acta Anaesthesiol Scand* 37:454–457, 1993.)

were followed by mediastinoscopy. The active drugs were compared with one another and with placebo.

Findings.—Given intramuscularly 30 minutes before anesthesia, the 2 drugs were equally potent in their antisialogogic effect. The same increase in heart rate was noted before induction. During anesthesia, the heart rate increased to the same level in the placebo group as in the active drug groups. Blood pressure during anesthesia was lowest in the atropine group. There were no between-group differences in cardiac arrhythmias (Fig 5–9).

Conclusion.—There appears to be no reason for preferring glycopyrrolate rather than atropine in patients undergoing direct laryngoscopy or bronchoscopy. The excellent drying effect of both drugs was the only reason for using any anticholinergic drug.

▶ One possible advantage of glycopyrrolate is its limited ability to cross lipid membranes such as the blood-brain barrier. In this regard, glycopyrrolate is less likely than atropine to cause CNS excitation in the rare susceptible patient.—R.K. Stoelting, M.D.

Esmolol

Defining the Dose Range for Esmolol Used in Electroconvulsive Therapy Hemodynamic Attenuation
Howie MB, Hiestand DC, Zvara DA, Kim PY, McSweeney TD, Coffman JA
(Ohio State Univ Hosps, Columbus)
Anesth Analg 75:805–810, 1992   101-94-5–47

Objective.—Patients undergoing electroconvulsive therapy (ECT) experience sinus tachycardia and increased arterial blood pressure, with the potential for cardiovascular stress in patients with heart disease. The ultrashort-acting β-adrenergic receptor blocker esmolol has been shown to decrease seizure duration in large doses; however, dose-response studies of hemodynamic response and seizure duration have been lacking.

Methods.—The double-blind, randomized Latin-Square study included 20 adult psychiatric inpatients, American Society of Anesthesiologists (ASA) physical status I to III, scheduled for ECT. Two matched-pair trials were done of placebo vs. esmolol, a 500-μg/kg bolus followed by 300, 200, or 100 μg/kg^{-1}/min^{-1}. Patients acted as their own controls during a total of 160 ECT procedures. Anesthesia was induced with methohexital and succinylcholine, followed 90 seconds later by ECT, followed 3 minutes later by discontinuation of placebo or esmolol.

Results.—The mean heart rate decreased significantly from minute 3 to minute 7. The maximum heart rate decreased as well (Fig 5–10). The mean maximum heart rate postseizure decreased from 146 beats/min in the placebo group to 112 beats/min in the high-dose group, 121 beats/min in the medium-dose group, and 124 beats/min in the low-dose

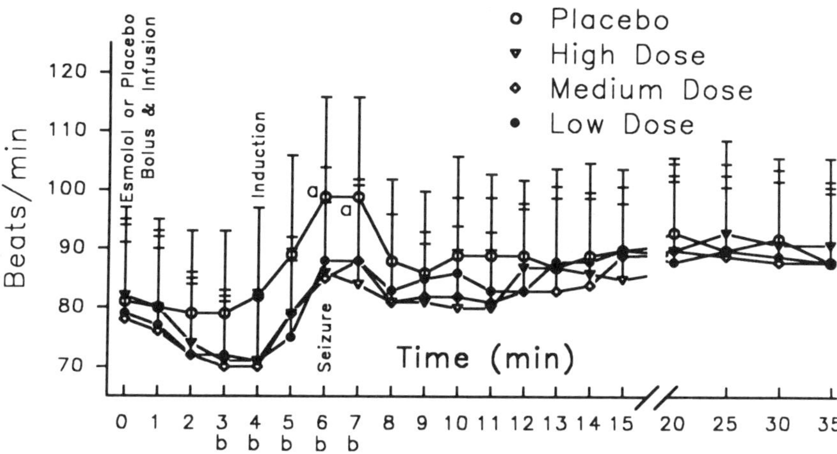

Fig 5–10.—Mean values ± SD for heart rate (beats/min) for all 20 patients given either placebo or esmolol at high dose (300 $\mu g/kg^{-1}/min^{-1}$), medium dose (200 $\mu g/kg^{-1}/min^{-1}$), and low dose (100 $\mu g/kg^{-1}/min^{-1}$) during electroconvulsive therapy. $a = P < .05$, significantly greater than placebo baseline. $b = P < .05$, significantly less than placebo heart rate. (Courtesy of Howie MB, Hiestand DC, Zvara DA, et al: *Anesth Analg* 75:805–810, 1992.)

group. The high-dose group had a mean arterial pressure of 100 mm Hg, compared with 122 mm Hg in the placebo group. Seizure length, as determined by clinical criteria, was 42 seconds in the placebo group, compared with 36 seconds in the high-dose esmolol group and 34 seconds in the medium-dose group.

Conclusion.—Esmolol, given in a 100-$\mu g/kg^{-1}/min^{-1}$ infusion after a 500-$\mu g/kg$ bolus, can control the hyperdynamic cardiovascular response to ECT without changing the duration of the induced seizure. This dose is as effective as higher doses. It remains to be seen whether seizure duration has any important effect on the efficacy of ECT.

▶ I do not believe that every patient undergoing ECT needs pharmacologic protection from seizure-induced sinus tachycardia. When this protection is deemed useful, the onset and duration characteristics of esmolol are very useful.—R.K. Stoelting, M.D.

Amiodarone

Postoperative Amiodarone Pulmonary Toxicity
Morrow B, Shorten GD, Sylvester W (Royal Perth Hosp, Australia; Sir Charles Gairdner Hosp, Perth, Australia)
Anaesth Intensive Care 21:361–362, 1993   101-94-5-48

Background.—Amiodarone is an iodinated benzofuran derivative and class III antiarrhythmic commonly used to treat and prevent ventricular and supraventricular tachyarrhythmias. A case was studied in which a life-threatening amiodarone pulmonary toxicity (APT) occurred immediately after an automatic implantable cardioverter/defibrillator was placed under general anesthesia.

Case Report.—Man, 61, underwent automatic implantable cardioverter/defibrillator placement. He had a 2-year history of syncope from ventricular tachycardia; significant coronary artery disease; and myocardial infarctions 10 and 18 years previously. Two years before the current admission, cardiac catheterization and angiography showed proximal occlusion of the right coronary artery, moderate left ventricular dysfunction, and a small inferior wall aneurysm. Amiodarone treatment was begun. After 6 months at a dose of 600 mg daily, the patient complained of increasing fatigue and dyspnea. The dose was reduced to 400 mg daily, resulting in symptom resolution.

For the current procedure, anesthesia was induced with sodium thiopentone and fentanyl and maintained with nitrous oxide, enflurane, and increments of fentanyl and papaveretum. The pericardium was opened and patches were placed on the anterior and inferior surfaces of the right and left ventricles. Just after extubation, the patient was tachypneic and febrile. Arterial blood gas analysis demonstrated a partial pressure of oxygen of 60 mm Hg. Diffuse bilateral pulmonary infiltrates were seen on chest radiographs. Pulmonary edema caused by left ventricular failure was diagnosed provisionally. The patient was taken to the intensive care unit, and frusemide and captopril treatment was begun. Fluids were restricted, and oxygen therapy with a continuous positive airway pressure mask was continued to maintain pulse oximetry of more than 90%. However, there was no improvement. On the fourth postoperative day, a pulmonary artery catheter was inserted, and a pulmonary artery wedge pressure of 10 mm Hg was revealed. Diuretic therapy was discontinued. The diagnosis of APT was then considered, and amiodarone treatment was stopped. Methylprednisolone treatment was begun. Assessment of a specimen obtained at open lung biopsy showed a low-grade pneumonitis and lipid-containing histiocytes. Findings on electron microscopy were consistent with APT. During the next 4 days, pulmonary gas exchange gradually improved, and the patient was successfully extubated. At discharge 4 weeks after the operation, the patient's respiratory function had almost normalized.

Conclusion.—Postoperative respiratory failure from APT may occur in patients taking amiodarone, even when respiratory function is adequate before surgery. Anesthetists need to be aware of this potential serious complication.

▶ I included this paper because when I teach my residents about various preoperative conditions or drugs, I use the concept of "red flags." When I see a patient who is taking amiodarone, I walk over to my mental flag box and pull out all the red flags possible and run them up the pole. This is one of the scariest drugs we have ever given to human beings. Its potential for disastrous interaction with anesthetics and its potential for various kinds of trouble including pulmonary toxicity postoperatively mean that all anesthesiologists should be very concerned when they see this drug listed as being taken by the patient. Frankly, most drugs that are or were "scary" to anesthesiologists have proven, with time, to be more benign than originally thought, in the presence of modern anesthesia, equipment, monitors, and anesthetic drugs. Amiodarone *still* raises all my red flags up the pole.—J.H. Tinker, M.D.

6 Studies of Neuromuscular Blocking Drugs

Mivacurium

Mivacurium-Induced Neuromuscular Blockade in Patients With Atypical Plasma Cholinesterase

Østergaard D, Jensen FS, Jensen E, Skovgaard LT, Viby-Mogensen J (Univ of Copenhagen)

Acta Anaesthesiol Scand 37:314–318, 1993
101-94-6-1

Purpose.—The neuromuscular blocking effect of mivacurium chloride, a new, short-acting, nondepolarizing neuromuscular blocking agent, was determined. Seventeen patients heterozygous and 5 patients homozygous for the atypical plasma cholinesterase (pChe) gene were evaluated during a modified neurolept anesthesia.

Methods.—Patients were assigned to 1 of 3 groups. Group 1 comprised 5 heterozygous patients, all of whom received a small intravenous dose of mivacurium, .03 mg/kg/bw^{-1}. The remaining 12 heterozygous patients (group 2) were given mivacurium, .2 mg/kg/bw^{-1} (2.5 × ED$_{95}$). Group 3 comprised the 5 homozygous patients, all of whom received mivacurium, .03 mg/kg/bw^{-1}. The response of the adductor pollicis muscle to train-of-four nerve stimulation was recorded with a Myograph 2000.

Results.—In group 1 patients, the mean suppression of the first twitch in the train-of-four responses (T$_1$) was 91%, with a range of 69% to 100%. The average time to 90% T$_1$ recovery was 23.9 minutes. In group 2 patients, the average time to 100% T$_1$ suppressions was 1.4 minutes. In addition, the time to reappearance of the T$_1$ response, to 90% T$_1$ recovery, and the recovery index was 25.3 minutes, 45.5 minutes, and 9.8 minutes, respectively—all of which were significantly longer than reported in phenotypically normal patients. In group 3 patients, the time to reappearance of T$_1$ response ranged from 26 to 128 minutes after receipt of the low mivacurium dose. In these patients, the neuromuscular blockade was effectively antagonized with neostigmine, preceded by atropine.

Conclusion.—Mivacurium-induced neuromuscular blockade was moderately prolonged in patients heterozygous for the usual and atypical pChe gene, whereas patients homozygous for the atypical pChe gene were exceptionally sensitive to this agent. In both groups of patients, antagonism with neostigmine is effective from T_1 recovery greater than 10%.

▶ This is an important mechanism for the anesthesiologist to consider should a patient experience an unexpected prolonged duration of action after administration of mivacurium or give a history of a similar experience after succinylcholine. It has also been observed that patients with chronic renal failure may experience prolonged neuromuscular blockage after administration of mivacurium (1).—R.K. Stoelting, M.D.

Reference

1. *Anesth Analg* 76:866, 1993.

Depth of Block After Divided Doses of Mivacurium Spaced 60 Seconds Apart

Silverman DG, Brull SJ (Yale Univ, New Haven, Conn)
Anesth Analg 77:164–167, 1993   101-94-6–2

Background.—In obtaining a nondepolarizing neuromuscular block at the diaphragm, large doses of the muscle relaxant mivacurium can induce significant histamine release. This can be overcome by giving the drug in 2 divided doses or giving it as a slow infusion. In one experience, however, divided doses do not achieve consistent loss of the adductor pollicis twitch response.

Methods.—This prospective, controlled study compared divided- and single-dose mivacurium for depth of block. The subjects were 30 patients undergoing anesthesia with midazolam, fentanyl, thiopental, and nitrous oxide. All had adductor pollicis contraction measured in response to train-of-four stimulation at 12-second intervals. They were then randomized to receive mivacurium either as a single .15-mg/kg bolus or in 2 boluses of .075 mg/kg each given 60 seconds apart.

Results.—All patients in the single-dose group had 95% or greater depression of twitch, and two thirds had 100% depression. Average maximum depression was 99%. In comparison, only about half of the divided-dose patients achieved 95% or greater depression, and only one fourth achieved 100% depression. The average maximum depression in this group was 92%.

Conclusion.—Divided doses of mivacurium do not achieve the same depth of neuromuscular block as does a single bolus, even though the total dosage is the same. This may be related to the rapid metabolism of mivacurium by plasma cholinesterases.

▶ I agree that the most likely explanation for the author's findings is the rapid enzymatic hydrolysis of mivacurium. Should histamine release be a concern and mivacurium the muscle relaxant selected, it is more logical to limit the dose to less than $3 \times ED_{95}$ and inject this dose over 30 seconds.—R.K. Stoelting, M.D.

Influence of Plasma Cholinesterase Activity on Recovery From Mivacurium-Induced Neuromuscular Blockade in Phenotypically Normal Patients

Østergaard D, Jensen FS, Jensen E, Skovgaard LT, Viby-Mogensen J (Univ of Copenhagen)
Acta Anaesthesiol Scand 36:702–706, 1992   101-94-6–3

Background.—Mivacurium chloride, a new, short-acting, nondepolarizing neuromuscular blocking agent, has an in vitro half-life that increases as plasma cholinesterase (pChe) activity decreases. Thus, its neuromuscular blocking effect may be prolonged in the presence of low pChe.

Patients and Methods.—Ten patients with normal pChe, composing group 1, and 5 with reduced pChe activity, composing group 2, were given a small test dose of mivacurium. After spontaneous recovery from this small dose, .1 mg of mivacurium per kg^{-1} was administered. In another 20 patients with normal or reduced pChe activity, composing group 3, a dose of .2 mg/kg^{-1} was administered.

Findings.—The mean suppression of the height of the first (T_1) of the train-of-four responses after the test dose in groups 1 and 2 was 40% and 56%, respectively. In both groups, the mean T_1 suppression after mivacurium, .1 mg/kg^{-1}, was 100%. Groups 1 and 2 did not differ in their times to different levels of twitch height recovery after the .1-mg/kg^{-1} dose. In group 3, the mean time to maximum block was 1.4 minutes. The time to reappearance of the T_1 response was 15 minutes. There was an inverse relationship between pChe activity and the time to the first response.

Conclusion.—In patients with normal pChe phenotype and normal or low-normal pChe activity, mivacurium is short-acting. However, a prolonged response to mivacurium may be expected in patients with very low pChe activity, a group not included in the current study.

▶ See the comment for Abstract 101-94-6–1.—R.K. Stoelting, M.D.

Atracurium, Vecuronium, Rocuronium

Severe Anaphylactic Shock After Atracurium

Kumar AA, Thys J, Van Aken HK, Stevens E, Crul JF (Universitaire Ziekenhuizen, Leuven, Belgium)
Anesth Analg 76:423–425, 1993

101-94-6–4

Background.—Several factors determine the sensitivity to muscle relaxants. One such factor is interaction with other drugs. One patient had a severe allergic reaction after administration of atracurium.

Case Report.—Woman, 23, obese, was undergoing a tympanoplasty for recurrent cholesteatoma. One month earlier, after taking a sulfamethoxazole-trimethroprim combination, she had an allergic reaction for which she was hospitalized. In the current procedure, anesthesia was induced with alfentanil and propofol. After establishing that ventilation was possible, 40 mg of atracurium was administered intravenously. After an easy endotracheal intubation, her skin color turned gray, and her sinus cardiac rhythm was 110 beats/min. The arterial blood pressure was not recordable. Asystole then occurred, and external cardiac massage was begun. Lactated Ringer's solution and a total dose of 6 mg of epinephrine, 2 g of methylprednisolone, and 50 mg of promethazine hydrochloride was given for 5 minutes through a subclavian deep vein catheter inserted during resuscitation. A 100-kJ shock after ventricular fibrillation had no effect, but she converted to a sinus rhythm of 140 beats/min with 300 kJ. Despite rapid infusion of Ringer's solution and plasma protein, her central venous pressure remained low at -2 mm Hg. Blood gases were pH_α, 7.32; partial pressure of CO_2 in arterial blood, 55.8 mm Hg; and partial pressure of oxygen in arterial blood, 279 mm Hg. After 45 minutes of cardiopulmonary resuscitation and a 40-mg dose of epinephrine, an epinephrine infusion was started, and a weak femoral pulse became palpable. Surgery was cancelled, and the patient was taken to the intensive care unit. The catecholamine infusion was stopped after 10 hours, and controlled ventilation was stopped 24 hours later. Her subsequent recovery was uneventful, with no neurologic damage. Prick tests were later performed, and the patient reacted to atracurium 10^{-2}. Her anaphylactic reaction was therefore attributed to the atracurium.

Conclusion.—Although atracurium is an excellent neuromuscular blocker, it may cause severe anaphylactic reactions. Large doses of epinephrine were needed in this case for resuscitation.

▶ All muscle relaxants are capable of evoking life-threatening allergic reactions. Indeed, the most likely offending drug is the muscle relaxant when an allergic reaction follows a rapid-sequence induction of anesthesia that may include injection of several drugs (opioids, barbiturates, and benzodiazepines). Postmarketing surveillance surveys do not show an increased incidence of bronchospasm or allergic reactions in patients receiving atracurium compared with other muscle relaxants (1). However, some case reports described profound bronchospasm after small doses of atracurium were administered to patients with a history of bronchial asthma (2).—R.K. Stoelting, M.D.

References

1. Lawson DH, et al: *Br J Anaesth* 62:596, 1989.
2. Oh TE, et al: *Br J Anaesth* 62:467, 1989.

A Comparison Between Vecuronium and Atracurium in Myasthenia Gravis

Chan KH, Yang MW, Huang MH, Hseu SS, Chang CC, Lee TY, Lin CY (Veterans Gen Hosp, Taipei, Taiwan, Republic of China; Natl Yang Ming Med College, Taipei, Taiwan, Republic of China; Univ of Chicago Hosps)
Acta Anaesthesiol Scand 37:679–682, 1993   101-94-6–5

Background.—The neuromuscular effects of nondepolarizing muscle relaxants are prolonged in individuals with myasthenia gravis (MG). Vecuronium and atracurium have become popular in the management of muscle relaxation during anesthesia in such patients, but there are few studies on the spontaneous recovery of train-of-four (TOF) response during recovery.

Methods.—The effects of vecuronium bromide, .04 mg/kg^{-1}, and atracurium besylate, .2 mg/kg^{-1}, on TOF response in muscle relaxation management in 20 patients with MG were studied. All patients were undergoing thymectomy.

Findings.—The clinical duration of vecuronium was shorter than that of atracurium. Patients receiving vecuronium had a shorter recovery time than those receiving atracurium. However, vecuronium was associated with a longer time until onset of neuromuscular blockade. During spontaneous recovery from neuromuscular relaxation, TOF fade with vecuronium was significantly higher than with atracurium, indicating that vecuronium may have a greater prejunctional effect.

Conclusion.—These data provide further evidence that both atracurium and vecuronium are safe in patients with MG. Vecuronium appears to have a more marked prejunctional effect.

▶ The response of the patient with MG to muscle relaxants is difficult to predict, although increased sensitivity to these drugs is assumed. In this regard, the drug with the most efficient clearance mechanism would be the logical choice. For that reason, I would select mivacurium rather than an intermediate-acting muscle relaxant for patients with MG.—R.K. Stoelting, M.D.

Continuous Intravenous Infusion of Rocuronium (ORG 9426) in Patients Receiving Balanced, Enflurane, or Isoflurane Anesthesia

Shanks CA, Fragen RJ, Ling D (Northwestern Univ, Chicago)
Anesthesiology 78:649–651, 1993   101-94-6-6

Background.—Rocuronium (ORG 9426), a new nondepolarizing neuromuscular blocking agent, has a rapid onset and an intermediate duration of action. The infusion requirements of rocuronium were studied in a group of patients in whom anesthesia was maintained with barbiturate-nitrous oxide–opioid, nitrous oxide and enflurane, or nitrous oxide and isoflurane.

Methods.—In 30 patients, anesthesia was induced with intravenous thiopental and fentanyl followed by rocuronium, .45 mg/kg. By random assignment, patients received nitrous oxide in 40% oxygen supplemented with fentanyl, thiopental, and droperidol (balanced anesthesia), 1.25 minimum alveolar concentration (MAC) enflurane–nitrous oxide; or 1.25 MAC isoflurane–nitrous oxide. After blockade recovered to 95% depression of twitch height, muscle relaxation was maintained by continuous infusion of rocuronium adjusted to maintain the mechanical twitch response at 95% depression.

Findings.—At 90 and 120 minutes, patients receiving enflurane and isoflurane had lower infusion requirements than patients receiving barbiturate–nitrous oxide–opioid anesthesia; however, these did not differ significantly between the 2 volatile agents. The final mean infusion requirements were 9.8 µg/kg/min for patients given barbiturate–nitrous oxide–opioid, 5.9 µg/kg/min for patients given enflurane, and 6.1 µg/kg/min for patients given isoflurane anesthesia. Spontaneous recovery began soon after the infusion was stopped. Twitch tension equaled 10% of control values in all cases within 5 minutes.

Conclusion.—During barbiturate–nitrous oxide–opioid anesthesia, the infusion requirement to maintain 95% twitch depression was about 10 µg/kg/min. Anesthesia with enflurane or isoflurane reduced this requirement by 40%.

▶ The unique advantage of rocuronium will be its more rapid onset than any other nondepolarizing muscle relaxant. Continuous-infusion techniques of rocuronium are not likely to enjoy any more or less enthusiasm than that already used for mivacurium, atracurium, or vecuronium.—R.K. Stoelting, M.D.

Edrophonium Antagonism of Vecuronium at Varying Degrees of Fourth Twitch Recovery

Salib YM, Donati F, Bevan DR (Royal Victoria Hosp, Montreal; McGill Univ, Montreal)
Can J Anaesth 40:839–843, 1993   101-94-6-7

Background.—Edrophonium has a faster onset of action and produces fewer muscarinic side effects than neostigmine. The evidence suggests that edrophonium may be effective in relatively small doses when blockade is not intense. The dose of edrophonium needed for successful antagonism of vecuronium-induced blockade when all 4 twitches were clearly visible in response to indirect train-of-four (TOF) stimulation was studied.

Methods.—The study subjects were 40 patients scheduled for elective surgery not exceeding 120 minutes. Vecuronium, .08 mg/kg^{-1}, was given during thiopentone-N$_2$ 0-isoflurane anesthesia. Then TOF stimulation was applied every 20 seconds, and the force of contraction of the adductor pollicis muscle was recorded. Increments of vecuronium, .015 mg/kg^{-1}, were given as needed. At the end of surgery, if neuromuscular activity had recovered to 4 visible twitches, edrophonium, .1 mg/kg^{-1}, was administered. If T$_4$/T$_1$ did not reach .7, edrophonium, .1 mg/kg^{-1}, was given 2 minutes later. After another 2 minutes, if T$_4$/T$_1$ did not reach .7 or more, edrophonium, .2 mg/kg^{-1}, was given. Finally, a dose of .4 mg/kg^{-1} was given if T$_4$/T$_1$ was still less than .7.

Findings.—Seventeen patients (42.5%) needed edrophonium, .1 mg/kg^{-1}, for successful reversal. Sixteen (40%) needed a cumulative dose of .2 mg/kg^{-1}, and 6 (15%) needed a dose of .4 mg/kg^{-1}. Only 1 patient received an edrophonium dose of .8 mg/kg^{-1}. The correlation between T$_4$/T$_1$ 2 minutes after the first dose of edrophonium and prereversal T$_4$/T$_1$ was good. All patients with prereversal T$_4$/T$_1$ of greater than .23 needed at most a .2-mg dose of edrophonium per kg^{-1} for successful reversal.

Conclusion.—When all 4 twitches are clearly visible after TOF stimulation, small doses of edrophonium may be enough to antagonize vecuronium neuromuscular blockade. With low doses, there are fewer side effects, the effect is manifest within 2 minutes, and the cost is lower.

▶ It is important to appreciate the importance of spontaneous recovery when evaluating the response to drug-assisted antagonism of nondepolarizing muscle relaxants. Edrophonium in doses of .25 to .5 mg/kg is an acceptable antagonist for short- and intermediate-acting muscle relaxants considering the added protection provided by the simultaneous elimination or hydrolysis of these drugs. A similar protection would be less apparent with long-acting muscle relaxants such as pancuronium.—R.K. Stoelting, M.D.

Succinylcholine

A Very Small Dose of Suxamethonium Relieves Laryngospasm
Chung DC, Rowbottom SJ (Prince of Wales Hosp, Shatin, Hong Kong)
Anaesthesia 48:229–230, 1993   101-94-6–8

Background.—Suxamethonium, given intravenously, is the drug of choice for severe laryngospasm. Typically, a dose of 25 mg or more is used, but doses as small as .1 mg/kg^{-1} have been used successfully. However, there is no evidence that the vocal cords are the target of action of such a small dose. The effect of a very small dose of suxamethonium on spastic vocal cords during laryngoscopy was observed.

Case Report.—Man, 67, underwent excision of a laryngeal tumor by carbon dioxide laser. Topical anesthesia of the nostrils and oropharynx was achieved by using 10% lidocaine spray. General anesthesia was induced by using alfentanil, .5 mg, and propofol, 60 mg, intravenously and maintained with an infusion of 1.5 mg of alfentanil in 40 mL of 1% propofol set to deliver 40 mL/hr. During laryngoscopy, the larynx was displayed on a television monitor. Additional 10% lidocaine was sprayed onto the laryngeal inlet, which resulted in a marked spasm of the vocal cords and paradoxical respiratory movements. The laryngeal spasm was not relieved by administration of propofol. Suxamethonium, 5 mg, was given intravenously, and vocal cord relaxation was clearly seen on the monitor. The spontaneous ventilatory effort was not interrupted. The patient did not become hypoxemic or experience cardiac arrhythmias.

Conclusion.—This experience visually confirmed the efficacy of low-dose suxamethonium for treating laryngeal spasm. The intravenous administration of suxamethonium, .1 mg/kg^{-1}, resulted in a relaxation of about 2 minutes. During this time the depth of anesthesia could be increased by assisting ventilation with a volatile agent or by giving supplementary intravenous agents. A small dose of suxamethonium apparently has little effect on spontaneous ventilatory effort.

▶ These observations should be reassuring to the anesthesiologist confronted with a patient with complete laryngospasm that has progressed to cyanosis and bradycardia. Nevertheless, the value of giving 5 to 10 mg vs. a larger paralyzing dose may not seem important in this potentially life-threatening situation. Conversely, a small nonparalyzing dose of succinylcholine that relaxes the vocal cords without altering spontaneous breathing may be useful for early intervention where recommended treatment has traditionally been positive-pressure mask oxygen.—R.K. Stoelting, M.D.

Anaphylaxis to Relaxants

Platelet Serotonin Is a Mediator Potentially Involved in Anaphylactic Reaction to Neuromuscular Blocking Drugs
Bermejo N, Guéant JL, Mata E, Gérard P, Moneret-Vautrin DA, Laxenaire MC (INSERM U 308, Med Faculty and Univ Hosp of Nancy, France)
Br J Anaesth 70:322–325, 1993   101-94-6–9

Objective.—When allergens bind IgE during an anaphylactic reaction, several mediators are released by blood cells. The IgE-dependent release of platelet serotonin in patients who previously had an anaphylactic reaction to a neuromuscular blocker was examined in vitro.

Patients and Methods.—A platelet serotonin release (PSR) test was performed on blood from 10 patients who had had an IgE-dependent allergic reaction to a neuromuscular blocking drug. The patients, 9 women and 1 man aged from 18 to 54 years, most often had reacted to suxamethonium. Eight control participants were also examined. A specific enzyme-linked immunosorbent assay for serotonin was used. The normal upper limit of serotonin release by neuromuscular blockers was estimated as 2.3%. The results were compared with those of the leukocyte histamine release test.

Results.—Six of the 10 patients had a positive test result. As much as 25% of total platelet serotonin was released by neuromuscular blockers in vitro. Histamine release was evident in 5 of the 6 patients who had a positive PSR test.

Conclusion.—Serotonin seems to be 1 of the mediators associated with histamine release during anaphylactic reactions to neuromuscular blocking agents. The PSR test may prove useful in investigating these reactions.

▶ Laboratory confirmation of the clinical impression that an allergic reaction occurred and determination of the specific drug responsible for the allergic reaction are of obvious value. In addition to serotonin, another chemical marker for the occurrence of an allergic reaction is the presence of tryptase in the plasma. This protease is only released in response to drug-induced degranulation of mast cells, thus verifying the occurrence of an allergic reaction.—R.K. Stoelting, M.D.

Call Mosby Document Express at **1 (800) 55-MOSBY** to obtain copies of the original source documents of articles featured or referenced in the YEAR BOOK series.

7 Malignant Hyperthermia

Delayed Onset of Malignant Hyperthermia Induced by Isoflurane and Desflurane Compared With Halothane in Susceptible Swine
Wedel DJ, Gammel SA, Milde JH, Iaizzo PA (Mayo Med School, Rochester, Minn; Mayo Graduate School of Medicine, Rochester, Minn; Univ of Minnesota, Minneapolis)
Anesthesiology 78:1138–1144, 1993   101-94-7–1

Introduction.—Desflurane, a new inhalational anesthetic, is capable of triggering malignant hyperthermia (MH) in susceptible swine. The ability of desflurane, isoflurane, and halothane to induce MH was compared in both purebred and mixed-bred Pietrain swine susceptible to the disorder.

Methods.—Susceptibility to MH was confirmed by in vivo exposure to succinylcholine and by the in vitro contracture test. Animals were exposed to 1 and, if necessary, to 2 minimum alveolar concentration doses of each of the volatile anesthetics in random order at 7–10-day intervals.

Results.—Malignant hyperthermia episodes developed most rapidly after exposure to halothane—in an average of 20 minutes. The mean interval was 48 minutes for isoflurane and 65 minutes for desflurane. The time needed for MH to develop with a given anesthetic did not differ in the 2 types of swine. The criterion for MH was a partial pressure of carbon dioxide in arterial blood of 70 mm Hg.

Conclusion.—Halothane exposure leads to MH more rapidly than exposure to either isoflurane or desflurane in this porcine model. The findings may help explain observations of delayed and variable triggering of MH in patients not known to be susceptible.

▶ In addition to giving us the not-unexpected news that desflurane also acts as a trigger for MH, at least in swine, I selected this paper because it also reminds us that MH triggering can be delayed in onset in humans as well. Indeed, I know of 1 devastating case where the patient did not trigger until at least an hour had gone by in the recovery room.—J.H. Tinker, M.D.

False-Negative Results With Muscle Caffeine Halothane Contracture Testing for Malignant Hyperthermia

Isaacs H, Badenhorst M (Witwatersrand Univ, Parktown, South Africa)
Anesthesiology 79:5–9, 1993   101-94-7-2

Background.—In muscle strip testing—the first reliable test for susceptibility to malignant hyperthermia (MH)—the degree of caffeine-induced contracture of muscle strips is more sensitive in MH-susceptible subjects. No previous report has mentioned false-negative results of this test.

Methods.—In the course of 350 muscle contracture studies performed during a 6-year period, four false-negative results were noted. The findings of these 4 cases were reported in detail. All muscle strip caffeine halothane tests followed the reliable protocol of the European Malignant Hyperthermia Society.

Results.—Overall, 36% of patients tested positive, 49% were normal, and 15% were equivocal. About half of the last group responded only to halothane and half only to caffeine. Of the 171 patients who tested normal, 4 experienced later clinical episodes of MH. One patient had 2 negative responses to muscle testing on 2 separate occasions.

Conclusion.—Patients in whom clinical and biochemical signs of MH develop in response to an anesthetic challenge should be considered to have MH, regardless of a negative test result. These results cannot be extrapolated to laboratories using the North American test protocol.

▶ In the case of muscle strip testing for MH, false-negatives are potentially more dangerous than false-positives, although false-positives create individuals who are forever after afflicted with a "disability" they do not really have. Nonetheless, I still think false-negatives are worse, as do the authors. The caffeine halothane muscle strip contracture test has always been controversial, but it is all there is at present . . . except for the rare but devastating unpredicted operating room disaster. This disease is still with us, and it is very important that we continue to try to achieve better diagnostic tests.—J.H. Tinker, M.D.

8 Monitoring

Studies of Pulse Oximetry

Randomized Evaluation of Pulse Oximetry in 20,802 Patients: I: Design, Demography, Pulse Oximetry Failure Rate, and Overall Complication Rate
Moller JT, Pedersen T, Rasmussen LS, Jensen PF, Pedersen BD, Ravlo O, Rasmussen NH, Espersen K, Johannessen NW, Cooper JB, Gravenstein JS, Chraemmer-Jørgensen B, Wiberg-Jørgensen F, Djernes M, Heslet L, Johansen SH (Univ of Copenhagen, Herlev, Denmark; Esbjerg Central Hosp, Denmark; Glostrup Hosp, Denmark; et al)
Anesthesiology 78:436–444, 1993   101-94-8-1

Background.—Even though the use of pulse oximetry is quite common, there is little research documenting improvement in patient outcome as a result of its use. The first large, prospective, random, multicenter study undertaken to document improvement in patient outcome was reported.

Patients and Methods.—A total of 20,802 patients who had surgical operations was randomized into 2 groups. One group of 10,312 patients received oximetry, and a control group of 10,490 patients did not. Data were gathered presurgically, during anesthesia, in the postanesthesia care unit, and up to the discharge day or the seventh postoperative day, whichever came first. Individual postsurgical events and/or complications were examined.

Results.—A slight intergroup difference was found in the distribution of age, duration of surgery, some types of surgery, and some types of anesthesia. The total failure rate was reported as 2.5%; however, it increased to 7.2% in patients with American Society of Anesthesiologists physical status 4. Of the total patient group, 13.5% sustained some event during the time they were in the operating room, and 14.9% experienced an event in the postanesthesia care unit. Some patients (2.78%) experienced a cardiovascular complication, and 3.5% had a respiratory complication; with the overall postoperative complication rate listed as 9.7%. Within the 7-day postoperative period, .47% of the patients died, but none of these deaths could be exclusively attributable to anesthesia.

Conclusion.—Even though few significant intergroup differences were found, the randomization was successful. The data collected were congruent with findings in other recent morbidity and mortality studies.

"

Randomized Evaluation of Pulse Oximetry in 20,802 Patients: II. Perioperative Events and Postoperative Complications

Moller JT, Johannessen NW, Espersen K, Ravlo O, Pedersen BD, Jensen PF, Rasmussen NH, Rasmussen LS, Pedersen T, Cooper JB, Gravenstein JS, Chraemmer-Jørgensen B, Djernes M, Wiberg-Jørgensen F, Heslet L, Johansen SH (Univ of Copenhagen, Herlev, Denmark; Esbjerg Central Hosp, Denmark; Glostrup Hosp, Denmark; et al)

Anesthesiology 78:445–453, 1993   101-94-8-2

Background.—Whether perioperative monitoring with a pulse oximeter reduces postoperative morbidity has not been established. Pulse oximetry and other monitoring modalities were evaluated.

Methods.—The effects of pulse oximetry monitoring on the frequency of unanticipated perioperative events, changes in patient care, and the rate of postoperative complications were assessed in a prospective, controlled, randomized, clinical study. In Denmark, 20,802 surgical patients were randomly assigned to monitoring or to no monitoring with pulse oximetry in the operating room (OR) and postanesthesia care unit (PACU).

Findings.—During anesthesia and in the PACU, significantly more monitored patients had at least 1 respiratory event than did unmonitored patients, resulting from a 19-fold increase in the incidence of diagnosed hypoxemia in the oximetry group than in the control group. In the OR, cardiovascular events occurred in similar numbers of patients in the 2 groups, except for myocardial ischemia, which occurred in 12 patients in the oximetry group and in 26 patients in the control group. Several changes in PACU care were associated with the use of pulse oximetry, including a higher flow rate of supplemental oxygen, increased use of supplemental oxygen at discharge, and increased use of naloxone. The rate of changes in patient care as a result of monitoring increased as physical status worsened. Ten percent of the monitored patients and 9.4% of the unmonitored patients had 1 or more postoperative complications, a nonsignificant difference. Cardiovascular, respiratory, neurologic, and infectious complications did not differ between groups. The length of hospitalization and mortality were also comparable between groups. Eighteen percent of the anesthesiologists experienced a situation in which a pulse oximeter helped avoid a serious event or complication. Eighty percent of the anesthesiologists felt more secure when pulse oximetry was used.

Conclusion.—Pulse oximetry can improve the ability of an anesthesiologist to detect hypoxemia and other events in the OR and PACU. The use of oximetry was associated with a significant reduction in the rate of myocardial ischemia. Although monitoring resulted in a number of management changes, the overall rate of postoperative complications was not reduced.

▶ Abstracts 101-94-8-1 and 101-94-8-2 say it all, but some comment is necessary. The editorial in the issue of *Anesthesiology* is also important, but we learn that it is often difficult to show benefits from changes in practice when anesthesia is already provided safely for the vast majority of patients. Furthermore, oximetry may provide benefits that cannot be captured by this outcome data because of what one learns from using it. In addition, other questions are raised by this study, such as, would the results have been the same if capnography were not used? Does oximetry provide for longer-lived faculty members because the duration of their coronary artery spasm during resident teaching is shorter? How much are the results of this study influenced by the low rates of complications already and the high rate of cause of those complications by postoperative factors? Maybe if oximetry were carried on into the postoperative period, the results would be different, or maybe the change in practice that has been accomplished because of pulse oximetry, such as use of oxygen from the operating room to the recovery room and better monitoring of and discharging of patients using pulse oximetry, needs to be evaluated as well.

By far the most conclusive result of this study is that anesthesiologists felt more secure when pulse oximetry was used. Are we just exposing our biases, or is there something real that cannot be quantified here? I feel like I have just seen propofol used for the first time again. There was something remarkable about its use, but no one could quantitate that something remarkable. It is probably still true that no one knows why propofol has gained such widespread acceptance, but clearly something about the drug makes it very special for patients. I think that there is also something about pulse oximetry that makes it very valuable for patients, and in addition to perhaps improving care, it lowers the cost of care, as we have shown (1).—M.F. Roizen, M.D.

Reference

1. Roizen MF, et al: *J Clin Monitor* 9:301, 1993.

Saturation by Pulse Oximetry: Comparison of the Results Obtained by Instruments of Different Brands
Thilo EH, Andersen D, Wasserstein ML, Schmidt J, Luckey D (Univ of Colorado, Denver; Children's Hosp, Denver)
J Pediatr 122:620–626, 1993   101-94-8-3

Introduction.—Pulse oximeters used to monitor oxygenation of arterial blood may give significantly different results under similar clinical circumstances. Observation that arterial oxygen saturation was generally lower when determined by the Ohmeda Biox 3700 pulse oximeter than when determined by the Nellcor N-100 device led to investigation of the reason for the discrepancy.

Methods.—The oximeters were placed simultaneously on 30 infants who required an umbilical artery catheter or posterior tibial artery catheter for clinical management. Both a Nellcor N-100 with an Oxisensor N-25 disposable probe and an Ohmeda Biox 3700 with a disposable Easy Probe were placed, 1 on each foot. They were then switched to the opposite foot halfway through the study period. Measurements were obtained of arterial partial pressure of oxygen, percentage of fetal hemoglobin, and complete co-oximetry, including arterial oxygen saturation with a Radiometer OSM-3 co-oximeter, with and without correction for fetal hemoglobin levels. Four samples of blood were taken from each infant during a 12-hour period.

Results.—Arterial oxygen saturation was consistently higher, by a mean of 1.61%, with the Nellcor than with the Ohmeda device. Nellcor readings correlated best with functional arterial oxygen saturation, and Ohmeda readings correlated best with fractional arterial oxygen saturation, indicating a basic difference in the calibration algorithms used in the 2 instruments.

Conclusion.—Debate exists as to whether functional or fractional arterial oxygen saturation is the more accurate standard. The important point, however, is that the oximeters are different, and this difference may be of clinical importance in predicting arterial partial pressure of oxygen on the basis of arterial oxygen saturation. A single range of "safe" arterial oxygen saturation cannot be applied to all brands of pulse oximeters.

▶ Functional hemoglobin saturation disregards the effects of methemoglobin and carboxyhemoglobin whereas fractional does not. Which is important for the neonate, or even the adult, is not clear. Nevertheless, what is impressive is that the range of 92% to 98% for the Nellcor had a 95% predictive positive value, whereas the range of 90% to 96% for the Ohmeda had a positive predictive value that was indistinguishable from that of the Nellcor or 94%. That is, by using functional oxygen saturation, the Nellcor has a reading that is 1.6% higher than the Ohmeda. Are the absolute values important? Maybe in a neonatal intensive care unit but probably not in an operating room. Both brands have about equal degree of accuracy of positive predictive value for abnormalities.—M.F. Roizen, M.D.

Reliability of a Pulse Oximeter in the Detection of Hyperoxemia
Poets CF, Wilken M, Seidenberg J, Southall DP, von der Hardt H (Medizinische Hochschule, Hannover, Germany; Univ of Keele, Stoke-on-Trent, Staffordshire, England)
J Pediatr 122:87–90, 1993   101-94-8-4

Introduction.—The pulse oximeter more accurately reflects arterial oxygenation than does the transcutaneous oxygen tension monitor. In addition, it responds faster and does not require calibration or heating of the skin. Nevertheless, pulse oximetry is, in theory, less sensitive to hyperoxemia because of the shape of the oxygen dissociation curve. This could be especially important in preterm infants because of the potential relationship between hyperoxemia and retinopathy of prematurity.

Patient Population.—Simultaneous estimates of the partial pressure of oxygen in arterial blood (PaO_2) and transcutaneous oxygen saturation ($tcSO_2$) were made in 50 patients (median age, 2.5 months) admitted to a pediatric intensive care unit who had indwelling arterial lines and received mechanical ventilation. Most were cardiac surgery patients, but 11 had prematurity-related illness.

Methods.—The Nellcor N200 pulse oximeter was used to detect hyperoxemia, defined as an oxygen tension more than 80 mm Hg. The oximeter was connected to a digital device recording both $tcSO_2$ readings from the oximeter and the photoplethysmographic waveforms from which saturation measurements were derived. A total of 213 simultaneous recordings was collected.

Results.—The PaO_2 exceeded 80 mm Hg in 137 of 202 evaluable measurements. In 130 instances, the $tcSO_2$ was 96% or more. None of the 7 false-positive pulse oximeter results were in patients with acidemia, hypercapnia, or anemia. Of 65 PaO_2 values of 80 mm Hg or less, 20% were associated with a $tcSO_2$ of 96% or more. About half of these false-positive pulse oximeter readings were from preterm infants. In all, the pulse oximeter was 95% sensitive and 80% specific for hyperoxemia at an upper alarm limit of 95%.

Conclusion.—The Nellcor N200 pulse oximeter identifies hyperoxemia precisely enough to ensure that patients will not be exposed to unwarranted hypoxemia. Whether the frequency of retinopathy of prematurity can be lessened as a result remains to be determined.

▶ I am amazed that a pulse oximeter was this good in detecting hyperoxemia, which is obviously an important concern for newborn infants. And remember, these were newborn infants in a neonatal intensive care unit and not in the operating room. Thus, it appears that the Nellcor pulse oximeter is sufficiently accurate to ensure detection of hypoxemia, that is, a PaO_2 greater than 90 mm Hg, while still permitting the PaO_2 to be kept greater than 60 mm Hg with a sensitivity of 95% and a specificity of 80%. Although these are not perfect readings, they are excellent, especially because we do not know how good the readings of the gold standard were against a true gold standard of what the oxygen saturation of the patient actually was.—M.F. Roizen, M.D.

Noninvasive Blood Pressure Monitoring

The Finapres 2300e Finger Cuff: The Influence of Cuff Application on the Accuracy of Blood Pressure Measurement

Jones RDM, Kornberg JP, Roulson CJ, Visram AR, Irwin MG (Univ of Hong Kong)

Anaesthesia 48:611–615, 1993   101-94-8–5

Introduction.—The Finapres model 2300e uses both oscillometry and a servo system controlling the inflation and deflation of a finger cuff to monitor blood pressure continuously and noninvasively. It appears to be at least as good as noninvasive oscillometric devices when both are compared with direct arterial pressure readings. The Finapres lacks precision, however, and is subject to drift. It has been difficult to apply the cuff because of the pneumatic transducer and the heavy connecting cable.

Objective and Methods.—Blood pressure was measured using the Finapres 2300e in 7 healthy individuals aged 29–43 years to ascertain the effects of varying the method of cuff application. In the control condition, an appropriately sized cuff was applied to the middle phalanx of the middle finger of the nondominant hand. Intra-arterial pressure was measured directly in the radial artery of the same extremity.

Results.—Correct application of the cuff yielded acceptably precise values for mean and diastolic pressures, and acceptable bias values. All systolic pressure readings in all cuff positions were outside the acceptable error range of 8 mm Hg. The largest errors occurred when too small a cuff was used and when the cuff was loose. Applying the cuff over the proximal interphalangeal joint also produced substantial errors. Excessively tight cuff application underestimated systolic, diastolic, and mean pressures, whereas a loose cuff most often overestimated the pressures.

Conclusion.—The Finapres is quite sensitive to small variations in application of the finger cuff. As a result, arterial pressure estimates are biased, and the instrument has limited clinical value.

▶ This is an excellent technology assessment that probably means this device should not be taken as useful for gaining absolute values of blood pressure. Whether changes in blood pressure are also subject to huge biases and errors was not determined, and before we relegate the Finapres to the scrap heap, such a study is needed.—M.F. Roizen, M.D.

Invasive Monitoring

Cannulation of the Internal Jugular Vein: The Very High Approach

Messahel FM, Al-Mazroa AA (King Khalid Univ Hosp, Riyadh, Saudi Arabia; King Abdulaziz Univ Hosp, Jeddah, Saudi Arabia)

Anaesthesia 47:842–844, 1992   101-94-8–6

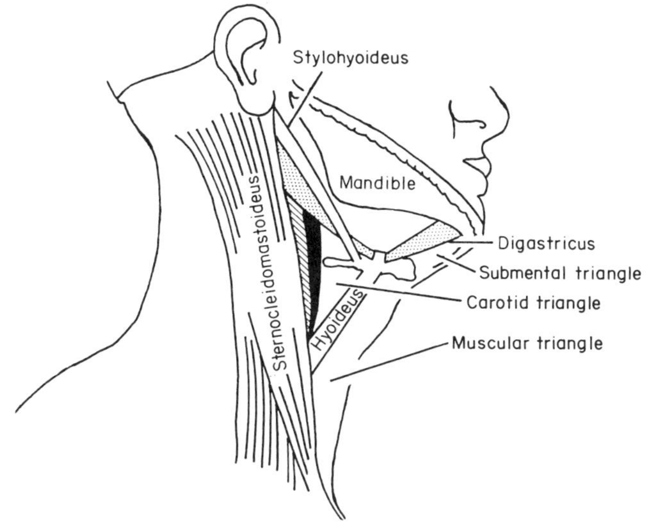

Fig 8–1.—Anatomy of the carotid triangle; *striped area,* internal jugular vein; *black area,* carotid artery. (Courtesy of Messahel FM, Al-Mazroa AA: *Anaesthesia* 47:842–844, 1992.)

Background.—Cannulation of large central veins is a common procedure, using either the internal jugular or the subclavian vein. The insertion of central venous lines carries the risk of complications and has stimulated the search for safer access routes. A new "very high" approach was investigated to measure its advantages over other methods currently used.

Methods.—Patients participating in the study were prepared as for other procedures of internal jugular cannulation. The patient's head was turned to the left, the anatomical carotid triangle was identified (Fig

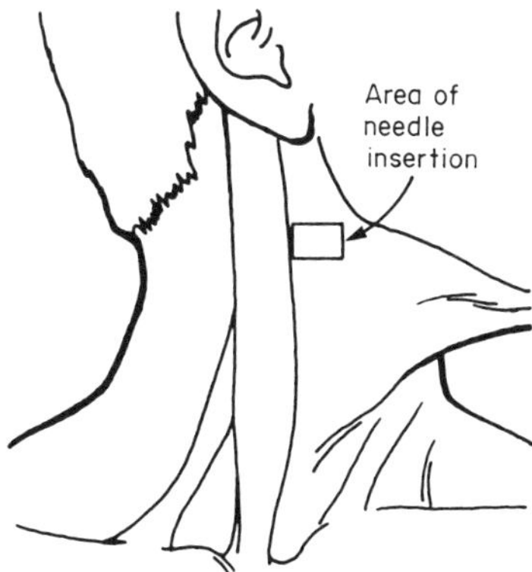

Fig 8–2.—Site of needle insertion. (Courtesy of Messahel FM, Al-Mazroa AA: *Anaesthesia* 47:842–844, 1992.)

8–1), and the internal carotid artery was located by palpation. The point lateral to the artery, as high as possible, was chosen for skin puncture (Fig 8–2). The tip of the introducing needle, attached to a 5-mL syringe, was passed in a caudad direction and adjusted to obtain an angle of 75 to 85 degrees to the coronal plane. Once venous blood was freely aspirated, the Seldinger technique was used to place the venous catheter. This was then attached to an extension tube, looped around the pinna of the ear.

Results.—During a 12-month period, 335 patients experienced the "very high" approach. In 85.4% of the patients, the first attempt at jugular venepuncture was successful. In the remainder, a second attempt through the same puncture proved successful. The point of skin puncture was 1–1.5 cm from the angle of the mandible. Once the needle was introduced, internal jugular venepuncture took place between .5 and 1 cm from the skin surface. All catheters were removed within 11 days, and no complications were observed.

Conclusion.—The "very high" method brought a number of advantages with no observable drawbacks. The approach is easy to learn and apply, it permits surgery to continue unhindered, and conscious patients are able to move their necks painlessly while the catheter is in place. The high site of venepuncture and the angle of needle insertion reduce the risk of pneumothorax, puncturing of major vessels, and injury to nerves. For these reasons, this new approach may become the preferred method.

▶ We have a low, middle, high, anterior, posterior, and now very high approach to the internal jugular vein. Most amazing is the 100% success rate in central line placement with no more than 2 attempts using this technique! It will be very interesting to see whether others who attempt this technique can reproduce these exceptional results.—D.M. Rothenberg, M.D.

A Controlled Trial of Scheduled Replacement of Central Venous and Pulmonary-Artery Catheters
Cobb DK, High KP, Sawyer RG, Sable CA, Adams RB, Lindley DA, Pruett TL, Schwenzer KJ, Farr BM (Univ of Virginia, Charlottesville)
N Engl J Med 327:1062–1068, 1992   101-94-8–7

Introduction.—Prolonged central venous catheterization increases the incidence of infection in patients who are critically ill. Some advocate changing catheters every 3 days to reduce the rate of infection, but it has not been conclusively demonstrated whether this helps. Neither is it known whether it is safer to change the catheter over a guidewire or insert it at a new site. The efficacy of replacing the central venous catheter every 3 days, using either a new puncture site or inserting it at a new site, was assessed in a randomized trial.

Methods.—The trial included 160 adult patients in the intensive care unit who required a central venous or pulmonary artery catheter for more than 3 days. After stratification by medical or surgical intensive care unit, patients were randomized into 4 groups. Group 1 had catheter replacement every 3 days by insertion at a new site, group 2 had replacement every 3 days by exchange over a guidewire, group 3 had replacement when indicated by insertion at a new site, and group 4 had replacement when indicated by exchange over a guidewire. A total of 523 catheters underwent semiquantitative culture.

Results.—There was a 5% rate of catheter-related bloodstream infection, a 16% rate of catheter colonization, and a 9% rate of major mechanical complications. Rates of bloodstream infection were 3 in 1,000 days in group 1, 6 in 1,000 days in group 2, 2 in 1,000 days in group 3, and 3 in 1,000 days in group 4. After the first 3 days, patients assigned to guidewire exchange had a 6% rate of bloodstream infection, compared with 0% in the other groups. However, the rate of mechanical complications in patients assigned to insertion at new sites was 5%, vs. 1% in the other groups.

Conclusion.—Replacing central venous catheters every 3 days does not prevent infection. Although using a guidewire increases risk of bloodstream infections, insertion at new sites increases the risk of mechanical complications. Pending further research, placing central venous catheters with optimal aseptic procedures and leaving them in place until a change is indicated is recommended. Indications include fever of unknown source and catheter malfunction.

▶ This important article looked at some of the complications of central venous pressure and pulmonary artery catheters in intensive care units and came to the very important conclusion that the mechanical and infectious complications dictate different strategies, but the common strategy is having experienced personnel replace them at a new site only when indications of colonization and bloodstream infection occur.—M.F. Roizen, M.D.

Does Radial Artery Pressure Accurately Reflect Aortic Pressure?
Pauca AL, Wallenhaupt SL, Kon ND, Tucker WY (Wake Forest Univ, Winston-Salem, NC)
Chest 102:1193–1198, 1992   101-94-8-8

Objective.—Because the radial artery is commonly used to monitor blood pressure in patients who are critically ill and those having surgery, an attempt was made to determine whether radial artery pressures accurately reflect pressures in the ascending aorta. Previous observations suggest that in awake humans and in dogs, systolic arterial pressure may be as much as 40 mm Hg higher in the radial artery than in the aorta.

Methods.—Fifty-one patients with atherosclerotic coronary artery disease were studied while in the narcotic-anesthetized state before cardiopulmonary bypass. Lorazepam and morphine were given an hour before fentanyl-pancuronium anesthesia. The radial artery was cannulated before induction, and the aorta was cannulated about 45 minutes later.

Results.—The mean systolic arterial pressure differed by 12 mm Hg in the radial artery and aorta. Differences in mean arterial pressure and diastolic pressure were much less marked. The radial systolic pressure was 10 to 35 mm Hg higher than the aortic pressure in half the patients.

Conclusion.—In these anesthetized patients, the radial systolic arterial pressure did not accurately reflect the ascending aortic pressure. Readings of the mean arterial pressure and diastolic pressure in the radial artery are relatively reliable, being within a mean of 3 mm Hg of aortic pressures in at least 90% of the patients.

▶ There is no compelling reason to expect that this finding in awake patients, which has been known since 1955, would be different in 1992 in the presence of general anesthesia that includes fentanyl. It would also be interesting to know whether blood pressure readings from a noninvasive blood pressure device confirmed a similar discrepancy.—R.K. Stoelting, M.D.

Blood Gases, Hematocrits

Clinical Performance of a Blood Gas Monitor: A Prospective, Multicenter Trial

Shapiro BA, Mahutte CK, Cane RD, Gilmour IJ (Northwestern Univ, Chicago; Univ of California, Irvine; Univ of South Florida, Tampa; et al)
Crit Care Med 21:487–494, 1993   101-94-8–9

Background.—The clinical feasibility of a prototypical fluorescent optode intra-arterial blood gas monitor was demonstrated, but it was judged impractical for routine use because of a number of patient interface problems. More recently, an extra-arterial fluorescent optode system was developed to circumvent these problems. The pH, partial pressure of carbon dioxide (PCO_2), and the partial pressure of oxygen (PO_2) fluorescent optodes are located within a sensor cassette inserted in series with the arterial catheter tubing system near the wrist.

Study Design.—A prospective study at 4 intensive care units (ICUs) with varying patient populations compared the new blood gas monitoring system with modern blood gas analyzer measurements. A total of 117 adults with a radial arterial catheter in place was included in the study.

Results.—A total of 1,341 concurrent blood gas analyzer and monitor measurements was available. Linear regression analysis revealed correlational values of .85 for arterial pH, .92 for PCO_2, and .94 for PO_2. The respective values for performance bias—the mean difference between the analyzer and monitor values—were −.004, −.8 torr, and −2.2 torr.

The presence of the blood gas monitoring system did not significantly alter arterial pressure values.

Conclusion.—The blood gas monitoring system can replace the blood gas analyzer when evaluating patients in the ICU with an arterial catheter in place.

▶ Cost-effectiveness data stimulated by this article are important considerations. Like pulse oximetry, which we have recently shown to decrease costs (1) and others have shown to possibly improve quality, this new technology might also decrease cost (whether or not it improves quality we will not know for some time). Thus, new technology may improve quality and reduce costs.—M.F. Roizen, M.D.

Reference

1. Roizen MF, et al: *J Clin Monit* 9:301, 1993.

Evaluation of STAT-CRIT® Hematocrit Determination in Comparison to Coulter and Centrifuge: The Effects of Isotonic Hemodilution and Albumin Administration
McNulty SE, Sharkey SJ, Asam B, Lee JH (Thomas Jefferson Univ, Philadelphia)
Anesth Analg 76:830–834, 1993   101-94-8–10

Background.—Conductivity-based measurements of the electrical resistance of whole blood using the STAT-CRIT method are useful for rapidly estimating hematocrit, but it is not clear whether or how the results should be corrected for electrolyte and protein levels.

Objective and Methods.—The accuracy of the STAT-CRIT was compared with that of the Coulter counter and centrifuge methods of estimating hematocrit in 31 patients having elective cardiac surgery. Studies were done before induction of anesthesia, during the rewarming phase of cardiopulmonary bypass, and after transfusing all available cell-saver blood after bypass. Twenty-eight patients were randomized to receive either 5% albumin or isotonic crystalloid after the end of cardiopulmonary bypass.

Results.—The Coulter hematocrit and microhematocrit by centrifuge correlated at a level of .95. Differences between the Coulter and STAT-CRIT results were most closely related to the protein, chloride, and sodium concentrations. A decrease of 1 g/dL in total protein produced a 1% decline in hematocrit. A chloride change of 10 mmol/L altered the accuracy of the STAT-CRIT by 3.5%, and a comparable change in sodium altered it by 2.5%. The Coulter and STAT-CRIT methods agreed more when albumin, rather than crystalloid, was used for postoperative fluid volume replacement.

Conclusion.—The STAT-CRIT provides accurate estimates of hematocrit if the results are adjusted for changes in serum sodium, serum chloride, and total protein.

▶ This wonderfully done technology assessment article shows how you can make even something that is relatively boring, such as a technology assessment article, very interesting to read.—M.F. Roizen, M.D.

Neuromuscular Blockade Monitoring

The Orbicularis Oculi and the Adductor Pollicis Muscles As Monitors of Atracurium Block of Laryngeal Muscles

Ungureanu D, Meistelman C, Frossard J, Donati F (Institut Gustave Roussy, Villejuif, France; McGill Univ, Montreal)
Anesth Analg 77:775–779, 1993   101-94-8–11

Introduction.—The adductor pollicis muscle is usually monitored as an indicator of laryngeal relaxation in patients undergoing neuromuscular block (NMB). The orbicularis oculi, however, may be preferred to the adductor pollicis for this purpose. Whether atracurium-induced NMB at the laryngeal adductor muscles could be predicted by visual inspection of either adductor pollicis or orbicularis oculi responses was examined.

Methods.—Twenty-one patients undergoing gynecologic, breast, or peripheral limb surgery were anesthetized with propofol (2–2.5 mg/kg)

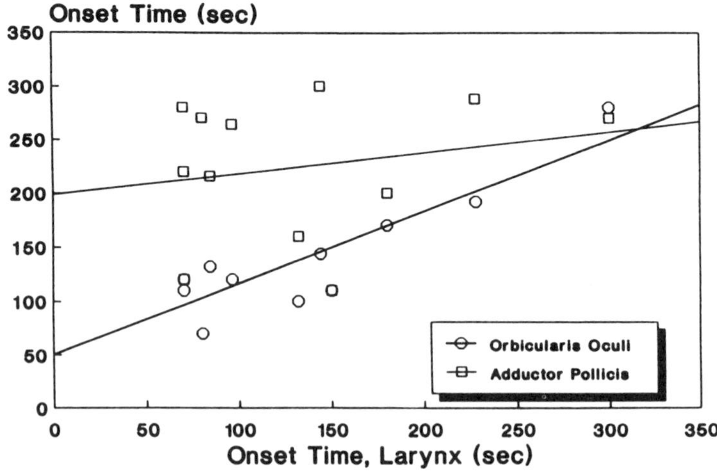

Fig 8–3.—Onset time to loss of visible detectable response in the orbicularis oculi and adductor pollicis, vs. measured onset time to 100% depression of response in laryngeal muscles. No correlation was found between the onset time of the adductor pollicis and laryngeal muscles. Orbicularis oculi correlated significantly with laryngeal muscle onset time (P < .001). (Courtesy of Ungureanu D, Meistelman C, Frossard J, et al: *Anesth Analg* 77:775–779, 1993.)

and fentanyl (2–5 μg/kg). Laryngoscopy and tracheal intubation were performed without neuromuscular blocking drugs. Patients were randomized to receive .3 or .5 mg of atracurium per kg intravenously. Laryngeal response was measured as the pressure change in the tracheal tube cuff positioned between the vocal cords. Two observers not involved in the study visually evaluated the time when all 4 responses to train-of-four stimulation were abolished completely, indicating NMB.

Results.—Complete laryngeal block was observed in only 2 of the 11 patients who received .3 mg of atracurium per kg. These 2 patients also had complete block at the adductor pollicis and orbicularis oculi muscles. However, 4 of the 9 patients with incomplete laryngeal block had complete block at the adductor pollicis. Only 1 patient with the .5-mg dose of atracurium per kg did not have complete NMB of the laryngeal adductor muscles. In this patient, maximum block reached 91%. The onset time was significantly shorter for the laryngeal adductor and orbicularis oculi muscles than at the adductor pollicis.

Conclusion.—After a bolus dose of atracurium, complete laryngeal adductor block corresponded more closely to orbicularis oculi than adductor pollicis paralysis, as detected visually (Fig 8–3). Thus, in terms of both quality and time course, orbicularis oculi monitoring appears to be a good predictor of adequate endotracheal intubating conditions.

▶ There is increasing awareness that adductor pollicis block may not parallel laryngeal relaxation, especially after administration of mivacurium. Nevertheless, I think that attempts to intubate the trachea in the absence of adequate skeletal muscle relaxation may increase the risk of aspiration owing to tensing of the patient's abdominal muscles or attempts to breathe. For this reason, skeletal muscle relaxation beyond paralysis of the laryngeal muscles remains, in my opinion, a desirable goal in many patients.—R.K. Stoelting, M.D.

Monitoring for Water Intoxication During Transurethral Resection of the Prostate

Ethanol Monitoring of Transurethral Prostatic Resection During Inhaled Anesthesia
Stalberg HP, Hahn RG, Jones AW (Huddinge Univ Hosp, Sweden; Natl Lab of Forensic Chemistry, Linköping, Sweden)
Anesth Analg 75:983–988, 1992   101-94-8–12

Background.—Typically, regional anesthesia is used for transurethral resection (TUR) of the prostate. In 5% to 10% of the patients, symptoms associated with irrigating fluid absorption may develop into the TUR syndrome, which can be life threatening. The precision of ethanol monitoring in patients undergoing TUR of the prostate with inhaled anesthesia was investigated.

Methods.—Forty-five patients were included in the study. A breath-alcohol analyzer was placed between the endotracheal tube and the Bains'

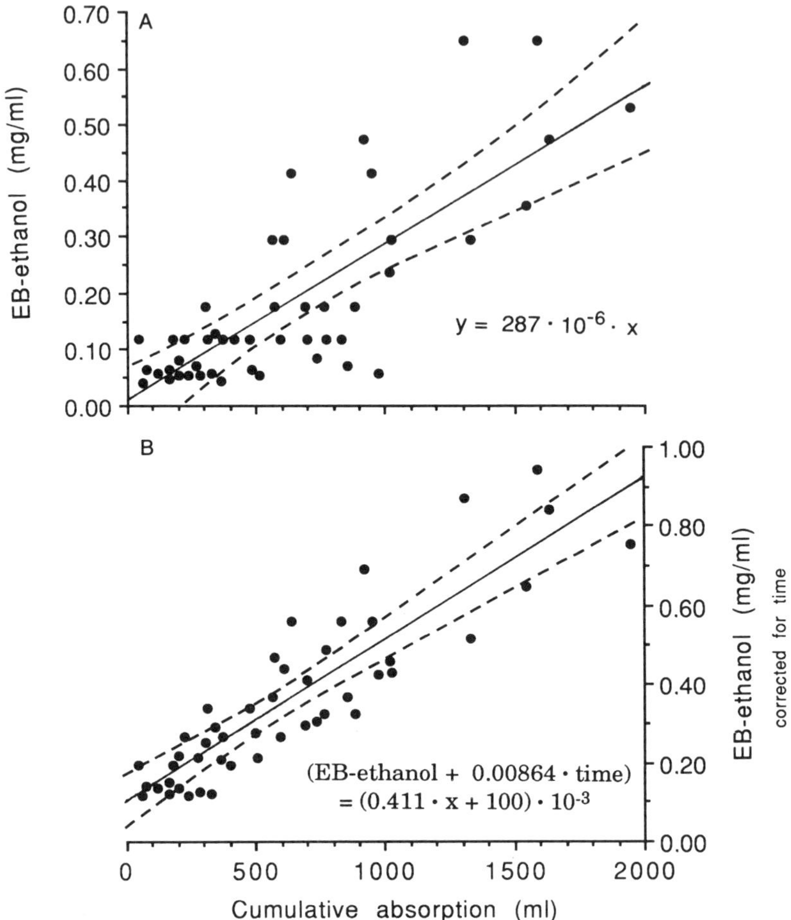

Fig 8–4.—Relationship between concentration of ethanol in expired breath (*EB-ethanol*) and cumulative volumetric fluid balance at end of all 10-minute periods of TURP with intravascular absorption of irrigating fluid (**A**). Same relationship but with EB-ethanol corrected for time required for absorption to occur (**B**). When absorption time was taken into account, the relationship was strengthened. *Dashed lines* indicate ± 1 SD. (Courtesy of Stalberg HP, Hahn RG, Jones AW: *Anesth Analg* 75:983–988, 1992.)

circuit, and the concentration of ethanol in the breath, the serum concentration of sodium, and the volumetric fluid balance were assessed every 10 minutes during 38 operations. The irrigating fluid contained 1.5% glycine and 1% ethanol.

Findings.—The mean absorption rates exceeding 14 mL/min were detected. The volume of irrigating fluid absorbed could be predicted from a single expired-breath test with a standard error of 325 mL in 17 patients who had hyponatremia with absorption. The standard error was 215 mL when the alcohol measures were corrected for absorption time.

Another 7 patients were given glycine, 2.2% wt/vol, as irrigating fluid, and ethanol, .35 g/kg, was given by intravenous infusion. Direct and indirect measures of the blood-alcohol concentration agreed well (Fig 8–4).

Conclusion.—Ethanol monitoring is a viable method for patients undergoing TUR of the prostate with inhaled anesthesia. This form of monitoring is precise enough to permit detection of absorption of irrigating fluid in amounts that may be clinically important for the safety of the patient.

▶ Seldom does a really exciting new idea come along, but this may be one. These authors have come far toward being able to quantitate the actual amount of water absorption during TURP. This really seems like a great idea to me! The only problem with any of this is that TURPs are becoming less and less common as we find out more and more that these are relatively high-risk operations from the standpoint of postoperative surgical complications.—J.H. Tinker, M.D.

Call Mosby Document Express at **1 (800) 55-MOSBY** to obtain copies of the original source documents of articles featured or referenced in the YEAR BOOK series.

9 Risk, Outcome, and Cost Studies

Risk: Pediatric vs. Adults (American Society of Anesthesiologists Closed Claims)

A Comparison of Pediatric and Adult Anesthesia Closed Malpractice Claims

Morray JP, Geiduschek JM, Caplan RA, Posner KL, Gild WM, Cheney FW
(Univ of Washington, Seattle; Virginia Mason Med Ctr, Seattle)
Anesthesiology 78:461–467, 1993   101-94-9–1

Introduction.—Past studies of anesthetic morbidity and mortality indicate a greater risk for children than for adults. The Committee on Professional Liability of the American Society of Anesthesiologists (ASA) has, since 1985, evaluated closed anesthesia malpractice claims using a standardized form and method.

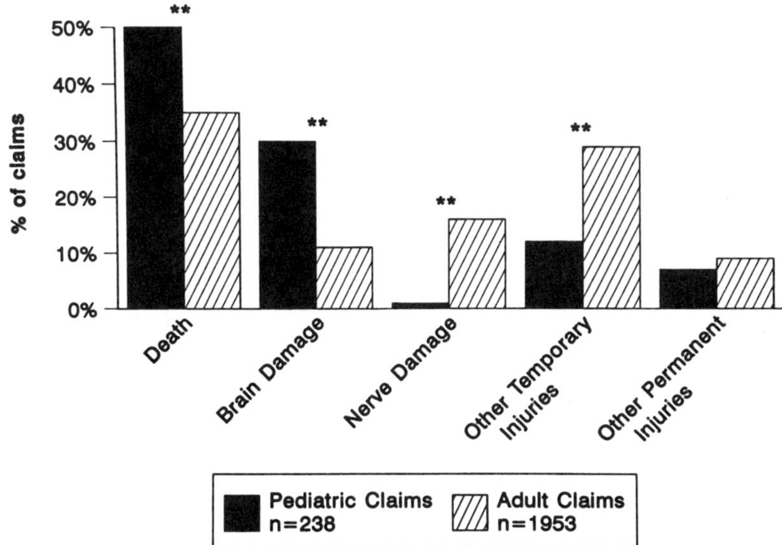

Fig 9–1.—Comparison of patient injury in pediatric and adult closed malpractice claims. **$P \leq$ .01. (Courtesy of Morray JP, Geiduschek JM, Caplan RA, et al: *Anesthesiology* 78:461–467, 1993.)

Data Base.—The ASA Closed Claims Project is a structured evaluation of closed anesthesia malpractice claims obtained from 28 insurance carriers throughout the United States. Of 2,400 claims reviewed, 238 involved children, aged 15 years and younger. Twenty-eight percent of the pediatric claims involved children younger than age 1 year, and 55% involved children aged 3 years and younger.

Findings.—Respiratory events were more frequent among pediatric than adult claims. Half of the pediatric patients and 35% of the adults died (Fig 9–1). In 54% of the pediatric and 44% of the adult claims, anesthetic care was judged to be less than appropriate. In 45% and 30% of cases, respectively, complications were considered to have been preventable through better monitoring. Inadequate ventilation was alleged in 20% of the pediatric claims and 9% of the adult claims. Cyanosis and/or bradycardia frequently preceded cardiac arrest in pediatric claims related to inadequate ventilation. There were no differences in the proportion of claims leading to payment, but the median payment was higher for pediatric than for adult claims.

Conclusion.—A review of pediatric anesthesia malpractice claims shows that respiratory-related damaging events are frequent and often are related to inadequate ventilation. Many claims appear to be preventable by pulse oximetry and/or end-tidal carbon dioxide measurements.

▶ The ASA Closed Claims Study is one of the finest efforts ever mounted by that organization. I have been privileged to write up some of the data, but the unsung heroes are the clinical anesthesiologists who have given so unstintingly of themselves in case review to make this possible.

In this particular report, the mortality rate in the pediatric claims was greater than for adults. I thought it was most interesting that anesthetic care was more often judged substandard than in the adult claims. Are we more critical of ourselves when children are involved? Was the anesthetic care really more substandard? Perhaps children are simply more difficult to anesthetize?

As the authors readily agreed, this study cannot tell us whether, in general, a pediatric anesthetic is more risky than an adult anesthetic. This study complements the famous 1985 study by Keenan and Boyan (1) of intraoperative anesthesia-related risk in which pediatric cases also had a higher incidence.—J.H. Tinker, M.D.

Reference

1. Keenan RL, Boyan CP: JAMA 253:2373, 1985.

Outcome Studies

Clinical Significance of Pulmonary Aspiration During the Perioperative Period

Warner MA, Warner ME, Weber JG (Mayo Med School, Rochester, Minn; Mayo Graduate School of Medicine, Rochester, Minn)
Anesthesiology 78:56–62, 1993   101-94-9–2

Objective.—Aspiration of gastric contents in the perioperative period may lead to pulmonary morbidity or even operative death. Thus, the frequency and course of aspiration were examined in a consecutive series of 172,335 patients aged 18 years and older who received 215,488 general anesthetics at the same center during a 6-year period. The series included 13,427 emergency surgical or diagnostic procedures.

Definition.—Pulmonary aspiration was defined as either the presence of bilious secretions or particulate matter in the tracheobronchial tree, or the finding of a new pulmonary infiltrate on the postoperative chest roentgenogram.

Risk of Aspiration.—Pulmonary aspiration occurred in 67 patients and in 1 of every 3,216 anesthetics. Aspiration complicated 1 in 895 emergency operations and 1 in 3,886 elective procedures. Worsening American Society of Anesthesiologists (ASA) physical status also correlated with a higher risk of aspiration. Factors predisposing to aspiration were identified in 24 of 52 patients having elective procedures and in all 15 patients having emergency procedures. The most frequent factor was gastrointestinal obstruction. More than two thirds of the episodes occurred during tracheal extubation or laryngoscopy.

Outcome.—One patient who aspirated before induction of anesthesia died of exsanguination during emergency repair of a ruptured aortic aneurysm. Of the 66 surviving patients with aspiration, 45 had no respiratory sequelae; 13 others required mechanical ventilatory support for longer than 6 hours. All 6 patients who required ventilation for longer than 24 hours had adult respiratory distress syndrome develop, and 3 of them died of pulmonary insufficiency. The overall mortality was 1 death in 71,829 anesthetics.

Conclusion.—Serious morbidity from pulmonary aspiration did not develop in the immediate perioperative period in ASA physical status I and II patients in this series. Aspiration is more frequent and the outcome more serious when comorbidity is present and procedures are done on an emergent basis. Patients who appear well 2 hours after aspiration or after the end of the procedure are not likely to have respiratory sequelae.

▶ This study is important because it showed that aspiration is a relatively infrequent event, but even with appropriate precautions, it will occur to a greater degree in high-risk patients. There is clearly an increased risk with comorbidity with ASA III and IV patients (1 in 3,000) compared with patients without risk factors or comorbidities (1 in 40,000). In addition, the mortality rate for high-risk patients is 1 in 5,000 as opposed to no mortality in patients without comorbidities.

Furthermore, this study showed that symptoms of cough, wheeze, and/or decreased oxygen saturation of 10% from preoperation to within 2 hours postoperatively predict morbidity, and lack of symptoms within 2 hours predicts patients you can discharge home.—M.F. Roizen, M.D.

The Incidence of Perioperative Myocardial Infarction in Men Undergoing Noncardiac Surgery

Ashton CM, Petersen NJ, Wray NP, Kiefe CI, Dunn JK, Wu L, Thomas JM (Veterans Affairs Med Ctr, Houston)
Ann Intern Med 118:504–510, 1993   101-94-9-3

Introduction.—The incidence of perioperative myocardial infarction in men undergoing noncardiac surgery was determined. In addition, the accuracy of a preoperative risk stratification scheme that classifies patients according to the probability of having coronary artery disease was evaluated.

Setting.—A total of 1,487 men older than age 40 years undergoing major, nonemergent, noncardiac surgery in a large urban Veterans Affairs hospital was evaluated within a prospective cohort design (Fig 9–2). Myocardial infarction was diagnosed in the presence of at least 2 of the following: development of new Q waves; typical change in creatine kinase MB; and positive technetium pyrophosphate scintigraphy. The risk stratification scheme was based on the premise that coronary atherosclerosis was a necessary precondition for perioperative infarction. Patients were stratified preoperatively into high-, intermediate-, low-, and negligible-risk strata based on clinical markers corresponding to different levels of coronary artery disease prevalence.

Results.—The overall incidence of perioperative myocardial infarction was 1.8%. The incidence of infarction decreased from 4.1% among patients with coronary disease (high-risk stratum) to .8% among patients with peripheral vascular disease but no evidence of coronary disease (intermediate-risk stratum), and to 0% among patients with high atherogenic risk factor profiles but no clinical atherosclerosis. No cardiac deaths occurred in men who had no atherosclerosis and with low atherogenic risk profiles (negligible-risk stratum). Multivariate analysis indicated that age older than 75 years, signs of heart failure on the preoperative examination, coronary artery disease, and a planned vascular operation were independently associated with myocardial infarction (table).

Conclusion.—Coronary artery disease is a powerful risk factor for perioperative myocardial infarction in men undergoing noncardiac sur-

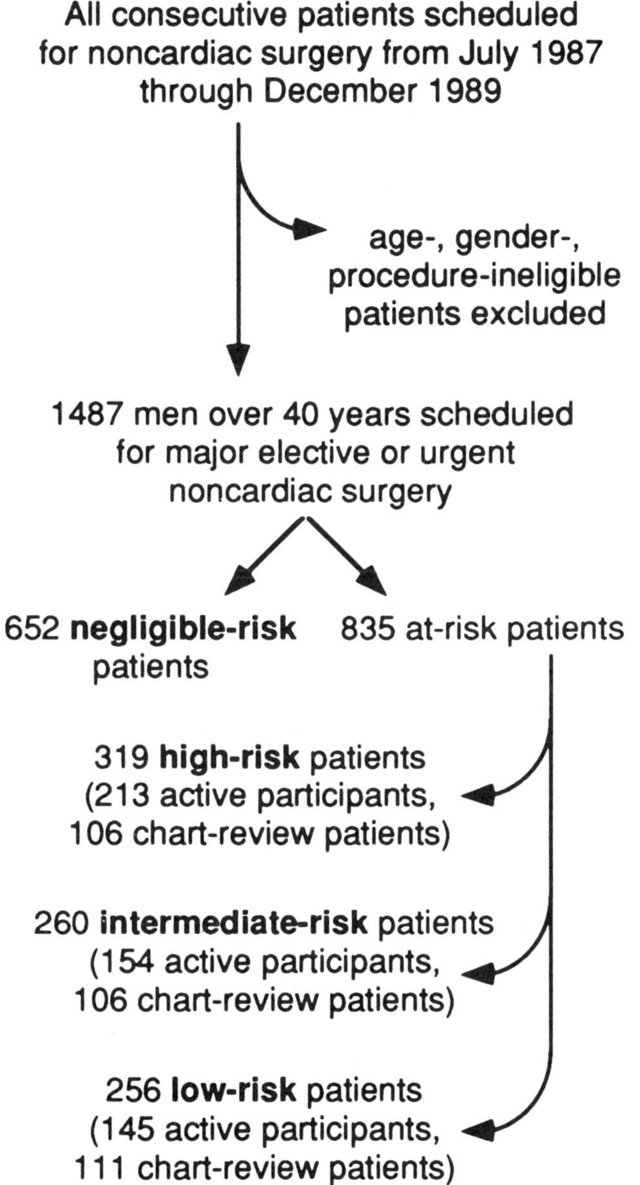

Fig 9–2.—Study population. Chart review patients are patients who declined to undergo a structured preoperative evaluation and postoperative testing for infarction or who were missed by the study team. (Courtesy of Ashton CM, Petersen NJ, Wray NP, et al: *Ann Intern Med* 118:504–510, 1993.)

Clinical Prediction Logistic Model (.15 Level to Remove)

Variable	Coefficient	P Value	Adjusted Odds Ratio (95% CI)
Age ≥ 75 years	1.56	0.03	4.77 (1.17 to 19.41)
Heart failure signs	1.20	0.06	3.31 (0.96 to 11.38)
Coronary artery disease	2.34	0.00	10.39 (2.27 to 47.46)
Vascular operation	1.31	0.03	3.72 (1.12 to 12.37)
Intercept	− 6.64		

Note: Goodness of fit, chi square = 9.46, P = .4.
(Courtesy of Ashton CM, Petersen NJ, Wray NP, et al: *Ann Intern Med* 118:504–510, 1993.)

gery. The risk stratification scheme allows rapid, inexpensive differentiation of levels of risk for perioperative infarction and may be useful in deciding which patients need further evaluation.

▶ The predictive value for postoperative myocardial infarction (MI) is best stratified by clinical signs: age older than 70 years had a risk ratio of 4.8; congestive heart failure signs or symptoms on preoperative examination had a relative risk ratio of 3.3; and prior vascular operation had a risk ratio of 3.72. But the most prominent was the diagnosis of coronary artery disease, which had a risk ratio of 10.4, meaning that 10.4 patients would have a MI if they had the disease compared with 1 who would have it if they did not have the finding. The problem with this report is that you can only guess as to what the authors mean by a history of coronary artery disease. Although the authors mean people with a prior MI, prior ECG evidence of a MI, and typical history of angina, do they also mean those who had prior abnormal coronary angiograms or prior coronary artery surgery? It is unclear from the article, but my guess is yes. Nevertheless, once again, history is the best predictor of poor outcome rather than all the expensive tests that we use too frequently.—M.F. Roizen, M.D.

Chance, Continuity, and Change in Hospital Mortality Rates: Coronary Artery Bypass Graft Patients in California Hospitals, 1983 to 1989

Luft HS, Romano PS (Univ of California, San Francisco; Univ of California, Davis)
JAMA 270:331–337, 1993   101-94-9–4

Background.—It is not clear whether routinely collected data help in identifying quality-of-care problems in hospitals. One theory is that much of what appears to be outlier status can actually be attributed to chance and the failure to adequately adjust for severity.

Study Design.—In an attempt to determine whether risk-adjusted mortality rates mainly reflect chance variation, data were collected on 132,750 adult patients having coronary bypass surgery at 115 California hospitals from 1983 to 1989. Data were taken from routinely collected discharge abstracts. Using the quartile of patients at highest predicted risk, with an average mortality of 10%, high- and low-outlier hospitals were identified from data collected in 2 consecutive years. The outcomes were examined 2 years later.

Findings.—Some hospitals had inpatient mortality rates consistently below those expected. Others had periods of mortality significantly higher than expected, followed by corrective periods. High-outlier hospitals selected on the basis of 2 years of data had mortality rates 2 years later that averaged 31% above those expected. Rates for low-outlier hospitals averaged 28% below what was expected. Survivors at high-outlier hospitals remained hospitalized longer, and these hospitals had proportionately more transfers to other acute care hospitals.

Conclusion.—Routinely collected data can help identify hospitals in which mortality after coronary bypass surgery is consistently higher than expected. At least for high-risk patients, outcomes better than expected are predictive of similar outcomes 2 years later. Data indicating poorer-than-average outcomes have less predictive value.

▶ As near as I can tell, these authors have found that there are "high-outlier" hospitals and "low-outlier" hospitals. When you stratify patients by alleged preoperative risk factors, in the lower-risk categories, the hospitals do not stratify themselves, but in the high-risk categories, they do. Translated, this means that some hospitals do not have good results when high-risk coronary artery bypass grafts (CABGs) are done in them.

The conclusion of this paper is startling. The authors concluded that the best thing would be to not send the high-risk CABG patients to the "high-outlier" hospitals. This seems way too soft for me. Why perform coronary bypasses at all in these hospitals?—J.H. Tinker, M.D.

Major Morbidity and Mortality Within 1 Month of Ambulatory Surgery and Anesthesia

Warner MA, Shields SE, Chute CG (Mayo Med School, Rochester, Minn; Mayo Graduate School of Medicine, Rochester, Minn)
JAMA 270:1437–1441, 1993   101-94-9–5

Introduction.—The demonstrated safety of ambulatory surgical procedures has led to an extension of these services to older and less healthy patients. There is concern that such patients are at greater risk of increased peri- and postoperative morbidity and mortality. The 30-day outcomes of a large population of adult patients who received anesthesia during ambulatory surgery procedures were assessed.

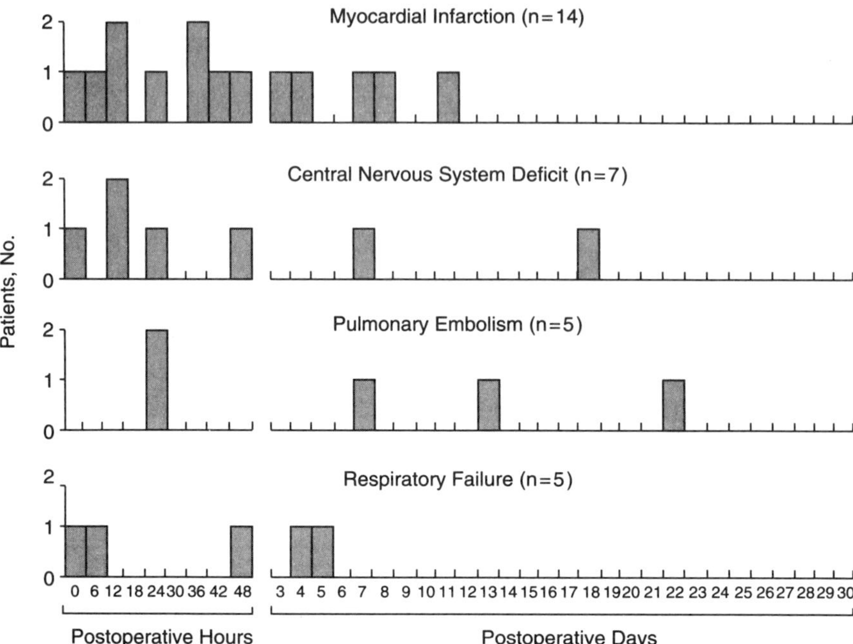

Fig 9–3.—Time sequence within 30 postoperative days of the 31 morbid events associated with 45,090 consecutive ambulatory procedures and anesthetics. The first 2 postoperative days are depicted in hours, and the remaining period is shown in postoperative days. (Courtesy of Warner MA, Shields SE, Chute CG: *JAMA* 270:1437–1441, 1993.)

Patients and Methods.—A total of 38,598 patients aged 18 years and older received 45,090 consecutive anesthetics in conjunction with ambulatory surgical procedures. Postoperative contacts were made by unbiased observers at 72 hours and 30 days. Contact rates for those periods were 99.94% and 95.9%, respectively. The patients were followed for mortality and morbidity, including myocardial infarction, CNS deficit, pulmonary embolism, and respiratory failure. Other data collected included age, gender, type of procedure and anesthetic, and American Society of Anesthesiologists physical status (ASA PS) classification.

Results.—The mean age of the patients was 57.8 years; 68% underwent general anesthesia. All patients were in ASA PS classes I–III. Thirty-three (1 in 1,366) patients experienced major morbidity or died. Two of the 4 deaths were accidental, and 2 were from myocardial infarction (MI). Neither patient who died of MI had a history or symptoms of coronary artery disease. Of 31 events classified as major morbidity, 4 occurred within 8 hours of surgery, 15 occurred in the next 40 hours, and 12 occurred in the next 28 days. Of the patients who experienced major morbidity, 23 were categorized as ASA PS I or II. Perioperative MI accounted for 45% of the morbidity, CNS deficits for 23%, pulmonary embolism for 16%, and respiratory failure for 16% (Fig 9–3).

Conclusion.—Overall, the incidence of mortality and major morbidity was low in this ambulatory surgery population. Both deaths from medical conditions and 39% of all major morbidity occurred more than 48 hours after the procedure but within a 30-day observation period. Ambulatory surgical procedures with concurrent anesthetic care have a good safety record, even in older patients with poorer health.

▶ I believe this report of more than 45,000 ambulatory surgical procedures and anesthetics is useful because it is based on a remarkable rate of follow-up, namely 99.94% at 72 hours and 95.9% at 30 days. I cannot imagine how they achieved that level of follow-up, but they did. No patient died within a week of surgery, and the overall complication rates related to major morbidity were extraordinarily low. I think this study will serve as a benchmark for ambulatory anesthesia and surgery. For me, it does one other thing. I clearly remember how horrified many of us were when we began to be pressured to do surgery with general anesthesia in outpatients. How quickly the dogma of the past fades when faced with economic reality.—J.H. Tinker, M.D.

Exercise Testing, 6-Min Walk, and Stair Climb in the Evaluation of Patients at High Risk for Pulmonary Resection

Holden DA, Rice TW, Stelmach K, Meeker DP (Cleveland Clinic Found, Ohio)
Chest 102:1774–1779, 1992   101-94-9–6

Background.—In patients undergoing lung resection, exercise testing may aid in better predicting successful outcome because a broader assessment of the cardiopulmonary axis can be obtained. The relative value of the 6-minute walk, stair climb, and cycle ergometry cardiopulmonary exercise test—in conjunction with more traditional parameters including the forced expiratory volume in 1 second (FEV_1), forced vital capacity, diffusing capacity for carbon monoxide, and their predicted postoperative values—was assessed.

Methods.—Sixteen patients were evaluated before lung resection. Patients underwent resting spirometry and then exercised on a cycle ergometer and walked 6 minutes on a cardiopulmonary stress-testing unit. On a separate day, patients performed timed, symptom-limited stair climb at their own pace. Cardiovascular and pulmonary measurements were taken before and during the exercises. Quantitative perfusion pulmonary scintigraphy was also performed.

Results.—Patients were divided into 2 groups. In group 1, 6 patients had no complications, and 5 had minor complications. All 5 of the group 2 patients died. Before death, the group 2 patients spent significantly more time in the intensive care unit. No patients in group 1 had died during the 18-month follow-up. The group 1 patients had longer 6-minute walking distance and a higher stair climb rate than the patients in group 2. There was no significant difference between the 2 groups in the maximum oxygen uptake on the cycle ergometer.

Conclusion.—There is considerable promise for preoperative exercise testing as a means of predicting the surgical outcomes of morbidity and mortality for patients with lung cancer. However, to demonstrate validity of the 6-minute walk distance of 1,000 ft and a stair climb in excess of 44 steps, additional prospective evaluation is necessary.

▶ This is an example of how we sometimes go about our "science" backward. These authors had 16 patients who underwent pulmonary resection. Eleven did reasonably well and 5 died within 90 days of surgery. This retrospective division of these patients into 2 groups, i.e., death or no death, was then traced backward to see what preoperative tests might have had predictive ability. It turned out that the 6-minute walk test and a standardized stair climb test were both predictive. What is wrong with this study is that these tests were *retrospectively* predictive. The authors then did not turn around and use their newly (retrospectively) obtained so-called predictive data to see whether these tests actually predicted anything prospectively. With all due respect to the authors, they are not even remotely justified, by this study, in stating that "preoperative exercise testing is a useful adjunct to traditional spirometric testing in evaluation of the high-risk surgical patient" until and unless they can show that their retrospectively derived tests actually predict anything in the way of successful or unsuccessful surgical outcome when these tests are administered prospectively to another group of similar patients.—J.H. Tinker, M.D.

Pneumococcal Polysaccharide Vaccine Efficacy: An Evaluation of Current Recommendations
Butler JC, Breiman RF, Campbell JF, Lipman HB, Broome CV, Facklam RR (Ctrs for Disease Control and Prevention, Atlanta, Ga)
JAMA 270:1826–1831, 1993   101-94-9–7

Objective.—There is still controversy regarding the efficacy and duration of protection afforded by the pneumococcal polysaccharide vaccine. An indirect cohort analysis was conducted to determine the efficacy of the pneumococcal polysaccharide vaccine in selected populations at risk for serious pneumococcal infection and to examine the duration of protection after vaccination.

Methods.—Data were obtained from hospital laboratories in the United States that submitted pneumococcal isolates to the Centers for Disease Control and Prevention from May of 1978 to April of 1992. The proportion of pneumococcal infections caused by serotypes included in the 14-valent and 23-valent vaccines was compared in vaccinated and unvaccinated individuals.

Results.—During the 14-year surveillance, 2,837 patients older than age 5 years had pneumococcus isolated from blood or CSF. The overall efficacy for preventing infection caused by vaccine-type serotypes was 84% in patients with diabetes mellitus, 73% in patients with coronary vascular disease, 69% for patients with congestive heart failure, 65% for patients with chronic pulmonary diseases, and 77% for patients with anatomical asplenia. Efficacy was not documented for patients with alcoholism or cirrhosis, sickle cell disease, chronic renal failure, lymphoma leukemia, or multiple myeloma, but the sample sizes were small for these groups. Efficacy was 75% for immunocompetent patients older than age 65 years. Vaccine efficacy did not decline with increasing time since vaccination. In fact, point estimates of efficacy increased with time: 71% at 5–8 years after vaccination and 80% at 9 years or more after vaccination.

Conclusion.—The efficacy of the pneumococcal polysaccharide vaccine among patients considered at high risk for invasive pneumococcal infection was confirmed. Efforts to improve pneumococcal vaccine coverage in these populations for whom vaccination is currently recommended should be intensified. Because the efficacy of the vaccine remains relatively constant with an increasing interval since vaccination, universal revaccination is not indicated.

▶ To me, one of the amazing things is that when we survey patients in our preoperative clinic, more than 80% of those who should receive pneumococcal vaccine have not received it. Should we, as anesthesiologists, be doing this in the preoperative clinic? Will this decrease or increase the morbidity associated with surgery? We are currently studying that, but this article brings up the point that it is a very efficacious vaccine for high-risk groups, and it only needs to be given once in a long period of time to maintain its efficacy.—M.F. Roizen, M.D.

Cost-Efficacy Studies

Low-Flow Isoflurane-Nitrous Oxide Anaesthesia Offers Substantial Economic Advantages Over High- and Medium-Flow Isoflurane-Nitrous Oxide Anaesthesia

Pedersen FM, Nielsen J, Ibsen M, Guldager H (Univ of Copenhagen, Herlev, Denmark)
Acta Anaesthesiol Scand 37:509–512, 1993   101-94-9–8

Background.—Although isoflurane is better than halothane and enflurane in many ways, its costliness has limited its use in many anesthesiology departments. The use of low fresh gas flows (FGFs) may substantially reduce the cost of isoflurane.

Methods.—Isoflurane consumption in 3 different FGFs using a partial rebreathing system without carbon dioxide absorption or a circle system with carbon dioxide absorption was studied. Thirty patients undergoing major elective abdominal, urologic, or gynecologic surgery were randomly assigned to the different FGF conditions. Anesthesia consisted of isoflurane in 40% oxygen and 60% nitrous oxide.

Findings.—The total consumption of liquid isoflurane in the first 2 hours was a mean 40.8 mL in patients given high-flow anesthesia using the partial rebreathing system without carbon dioxide absorption, 18.5 mL in patients given medium-flow anesthesia using a circle system with carbon dioxide absorption, and 7.9 mL in patients given low-flow anesthesia in a circle system with carbon dioxide absorption. The low-flow method resulted in substantial cost savings over high- and medium-flow isoflurane–nitrous oxide anesthesia.

Conclusion.—Low FGF in the circle system reduces isoflurane consumption by 81% compared with high FGF in the partial rebreathing system. Compared with medium FGF in the circle system, low FGF reduced isoflurane consumption by 57%. Low-flow anesthesia has several advantages over other anesthetic techniques, including cost-effectiveness.

▶ These authors found that their version of low-flow anesthesia costs about $6 for 2 hours of anesthesia, and medium-flow isoflurane anesthesia costs about $14 for 2 hours of anesthesia. Is this difference really worth the added risk of low-flow anesthesia? What are the risks of low-flow anesthesia? I think we need to ask why low-flow anesthesia has never really "caught on" in most areas of practice. Is it more dangerous? Is it *perceived* to be more dangerous? Do we as anesthetists simply feel less comfortable in its administration? I am certain that the last statement is true even if I am less certain about the others.—J.H. Tinker, M.D.

Anaesthesia: Cheap at Twice the Price?: Staff Awareness, Cost Comparisons and Recommendations for Economic Savings
Bailey CR, Ruggier R, Cashman JN (St Georges Hosp, London)
Anaesthesia 48:906–909, 1993   101-94-9–9

Background.—Studies have shown that anesthetic staffs have a limited awareness of costs. A survey was conducted to test the present knowledge of anesthetic cost among 50 anesthetists of various grades.

Methods and Findings.—The questionnaire administered elicited estimates of the cost of 28 drugs, fluids, and disposable items. Forty-seven percent of all estimated costs were within 50% of the actual costs. Seventy-five percent were within 100%. The cost of fairly expensive items, such as blood, laryngeal mask airways, enflurane, and isoflurane, were consistently underestimated. The cost of cheaper products, such as disposable syringes and electrocardiograph electrodes, were consistently overestimated. Allowing for inflation, the cost associated with an hour-long anesthetic in 1992 was equivalent to the cost in 1959. There has been no consistent pattern in drug prices since 1980; some prices have remained the same, whereas others have decreased and others have increased.

Conclusion.—Staff knowledge of anesthetic product prices is better than that previously reported. Furthermore, drug costs have declined in the past 30 years. Cost savings may be possible by using propofol and the newer muscle relaxants judiciously and by using low-flow closed-circuit systems.

▶ It is amazing to me that the costs of anesthesia have actually decreased, despite the improvements in drugs and the use of newer drugs that are clearly high-priced. We as anesthesiologists appear to have some awareness of what is high-priced and what is not and to have found ways such as low-flow systems to decrease the cost of anesthesia per se. I think we have even gone further than that because of our reduction in recovery room stays, preoperative testing, etc., and have decreased anesthesia costs more than these authors realize. Maybe our specialty should have a new motto: Improve quality and reduce costs, and do so before government bureaucrats tell us to.—M.F. Roizen, M.D.

Value and Cost of Teaching Hospitals: A Prospective, Multicenter, Inception Cohort Study

Zimmerman JE, Shortell SM, Knaus WA, Rousseau DM, Wagner DP, Gillies RR, Draper EA, Devers K (George Washington Univ, Washington, DC; Northwestern Univ, Evanston, Ill; APACHE Med Systems, Inc, Washington, DC)
Crit Care Med 21:1432–1442, 1993   101-94-9–10

Background.—The reduction in reimbursement and specific considerations that had been formerly provided for teaching services and the demands for graduate medical education present substantial burdens to many teaching hospitals. Precise measures of patients' health status were evaluated to objectively estimate the incremental value and cost of teaching hospitals through the delivery of intensive care.

Methods.—Patient characteristics, resource use, and structural and organizational features were compared in 20 teaching intensive care units (ICUs) at 18 hospitals and 17 nonteaching ICUs at 17 hospitals using a prospective inception cohort design. Outcomes were compared using ratios of observed to risk-adjusted predicted hospital death rates, length of ICU stay, and resource use. Information for an average of 415 patients at each ICU was used.

Results.—The case-mix in teaching ICUs was more complex than in nonteaching ICUs. Patients in teaching ICUs were significantly younger and more severely ill with a higher overall admission risk of death. The risk-adjusted length of ICU stay was similar, but resource use was greater in teaching ICUs because of increased use of diagnostic testing and invasive procedures. The estimated cost of an ICU admission was $20,070 at a nonteaching ICU and \$28,650 at a teaching unit. More than half (65%) of this cost was secondary to variations in patient characteristics, and about \$3,000 or 10.5% of the total cost represented the cost of teaching. Teaching ICUs were also more complex organizationally and had twice the number of physicians regularly involved in patient care. Despite these differences, risk-adjusted hospital death rates did not differ significantly between teaching and nonteaching ICUs. However, when compared with the average performance for all ICUs, 4 teaching ICUs had significantly better survival rates, compared with only 1 nonteaching ICU. Furthermore, an identical analysis involving 14 hospitals that were members of the Council of Teaching Hospitals demonstrated a significantly better risk-adjusted outcome in their 16 ICUs than all others.

Conclusion.—Teaching ICUs have a more complex case mix in a substantially more complex organizational structure. The best risk-adjusted survival rates occur at teaching ICUs, but production cost is higher with increased testing and therapy. Furthermore, teaching ICUs are training individuals who can provide these services with equivalent results at lower cost in nonteaching ICUs.

▶ This article, supported by the Health Care Financing Administration, delineated outcome relative to economic cost in critically ill patients. The importance of this study is not that teaching hospitals administer better care than nonteaching hospitals, but rather that with proper training, future intensivists will hopefully be able to deliver high-quality, cost-efficient intensive care.—D.M. Rothenberg, M.D.

Computerization Studies

Requiring Physicians to Respond to Computerized Reminders Improves Their Compliance With Preventive Care Protocols

Litzelman DK, Dittus RS, Miller ME, Tierney WM (Regenstrief Inst for Health Care, Indianapolis, Ind; Indiana Univ, Indianapolis; Richard L Roudebush VA Med Ctr, Indianapolis Ind)
J Gen Intern Med 8:311–317, 1993   101-94-9-11

Introduction.—Not all physicians comply with guidelines regarding preventive care, despite their agreement with such protocols. In some cases, a patient's presenting symptoms may distract from preventive care activities. A prospective trial tested the hypothesis that computer-generated reminders would improve physician compliance in performing fecal occult blood testing (FOBT), mammography, and cervical Papanicolaou testing.

Methods.—The study was conducted in an academic primary care general internal medicine practice during 1989. The General Medicine Practice (GMP) of the center is staffed by residents, fellows, and faculty members. While practicing in the GMP, all physicians deliver primary care for an assigned panel of patients. Each of the 4 separate practices of the GMP meets for 8 half-day sessions each week, yielding 32 sessions. Of the 32 practice sessions, 16 were randomly assigned to intervention status and 16 to control status. Intervention physicians received computer reminders that required 1 of 4 responses to be circled: "done/order today," "not applicable to this patient," "patient refused," or "next visit." Reminders given the control group did not require a response.

Results.—During the 6-month study, 5,407 patients with scheduled visits were eligible for any of the 3 cancer screening protocols. Intervention physicians complied more frequently (46%) than did control physicians (38%) with all reminders combined. The intervention group also complied significantly more frequently than the control group for FOBT (61% vs. 49%) and mammography (54% vs. 47%). For all reminders together and separately for FOBT, compliance rates for control faculty were significantly higher than the rates for control residents. The greatest effect of intervention was observed for patients age 70 years or older seen by residents. This finding was encouraging, for many older patients had never had any of the targeted screening tests. In 21% of cases, intervention physicians thought that the reminders were not applicable.

Conclusion.—Computer-generated reminders that require physicians to respond and justify noncompliance should improve adherence to preventive care protocols. But because of incomplete data and patient refusal, total compliance with cancer screening reminders may never be achieved.

▶ At first this article may look like it does not pertain to us, but it does, in 2 ways. First, it shows that to change physician behavior often requires responses to protocols; that is, computer responses to a computer reminder before you can go on. Although one wishes that we could just educate ourselves about what we should do right, the myriad of things we have to do right and the specificness of them based on patient risk groupings mean that it is very tough for the human mind to comply with protocols without help from technology. This system may in fact be adaptable to anesthesia providers to give us help with protocol compliance such as appropriate management of the diabetic in the operating room.

The second aspect of this study that deserves comment is that perhaps we should be doing more preventive care in the preoperative clinic. It may prove to be a way of providing preventive care to 27 million patients in North America each year at a time when health-care concerns are high. It is also a way that we can reduce testing, improve preventive care, and justify the existence of preoperative clinics to the managed care providers.—M.F. Roizen, M.D.

Physician Inpatient Order Writing on Microcomputer Workstations: Effects on Resource Utilization

Tierney WM, Miller ME, Overhage JM, McDonald CJ (Indiana Univ, Indianapolis; Richard L Roudebush Veterans Affairs Med Ctr, Indianapolis, Ind)
JAMA 269:379–383, 1993   101-94-9-12

Introduction.—The adoption of a system of electronic medical records (EMRs) is proposed as a means of lowering health-care costs. As yet, however, no controlled trials have shown that any kind of EMR results in cost savings. Patient charges and hospital costs using a network of microcomputer workstations for writing inpatient orders were compared with those of the traditional system of paper charts.

Methods.—The study setting was the medical service of an urban public hospital with an average daily inpatient census of 100. More than 75% of patients are admitted from the emergency department. During the study period, April of 1990 through October of 1991, there were 5,219 eligible admissions and 68 teams of faculty internists, house officers, and medical students who cared for them. Using the network of workstations, physicians can select orders from menus or type them freehand. All menus are designed to encourage cost-effective ordering. In a formal time-motion study, trained observers noted all activities for 24 randomly selected interns, 12 from the intervention group and 12 from the control group. Total charges per hospital admission was the main outcome variable.

Results.—The time-motion study determined that interns in the intervention group spent an average of 33 more minutes writing orders between 10 A.M. and 8 P.M. than did interns in the control group. On average, admitting drug orders were filled 63 minutes sooner for patients of intervention interns and daily drug orders were filled 34 minutes sooner than for the patients of control interns. The intervention teams generated charges that were $887 (12.7%) lower per admission than the charges of control teams. Intervention also resulted in significantly lower hospital costs, bed charges, drug charges, and diagnostic test charges (table).

Conclusion.—Patient charges and hospital costs were significantly reduced when a network of microcomputer workstations was used for writing all inpatient orders. In this hospital's medical service, annual savings would exceed $3 million. The system did require more physician time than did the system using the paper charts.

▶ This article again shows the future of medicine: using computerized systems can reduce the cost of care and improve its quality. I believe that microcomputer stations will help us reduce the cost of care and improve its quality by helping us follow efficient protocols.—M.F. Roizen, M.D.

Differences Between Intervention and Control Resident Teams' Hospital Charges and Length of Stay Per Admission

Outcome Variable	Control Resident Teams (n=46)	Intervention Resident Teams (n=22)	Absolute Difference	% Reduction	P
Charges, $					
Total					
Mean (SE)	6964 (242)	6077 (210)	887	12.7	.02
Median	3984	3669	...	...	...
Bed					
Mean (SE)	2551 (81)	2283 (69)	268	11.9	.04
Median	1550	1450	...	...	...
Test					
Mean (SE)	1852 (53)	1621 (58)	231	12.5	.006
Median	1143	992	...	...	...
Drug					
Mean (SE)	1181 (47)	1001 (42)	180	15.3	.008
Median	546	505	...	...	...
Other					
Mean (SE)	1381 (83)	1171 (63)	210	15.2	.81
Median	533	541	...	...	...
No. of days in hospital					
Mean (SE)	8.49 (0.24)	7.60 (0.20)	0.89	10.5	.11
Median	6	5	...	...	...

(Courtesy of Tierney WM, Miller ME, Overhage JM, et al: JAMA 269:379–383, 1993.)

Accuracy of a Computer-Based Anaesthetic Audit System

Lillywhite N, Ward P (Parkside, London)
Anaesthesia 48:885–886, 1993

101-94-9–13

Background.—Many anesthetic departments have computer-based auditing systems that can be used to make clinical, financial, or management decisions. The accuracy of the computer-based anesthetic audit system in one department was studied.

Methods and Findings.—Retrospective and prospective surveys were performed. In an attempt to access data on operations performed 4 months previously, only 50% of the patients' notes could be found. Forty percent of these notes did not contain an anesthetic chart. In the prospective survey, the accuracy with which the computer output reflected the anesthetic technique was only 33%. In the retrospective survey, its accuracy was 52%.

Conclusion.—The computer-based audit system at this institution had an overall accuracy of 33% to 52%. Although these findings cannot be generalized to other institutions, audit systems should be audited before their data are used for decision making.

▶ Bravo! An article that finally says it all. *Garbage in equals garbage out, even in medical informatics.* Clearly, better systems for keeping track of records are needed, and the paper-based record is long overdue for replacement by an electronic record where the information can be accurately collected, tabulated, and audited.—M.F. Roizen, M.D.

Data Torturing

Mills JL (Natl Inst of Child Health and Human Development, Bethesda, Md)
N Engl J Med 329:1196–1199, 1993

101-94-9–14

Introduction.—Manipulation of data can often be done in such a way that whatever the investigator wants to prove can be proved. Data "torturing" occurs when the presentation of facts goes beyond what is a reasonable interpretation. Some of the telltale signs of data torturing were described in the hope that this process can be recognized and eradicated.

Opportunistic Data Torturing.—In this type of data torturing, the perpetrator pores over the data to find a "significant" association, then devises a hypothesis to fit the association. By making multiple comparisons, the data torturer can find significant results when none exist. For 2 tests, for example, the probability that the "significant" differences found by the investigator will reflect true differences is 90%; for 20 tests, it is only 36%. When this type of data torturing is practiced, it may be difficult for readers to tell that the positive association was derived from an a priori hypothesis.

Procrustean Data Torturing.—Procrustes, a robber in Greek mythology, stretched or cut off the legs of his victims so that they would fit his bed. In Procrustean data torturing, the investigator makes the data fit the hypothesis. Study subjects may be dropped because their experiences do not fit the hypothesis; the exposure may be redefined to strengthen the association; disease outcomes may be lumped together, split, or dropped altogether; and normal ranges for laboratory values might be altered. Procrustean data torturing is more difficult to accomplish than opportunistic data torturing and may be more destructive, for the results "produced" may appear to be definitive proof of the hypothesis.

Means of Identifying Data Torturing.—To identify these types of data manipulation, the reader must question the study methods. The P values and confidence intervals need to be examined for evidence that they are being misused. Many of the techniques of data manipulation have been known for years, but little has been done to alert the medical community. Editors, reviewers, and readers need to know the rationale for excluding various subjects from analysis, the number of statistical tests performed, whether both P values and confidence intervals are reported, and whether data are included for all subgroups and at all follow-up points.

▶ Two things in this article deserve much emphasis. One is that there are ways of finding out whether an article has tortured data, and for some of the articles, it is quite easy. First, if dose-related effects and confidence intervals are reported, it is unlikely that data torturing has occurred. Second, to find out whether data torturing is likely, see whether, for example, multiple comparisons have been made. For instance, if 2 comparisons have been done, there is only a 10% chance that significant findings occurred by chance, whereas if 20 comparisons have been done, there is a 64% chance that a significant difference at the P values less than .05 was found by chance 1 − $(.95)^{20}$. It is also interesting that the Food and Drug Administration is very cognizant of this and insists that the manufacturer state what 3 variables it will test for efficacy before starting an efficacy study and what 3 secondary variables, thus allowing at most 6 statistical tests. Similarly, the manufacturer must also implement the side effect likelihoods for routine (that is, nonallergic, nonidiosyncratic) toxicities. I urge you to read this article if you read medical literature at all for changing your practices.

I think we should be really cognizant of data torturing now when publicity is more commonly used to gain prominence and publicity for both federally and nonfederally funded grants that require *New York Times*-type reporting to obtain. In fact, I think data torturing is more common now than in the past because of the influence of the press in trying to get medically sensational research reported.—M.F. Roizen, M.D.

10 Operating Room Environment: Safety, Infection Prevention

Laser Fires

A Comparison of CO$_2$ Laser Ignition of the Xomed, Plastic, and Rubber Endotracheal Tubes

Sosis MB, Dillon FX (Rush-Presbyterian-St Luke's Med Ctr, Chicago; Midwest Med Ctr, Indianapolis, Ind)

Anesth Analg 76:391–393, 1993   101-94-10–1

Introduction.—Lasers are increasingly used in medicine and surgery. When a high-energy density surgical laser is used close to a combustible endotracheal tube during airway surgery, it can be converted into a "blow torch" and cause extensive burn injury. The xomed LaserShield endotracheal tube was touted as being "resistant" to the carbon dioxide (CO$_2$) laser.

Methods.—The combustibility of xomed LaserShield endotracheal tubes was compared with that of polyvinyl chloride (PVC) and rubber tubes when a CO$_2$ laser was operated at power levels of 15, 17, and 20 W. Oxygen passed through the tubes at a flow rate of 5 L per minute. The laser was aimed perpendicularly at the endotracheal tube shaft and actuated until an intraluminal fire began.

Results.—The PVC tubes caught fire after 1.5–1.8 seconds of laser exposure, and the rubber tubes caught fire after 22–25 seconds. In contrast, the xomed tubes did not ignite until 86 seconds after the start of exposure to 15 W of laser power. The interval was 42.5 seconds at the intermediate-power level, and 20 seconds at the highest level of 20 W.

Conclusion.—None of these endotracheal tubes provides adequate protection from combustion by actuation of a CO$_2$ laser. It is suggested that the tube be wrapped with metallic foil tape; that the Laser-Guard protective coating be used; or that the Mallinckrodt Laser-Flex endotracheal tube be used instead.

▶ I guess the phrase "buyer beware" is appropriate here. The xomed and other tubes are much more expensive and are only laser "resistant." The appropriate way, it appears, to have more resistance to fires when CO$_2$ laser is being used is wrapping a standard endotracheal tube with the appropriate metallic foil tape, using the Laser-Guard protective coating, or using the Mallinckrodt Laser-Flex endotracheal tube. Is wrapping a standard tube with tape the most inexpensive and efficient form of providing such protection if you do it in otherwise-down time?—M.F. Roizen, M.D.

Infection Prevention (Including HIV)

HIV Risk Factors and Seroprevalence in Surgical Patients

Reid CBA, Kaldor JM, Lord RSA, Cooper DA (Univ of New South Wales, Darlinghurst, Australia)
Med J Aust 158:21–23, 1993   101-94-10-2

Objective.—The prevalence of risk factors for HIV infection and of antibody to HIV-1 were determined in a prospective series of 1,292 adult surgical patients in Australia. Antibody testing was completed for 1,171 patients who had not received a previous diagnosis of HIV-1 infection.

Findings.—Twenty-seven patients (2.1%) had HIV-1 infection previously diagnosed. Among the remaining patients, 17% of men and 12% of women had received a blood transfusion in the past 5 years, had injected a nonprescription drug, or reported homosexual contact. The proportions of previously unexposed patients who reported various risk factors are given in Tables 1 and 2. Only one third of transfused patients had had an HIV-1 antibody test previously. More than a third of the men reporting homosexual contact had not been tested for HIV-1 antibody, and the same was true for 30% of the drug users. Three patients, all men, were newly found to have HIV-1 infection, for a prevalence of .26%.

TABLE 1.—Surgical Patients Not Previously Known to Have HIV-1 Infection, by Age Group—Men

| | | | | Risk factors for HIV infection | | |
Age group (years)	Patients approached	Responded to questionnaire	Previous HIV-1 test	Male homosexual contact	Injecting drug use	Blood transfusion 1980–1985
<20	15	15	2	1	0	1
20–29	79	78	20	4	9	3
30–39	98	96	29	6	11	7
40–49	100	99	24	6	3	8
50–59	136	134	20	3	0	15
>60	359	359	37	4	0	52
Total	787	781	132 (17%)	24 (3.1%)	23 (3%)	86 (11%)

(Courtesy of Reid CBA, Kaldor JM, Lord RSA, et al: *Med J Aust* 158:21–23, 1993.)

TABLE 2.—Surgical Patients Not Previously Known to Have HIV-1 Infection, by Age Group—Women

| | | | | Risk factors for HIV infection | |
| | | | | | Blood |
Age group	Patients approached	Responded to questionnaire	Previous HIV-1 test	Injecting drug use	transfusion 1980–1985
<20	8	8	2	2	0
20–29	36	36	15	1	2
30–39	39	39	15	4	6
40–49	62	61	13	0	9
50–59	73	72	9	0	5
>60	260	260	18	0	30
Total	478	476	72 (15%)	7 (1.5%)	52 (11%)

(Courtesy of Reid CBA, Kaldor JM, Lord RSA, et al: *Med J Aust* 158:21–23, 1993.)

Conclusion.—It is fairly common for surgical patients to describe factors associated with an elevated risk of HIV infection, but the prevalence of undiagnosed infection in this series was very low.

▶ In this inner-city hospital, approximately 17% of men and 12% of women reported a risk factor for HIV infection. Nevertheless, very few had an HIV infection by double blood test; that is, enzyme-linked immunosorbent assay and western blot testing on 2 blood samples. I think it is important to note that we do not know the adverse effect that testing would have were a different strategy for testing patients not at risk used, but one individual with an HIV diagnosis in this series had no known risk factors and answered negative to all the risk factor questions. Thus, we do not know the adverse effect of false-positive tests on a patient, but we have patients who are at risk who do not divulge so in this questionnaire. Would better results be obtained if a more confidential, i.e., computer-linked, questionnaire were used? (Computer-linked questionnaires have been found to be able to obtain more accurate information in socially difficult areas.) We do not know the answer to that question, but this study certainly stimulates a lot of important questions.—M.F. Roizen, M.D.

Surgical Glove Punctures During Cardiac Operations

Wong PS, Young VK, Youhana A, Wright JE (London Chest Hosp)
Ann Thorac Surg 56:108–110, 1993
101-94-10–3

Background.—Occult glove punctures can result in the transmission of infectious diseases and potential contamination of implanted cardiac prostheses. A new technique for detecting occult glove punctures has been developed to determine its frequency during cardiac surgery.

Methods.—Forty-eight adults undergoing open heart surgery were enrolled in a study of surgical glove punctures. Gloves worn by surgeons and nurses were collected and tested after each procedure. In 22 cases, the principal operating room personnel changed their gloves at 3 different stages: skin incision to commencement of cardiopulmonary bypass, cardiopulmonary bypass to sternotomy closure, and sternotomy closure to skin closure.

Findings.—Thirty-two percent of the gloves had 1 or more punctures. Only 20 of the 162 punctures were noticed at the time of or at the end of the operation. One hundred eighty-five occult glove punctures were identified. Sixty percent of the punctures were on the nondominant hand. Thirty percent of the perforations were located in the nondominant index finger. No significant differences were found among glove perforation rates for the principal operators at stages I, II, and III. Sixty-one percent of gloves worn by scrub nurses had 1 or more punctures, compared with 23.6% of those worn by surgeons.

Conclusion.—Glove damage during cardiac surgery is frequent but not easily detected. The rate of occult glove punctures is surprisingly high, especially among those worn by scrub nurses.

▶ This study determined glove holes by inflation of the gloves with air and submersion under water to find air bubble leakage through the glove. Interestingly, the scrub nurses had more punctures than the surgeons, and even had punctures in the same nondominant index finger as the surgeons. I guess double gloving should be routine for everyone, surgeons and nurses, and maybe even anesthesia personnel.—M.F. Roizen, M.D.

Bacterial Filters Protect Anaesthetic Equipment in a Low-Flow System

Luttropp HH, Berntman L (Univ Hosp, Lund, Sweden)
Anaesthesia 48:520–523, 1993   101-94-10–4

Background.—Recently, a system for mechanical ventilation during low-flow anesthesia was studied. In this system, the circle is separated from the ventilator by a large-bore corrugated hose, which produces a route for possible bacterial contamination of the hose and ventilator. Bag-in-bottle low-flow system contamination has not been thoroughly studied. The temperature, humidity, and degree of rebreathing are higher in such systems than in conventional systems; thus, the risk of bacterial growth and spread may be significant.

Methods.—The low-flow system had 3 parts: an anesthesia circle with a disposable absorber and an excess valve, a ventilator, and a large hose connecting the circle and ventilator. Bacterial contamination was assessed with and without bacterial filters between the patient and Y-piece and between the circle system and corrugated hose. These 2 filters were designated A and B, respectively.

Findings.—Despite the use of filters, 17 of 27 expiratory and 14 of 27 inspiratory tubings had positive cultures. Positive cultures occurred at the patient side of filter A. None of the cultures from the circle side of any filter was positive. Most commonly found organisms were *Staphylococcus epidermidis, Propionibacterium acnes,* and *Micrococcus* and *Bacillus* species. Cultures from both sides of the B filter were positive on 1 occasion after 7 days of use. The positive culture, showing *S. epidermidis,* was from the circle side of the filter. No bacteria were found after 1 month.

Conclusion.—Although filters between the tracheal tube and circle are effective barriers, their absence was not associated with increased contamination of the circle or ventilator. Some filters are effective as heat and moisture exchangers when located at the tracheal tube. Bacterial contamination was not found in this study, suggesting that a prolonged interval between disinfection of the open connection and ventilator is acceptable. This will reduce cost and wear.

▶ I suppose that using a volatile anesthetic would be even more protective than the filter. It might even be better for the patient. Most of us use disposable corrugated tubing as well as anesthetic gases that do prevent bacterial contamination. In the article by Feeley et al. (1) that they quoted, this problem was shown to be a nonproblem with such an anesthetic, and disposable equipment was not needed to prevent the bacterial contamination when volatile anesthetics were used as the main form of anesthesia.—M.F. Roizen, M.D.

Reference

1. Feeley TW, et al: *Anesthesiology* 54:369, 1981.

Inhibition of Interferon Stimulation of Natural Killer Cell Activity in Mice Anesthetized With Halothane or Isoflurane

Markovic SN, Knight PR, Murasko DM (Med College of Pennsylvania, Philadelphia; Univ of Michigan, Ann Arbor)
Anesthesiology 78:700–706, 1993   101-94-10-5

Background.—A variety of transient immunologic defects have been described in patients recovering from surgery or trauma. They include altered basal cytotoxic activity of natural killer (NK) cells, the lymphocytes involved in nonspecific immune responses to micro-organisms, and tumors.

Objective and Methods.—The effects of halothane and isoflurane on interferon-induced enhancement of NK cell cytotoxicity were examined in mice. The animals were exposed to either anesthetic the day before interferon treatment or 1, 5, or 10 days afterward, and NK cytotoxicity was evaluated 24 hours later. In addition, splenic mononuclear cells including NK cells were treated with interferon before and after in vitro exposure to halothane or isoflurane.

Results.—Exposure to isoflurane inhibited subsequent interferon-induced NK cell stimulation by more than 90% and exposure to halothane by 67%. Significant inhibition was seen 11 days after anesthesia. No inhibition was evident when interferon was given before anesthetic exposure. Both anesthetics inhibited subsequent stimulation of NK cytotoxicity by interferon in vitro, but no change was seen when cells were pretreated with interferon.

Interpretation.—Halothane and isoflurane might prevent NK cells from responding to interferon, or they might act indirectly by altering other mononuclear cells (e.g., T cells or macrophages), which then inhibit the induction of NK cells.

▶ Interest in the possibility that anesthetics might inhibit patient resistivity to infection goes back several decades. In this study, there was interference with a particular kind of immune response, namely interferon-induced stimulation of NK cell cytotoxicity. Furthermore, it lasted at least 24 hours. What does all this mean? In my opinion, if anesthetics had been doing anything very dramatic to decrease resistance to infection, we probably would have been aware of the problem before now. Nonetheless, in 1993, we are dealing with a pandemic the likes of which we have not seen in most of our professional lifetimes, namely the HIV virus. Therefore, it is reasonable to reopen these issues.—J.H. Tinker, M.D.

Anaesthetic Uptake and Washout Characteristics of Patient Circuit Tubing With Special Regard to Current Decontamination Techniques
Gilly H, Weindlmayr-Goettel M, Köberl G, Steinbereithner K (Univ of Vienna)
Acta Anaesthesiol Scand 36:621–627, 1992   101-94-10–6

Background.—Contamination of components of the anesthetic circuit is mainly determined by the solubility of anesthetics in the tubing, the concentration of the gas mixtures used, and the duration of exposure. Residual contamination carries a potential risk of triggering malignant hyperthermia in susceptible patients, but the actual amounts of volatile anesthetics retained in tubing after everyday use of routine anesthesia are unknown.

Methods.—Gas chromatography was used to quantify the amounts of halothane and isoflurane trapped in commonly used anesthesia circuit tubing after exposure at 2 minimum alveolar concentrations for as long as 3 hours. The efficacy of various decontaminating measures was examined, including flushing with oxygen, thermal disinfection, and routine storage.

Results.—Residual levels of halothane were higher in silicone than in electrically conductive latex, conductive rubber, polyethylene-vinyl-acetate, nonconductive corrugated and spiral tubes, and polysulfone. Levels of isoflurane were substantially lower but also were highest in silicone tubing. Decontamination procedures were variably effective. Levels were highest in conductive latex and rubber tubings after thermal disinfection and subsequent storage. Flushing with oxygen for 20 minutes lowered effluent gas concentrations to below 5 ppm in all tubings except silicone, where levels exceeded 8 ppm after 1 hour of flushing.

Conclusion.—If disposable tubing is not immediately available, "contaminated" tubings of conductive rubber, latex, or polysulfone may be used after a 20-minute flush with oxygen at 8 L/min. Silicone and disposable polyethylene-vinyl-acetate tubings should not be reused. Concentrations of 3 ppm may be taken as a safe lower limit.

▶ This paper clearly documented that a patient with a known or strongly suspected history of malignant hypothermia must be anesthetized either with a special anesthesia machine or with an anesthesia machine that has been stripped of all possible nooks and crannies into which halothane, isoflurane, or enflurane might have accumulated. This paper also debunks the notion that the more modern plastic tubing that has essentially replaced the old black rubber is somehow less of a reservoir for these agents. It just is not so according to this paper. In this cost-cutting era, there is much temptation to reuse equipment that is designed for single use. In fact, there is considerable cynicism among our rank and file about these "single use" items. Many anesthesiologists believe that the single-use designation has been obtained by the manufacturer more for commercial gain than because of scientific validity. This paper casts doubt on that cynicism, at least with respect to "storage" of these potential triggers of malignant hypothermia.—J.H. Tinker, M.D.

The Incidence of Bacteraemia Following Laryngeal Mask Insertion
Brimacombe J, Shorney N, Swainston R, Bapty G (Cairns Base Hosp, Queensland, Australia)
Anaesth Intensive Care 20:484–490, 1992   101-94-10-7

Background.—Transient bacteremia can occur with many types of procedures. Although insertion of the laryngeal mask airway (LMA) is considered relatively free of trauma, trauma and resulting infection can occur. The incidence of bacteremia after insertion of LMA has not been studied; therefore, its incidence was studied in 100 fit adult patients.

Study Design.—The study group consisted of 100 patients, aged 18–70 years, for whom LMA was considered appropriate. Before induction, a blood sample was taken during a 3-minute period and swabs were also taken. Another blood sample was taken for 3 minutes starting 30 seconds after insertion of the LMA. Samples were cultured both aerobically and anaerobically.

Results.—All insertions were successful. Four cultures were positive. Of these, 3 were contamination with skin flora. The other culture grew in an anaerobic culture bottle but could not be cultured from the throat swab and may also represent a contamination.

Conclusion.—Insertion of LMA does not result in significant bacteremia. Under these circumstances, antibiotic prophylaxis is not necessary.

▶ My bias is that the risk of bacteremia after atraumatic use of a LMA should be no greater than that associated with use of an oropharyngeal airway. This bias is not altered by the observations described here.—R.K. Stoelting, M.D.

Equipment Safety

Anaesthesia Equipment Safety in Canada: The Role of Government Regulation

Gilron I (McGill Univ, Montreal)
Can J Anaesth 40:987–992, 1993 101-94-10–8

Objective.—Problems with anesthesia equipment were surveyed by reviewing data collected during 1987–1992 by the Health Protection Branch of Health and Welfare Canada.

Data Sources.—A Medical Devices Notification Database contains all notifications for newly marketed medical devices in Canada. In addition, a reporting system records all problem reports and manufacturer recalls along with their designated safety priority status. When a significant safety hazard is recognized, an alert may be issued to inform hospitals and health-care professionals.

Findings.—Anesthesia devices constituted 2.3% of all newly marketed devices during the review period. A total of 471 problem reports and recalls involved anesthesia devices, 8.6% of the total. Six anesthesia device–related problems prompted issuance of an alert, representing 37.5% of all marketed devices leading to an alert. Ten percent of all problem reports and recalls for anesthesia devices were class I priority situations—the highest safety priority—compared with 4.9% of those relating to nonanesthesia devices. Only 1% of all problem reports were from anesthetists.

Conclusion.—Anesthesia equipment is over-represented among devices causing safety problems in Canada. How these devices are used is more important than equipment failure. In the future, anesthetists may assume a more prominent role in postmarketing surveillance of anesthesia equipment.

▶ For those of us who believe in small government and that private enterprise usually does things better, this article points up a role for government— as a clearing house for individuals to send data about problem equipment. Like the Food and Drug Administration in this country, government regulators in Canada appear to have an important role as a database collection and distribution point for problems.—M.F. Roizen, M.D.

Association of Anaesthetist's Checklist for Anaesthetic Machines: Problem With Detection of Significant Leaks
Jackson IJB, Wilson RJT (York District Hosp, England)
Anaesthesia 48:152–153, 1993   101-94-10–9

Background.—The Association of Anaesthetists' Checklist for Anaesthetic Machines includes no formal check for leaks, aside from occlusion of the common gas outlet and checking for "bobbin bounce" on machines with a pressure-relief valve. Page has suggested a simple technique of checking for leaks in which the system is subjected to a pressure of 120 mm Hg and the oxygen Rotameter is slowly turned on. The machine is rejected if the flow required to maintain pressure exceeds 400 mL/min^{-1}. Whether anesthetists following the association's guidelines would be able to detect a significant leak from an anesthetic machine was investigated.

Methods and Results.—A significant leak—3 L/min^{-1} at a pressure of 120 mm Hg—was created in a Boyle-type anesthetic machine by loosening the nut on the side of the Rotameter block. Eight experienced anesthetists were asked to check the machine according to the association guidelines. Just 1 anesthetist was able to detect the leak, and only because the leak was audible when the common gas outlet was occluded. The other 7 subjects said they would use the machine in the operating room. Using this machine with a minute volume divider ventilator produced an inspired oxygen concentration of only 6%.

Conclusion.—The "cockpit drill" recommended by the Association of Anaesthetists is insufficient for detection of a significant leak in a commonly used anesthetic machine. The technique recommended by Page to check for leaks should be included in the standard protocol.

▶ I guess all checklists should be checked before they become standards. This one has some obvious flaws that were highlighted here by Jackson and Wilson.—M.F. Roizen, M.D.

Safety of Fibreoptic Endoscopy: Analysis of Cardiorespiratory Events
Thompson AM, Park KGM, Kerr F, Munro A (Raigmore Hosp, Inverness, Scotland)
Br J Surg 79:1046–1049, 1992   101-94-10–10

Background.—Although fiberoptic endoscopy has been commonly used for many years, only recently have the potential cardiorespiratory complications received attention in the literature. These complications

Effects of Sedation and Endoscopy on Cardiorespiratory Function

	Upper gastrointestinal endoscopy ($n = 66$)	Colonoscopy ($n = 74$)
Oxygen saturation <90%	10 (15)	29 (39)
Systolic blood pressure <100 mmHg	4 (6)	23 (31)
Heart rate <50 beats/min	1 (2)	7 (9)
Heart rate >100 beats/min	19 (29)	20 (27)
Electrocardiographic changes	15 (23)	12 (16)
Ventricular ectopic beats	14	10
ST segment changes alone	1	1
Atrial fibrillation	0	1

Note: Values in parentheses are percentages.
(Courtesy of Thompson AM, Park KGM, Kerr F, et al: *Br J Surg* 79:1046–1049, 1992.)

remain a topic of controversy, as no study has prospectively monitored the ECG, pulse rate, blood pressure, and oxygen saturation during the procedure or tried to differentiate the effects of sedation from those of the endoscopy itself.

Patients and Methods.—Such a study was conducted in 164 patients undergoing gastrointestinal endoscopy. Included were 78 patients undergoing upper gastrointestinal endoscopy and 86 patients undergoing colonoscopy. The mean patient ages were 63 and 60 years, respectively. All patients were monitored for the occurrence of oxygen saturation less than 90%, ECG changes, and heart rate less than 50 or greater than 100 beats/min.

Results.—By these criteria, cardiorespiratory events occurred in 111 patients. Twenty-four of those events were deemed to result solely from the use of intravenous sedation. Excluding those patients, cardiorespiratory events were recorded in 34% of patients undergoing upper gastrointestinal endoscopy and 72% of those undergoing colonoscopy (table). A patient in the colonoscopy group sustained a myocardial infarction; this was the only instance of morbidity, for a rate of .6%. Patients with a history of cardiac disease were more likely to exhibit cardiorespiratory events. Events were also more common with esophageal dilation than with diagnostic endoscopy.

Conclusion.—This prospective study shows a high incidence of cardiorespiratory events during fiberoptic endoscopy. The corresponding morbidity rate is low, however. Close monitoring of all patients with a history of cardiac problems and of those undergoing therapeutic endoscopy is recommended. Oxygen should be given routinely.

▶ This article implies that the anesthesiologist may have a role in stress reduction and maybe even in preoperative counseling for patients undergoing endoscopy. Should there be an expanding role for anesthesia in this field as the degree of sickness of patients increases? I do not think we have the answer to this question, but it again gives an impetus for increasing the education of all medical students about anesthesia pain relief and stress blockade in the perioperative and periprocedure period to try to decrease the adverse consequences of things internists, primary care physicians, obstetricians, and gynecologists, etc., do routinely.—M.F. Roizen, M.D.

Liquid Full Nitrous Oxide Cylinders

Meyer RM, Ferderbar PJ (Northwestern Univ, Chicago)
Anesthesiology 78:584–586, 1993   101-94-10–11

Introduction.—High readings on the nitrous oxide (N_2O) cylinder pressure gauges of several anesthesia machines prompted the question of how the contents could exceed their saturated vapor pressure. An investigation showed that the E cylinders were entirely filled with liquid N_2O. Chemists know that cylinders can become "liquid full," but this potentially hazardous situation has not been described in the past 25 years of medical literature.

Investigation.—When the hospital changed suppliers of medical gases, fresh E cylinders were installed at 13 anesthesia sites. The N_2O pressure gauges of some of the cylinders read in the 900–950-psig range, and the high-pressure system took several minutes to empty at a rate of 9 L/min rather than the expected 15 seconds. Of 14 cylinders, 4 had pressures that were 50 psi or more above the vapor pressure of N_2O at the ambient temperature. Analysis of the 3 cylinders with the highest pressures showed that each contained more than 99% N_2O and only trace contaminants. The overpressurized cylinders were removed from service. They may have been nearly completely filled with liquid N_2O.

Risks.—This situation becomes dangerous if a liquid full cylinder with a rupture-disk pressure-relief device vents into a confined space with personnel present, or if 1 with a combined rupture-disk–fusible-alloy pressure-relief device becomes warm and reaches the bursting pressure at a temperature below the melting point of the fusible plug. The latter devices are being phased out.

▶ In these days of intense concern about "quality," a real question here is how these cylinders became so grossly overfilled that they became liquid full. This is an extraordinarily worrisome case not only because we have not heard of it before but because, on warming, this could theoretically result in extraordinarily high pressures inside these cylinders, which could rupture them. If you fill a cylinder completey liquid full with a cold enough liquid, then let it warm up to room temperature, I hope you do it behind an earthen dike, because that cylinder's weakest point could make it into a rocket that Werner Von Braun would have been proud to have in his arsenal at Peenemunde.—J.H. Tinker, M.D.

Identification/Labeling Problems

Illegibility of Drug Ampoule Labels

James RH, Rabey PG (Leicester Royal Infirmary, England)
BMJ 307:658–659, 1993   101-94-10-12

Introduction.—Both published research and anecdotal experience suggest that it often is difficult to read the labels on drug ampules, even though labels are supposed to be clear and readily legible.

Study Plan.—The labels on 33 drug ampules were examined using calipers with a vernier scale to measure the length of the drug names and dosage.

Findings.—Six of 7 labels on ampules of less than 2 mL had names written in type no larger than that used in the phone directory. Several proprietary drug labels had generic names printed in letters the size of share prices in the newspaper. Even some larger ampules inexplicably used small type. Nearly half of the ampules examined had poor contrast because both the typeface and background were dark or light; the print was very thin; or details on the other side of the container obscured the writing on a clear label.

Conclusion.—Standards for the size and clarity of drug ampule labels are urgently needed in Britain.

▶ I heartily agree. We need some way for those of us whose eyes are getting "senile" to be able to read the drug ampules easily, and it is not by putting more data on them with smaller and smaller print, or by making them all look alike with the same size, shape, and color, as seems to happen on many generic-drug vials manufactured by United States companies. The similarity of shapes of vials for drugs that have opposite action or serious action could be a detriment to the patient, and the potential for errors is too great to not have standardized labels, with big print, different sizes, and different shapes for different therapeutic classes of drugs.—M.F. Roizen, M.D.

Wristband Identification Error Reporting in 712 Hospitals: A College of American Pathologists' Q-Probes Study of Quality Issues in Transfusion Practice

Renner SW, Howanitz PJ, Bachner P (Veterans Affairs Med Ctr, West Los Angeles; Univ of California at Los Angeles; United Hosp, Port Chester, NY)
Arch Pathol Lab Med 117:573–577, 1993   101-94-10-13

Background.—Patient safety relies on correct identification of patients in the hospital, a process that begins with the wristband. Reviews of incompatible transfusions show that more than three fourths of preventable deaths resulted from clerical errors involving patient identification.

Many deaths resulted from the failure to follow established procedures for matching blood labels with wristband identification.

Objective.—The nature of the clerical errors leading to incompatible transfusions was examined by reviewing wristband identification errors in 712 North American hospitals.

Findings.—Phlebotomists checked patient wristbands on nearly 2.5 million occasions and found a total of 67,289 errors. In about half of these cases, the wristband was missing altogether. The overall error rate was 2.2%, but 10% of the participants had error rates exceeding 10%. Absence of a wristband was by far the most frequent type of error, followed by patients wearing more than 1 wristband containing different information and wristbands bearing incomplete data. At more than half the participating hospitals, wristbands are initially placed by admissions clerks. Error rates were higher when the nursing staff placed wristbands. Phlebotomy staffs at more than 60% of the participating hospitals continuously monitor for wristband errors. Written protocols were associated with lower error rates. Nearly all phlebotomists immediately notify the hospital nursing service or a ward clerk/secretary about wristband errors.

Recommendations.—Phlebotomy should be delayed until a wristband error is corrected. Each error should lead to an incident report, and periodic reports should go to the appropriate hospital services and committees. Wristbands should be placed by admissions personnel. The ankle should be designated a standard alternative site for band placement. The removal of bands at any time—especially at the time of surgery—should be strongly discouraged.

▶ Well, here is another preaching article without any data to support the supposition that what they recommend would cut down on the errors of transfusion. In fact, not cutting a wristband off in patients who have surgery on that arm or not cutting it off when they are going to require a radial artery line or some other procedure could result in a more severe problem. Nonetheless, this article does remind us that if we do cut off a wristband, or when patients come in for day surgery (come-and-stay surgery) and require a transfusion, that clerical errors for blood transfusion are the most frequent type of errors in transfusion practice. Clearly, when such is done, alternate sites for identification should be used, and replacement of the wristband should be an immediate and constant practice. We need to get better at our hospitals, and hopefully this article will trigger such action. I wish better data existed to substantiate that such action will decrease clerical errors, but logic dictates it will. However, logic is often found wanting when subjected to vigorous scientific testing.—M.F. Roizen, M.D.

11 Cardiopulmonary Resuscitation and Prehospital Care

Outcome, Prediction, and Cost Studies

Outcome of Cardiopulmonary Resuscitation in the Intensive Care Setting

Landry FJ, Parker JM, Phillips YY (Walter Reed Army Med Ctr, Washington, DC)

Arch Intern Med 152:2305–2308, 1992　　　　　　　　　101-94-11–1

Background.—Cardiopulmonary resuscitation (CPR) has been shown to be successful in a monitored setting. However, most research has concentrated on patients with acute cardiac events rather than chronic progressive disease. The outcome of CPR on patients with acute illness superimposed on chronic disease was investigated.

Method.—A retrospective chart review of 114 patients receiving CPR in medical and surgical intensive care units was carried out during a 12-month period. The principal underlying diseases were malignancy, vascular disease, chronic liver disease, and chronic obstructive pulmonary disease.

Results.—Sixty-four patients died immediately after resuscitation. Fifteen more died within 24 hours. Twenty-nine patients died after an average hospital stay of 11.4 days after CPR. Six patients survived discharge, but 4 of these died within 1 year, and the 2 others sustained severe disabilities (table).

Conclusion.—Patients who are chronically ill rarely survive CPR. Therefore, the decision to resuscitate should take into account underlying chronic medical conditions, not simply the setting of the arrest.

Factors Affecting the Outcome of Resuscitation

Factor	Died Within 24 Hours (n=79)	Died After 24 Hours in Hospital (n=29)	Survivors to Discharge (n=6)
Duration of code * (time+SD)	36.8±31.3	18.3±12.1	12.0±10.0
Intubation status, % n			
Prior to code	57.7	53.6	0
During code	35.9	32.1	83.3
No intubation	6.4	14.3	16.7
Arrest mechanism † % n			
Respiratory or VT/VF	29.5	55.5	66.7
All other	70.5	44.5	33.3
ICU admission source, % n			
Emergency department	32.4	28.0	60.0
Inpatient ward	50.0	60.0	40.0
Other	17.6	12.0	0.0

Abbreviations: VT, ventricular tachycardia; *VF,* ventricular fibrillation; *ICU,* intensive care unit.
* $P = .001$.
† $P = .01$ comparing survivors with nonsurvivors.
(Courtesy of Landry FJ, Parker JM, Phillips YY: *Arch Intern Med* 152:2305–2308, 1992.)

Selective Application of Cardiopulmonary Resuscitation Improves Survival Rates

Schwenzer KJ, Smith WT, Durbin CG Jr (Univ of Virginia, Charlottesville)
Anesth Analg 76:478–484, 1993   101-94-11–2

Background.—Which patients benefit from cardiopulmonary resuscitation (CPR) and which do not was assessed. It is thought that if CPR were only offered to patients who can experience clear benefits, survival rates would be higher. Particularly evaluated were cases of patients with metastatic and other chronic diseases, as well as those involving the elderly.

Method.—A review of all patients who died without CPR or who experienced sudden cardiopulmonary arrest in the hospital and received CPR during a 2-year period was done. Patients with ongoing CPR initiated before admission to the emergency department were not excluded.

Results.—A total of 550 patients who experienced sudden cardiopulmonary arrest received CPR. Of these, 390 survived the procedure initially, but only 138 lived to be discharged from the hospital. A "do not resuscitate" record was entered in the charts of a further 1,206 patients who later died in the hospital.

Discussion.—The high survival rate seen here probably reflects a selection procedure whereby CPR was withheld in patients in whom it would seem futile. Selected patients with multiple medical problems as well as patients of advanced age appear to have a reasonable chance of survival after CPR. Therefore, the decision to withhold the procedure should be made on an individual basis, rather than by diagnostic classification or age.

▶ These articles (Abstracts 101-94-11–1 and 101-94-11–2) reiterated the importance of applying CPR to only those patients in whom the arrest is not heralding the end of the dying process. The use of CPR is not intended to prolong the dying process and should therefore be considered futile care in selected patient populations.—D.M. Rothenberg, M.D.

Predicting the Outcome of Unsuccessful Prehospital Advanced Cardiac Life Support
Kellermann AL, Hackman BB, Somes G (Univ of Tennessee, Memphis)
JAMA 270:1433–1436, 1993   101-94-11–3

Background.—Research has shown that prompt prehospital cardiac care markedly increases rates of resuscitation and survival compared with rapid transport to the hospital, but it is not certain whether patients remaining in cardiac arrest should be transported. Patients who received prehospital advanced cardiac life support (ACLS) were studied to determine whether failure to obtain return of spontaneous circulation after ACLS merits termination of efforts at the scene.

Methods.—Adult victims of out-of-hospital cardiac arrest from heart disease in Memphis were studied retrospectively. After prehospital ACLS, patients were taken to the nearest hospital emergency department, whether or not a pulse was restored at the scene.

Findings.—The Memphis Fire Department attended to 1,068 persons with out-of-hospital cardiac arrest during the 39-month study. Of these patients, 29% had return of spontaneous circulation before transport, and 71% never regained a pulse. This latter group was transported with ongoing cardiopulmonary resuscitation. Sixty-nine percent of patients with return of spontaneous circulation before transport and only 7% without return of spontaneous circulation before leaving the scene were hospitalized. Of the former group, 27% were discharged alive, compared with only .4% of the latter group. Three patients surviving to hospital discharge despite the failure to achieve return of spontaneous circulation before emergency transport sustained cardiac arrest after the paramedics arrived. All 3 of these patients were discharged from the hospital with moderate to severe cerebral disability.

Conclusion.—Rapidly transporting victims of out-of-hospital cardiac arrest who did not respond to an adequate trial of prehospital ACLS is not associated with meaningful survival rates. Emergency medicine physicians should authorize paramedics to cease efforts on the scene in such cases.

Prehospital Traumatic Cardiac Arrest: The Cost of Futility

Rosemurgy AS, Norris PA, Olson SM, Hurst JM, Albrink MH (Univ of South Florida, Tampa)

J Trauma 35:468–474, 1993   101-94-11–4

Background.—Despite desperate attempts to save the lives of victims sustaining traumatic cardiopulmonary arrest, it is becoming more obvious that chances of survival are few, whereas the cost of extreme resuscitative measures is high. Such treatment in a large number of trauma patients was reviewed, and the outcomes and cost were assessed.

Method.—During a period of 6 months, 12,462 patients cared for by prehospital services were monitored. Of these, 138 patients had cardiopulmonary resuscitation at the scene or in transport. Ninety-six had blunt trauma, whereas 42 had penetrating injuries. Sixty patients were transported by air.

Results.—None of the 138 patients who received cardiopulmonary resuscitation on scene or in transit survived, yet the total cost of their care amounted to $871,186.

Conclusion.—The cost of caring for trauma patients sustaining cardiopulmonary arrest at the scene or during transportation cannot be justified. We should question whether to continue allocating limited resources to "futile" cases and consider the risk of exposing health-care workers to the occupational health hazards they may bring.

▶ Failure to achieve restoration of spontaneous circulation at the scene again appears to justify terminating resuscitation efforts before transporting the victim to an emergency center. Risks of injury to pedestrians, motorists, or paramedical personnel coupled with the economic impact of further emergency and intensive care are further reasons to address our current practices. This appears to hold true for the trauma victim as well.—D.M. Rothenberg, M.D.

Resuscitation From Severe Acute Hypercapnia: Determinants of Tolerance and Survival

Potkin RT, Swenson ER (Cedars-Sinai Med Ctr, Los Angeles; Univ of Washington, Seattle)

Chest 102:1742–1745, 1992   101-94-11–5

Arterial Blood Gas Data During Successful Resuscitation From Severe Hypercapnia

Time	pH	$PaCO_2$, mm Hg*	PaO_2, mm Hg*	HCO_3^-, mEq/L	Base excess, mEq/L
Admission	6.60	375	40	34	-16
5 min of mask ventilation	6.91	151	244	29	-9
25 min of mechanical ventilation	7.08	68	56	25	-7
90 min of mechanical ventilation	7.19	58	65	21	-5

* Conversion of traditional units to SI: 1 mm Hg = .133 kPa.
(Courtesy of Potkin RT, Swenson ER: *Chest* 102:1742–1745, 1992.)

Introduction.—Severe chronic hypercapnia is tolerated in patients with end-stage lung disease in whom supplemental inspired oxygen maintains adequate arterial hemoglobin saturation and renal compensation affords remarkable pH homeostasis. In contrast, severe acute hypercapnia (partial pressure of carbon dioxide [P_{CO_2}] > 100 mm Hg) is associated with deleterious neurologic and cardiovascular consequences that may be fatal. However, complete functional recovery has also been reported after severe acute hypercapnia.

Case Report.—Man, 46 underwent cosmetic facial surgery with the use of general anesthesia. Because he could not be intubated, the patient was ventilated by mask with an oxygen-enriched gas mixture for 4–6 hours and monitored by pulse oximetry. Despite arterial saturation more than 90% during the procedure, the patient did not regain consciousness after termination of anesthesia. On transfer to an emergency facility, the patient was comatose, hypotensive, and hypothermic, with temperature-corrected values for pH of 6.6, partial pressure of carbon dioxide in arterial blood of 375 mm Hg, and a calculated base excess of −16 mEq/L. The patient was intubated and given mechanical ventilation. During the next 24 hours, the patient's respiratory acidosis improved (table) and he regained consciousness with no neurologic deficits.

Discussion.—Even with profound hypercapnia with P_{CO_2} greater than 150 mm Hg, survival is possible in acute severe respiratory acidosis provided oxygenation and tissue perfusion are maintained. Many vital tissues have remarkable ability to regulate their intracellular pH far greater than that observed in extracellular space. Tolerance to extreme respiratory acidosis results from an effective intracellular pH defense in critical tissues, such as the brain and heart, by active extrusion of protons into the extracellular space through the Na^+/H^+ exchange across the cell membrane or by direct proton extrusion mediated by membrane H^+ translocating adenosine triphosphatoses. Both these mechanisms are energy consuming and, as such, require adequate tissue oxygenation and perfusion.

▶ This case report demonstrated how much the human body can tolerate at the absolute lowest level of anesthetic care! Unbelievable reading!—D.M. Rothenberg, M.D.

New Techniques

Interposed Abdominal Compression–Cardiopulmonary Resuscitation and Resuscitation Outcome During Asystole and Electromechanical Dissociation

Sack JB, Kesselbrenner MB, Jarrad A (Seton Hall Univ, South Orange, NJ; St Joseph's Hosp and Med Ctr, Paterson, NJ; Univ of California at Los Angeles)
Circulation 86:1692–1700, 1992   101-94-11–6

	Breakdown of Outcome by Initial Arrest Rhythm	
Rhythm	ROSC	Survived 24 hours
Asystole	31/97 (32%)	17/97 (18%)
IAC-CPR	18/44 (41%)	11/44 (25%)
STD-CPR	13/53 (25%)	6/53 (11%)
Electromechanical dissociation	23/46 (50%)	15/46 (33%)
IAC-CPR	15/23 (65%)	11/23 (48%)
STD-CPR	8/23 (35%)	4/23 (17%)

(Courtesy of Sack JB, Kesselbrenner MB, Jarrad A: *Circulation* 86:1692–1700, 1992.)

Background.—Coronary perfusion pressure must be adequately maintained for the return of spontaneous circulation (ROSC) from cardiac arrest. Both human and animal models have shown an increase in coronary perfusion pressure after the addition of interposed abdominal compression (IAC) to otherwise standard (STD) cardiopulmonary resuscitation (CPR). Whether IAC-CPR could improve resuscitation outcome over STD-CPR in patients experiencing in-hospital cardiac arrest when the initial arrest rhythm was asystole or electromechanical dissociation was determined.

Methods.—The randomized, prospective study included 143 consecutive patients. The IAC-CPR method was performed in 67 resuscitation attempts and STD-CPR was done in 76 resuscitation attempts. All patients were unresponsive, apneic, and pulseless when CPR was administered. End points were the return of spontaneous circulation and 24-hour survival.

Results.—The mean age of the patients was 64 years; 69 patients were men and 74 were women. The overall rate of ROSC was 38%. Patients in the IAC-CPR group had a significantly higher rate of ROSC than patients in the STD-CPR group (49% vs. 28%). At 24 hours, significantly more patients were alive in the IAC-CPR group than in the STD-CPR group (33% vs. 13%). Neither age nor the presence of diabetes affected ROSC or 24-hour survival. No patient from either group survived to hospital discharge with intact neurologic function. Postmortem reports, available for 5 patients who received IAC-CPR, showed no evidence of abdominal organ damage.

Conclusion.—The addition of IAC to STD-CPR can improve resuscitation outcome of patients experiencing in-hospital cardiac arrest from asystole and electromechanical dissociation (table). This easily applied manual technique may work by providing hemodynamic augmentation similar to that provided by catecholamines or by priming the thoracic pump.

A Preliminary Study of Cardiopulmonary Resuscitation by Circumferential Compression of the Chest With Use of a Pneumatic Vest

Halperin HR, Tsitlik JE, Gelfand M, Weisfeldt ML, Gruben KG, Levin HR, Rayburn BK, Chandra NC, Scott CJ, Kreps BJ, Siu CO, Guerci AD (Johns Hopkins Med Institutions, Baltimore, Md)
N Engl J Med 329:762–768, 1993   101-94-11-7

Background.—Induced increases in intrathoracic pressure are known to produce blood flow during cardiac arrest. The effectiveness of circumferential compression of the thorax by inflation of a pneumatic vest was compared with manual techniques of cardiopulmonary resuscitation (CPR). It is thought that the vest may prevent some of the chest wall trauma and abdominal and thoracic visceral injury associated with manual resuscitation.

Methods.—A pneumatically cycled circumferential thoracic vest system was developed with the aim of producing periodic increases in intrathoracic pressure. The vest comprises a bladder that is inflated by the pneumatic system. Defibrillation can be achieved during chest compression through the flat defibrillator electrodes under the vest. Electrocardiogram recordings are made through the same electrodes (Fig 11-1). The use of this system was compared with that of manual CPR. In phase 1, aortic and right atrial pressures produced by the vest (at 60 inflations per minute) and manual CPR were compared in 15 patients in whom a mean of 42 ± 16 minutes of initial manual CPR had failed. Vest CPR was also given to a further 14 patients in whom such pressure measurements were not taken. In phase 2, short-term survival was examined in 34 additional patients who were randomly assigned vest CPR or manual CPR after initial manual CPR of 11 ± 4 minutes had failed.

Results.—In phase 1, vest CPR increased the peak aortic pressure from 78 ± 26 mm Hg to 138 ± 28 mm Hg. The coronary perfusion pressure increased from 15 ± 8 mm Hg to 23 ± 11 mm Hg (Fig 11-2). Despite the fact that prolonged manual CPR had proved unsuccessful, spontaneous circulation returned in 4 of the 29 patients after using the vest. In phase 2, spontaneous circulation returned in 8 of 17 patients experiencing vest CPR, compared with only 3 of 17 patients who underwent conventional manual treatment. More patients in the vest group were alive 6 hours after resuscitation than in the manual group (6 of 17 compared with 1 of 17). Twenty-four hours after resuscitation, the number of survivors was still higher in the vest group (3 of 17 compared with 1 of 17). However, none survived to be discharged.

Conclusion.—The vest CPR successfully increases aortic pressure and coronary perfusion pressure and is effective in restoring cardiac activity. If this method is used to restore spontaneous circulation early after arrest, it may prevent irreversible organ damage. However, the long-term effect of CPR on survival rates requires further examination.

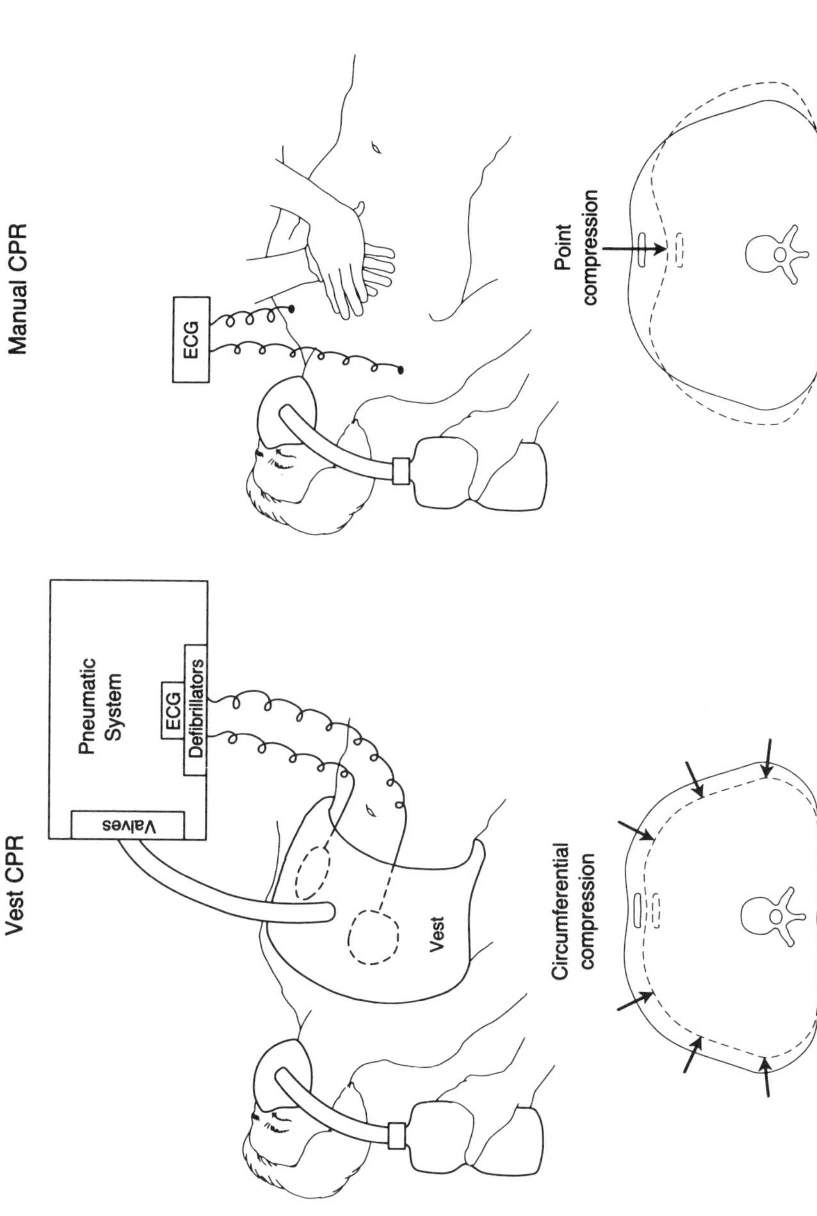

Fig 11-1.—Comparison of the thoracic-vest system for CPR with standard manual CPR. Flat defibrillator electrodes are indicated by *dashed circles*. (Courtesy of Halperin HR, Tsitlik JE, Gelfand M, et al: *N Engl J Med* 329:762–768, 1993.)

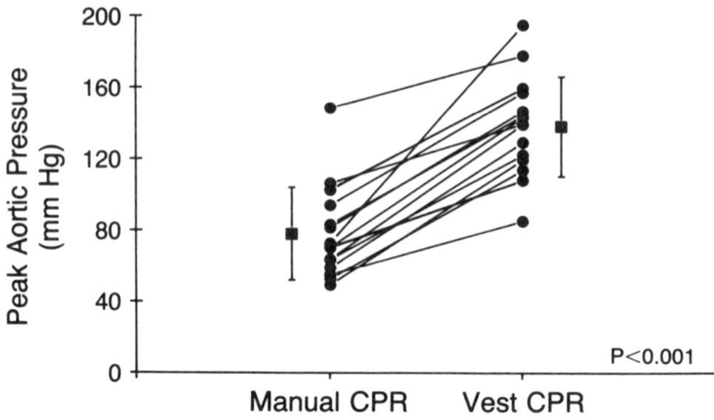

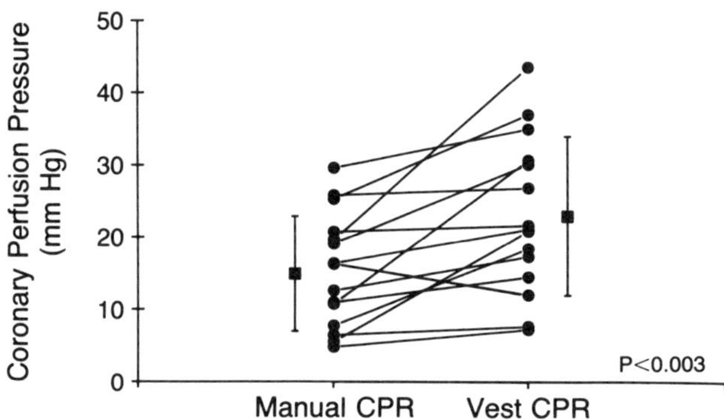

Fig 11–2.—Peak aortic pressure and coronary perfusion pressure measured in 15 patients during manual CPR and vest CPR in phase 1. The *vertical bars* and *squares* are the mean values ± standard deviation for the 2 types of CPR. There was a significant increase in each vascular pressure with the vest CPR as compared with manual CPR. (Courtesy of Halperin HR, Tsitlik JE, Gelfand M, et al: *N Engl J Med* 329:762–768, 1993.)

▶ Both of these articles (Abstracts 101-94-11–6 and 101-94-11–7) applied the thoracic pump theory of CPR to the clinical setting with statistical success. Unfortunately, return of spontaneous circulation as defined in the study by Sack et al. as a systolic pressure greater than 80 mm Hg and a palpable femoral arterial pulse does not equate with long-term survival. In both studies combined, there were only 2 survivors, neither of whom were neurologically intact on discharge from the hospital. These techniques will need to demonstrate improved neurologic outcome before they are adopted as standard methods of resuscitation.—D.M. Rothenberg, M.D.

Five-Year Experience in Prehospital Intraosseous Infusions in Children and Adults

Glaeser PW, Hellmich TR, Szewczuga D, Losek JD, Smith DS (Med College of

Wisconsin, Milwaukee; Milwaukee County Paramedic Training Inst, Wis)
Ann Emerg Med 22:1119–1124, 1993   101-94-11–8

Background.—The use of intraosseous infusions has been widely endorsed, and numerous communities have adopted the procedure for pediatric prehospital care. Pilot research suggests that emergency medical technician-paramedic (EMT-P) units can use intraosseous infusion lines safely and reliably. The 5-year (1987–1991) experience of Milwaukee County EMT-Ps with the intraosseous infusion technique was reported.

Methods.—The EMT-Ps were instructed in use of the disposable 18-gauge Jamshidi sternal intraosseous infusion needle that is placed in the proximal tibia bone marrow of patients requiring emergency vascular access for administration of fluid and/or medication. After the first year, during which all lines were placed by base physician order, intraosseous infusion became a standing order for pulseless nonbreathing patients; other patients still required base orders. Airway management remained the number 1 priority, and 1 or 2 attempts (depending on the child's age) were to be made at peripheral vein access before attempting the intraosseous infusion line. All run records and base physician reports generated during the 5 years were reviewed.

Results.—A total of 152 patients, ranging in age from newborn to 102 years, received 165 attempts at an intraosseous infusion line. The median age of the patients was 6 months. Successful placement was achieved in 115 patients. Success rates were significantly higher in young children (younger than 3 years) compared with older children and adults (table). Materials infused by the lines included epinephrine, atropine, bicarbonate, calcium chloride, lactated Ringer's solution, and dextrose in water. Proficiency in the technique was maintained by the EMT-Ps during the 5-year period. The most common complication, infiltration, occurred in 14 patients. Unsuccessful attempts to place the line were most often attributed to needle bending and errors in landmark identification.

Patient Age and Intraosseous Infusion Line Success Rates

	Patient Age				
	0–11 Months	1–2 Years	3–9 Years	≥ 10 Years	Total
No. of patients	109	20	9	14	152
No. of attempts	118	22	11	14	165
Success rate per patient (%)	78	85	67	50	76
Success rate per attempt (%)	72	77	70	50	70

(Courtesy of Glaeser PW, Hellmich TR, Szewczuga, et al: *Ann Emerg Med* 22:1119–1124, 1993.)

Conclusion.—The intraosseous infusion line technique is used infrequently relative to other EMT-P skills. Nevertheless, the success rate remained high. The time from arrival at the patient site to placement averaged 13 minutes. Intraosseous infusion line placement can be performed reliably by EMT-Ps in both children and adults.

▶ The use of intraosseous infusions for pediatric arrest situations has been well established although it is probably underutilized. Essentially, all cardioresuscitative agents may be administered by this route, including epinephrine, atropine, lidocaine, bretylium, naloxone, diazepam, and dopamine. Volume resuscitation may also be performed by this route. This technique may prove invaluable to the anesthesiologist who is faced with a pediatric arrest and impossible vascular access.—D.M. Rothenberg, M.D.

Ethics Related to Cardiopulmonary Resuscitation

Distinct Criteria for Termination of Resuscitation in the Out-of-Hospital Setting

Bonnin MJ, Pepe PE, Kimball KT, Clark PS Jr (City of Houston Ctr for Resuscitation and Emergency Med Services; Baylor College of Medicine, Houston)
JAMA 270:1457–1462, 1993   101-94-11–9

Background.—Most cases of cardiac arrest occur in the home or other settings outside the hospital. In most communities, victims of cardiac arrest who are not revived at the scene are transported quickly to an emergency department. Recently, however, it has been suggested that some of these persons should be pronounced dead at the scene. Criteria were established for appropriate on-scene termination of resuscitation efforts for out-of-hospital cardiac arrest when on-scene interventions do not restore spontaneous circulation.

Methods.—All cases of out-of-hospital cardiac arrest for 18 months were studied prospectively in a large municipality. Factors analyzed included survival to hospital discharge and established survival predictors such as age, gender, and presenting cardiac rhythm; whether it was a witnessed event; performance of basic cardiopulmonary resuscitation by bystanders; and interval to paramedic arrival and return of spontaneous circulation (ROSC).

Findings.—Of 1,461 consecutive primary cardiac arrests, 139 were witnessed by paramedics. Fifty-nine of these occurred en route to the hospital. Of the 1,322 unwitnessed events, ROSC was achieved at the scene in 370 patients. Only 6 patients (.6%) of the 952 without ROSC at the scene survived. Persistent ventricular fibrillation was readily identified in all 6 of these cases. Excluding patients with persistent ventricular fibrillation, ROSC was achieved in all survivors within 25 minutes of paramedic arrival (Table 1).

Conclusion.—Except in cases of persistent ventricular fibrillation, resuscitation efforts can be terminated at the scene when normothermic

TABLE 1.—Patient Characteristics and Results of Univariate and Logistic Regression Analyses of These Variables in 1,322 Consecutive, Unmonitored, Out-of-Hospital, Primary Cardiac Arrest Patients

	Nonsurvivors (n=1230)	Survivors (n=92)	Univariate *P*	Joint *P* (OR, 99% CI)*
Age, y	65±15	61±12	.02	.27 (0.9, 0.7-1.2)
Male gender, No. (%)	781 (64)	65 (71)	.18	.65 (1.1, 0.5-2.4)
Bystander CPR† performed, No. (%)	274 (22)	37 (40)	<.001	<.03 (1.9, 0.9-3.8)
Paramedic response interval, min‡	10.2±4.2	8.7±3.3	.002	.08 (0.9, 0.9-1.0)
On-scene interval, min§	28±9.3	26±8.6	...¶	...¶
Transport interval, min	7.9±4.3	8.4±5.1	...¶	...¶
ROSC, No. (%)‖	284 (23)	86 (93)	<.0001	<.0001 (32, 10-99)
Initial rhythm, No. (%)				
Ventricular fibrillation	471 (38)	79 (86)	<.0001	<.0001 (5.2, 2.1-12.3)
Asystole	506 (41)	5 (5)	<.0001	...
Idioventricular	191 (16)	7 (8)	...	...
Electromechanical dissociation	52 (4)	0	...	...
Ventricular tachycardia	6 (<1)	1 (1)	...	...
Other/unknown	4 (<1)	0	...	...

* Results of logistic regression analysis for the 6 predictors in the model: age, male gender, performance of bystander cardiopulmonary resuscitation, paramedic response interval, ROSC at the scene, and an initial ECG presentation of ventricular fibrillation.

† CPR, cardiopulmonary resuscitation.

‡ Interval from first 911 telephone ring until arrival at street location of patient.

§ Interval from paramedic arrival at street location until ambulance departure from location.

‖ ROSC at the scene for at least 5 minutes.

¶ Ellipses indicate not tested in logistic regression analyses.

(Courtesy of Bonnin MJ, Pepe PE, Kimball KT, et al: JAMA 270:1457–1462, 1993.)

adults with unmonitored, out-of-hospital, primary cardiac arrest do not regain spontaneous circulation with 25 minutes of standard advanced cardiac life support (Table 2). Studies in large centers with high survival rates are now needed to validate these criteria.

TABLE 2.—Criteria for Termination of Resuscitation
Efforts at the Scene After Unmonitored, Out-of-Hospital,
Adult, Primary Cardiac Arrest

1. Adult cardiopulmonary arrest (not associated with trauma, body temperature aberration, respiratory etiology, or drug overdose)
2. Standard advanced cardiac life support[5] for 25 min
3. No restoration of spontaneous circulation (spontaneous pulse rate of >60 beats per min for at least one 5-min period)
4. Absence of persistently recurring or refractory ventricular fibrillation/tachycardia or any continued neurological activity (eg, spontaneous respiration, eye opening, or motor response)

(Courtesy of Bonnin MJ, Pepe PE, Kimball KT, et al: *JAMA* 270:1457–1462, 1993.)

▶ The results of this study are substantiated by numerous other studies that document near 0% survival from out-of-hospital cardiac arrest in adults that is caused by anything other than ventricular fibrillation. In this sense, the ethics of medical futility should apply, and justification for on-sight termination of resuscitation may be warranted. I hope that the societal acceptance of such practice, however, will be based on the level of experience of each community's emergency medical system rather than on purely economic factors.—D.M. Rothenberg, M.D.

12 Cardiac Anesthesia

Preoperative Evaluation

Supplemental Oxygen Does Not Reduce Myocardial Ischemia in Premedicated Patients With Critical Coronary Artery Disease

Kavanagh BP, Cheng DCH, Sandler AN, Chung F, Lawson S, Ong D (Univ of Toronto)
Anesth Analg 76:950–956, 1993   101-94-12-1

Introduction.—The presence of myocardial ischemia definitely raises the risk of postoperative myocardial infarction. Premedication is often given before coronary bypass graft surgery to lessen the tachycardia and hypertension associated with perioperative anxiety, but narcotics have been associated with arterial hemoglobin desaturation.

Objective.—A randomized prospective trial determined the value of administering supplemental oxygen to premedicated patients having critical coronary artery stenosis. The study enrolled 104 patients who had continuous ECG monitoring and pulse oximetry before elective coronary bypass surgery.

Methods.—All patients received lorazepam sublingually in a dose of .03 mg/kg. Half the patients then received oxygen by nasal catheter at a rate of 4 L/min for 1 hour. All patients then received morphine, .15 mg/kg, and perphenazine, .05 mg/kg, intramuscularly.

Results.—Patients given supplemental oxygen had a 25% rate of arterial hemoglobin desaturation before premedication and a rate of 11.5% afterward. In contrast, in control patients, the incidence of desaturation increased from 25% to 57% after premedication. In both groups, the incidence of myocardial ischemia, as reflected by ST-segment depression, was less than 10% at most intervals, and there was no significant difference according to whether supplemental oxygen was administered. Ischemia was not associated temporally with arterial hemoglobin desaturation.

Conclusion.—Administering supplemental oxygen after premedication lessens the risk of arterial hemoglobin desaturation developing, but it does not reduce the risk of perioperative myocardial ischemia.

▶ I would like to find a problem with this article because it argues against 1 of my biases, but I cannot. If you find 1, write to me.—M.F. Roizen, M.D.

Preoperative Plateletpheresis Does Not Reduce Blood Loss During Cardiac Surgery

Boey SK, Ong BC, Dhara SS (Singapore Gen Hosp)
Can J Anaesth 40:844–850, 1993   101-94-12-2

Background.—Studies have shown that acute preoperative plateletpheresis effectively reduces blood loss and blood component transfusion while improving hematologic profiles in patients undergoing open heart surgery. In those studies, however, the concomitant use of cell saver methods may have been responsible for the benefits. These methods remove free hemoglobin and activated procoagulants and may therefore mask the deleterious effects of combined plateletpheresis and cardiopulmonary bypass (CPB).

Methods.—Forty patients undergoing primary myocardial revascularization were randomly divided into a control group, without plateletpheresis, and a treatment group, in which preoperative platelet-rich plasma, 10 mL/kg⁻¹, was collected and reinfused after heparin reversal. Standard surgery, anesthesia, and CPB were then done without concomitant cell saver methods.

Findings.—Blood transfusion was decreased in the treatment group compared with the control group. However, this reduction in transfusion was accompanied by lower postoperative hemoglobin levels. No between-group differences were found in blood loss, fresh frozen plasma, or platelet requirements. Reinfusion did not improve platelet count and function or coagulation tests. Fibrinogen levels were lower in the treatment group on the day of surgery, suggesting increased fibrinogen intake. More patients in the treatment group had low haptoglobin concentrations during CPB, indicating greater hemolysis.

Conclusion.—Preoperative plateletpheresis does not decrease blood loss or improve the hemostatic profiles of patients undergoing CAPBG with CPB but not concomitant cell saver methods. More research is needed to define the hematologic effects of cell saver and plateletpheresis techniques, individually and combined, in patients having cardiac surgery.

▶ The authors segregated plateletpheresis from salvage by cell saver use and found that the plateletpheresis without the salvage by cell saver use may not be as beneficial as using the 2 together. They attributed this synergy to the change in activation of procoagulants that washing with the cell saver discards. Once again, you have to test the hypotheses before you find out whether they are right. This innovative study looked at a problem and found a result that I would have bet against. Like all good science, it raises more questions than it answers.—M.F. Roizen, M.D.

MAO Inhibitors and Coronary Artery Surgery: A Patient Death

Noble WH, Baker A (St Michael's Hosp, Toronto; Univ of Toronto)
Can J Anaesth 39:1061–1066, 1992   101-94-12-3

Background.—The mechanisms of action of monoamine oxidase inhibitors (MAOIs) may produce hyper- or hypotension in patients undergoing coronary artery surgery. However, it is currently recommended that patients taking MAOIs may continue to do so before surgery. In this case report, MAOIs were continued until the time of surgery in a patient undergoing coronary artery bypass grafting (CABG). The patient subsequently died in the intensive care unit (ICU), and although the underlying cause of death was not firmly established, MAOIs may have played a role.

Case Report.—Man, 64, underwent CABG without problems. Fentanyl and midazolam were the anesthetic agents used. After surgery, ICU care was complicated by hypertension, hyperthermia, and severe shivering. Hypotensive episodes developed next. In spite of efforts to control these problems, the patient experienced an asystolic cardiac arrest, requiring 4 minutes of cardiopulmonary resuscitation. As the day progressed, cardiac output decreased, and blood pressure was difficult to maintain. The patient became asystolic the next morning. Postmortem examination was not allowed, but 2 results of blood cultures and a urine culture were negative. Diagnoses of pulmonary embolism and sepsis were not confirmed, but they may have played a role in this patient's death. The MAOIs might have been a causative factor as well.

Conclusion.—To date, there are only 5 reported instances in which patients taking MAOIs were given fentanyl during CABG surgery. Thus, until further information on using high-dose fentanyl in the presence of MAOIs is obtained, MAOIs should be discontinued, when possible, before surgeries that may require catecholamine use.

▶ The MAO inhibitors once were "absolutely contraindicated" for elective surgery. The dogma of not that many years ago indicated that they should be stopped for at least 2 weeks before surgery (no matter what happened to the patient who needed the MAO inhibitor). In more recent years, there has been a gradual softening of that request, to the point where we have begun to see papers that state that this old dogma can now be safely abandoned, i.e., patients taking MAOs should remain taking their MAOs right up to and through elective surgery. That is why I selected this article. Here is a case in which the presence of MAOs plus postoperative norepinephrine seemed to have combined to produce a severe reaction. It is also possible that the demerol derivative, namely fentanyl, played a role here in combination with the MAO inhibitor. Although this is only 1 case, it does make us wonder whether our senior colleagues, who were very much afraid of MAO inhibitors in combination with anesthesia, might have been right. There may be a price for modern-day iconoclasm.—J.H. Tinker, M.D.

Pharmacologic Studies

Magnesium Administration and Dysrhythmias After Cardiac Surgery: A Placebo-Controlled, Double-Blind, Randomized Trial

England MR, Gordon G, Salem M, Chernow B (Tufts Univ, Boston; Johns Hopkins Univ, Baltimore, Md)
JAMA 268:2395–2402, 1992   101-94-12-4

Purpose.—The frequency of hypomagnesemia after cardiac surgery suggests that magnesium supplementation might decrease postoperative morbidity and mortality related to magnesium deficiency.

Methods.—One hundred patients undergoing elective cardiac surgery involving cardiac bypass were studied. After the termination of bypass, half the patients received an intravenous infusion of magnesium chloride, 2 g, and 50 received placebo.

Results.—The postoperative dysrhythmia rate was 16% in the magnesium group vs. 34% in the placebo group. Of patients with normal postoperative magnesium levels, 17% had new supraventricular dysrhythmias, compared with 37% of those who were hypomagnesemic. The postoperative cardiac index in the intensive care unit was 2.8 L/min/m^2 in the magnesium group vs. 2.5 L/min/m^2 in the placebo group. Postoperative ventricular dysrhythmias requiring prolonged mechanical ventilatory support were also more common in patients with hypomagnesemia.

Conclusion.—In cardiac surgery patients, postoperative hypomagnesemia carries potentially serious morbidity. The occurrence of ventricular dysrhythmias is decreased and stroke volume and cardiac index are increased with magnesium supplementation in the early postoperative period.

▶ This study, as well as many others, confirmed the use of intravenous magnesium as an effective antidysrhythmic agent. This effect appears to occur irrespective of serum magnesium levels. I suspect that had a dose-response curve been performed, an even greater antidysrhythmic effect would have been seen at higher doses (i.e., 4 g).—D.M. Rothenberg, M.D.

Effect of "Renal-Dose" Dopamine on Renal Function Following Cardiac Surgery

Myles PS, Buckland MR, Schenk NJ, Cannon GB, Langley M, Davis BB, Weeks AM (Alfred Hosp, Melbourne, Australia)
Anaesth Intensive Care 21:56–61, 1993   101-94-12-5

Objective.—The incidence of renal impairment after cardiac surgery ranges from 5% to 30%, with a mortality rate as high as 65%. The effect of renal-dose dopamine in renal function in patients undergoing cardiac surgery was evaluated.

Study Design.—In a prospective, double-blind, randomized trial, 49 patients undergoing elective coronary artery bypass surgery received for 24 hours either dopamine at 200 µg/min or placebo commenced at induction. No patient had preexisting renal failure. A standard general anesthetic and cardiopulmonary bypass were used. If a patient became oliguric, a protocol of diuretic administration was followed. The use of fluid therapy, inotropes, or vasodilators was not restricted.

Outcome.—No patient had renal failure or required dialysis or hemofiltration. Transient renal impairment, defined as a more than 25% increase in serum creatinine, occurred in 36% of the patients who received dopamine and 50% of the control patients; the difference was not significant. In addition, there were no significant differences between groups in urine output, daily serum creatinine, repeated creatinine, and free-water clearance estimations. The 7-day mortality rate was 0.

Conclusion.—Routine perioperative use of renal-dose dopamine is not associated with improvement in renal function and does not prevent transient renal impairment in patients undergoing elective coronary artery surgery.

▶ Unfortunately, the wrong group of patients was studied. It is of no surprise that patients with normal renal function would have been unlikely to benefit from this therapy (the mean estimated creatinine clearances in the dopamine and control groups were 91 and 96 mL/min, respectively). A better design would have been to study patients with preexisting renal insufficiency.—D.M. Rothenberg, M.D.

The Use of Esmolol to Attenuate the Haemodynamic Response When Extubating Patients Following Cardiac Surgery—A Double-Blind Controlled Study
O'Dwyer JP, Yorukoglu D, Harris MNE (St Thomas' Hosp, London)
Eur Heart J 14:701–704, 1993   101-94-12–6

Background.—There have been many efforts to lessen the tachycardia and hypertension that may accompany laryngoscopy and intubation, but less is known of the hemodynamic effects of extubation. The use of opioids to suppress these responses is limited by their dose-dependent respiratory depressant action. Now that early extubation of cardiac surgical patients is more widely practiced, the issue is particularly important.

Study Design.—Cardiovascular function was monitored in 14 coronary bypass surgery patients during emergence from anesthesia, the reversal of neuromuscular blockade, and extubation. The patients were randomly assigned to receive either esmolol, 500 µg/kg^{-1} in 1 minute, followed by an infusion of 100 µg/kg^{-1}/min, or placebo. The loading dose was given just before reversal of neuromuscular blockade.

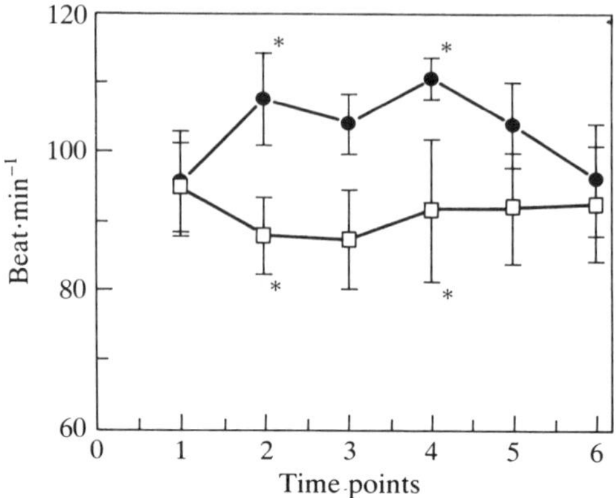

Fig 12–1.—Mean changes in heart rate. *Boxes* indicate esmolol group; *circles* indicate saline group. P ≤ .05. (Courtesy of O'Dwyer JP, Yorukoglu D, Harris MNE: *Eur Heart J* 14:701–704, 1993.)

Observations.—Heart rate increased only in placebo recipients (Fig 12–1). Systemic blood pressure increased significantly in placebo patients but not in those given esmolol. The mean arterial pressure increased 15% in the placebo patients (Fig 12–2). There were no significant group differences in the cardiac output or mean pulmonary artery pressure, and no patient had evidence of ischemic change. Three placebo recipients were given glyceryl trinitrate to control the blood pressure.

Conclusion.—Hypertension and tachycardia at the end of cardiac surgery may be prevented by the prior intravenous administration of esmolol.

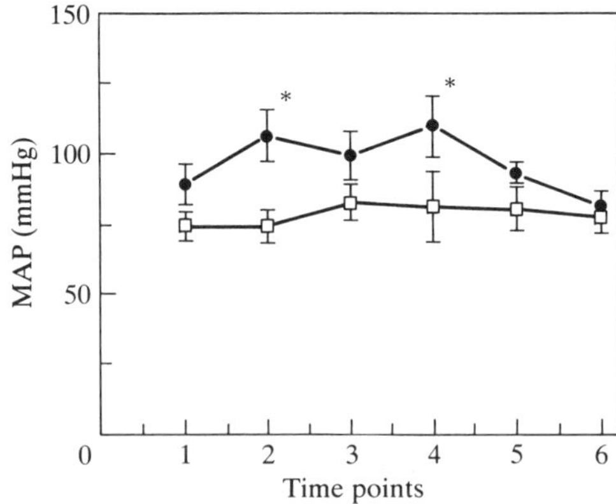

Fig 12–2.—Mean changes in arterial pressure. *Boxes* indicate esmolol group; *circles* indicate saline group. P ≤ .05. (Courtesy of O'Dwyer JP, Yorukoglu D, Harris MNE: *Eur Heart J* 14:701–704, 1993.)

▶ I am critical of this kind of study. The authors know perfectly well that es-molol will attenuate the hypertension and tachycardia associated with darn near any kind of stimulus, compared with placebo. So what? These authors contended that "tachycardia and hypertension are well documented complications of laryngoscopy and intubation . . ." but that "there is less information on the haemodynamic effects of extubation." The authors called these normal reflex responses "complications." I would strongly disagree unless they can show that these reflex responses have led to any negative outcomes, either short term or long term. Because they cannot show that, administration of a beta-blocker during intubation or extubation constitutes the use of a drug to do something that may seem logical but that is unproven to have real beneficial effect. We do this a lot in our medicine, and we will probably not be talked out of it often, but if the history of medicine shows nothing else, it shows that what seems logical today may not seem logical tomorrow and may not be able to withstand the test of time or scientific inquiry.—J.H. Tinker, M.D.

Effects of Low-Dose Adenosine on Myocardial Performance After Coronary Artery Bypass Surgery

Öwall A, Ehrenberg J, Brodin L-Å, Juhlin-Dannfelt A, Sollevi A (Karolinska Hosp, Stockholm)
Acta Anaesthesiol Scand 37:140–148, 1993   101-94-12-7

Background.—Adenosine acts as a potent vasodilator in most vascular beds and has exhibited a preferential coronary vasodilator effect. Non-hypotensive doses have markedly increased coronary graft flow and enhanced cardiac output when infused during coronary bypass surgery.

Study Design.—The effects of adenosine given at a rate of 30 µg/kg/minute (a nonhypotensive dose level) were examined in a blinded, placebo-controlled study in 16 patients with stable angina who were scheduled for elective coronary revascularization. Eight patients had adenosine infused into the right ventricle for 4 hours beginning after arrival in the intensive care unit.

Results.—Three patients in each group required labetalol to prevent hypertension and tachycardia. Left ventricular stroke work increased in the first hour of adenosine infusion. The cardiac index increased by about 50% during adenosine infusion. Systemic vascular resistance was lower in the adenosine group than in placebo recipients. Levels of arterial partial pressure of oxygen were lower in the adenosine-infused patients. There were no group differences in left ventricular end-diastolic area or area ejection fraction at any time. Four patients given adenosine and 3 given placebo had echocardiographic signs of myocardial ischemia. Myocardial infarction developed in 1 patient in each group.

Conclusion.—Adenosine induced peripheral vasodilatation and improved cardiac output in these cardiac surgery patients without compromising arterial blood pressure. Ventricular function remained intact.

▶ The key here is "low dose." It is critically important that the reader keep in mind that adenosine is a powerful inducer of coronary steal! These authors have made a critical assumption, namely that the worst coronary stenoses would be bypassed in these "postbypass" patients. That may be true, but, then again in many patients it may not because many stenoses are too small to be bypassable. There is no doubt that adenosine, in just a small increment of dosage above what was used here, can dilate normal coronaries, thus inducing coronary steal. The makers of this drug were acutely aware of the above facts, which is why adenosine has not been approved by the Food and Drug Administration for this use. I am very concerned about indiscriminate use of adenosine in postoperative patients for the purpose of increasing cardiac output or lowering blood pressure. Nonetheless, nitroprusside does more or less the same thing, and yet it is used for these purposes all the time. Perhaps it will work, but I remain skeptical and concerned about coronary steal here. Isoflurane does not induce coronary steal in very many, if any, patients because its tendency to produce coronary vasodilation is accompanied by considerable myocardial depression. Excellent work in recent years has clearly shown that nifedipine has a similar effect. Concomitant myocardial depression is the reason why nifedipine stays out of trouble in the coronary steal realm. There is no concomitant myocardial depression with adenosine, hence my concern about steal.—J.H. Tinker, M.D.

Fentanyl Plasma Concentrations Maintained by a Simple Infusion Scheme in Patients Undergoing Cardiac Surgery
Hall RI, Molderhauer CC, Hug CC Jr (Emory Univ, Atlanta, Ga)
Anesth Analg 76:957–963, 1993   101-94-12–8

Objective.—Pending the wider availability of computer-assisted continuous-infusion systems, a simple method of infusing fentanyl to achieve and maintain 1 of 2 target plasma concentrations was evaluated in 17 patients having cardiac surgery under moderate hypothermic cardiopulmonary bypass.

Management.—The patients received morphine, a benzodiazepine, and/or scopolamine as premedication. Six patients then received a priming infusion of fentanyl, 2.4 µg/kg/min, for 20 minutes and then .3 µg/kg/min for the duration of surgery, yielding plasma fentanyl levels of 20–25 ng/mL. The other 11 patients received the same priming infusion and a maintenance infusion of .15 µg/kg/min in an attempt to produce plasma levels of 12–15 ng/mL.

Results.—Peak plasma fentanyl levels were 67 ng/mL in the high-fentanyl group, declining to 27 ng/mL before the start of cardiopulmonary bypass. Levels remained at about 20 ng/mL for the duration of surgery.

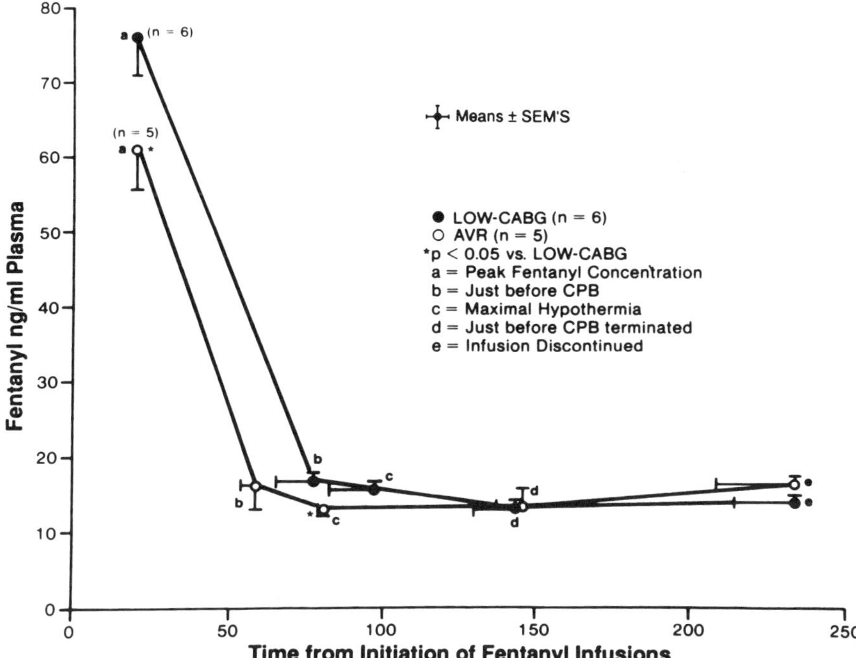

Fig 12–3.—Plasma fentanyl concentrations vs. time of intraoperative events in 6 patients having coronary artery bypass grafting (CABG) and 6 patients having replacement of the aortic valve (AVR). Each group received fentanyl as a priming infusion of 2.4 $\mu g/kg^{-1}/min^{-1}$ and a maintenance infusion of .15 $\mu g/kg^{-1}/min^{-1}$. Note that there was no difference in the concentration achieved by the infusion in either group apart from those measured at the completion of the priming infusion and during cardiopulmonary bypass (CPB) at the time of maximum cooling. (Courtesy of Hall RI, Molderhauer CC, Hug CC Jr: *Anesth Analg* 76:957–963, 1993.)

One patient in this group required a single dose of thiopental after bypass ended. Low-fentanyl patients had a peak level of 77 ng/mL and maintenance plasma levels of 13–15 ng/mL during surgery. Eight of the 11 patients required supplemental anesthesia before, and 10 after cardiopulmonary bypass. The results in patients having aortic valve replacement are shown in Figure 12–3. Eight other patients received a single bolus of 75 μg of fentanyl per kg for induction, and 7 of them required supplemental anesthesia.

Conclusion.—A simple infusion scheme may be used for administering fentanyl to patients having cardiac surgery.

▶ This technique suffers from the same problem it has faced for years, namely the inability to measure pharmacokinetics of fentanyl on line. Therefore, fixed-dosage regimens, however graded they might be, will lead to relatively wide ranges in resultant fentanyl plasma concentrations. Because it is known that we can use high-dose or moderate-dose fentanyl for "anesthesia" at wide ranges of blood levels, this may not be too critical. It probably does make sense to get away from the bolus technique that so many of us have used for so many years.—J.H. Tinker, M.D.

Vasodilation With Adenosine or Sodium Nitroprusside After Coronary Artery Bypass Surgery: A Comparative Study on Myocardial Blood Flow and Metabolism
Zäll S, Kirnö K, Milocco I, Ricksten S-E (Univ of Gothenburg, Sweden)
Anesth Analg 76:498–503, 1993   101-94-12–9

Background.—Many patients become hypertensive shortly after coronary artery bypass surgery. Ventricular function may decline as a result, and patients are at risk of hemorrhage, arrhythmia, and stroke. An increase in systemic vascular resistance is primarily responsible. Adenosine is a potent vasodilator in humans that lowers systemic arterial blood pressure without causing rebound hypertension, and without tachyphylaxis.

Objective and Methods.—The effects of adenosine and sodium nitroprusside (SNP) were compared in 10 patients with double- or triple-vessel coronary artery disease who underwent elective coronary artery bypass surgery. All had an ejection fraction exceeding 50%. Sodium nitroprusside was infused during two 15-minute periods at rates of .8 and .7 µg/kg/min, separated by a 15-minute infusion of adenosine at a rate of 8.9 µg/kg/min. The goal was to maintain the mean arterial pressure at about 80 mm Hg.

Results.—Pulmonary and central venous pressures tended to increase during adenosine infusion. The cardiac index increased 32% with no change in heart rate. Systemic vascular resistance declined 26% compared with SNP infusion. The intrapulmonary shunt fraction increased 57% during adenosine infusion compared with the initial SNP infusion, and the arterial partial pressure of oxygen declined 11%. Coronary perfusion pressure decreased 5% with adenosine compared with initial SNP infusion. Blood flow in both the coronary sinus and the great cardiac vein more than doubled during adenosine infusion. Coronary oxygen content increased by 51%, and the arterio-great cardiac vein oxygen content difference decreased by about the same degree. The ST segment was more depressed during adenosine infusion than with SNP. The drugs had similar effects on regional myocardial lactate extraction and uptake. One patient had myocardial ischemia while receiving adenosine.

Conclusion.—Adenosine infusion produced hyperperfusion of the left ventricular myocardium in these patients and increased the cardiac index. Systemic and coronary vasodilation are more marked with adenosine than with SNP infusion in patients having coronary artery bypass surgery.

▶ Adenosine has long been used in various animal models of coronary steal as the "positive control" drug. By this I mean that any model of coronary steal must be shown to actually produce coronary steal given a known global coronary vasodilating agent. For this, in the original paper by Becker (1), dipyridamole was chosen. A few years later, Chiariello et al. (2) showed that nitroprusside could do the same thing. Since that time, many investigators have used adenosine as the positive control. Thus, when adenosine was finally released for human use, it was not approved for treatment of hypotension or other vasodilator uses.

That is why this paper is so interesting. These authors have used adenosine to control postcardiac surgical hypertension. They compared it in an elegant study to nitroprusside. They encountered ST-segment depression with adenosine, and I think this study basically confirms our fears about adenosine. I do not think it should replace nitroprusside, even though I realize that many people are looking for a replacement for nitroprusside (and have been for years).—J.H. Tinker, M.D.

References

1. Becker LC: *Circulation* 57:1103, 1976.
2. Chiariello M, et al: *Circulation* 54:766, 1978.

Combined Inotropic Effects of Amrinone and Epinephrine After Cardiopulmonary Bypass in Humans
Royster RL, Butterworth JF IV, Prielipp RC, Zaloga GP, Lawless SG, Spray BJ, Kon ND, Wallenhaupt SL, Cordell AR (Wake Forest Univ, Winston-Salem, NC; du Pont Med Inst and Children's Hosp, Wilmington, Del)
Anesth Analg 77:662–672, 1993   101-94-12–10

Background.—The inotropic drugs amrinone and epinephrine are used during cardiac surgery to reverse myocardial depression after cardiopulmonary bypass. The combination of these drugs may have complementary actions in improving myocardial function.

Methods.—Amrinone, epinephrine, and the combination of the 2 were compared in a randomized, blinded, placebo-controlled study of 40 patients having coronary artery bypass grafting. After bypass separation, 20 patients were given placebo and 20 were given amrinone bolus, 1.5 mg/kg, at time 0. Subsequently, 20 patients were given placebo and 20 were given epinephrine, 30 ng/kg^{-1}/min^{-1}, at 5 minutes.

Findings.—Epinephrine, amrinone, and the combined agents significantly increased cardiac output, stroke volume, oxygen delivery, and left ventricular stroke work. The combined agents increased stroke volume as much as the sum of amrinone and epinephrine given individually. Systemic vascular resistance and pulmonary vascular resistance declined with amrinone and the combined drugs, but not with epinephrine. The mean arterial and pulmonary arterial pressures were increased with epi-

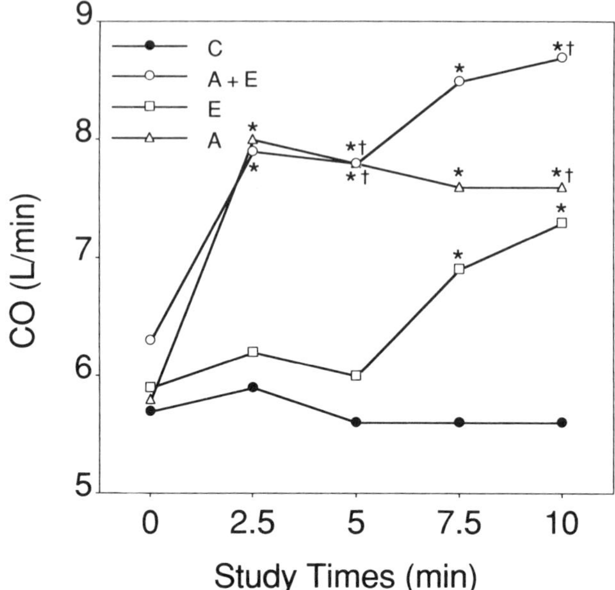

Fig 12–4.—Cardiac output (CO) changes for control (C, placebo), epinephrine (E), amrinone (A), and amrinone + epinephrine (A + E) groups. The *asterisk* denotes all 3 groups significantly increased CO compared with placebo ($P < .05$). The *dagger* denotes A and A + E groups were significantly different from C at 5 minutes and 10 minutes. (Courtesy of Royster RL, Butterworth JF IV, Prielipp RC, et al: *Anesth Analg* 77:662–672, 1993.)

nephrine. Amrinone and the combination but not epinephrine significantly increased right ventricular ejection fraction (Fig 12–4).

Conclusion.—During cardiac surgery, amrinone and epinephrine effectively increase myocardial performance. Right ventricular function was particularly improved with amrinone and the 2 agents combined. The combined effects of amrinone and epinephrine may be of benefit in patients recovering from ischemia and reperfusion injury from coronary artery bypass grafting.

▶ Lots of people think that amrinone has a different mechanism of action than epinephrine. Strictly speaking, this is not so. Epinephrine stimulates adenyl cyclase to generate cyclic adenosine monophosphate (AMP). Cyclic AMP is then the "second messenger" that stimulates or causes the cellular effect. Cyclic AMP is then broken down to AMP by cardiac or other tissue phosphodiesterases. Amrinone is a selective inhibitor of cardiac phosphodiesterase, allowing the second messenger to stay around longer. Therefore, both epinephrine and amrinone are working on the same intracellular mechanism, namely the cyclic AMP second messenger system for catecholamine-related inotropic stimulation. They can be either additive or synergistic. This is so because of the actual receptor for epinephrine itself and the possibility of its "down regulation," plus the peripheral vasodilation often seen with addition of amrinone. Thus, these drugs, when used in combination, may have beneficial effects as described in this paper. It is important, I think, to understand that when used alone, in this situation, amrinone is often a potent peripheral vasodilator. It probably makes the most sense to usually use amrinone with epinephrine, the way the authors have in this study.—J.H. Tinker, M.D.

Myocardial Metabolic and Hemodynamic Changes During Propofol Anesthesia for Cardiac Surgery in Patients With Reduced Ventricular Function

Hall RI, Murphy JT, Landymore R, Pollak PT, Doak G, Murray M (Dalhousie Univ, Halifax, NS, Canada)
Anesth Analg 77:680–689, 1993   101-94-12–11

Background.—Early tracheal extubation may permit some patients to be moved to intermediate care units sooner after cardiac surgery, thus freeing up scarce intensive care unit resources. The use of propofol for inducing and maintaining anesthesia in patients with reduced ejection fraction who are undergoing coronary artery revascularization may not be associated with a higher degree or incidence of myocardial ischemia than a moderate-dose sufentanil-enflurane anesthetic method.

Methods.—By random assignment, 21 patients in group 1 were given propofol, 1–2 mg/kg, as the induction drug and sufentanil, .03 $\mu g/kg^{-1}/min^{-1}$, plus propofol, 50–200 $\mu g/kg^{-1}/min^{-1}$, infusions for anesthesia maintenance. Twenty-one patients in group 2 were given sufentanil, 5 $\mu g/kg$, for induction and infusion of propofol, 50–200 $\mu g/kg^{-1}/min^{-1}$, for maintenance. Eighteen patients in group 3 received sufentanil, 5 $\mu g/kg$, for anesthesia induction and enflurane maintenance.

Findings.—The patients in group 2 had a lower incidence of myocardial lactate production than those in group 3 (Fig 12–5). As surgery progressed, myocardial lactate flux decreased in all groups. Except for the reduction in flux seen in group 3 compared with group 2 after induction, there were no differences between groups. There were also no differences between groups in hemodynamics, inotropic requirements to separate from cardiopulmonary bypass, complications, or changes in laboratory factors before compared with after surgery. Compared with group 1 but not group 3, recovery in group 2 was prolonged.

Conclusion.—The use of propofol in patients with reduced ejection fractions having coronary artery revascularization results in satisfactory anesthetic control of hemodynamics. This method was not associated with an increased incidence or degree of myocardial ischemia.

▶ In the past, physicians have shied away from propofol anesthesia in patients with severe coronary artery disease because of the peripheral dilation that propofol generates and the worry that cardiac hypoperfusion would produce myocardial ischemia or worse. These authors have shown that propofol

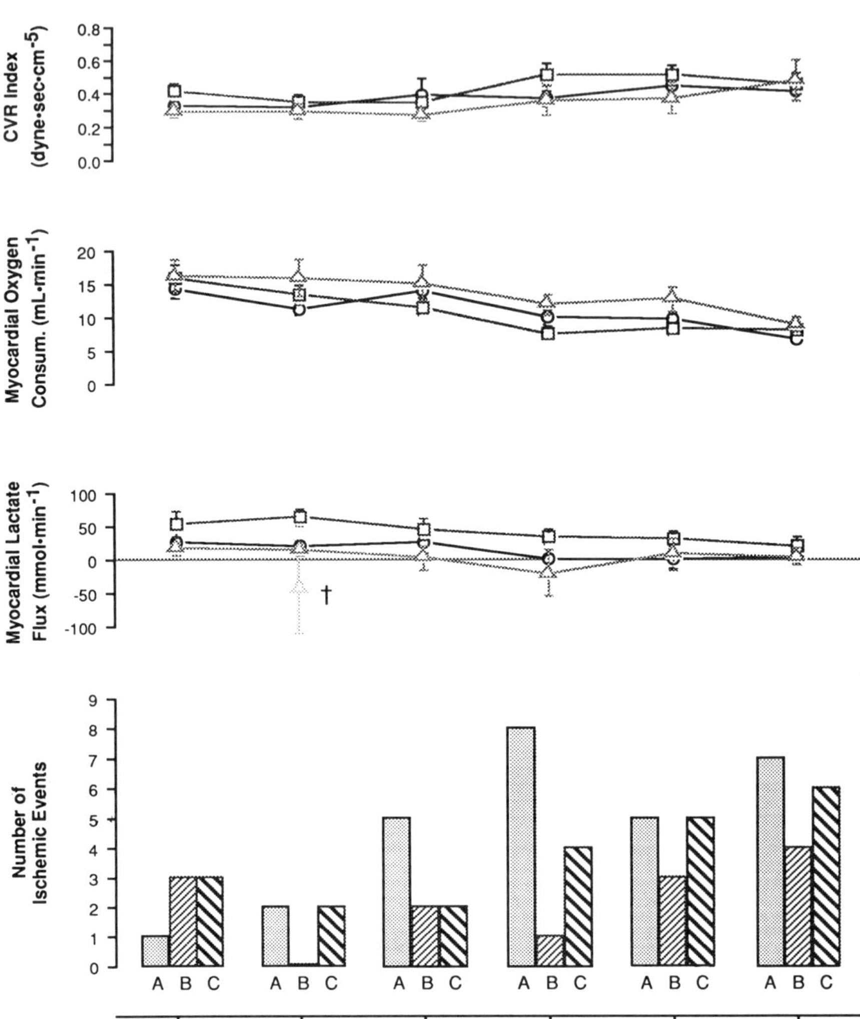

Fig 12–5.—Mean ± SE for coronary vascular resistance index, myocardial oxygen consumption, myocardial lactate flux, and number of events during which myocardial lactate production (e.g., ischemia) was seen at the indicated intraoperative periods. The number of events denotes the number of patients with ischemic indices at the time the measurement was taken. Group A ($n = 21$, *circles*) received propofol for induction of anesthesia, which was maintained with propofol and sufentanil infusions. Group B ($n = 21$, *squares*) received sufentanil for induction of anesthesia, which was maintained with a propofol infusion. Group C ($n = 18$, *triangles*) received sufentanil for induction of anesthesia, which was maintained with enflurane. One patient in group C who had a myocardial infarction during surgery had a myocardial lactate flux of −1,725 mmol/min at induction. When this outlier is included in the mean, the point marked by the *cross* is produced. When it is not included, the more normal value indicated by the *triangle above the error bar* is produced. (Courtesy of Hall RI, Murphy JT, Landymore R, et al: *Anesth Analg* 77:680–689, 1993.)

plus sufentanil can be successfully used to produce cardiac anesthesia, either with or without enflurane added in small amounts. This is not surprising, nor is it the first peripheral vasodilating anesthetic that has been shown to be reasonable for cardiac patients. Remember how terrible isoflurane was supposed to be in these patients? Not so, with good hemodynamic management.—J.H. Tinker, M.D.

Topical Nitroglycerine Prevents the Pressor Response to Tracheal Intubation and Sternotomy in Patients Undergoing Coronary Artery Bypass Graft Surgery
Mahajan RP, Ramachandran R, Saxena N (All India Inst of Med Sciences, New Delhi)
Anaesthesia 48:297–300, 1993   101-94-12–12

Background.—Reflex hypertension and tachycardia are observed at the time of tracheal intubation or midline sternotomy and, in patients with ischemic heart disease, may cause serious problems including myocardial ischemia and left ventricular failure. Nitroglycerin has lessened the pressor response to tracheal intubation in healthy persons having minor surgery.

Study Plan.—Thirty patients aged 40–60 years scheduled for coronary bypass surgery were randomly assigned, in a double-blind manner, to have either 2% nitroglycerin or a placebo ointment applied topically over a 5- × 10-cm area of the forehead 1 hour before induction of anesthesia. The patients were given oral diazepam and intramuscular morphine and promethazine as premedication and were induced with morphine and thiopentone. Anesthesia was maintained with .5% halothane and 40% oxygen in nitrous oxide.

Observations.—The heart rate increased to a similar extent in the nitroglycerin-treated patients and placebo recipients during and after laryngoscopy and after sternotomy. However, the increase in arterial pressure was significantly greater in the placebo patients. All but 3 of 15 control patients required added halothane to control their blood pressure, but this was not the case for any of the patients given nitroglycerin. The rate-pressure product remained significantly lower in the treated patients. No patient had evidence of ischemia or had arrhythmia develop.

Conclusion.—Applying a nitroglycerin ointment to a limited area of skin before anesthetic induction is an effective and safe means of preventing an increase in blood pressure in conjunction with intubation and sternotomy in patients having coronary bypass surgery.

▶ Again, as with the paper by O'Dwyer et al. (Abstract 101-94-12–6), I am critical of comparing a drug with well-known hemodynamic effects against a placebo and coming up with the not-very-surprising conclusion that the drug works better than nothing. Again, the trouble is that we do not know whether preventing these hemodynamic responses makes the slightest difference in the outcome of the patient.—J.H. Tinker, M.D.

CNS Complications and Protection

Brain Protection Via Cerebral Retrograde Perfusion During Aortic Arch Aneurysm Repair

Safi HJ, Brien HW, Winter JN, Thomas AC, Maulsby RL, Doerr HK, Svensson LG (Baylor College of Medicine, Houston; Methodist Hosp, Houston)
Ann Thorac Surg 56:270–276, 1993   101-94-12-13

Introduction.—A safe duration of circulatory arrest has not been established for surgery to correct aneurysms of the ascending aorta and transverse aortic arch. The risk of stroke increases after 45 minutes of cerebral ischemia; the risk of death increases after 65 minutes. Retrograde continuous perfusion (RCP) of the brain via the superior vena cava, as an adjunct to profound hypothermia, has safely extended circulatory arrest time in animals. The degree of cerebral protection provided by RCP in humans was investigated in a prospective study.

Methods.—Retrograde continuous perfusion was administered through the superior vena cava as an adjunct to systemic hypothermia in 11 patients undergoing resection and graft replacement of ascending aortic and aortic arch aneurysms. The systemic circulation was stopped on attainment of an isoelectric electroencephalogram. Superior vena cava pressure was maintained below 25 mm Hg. Blood samples were drawn from the innominate and left carotid arteries after 1 and 5 minutes and, subsequently, at 10-minute intervals; the total creatine kinase and creatine kinase BB fraction were analyzed as possible markers of brain damage.

Results.—All 11 patients survived the procedure; an apparent embolic stroke occurred in 1 patient. All creatine kinase BB levels remained normal throughout surgery; increases observed in the total creatine kinase were attributable to the MM fraction. The cerebral ischemic time ranged from 11 to 71 minutes. The early mean awake time was 4 hours; both patients whose circulatory ischemia exceeded 70 minutes awoke within 6 hours. Vocal cord paralysis, acute renal failure, acute cholecystitis, premature atrial contractions, myasthenia gravis, dysphasia, and atrial fibrillation were the reported postsurgical complications.

Conclusion.—Retrograde continuous perfusion via the superior vena cava appears to be a safe, protective adjunct to hypothermia in repair of transverse aortic arch aneurysm. However, intraoperative cerebral monitoring is necessary because creatine kinase is not a good marker of brain injury. Further study in larger numbers and the development of a reliable marker for brain injury are needed to more clearly define the cerebroprotective role for RCP in repair of transverse aortic arch aneurysm.

▶ This YEAR BOOK OF ANESTHESIOLOGY AND PAIN MANAGEMENT abstract says it all, save that the quality of the surgeon and quality of perfusion cannulation are vitally important. Is there a role for echocardiography to predict smooth takeoffs of the arteries so that cannulation and perfusion can proceed more easily? A lot of answers are needed, but I doubt that anecdotal reports from the group of investigators at Baylor will provide such. Solid science is needed in addition to good surgery if we are to get results that are meaningful to generalize to the rest of the world's population.—M.F. Roizen, M.D.

Central Nervous System Complications After Cardiac Surgery: A Comparison Between Coronary Artery Bypass Grafting and Valve Surgery

Kuroda Y, Uchimoto R, Kaieda R, Shinkura R, Shinohara K, Miyamoto S, Oshita S, Takeshita H (Yamaguchi Univ Hosp, Japan; Kokura Mem Hosp, Kitakyushu, Fukuoka, Japan)
Anesth Analg 76:222–227, 1993   101-94-12–14

Objective.—The frequency of CNS complications was determined in 638 patients undergoing coronary bypass graft surgery and in 345 having cardiac valve operations in 1985–1989.

Management.—When ventricular function was adequate, anesthesia was induced with fentanyl and also thiamylal. Anesthesia was maintained with nitrous oxide and, if needed, halothane or enflurane. A median sternotomy was used in all cases. Bubble oxygenators were used in patients aged 65 years and younger; membrane oxygenators were used in older patients and if a bypass time exceeding 3 hours was expected. Perfusion flow rates were maintained at 2.2–2.6 L/min/m², and perfusion pressures were maintained at 40–90 mm Hg.

Results.—Complications of the CNS developed in 11% of patients having bypass surgery and in 7% of the group having valve surgery. Both preexisting cerebrovascular disease and prolonged cardiopulmonary bypass predisposed to CNS complications. The most frequent complications were disturbed consciousness, seizures, and focal motor deficits.

Discussion.—Complications of the CNS occur significantly more often in the setting of coronary bypass surgery than in valve surgery. Existing cerebrovascular disease and a prolonged bypass time most likely increase the risk of cerebral embolism or cerebral hypoperfusion. Measures for minimizing the risk of embolism, new methods of protecting the brain, and shorter cardiopulmonary bypass times will hopefully lower the risk of CNS complications.

▶ Most anesthesiologists would opine that neurologic complications after cardiopulmonary bypass should be more common after valvular surgery than after coronary bypass. Indeed, the older literature indicated that that was so. More recent prospective studies of barbiturate "protection" during cardiopulmonary bypass used patients undergoing valvular surgery, because the authors believed that these patients were at greatest risk. Now comes this elegant study from Japan that calls into question the idea that patients undergoing valvular surgery are the worst risks for neurologic dysfunction. When you think about it, it makes sense that today's patients undergoing coronary artery bypass graft surgery, who are often very old with diabetes and extensive atherosclerosis, may be at great risk. The coronary bypass patients we are doing today are clearly not the same kinds of patients we did just a few years ago. The idea that coronary bypass is "routine" must now be rethought.—J.H. Tinker, M.D.

Myocardial Ischemia

Intraoperative Hemodynamic Changes Are Not Good Indicators of Myocardial Ischemia

Urban MK, Gordon MA, Harris SN, O'Connor T, Barash PG (Yale Univ, New Haven, Conn)
Anesth Analg 76:942–949, 1993   101-94-12–15

Introduction.—Patients having coronary bypass surgery in whom myocardial ischemia develops during surgery are at risk of perioperative myocardial infarction. If physiologic indicators of ischemia could be found, it might be possible to institute treatment early enough to prevent cardiac morbidity.

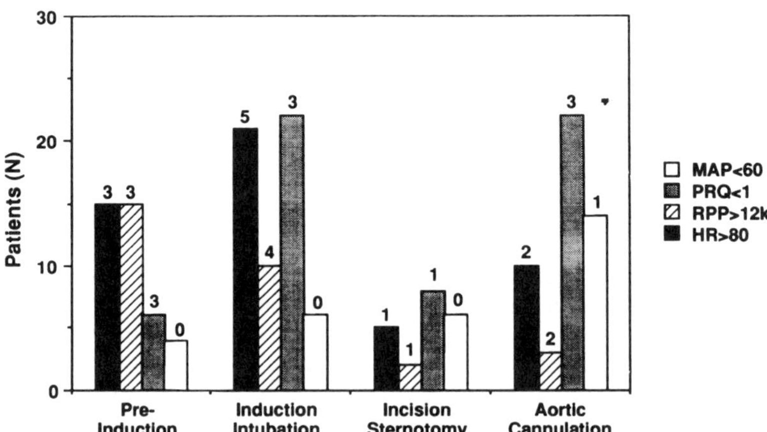

Fig 12–6.—*Abbreviations: MAP*, mean arterial blood pressure; *PRQ*, pressure rate quotient; *RPP*, rate pressure product; *HR*, heart rate. Number of patients exhibiting hemodynamic variables suggestive of myocardial ischemia at various anesthetic or surgical periods before cardiopulmonary bypass. *Numbers above the bars* represent the number of ischemic patients at each surgical period with that particular hemodynamic variable. (Courtesy of Urban MK, Gordon MA, Harris SN, et al: *Anesth Analg* 76:942-949, 1993.)

Objective.—The relationships among fixed cardiac risk factors, reversible intraoperative hemodynamic variables, myocardial ischemia, and perioperative infarction were examined prospectively in 100 consecutive patients having elective coronary bypass surgery. Ischemia was defined as new ST-segment deviation of 1 mm or more from the baseline ECG that lasted at least 2 minutes.

Results.—Intraoperative myocardial ischemia developed in 16 patients before the onset of cardiopulmonary bypass. Of the 5 patients who were ischemic on arrival at the operating room, 2 responded to treatment. Only 1 patient had further ischemia after the initial episode, and, in most cases, ischemia lasted less than 10 minutes. Nitroglycerin and esmolol were administered as needed. Most hemodynamic events occurred at the same time as most ischemic events—during anesthetic induction and aortic cannulation (Fig 12–6). No hemodynamic index was highly predictive of myocardial ischemia, but all had a high negative predictive value. No significant association was evident between prebypass ischemia and any fixed cardiac risk factors. Nine of the 100 patients sustained perioperative myocardial infarction, which in 4 cases was transmural. Infarction occurred in 4 of the 16 patients with prebypass ischemia and in 6% of those without ischemia. Prebypass ischemia on the ECG was the only significant correlate of perioperative infarction.

Conclusion.—This study failed to identify a sensitive, clinically convenient hemodynamic indicator of myocardial ischemia in patients having coronary bypass surgery.

▶ In the movie "Casablanca," the police chief orders, "Haul out the usual suspects." In this paper, the authors studied "the usual suspects," namely tachycardia, hypertension, elevated pulmonary artery diastolic pressures, and elevated rate pressure products. None of these hemodynamic occurrences accurately predicted either the incidence or the severity of myocardial ischemia or perioperative myocardial infarction. Whether or not this is because these hemodynamic perturbations were generally rapidly treated is the question I must ask of this work. Certainly these perturbations were not left untreated, so we cannot know whether any of them would lead to myocardial ischemia or perioperative myocardial infarction had they been left untouched.—J.H. Tinker, M.D.

Coronary Artery Bypass in Patients With Severely Depressed Ventricular Function

Milano CA, White WD, Smith LR, Jones RH, Lowe JE, Smith PK, Van Trigt III P (Duke Univ, Durham, NC)
Ann Thorac Surg 56:487–493, 1993   101-94-12–16

Background.—Patients with coronary artery disease (CAD) and severe generalized left ventricular dysfunction have been at increased risk for operative mortality when undergoing coronary artery bypass grafting

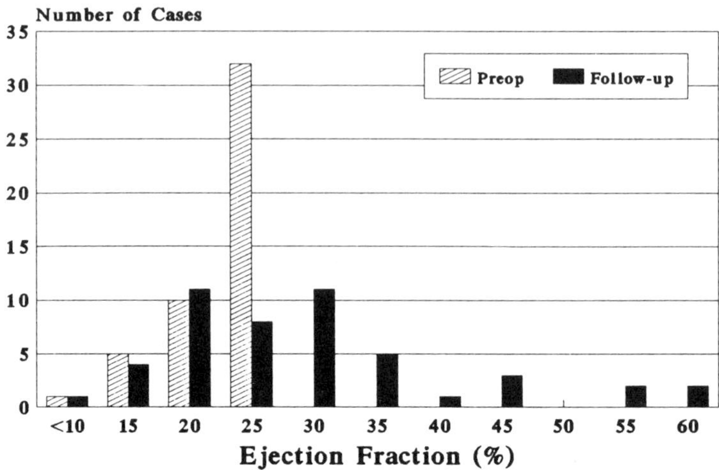

Fig 12–7.—Distribution of preoperative and follow-up EFs in 48 survivors. Preoperative vs. follow-up: $P < .003$ by paired t-test. (Courtesy of Milano CA, White WD, Smith LR, et al: *Ann Thorac Surg* 56:487–493, 1993.)

(CABG). However, improvements in this procedure suggest that such patients may now benefit from bypass. The results of CABG in patients with an ejection fraction (EF) of .25 or less during 10 years were examined and survival after CABG was compared with the estimated survival with medical therapy alone.

Methods.—From 1981 to 1991, 118 patients with a preoperative EF ≤.25 underwent CABG at Duke University Medical Center, Durham, North Carolina. All but 2 patients were available for evaluation; the median duration of follow-up was 26.5 months. The medical records of these patients were examined for 22 preoperative and operative variables. Survival estimates for medical therapy alone were calculated from data of patients who had received cardiac catheterization and treatment for CAD between 1970 and 1985.

Results.—The patient group was predominantly male (105 of 118); 64% were aged 60 years or older, 58% had hypertension, and 61.5% had recent myocardial infarction. Twelve patients died in the hospital, and 1 died after discharge but within 30 days of surgery. Survivors were hospitalized for a median of 9 days. The most common postoperative complications were ventricular arrhythmia requiring treatment (27%) and low cardiac output state (22%). The Kaplan-Meier estimates of survival at 1 year and 5 years, 77.2% and 57.5%, respectively, were better than the estimated survival with medical therapy alone. Patients who survived had significant improvement in angina class, congestive failure class, and follow-up EF (Fig 12–7). A multivariate Cox model showed 3 variables associated with increased mortality: time on cardiopulmonary bypass, acute presentation, and female sex.

Review of the Literature for CAD Patients With Severely Reduced EF Treated With CABG

First Author	No. of Patients	Years	EF	30-Day Mortality	Late Mortality
Vlietstra	10	1966–72	<0.25		60% (2 y)
Manley	183	1968–71	mean 0.22	16.0%	43% (5 y)
Yatteau	24	1968–72	<0.25	42.0%	50% (2 y)
Oldham	11	1969–72	≤0.25	55.0%	
Zubiate	140	1969–75	<0.20	22.0%	41% (6 y)
Faulkner	46	1969–75	mean 0.21	4.0%	17% (2 y)
Mitchel	9		<0.20	0.0%	11% (1 y)
Fox	7	1971–74	<0.20	0.0%	14%
Jones	41	1973–77	<0.20	2.5%	10% (1 y)
Alderman	82	1975–79	≤0.25	8.0%	37% (5 y)
Mochtar	62	1975–83	mean 0.25	4.8%	30% (5 y)
Zubiate	93	1976–81	<0.20	5.0%	50% (5 y)
Hochberg	51	1976–82	0.20–0.24	12.0%	42% (3 y)
Hochberg	41	1976–82	<0.20	37.0%	85% (3 y)
Sanchez	23	1982–89	mean 0.28	9.0%	24% (2 y)
Kron	39	1983–88	<0.20	2.6%	17% (3 y)
Blakeman	20	1984–88	mean 0.18	15.0%	30% (1 y)
Wong	22	1986–89	mean 0.25	9.0%	23% (3 y)
Christakis	487	1982–90	<0.20	9.8%	
Hammermeister	251	1987–90	<0.20	9.2%	

(Courtesy of Milano CA, White WD, Smith LR, et al: *Ann Thorac Surg* 56:487–493, 1993.)

Conclusion.—Patients with CAD and severely depressed ventricular function benefit from CABG. In an evaluation of the literature (table), more recent studies show that such patients have an operative mortality of approximately 10% and that surgical treatment offers improved survival relative to medical therapy. With attention to preoperative risk factors and careful patient selection, CABG may be offered to patients with very low EFs.

▶ Past dogma has dictated that patients with severely depressed myocardial function, i.e., EF less than 25%, have not benefited from the standpoint of longevity or quality of life from CABG surgery. In this study, despite the operative mortality of 11%, the overall survival does seem to have been improved by coronary bypass surgery. On the other hand, the "control group" was not really more than a computer estimate of survival with medical therapy alone. Nonetheless, I included it because the table is an extensive compilation of the literature on this subject. I also included it because surgeons are still reporting these kinds of studies, with no valid control group, to justify their operations in 1993.—J.H. Tinker, M.D.

Effects of Steal-Prone Anatomy on Intraoperative Myocardial Ischemia

Leung JM, Hollenberg M, O'Kelly BF, Kao A, Mangano DT, the Study of Perioperative Ischemia Research Group (Univ of California, San Francisco)
J Am Coll Cardiol 20:1205–1212, 1992   101-94-12–17

Background.—Coronary steal occurs when blood flow to the nonischemic myocardium increases at the expense of collateral flow to ischemic regions. Patients with total occlusion of a coronary vessel that is supplied distally by collaterals from a significantly stenosed artery are said to have "steal-prone" anatomy and may be at risk of intraoperative myocardial ischemia when the anesthetic used has vasodilator properties.

Objective.—The risk of myocardial ischemia was examined in relation to the coronary artery anatomy in 186 patients who were scheduled for elective coronary bypass surgery with isoflurane or sufentanil anesthesia. Myocardial wall motion was assessed by transesophageal echocardiography.

Findings.—Hemodynamic status was quite stable during bypass surgery. At least 1 major coronary artery was totally occluded in 103 patients, and 62 of them had steal-prone anatomy. About half these patients had collaterals supplied by a coronary artery that was at least 90% stenosed. Myocardial ischemia was similarly frequent in patients with and without steal-prone anatomy and also in those given isoflurane and sufentanil anesthesia. In both anesthetic groups, roughly one third of the patients with steal-prone anatomy had evidence of ischemia. The concentration of isoflurane was not a risk factor. Eight percent of the pa-

Surgical and Outcome Data in 186 Patients

	Patients With Steal-Prone Coronary Anatomy (n = 62)	Patients Without Steal-Prone Coronary Anatomy (n = 124)
Surgical data		
Grafted vessels		
No.	3	3
Range	1 to 5	1 to 5
Aortic cross-clamp time (min)	57 ± 16	60 ± 17
Cardiopulmonary bypass time (min)	97 ± 27	106 ± 31
Surgical assessment		
Grade 4 (excellent)	18 (32)	24 (21)
Grade 3 (good)	25 (45)	61 (52)
Grade 2 (fair)	12 (21)	30 (26)
Grade 1 (poor)	1 (2)	2 (2)
Outcome data		
Myocardial infarction	3 (5)	8 (6)
Ventricular failure	1 (2)	3 (2)
Cardiac death	1 (2)	3 (2)
Total outcome	5 (8)	14 (11)

Note: Data are expressed as mean value ± 1 SD or number (%) of patients in each subgroup.

(Courtesy of Leung JM, Hollenberg M, O'Kelly BF, et al: *J Am Coll Cardiol* 20:1205–1212, 1992.)

tients with steal-prone anatomy and 11% of the others had an adverse cardiac outcome (table).

Conclusion.—Under conditions of hemodynamic stability, a steal-prone coronary artery anatomy does not increase the risk of intraoperative myocardial ischemia or that of an adverse cardiac outcome after coronary bypass surgery. In addition, the use of an anesthetic with vasodilator properties, such as isoflurane, is not a risk factor.

▶ The term steal-prone anatomy is a buzzword, no more than that. It is sort of like a slogan, e.g., "Live free or die." Just like most slogans, although it may have some emotional "logic," it has no real validity. Steal-prone anatomy is really anatomy that bears resemblance to the experimental anatomy created by Becker in 1978 in his original report (1) on the production of coronary steal in dogs. This elegant paper exists because of our propensity to create buzzwords and "straw men."—J.H. Tinker, M.D.

Reference

1. Becker LC: *Circulation* 57:1103, 1978.

Early Extubation After Cardiac Surgery

Early Extubation of the Trachea After Repair of Secundum-Type Atrial Septal Defects in Children
Burrows FA, Taylor RH, Hillier SC (Univ of Toronto)
Can J Anaesth 39:1041–1044, 1992   101-94-12–18

Introduction.—The results of early tracheal extubation were examined in 36 children having surgical closure of an isolated secundum-type atrial septal defect.

Study Design.—All children in the study were classified as American Society of Anesthesiologists physical status II. Nineteen children were extubated immediately after surgery, whereas 17 remained intubated and had their lungs ventilated in the intensive care unit. The former group received humidified oxygen by open-face mask to maintain the partial pressure of oxygen in arterial blood at 80 mm Hg or less. The groups were similar in age and body weight, but those having early extubation were on cardiopulmonary bypass for a shorter time. Aortic cross-clamp times were comparable. The total dose of fentanyl was lower in the early extubation group.

Results.—Hemodynamic function remained adequate in both groups. There were no contraindications to early extubation in any case. Children having early extubation had lower arterial pH values and a higher partial pressure of carbon dioxide in arterial blood values than those who remained intubated. Morphine requirements were less for the extubated patients, and they were discharged earlier from the intensive care unit. No child required reintubation of the trachea.

Conclusion.—Selected children may be safely extubated immediately after cardiac surgery as long as close monitoring is assured and facilities for cardiorespiratory support are available.

▶ For some reason, in cardiac anesthesia, the time of extubation of the trachea has undergone many cycles. Just after halothane was introduced, early extubation of the trachea was routine. Then we went through the long period of "large-dose narcotics," which necessitated longer times to extubation. Some individuals believed that "resting the lungs" by paralysis and ventilation overnight somehow made things better. Now we are in a new cycle when early extubation is popular again. Some of this popularity is undoubtedly related to economics, but, from the standpoint of physiology, quite frankly, it makes an enormous amount of sense (and always did).—J.H. Tinker, M.D.

Cardioplegia

Warm Versus Cold Blood Cardioplegia—Is There a Difference?
Matsuura H, Lazar HL, Yang X, Rivers S, Treanor P, Bernard S, Shemin RJ

(Boston Univ)
J Thorac Cardiovasc Surg 105:45–51, 1993   101-94-12–19

Background.—Although cold blood cardioplegia allows safe, reliable myocardial protection and optimal visualization of the operative field in cardiac operations, it can result in periods of ischemia and subsequent reperfusion injury. The alternative—warm blood cardioplegia—avoids ischemia, but it can reduce visualization, and the safe period for its interruption is unknown. No prospective studies have compared warm with cold blood cardioplegia.

Methods.—Experiments in pigs were conducted to compare the effectiveness of the 2 techniques of cardioplegia in protecting areas of ischemic myocardium during urgent coronary revascularization. Forty pigs underwent snare occlusion of the second and third diagonal vessels for 90 minutes. The snares were released during the subsequent 3 hours of reperfusion. The pigs received 4 different treatments during cardioplegic arrest. One group received antegrade continuous warm blood cardioplegic solution at 100 mL/min, 1 group received retrograde warm blood cardioplegic solution at the same rate, 1 group received intermittent antegrade cold blood cardioplegic solution, and 1 group received intermittent antegrade/retrograde cold blood cardioplegic solution.

Results.—The pH values in the area at risk were lowest with antegrade warm blood cardioplegia, 6.59, and highest with antegrade/retrograde cold blood cardioplegia, 6.85. The area of necrosis was also highest with antegrade warm blood cardioplegia, 42%, compared with 21% with antegrade/retrograde cold blood cardioplegia.

Conclusion.—This animal model of acute coronary occlusion with ischemic myocardium suggests that warm blood cardioplegic solution should be given in a continuous retrograde fashion. Still, this technique does not improve protection over that achieved with antegrade/retrograde cold blood cardioplegia. Adequate distribution of the cardioplegic solution appears to be more important than its temperature in achieving optimal myocardial protection.

▶ I included this paper because our readers should be aware that there still is controversy about cardioplegia, warm vs. cold, antigrade vs. retrograde, not to mention the composition, e.g., toad bladder extract and powdered bat wings. If I seem a little cynical about cardioplegia, I am.

One last point. For our readers who do not understand "retrograde" cardioplegia, it has been known since World War II that it is possible to perfuse some areas of myocardium by turning the veins into arteries and allowing the blood or other substances to flow "backward" in the veins. This can be done because the veins of the heart are valveless, and, amazingly enough, capillary perfusion does occur, presumably because there are capillary-venule connections to thebesian venous drainage into both ventricles. It is certainly possible to perfuse a beating heart via its venous system only and observe almost no change in ventricular function (I have done it for more than 5 hours in a pig). This is why cardiac surgeons use "retrograde" as well as "antigrade" cardioplegia.—J.H. Tinker, M.D.

13 Cardiopulmonary Bypass

Extracorporeal Life Support for Pediatric Respiratory Failure: Predictors of Survival From 220 Patients
Moler FW, Palmisano J, Custer JR (Univ of Michigan Hosps, Ann Arbor)
Crit Care Med 21:1604–1611, 1993   101-94-13-1

Background.—Extracorporeal life support for pulmonary support is effective in the pediatric neonatal population, with an overall cumulative survival rate for all respiratory diagnoses of 83%. The efficacy of extracorporeal life support in the nonneonatal pediatric population was evaluated.

Study Design.—Using the data base of the Extracorporeal Life Support Organization, a retrospective cohort study was conducted of all pediatric patients between 1 month and 18 years of age who received either venoarterial or venovenous extracorporeal life support for severe life-threatening pulmonary failure as of August of 1991. Patients with congenital heart disease and congenital gastrointestinal malformations were excluded.

Findings.—Of the 220 pediatric patients, 46% survived to hospital discharge; 56% of those who were treated after 1989 survived. The mean patient age was 36.8 months. The mean duration of mechanical support before extracorporeal life support was 6.3 days, and the mean duration of extracorporeal life support was 247 hours. For the 102 survivors, the mean time for decannulation from extracorporeal life support to extubation from mechanical ventilation was 6.5 days. The univariate analysis indicated that older patients, more days of mechanical ventilation before extracorporeal life, poorer oxygenation status, greater mechanical ventilation airway pressures, and early experience with the extracorporeal life support were significantly associated with a poorer prognosis. Stepwise logistic regression modeling identified 5 variables that were predictive of survival: age, duration of mechanical ventilation before extracorporeal life support, peak inspiratory pressure, alveolar-arterial oxygen gradient, and extracorporeal life support administered since December 31, 1988, were significant predictors of outcome.

Conclusion.—Extracorporeal life support may provide an effective rescue therapy for selected pediatric patients with severe respiratory failure who fail to improve with conventional mechanical ventilation support. By using patient age, duration of mechanical ventilation before extracorporeal life support, the degree of oxygen impairment, and amount of ventilation pressure required for ventilation, the probability of survival with extracorporeal life support can be estimated and may prove useful for individual prognostication and future prospective research.

▶ This retrospective study underwent a thorough statistical analysis to define predictors of survival in pediatric patients undergoing extracorporeal life support. One has to wonder, however, whether patients who were younger, with better oxygenation, lower airway pressures, and fewer days on mechanical ventilation would have done equally well with only conventional therapy. The answer to this question poses a significant dilemma when considering the application of these predictive variables to a large, multicenter, prospective clinical trial.—D.M. Rothenberg, M.D.

Effect of Acid-Base Management With or Without Carbon Dioxide on Plasma Phosphate Concentration During and After Hypothermic Cardiopulmonary Bypass

Kancir CB, Madsen T (Odense Univ, Denmark)
Scand J Thorac Cardiovasc Surg 26:151–155, 1992   101-94-13-2

Introduction.—The best way to manage acid-base status during hypothermic cardiopulmonary bypass remains uncertain. Some favor correcting blood gas readings for the patient's temperature to maintaining the arterial pH at 7.4. Because phosphate is the primary intracellular anion and critical to cellular energy metabolism, changes in plasma phosphate were compared in cardiac surgery patients undergoing hypothermic bypass who were managed by either the pH-stat or the alpha-stat method. The latter technique is designed to maintain ionization of the alpha-imidazole group of histidine, thereby preserving the intracellular milieu.

Study Plan.—Twenty-four patients who were scheduled for heart surgery with cardiopulmonary bypass were anesthetized with etomidate, fentanyl, and pancuronium. Bypass was instituted under generalized hypothermia. In the alpha-stat group, the oxygenator gas flow was adjusted to maintain a partial pressure of carbon dioxide in arterial blood ($PaCO_2$) of 40 mm Hg, as measured at 37°C. In the pH-stat group, carbon dioxide (CO_2) was added to the oxygenator gas mixture to maintain a $PaCO_2$ of 40 mm Hg when corrected for body temperature.

Results.—The pH declined significantly shortly after the start of perfusion (Fig 13–1). When the blood gases were analyzed at 37°C, the pH-stat patients were more acidic than the alpha-stat group during hypothermic bypass. The pH was lowest when the patients were most hypothermic, just before rewarming. The $PaCO_2$ remained much higher in the pH-stat group throughout the bypass period. Plasma phosphate levels decreased initially and then gradually increased, reaching higher levels in the pH-stat group at the end of perfusion (Fig 13–2). Values continued to increase in the alpha-stat group in the post-bypass period. Patients in

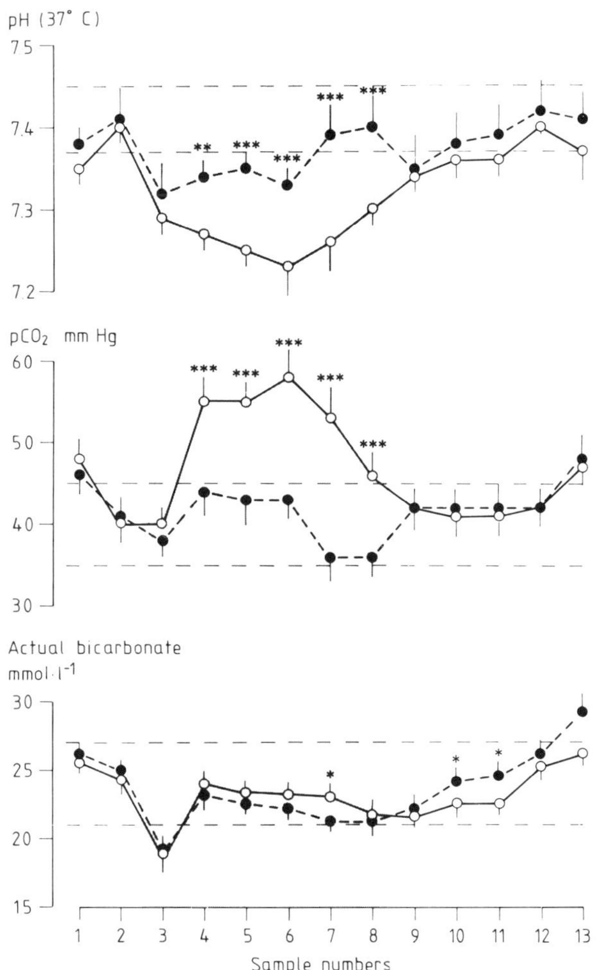

Fig 13–1.—Arterial pH, pCO$_2$, and actual bicarbonate values during and after hypothermic cardiopulmonary bypass in alpha-stat (*filled circles*) and pH-stat (*open circles*) patients. *Vertical line* at each sample represents 90% confidence for the mean. *Area between the horizontal dashed lines* is the reference interval. (* P < .05, ** P < .01, *** P < .001 between the 2 groups.) (Courtesy of Kancir CB, Madsen T: *Scand J Thorac Cardiovasc Surg* 26:151–155, 1992.)

both groups were slightly hypophosphatemic on the first postoperative day.

Conclusion.—Acid-base management may influence phosphate homeostasis in patients who undergo cardiac surgery under hypothermic

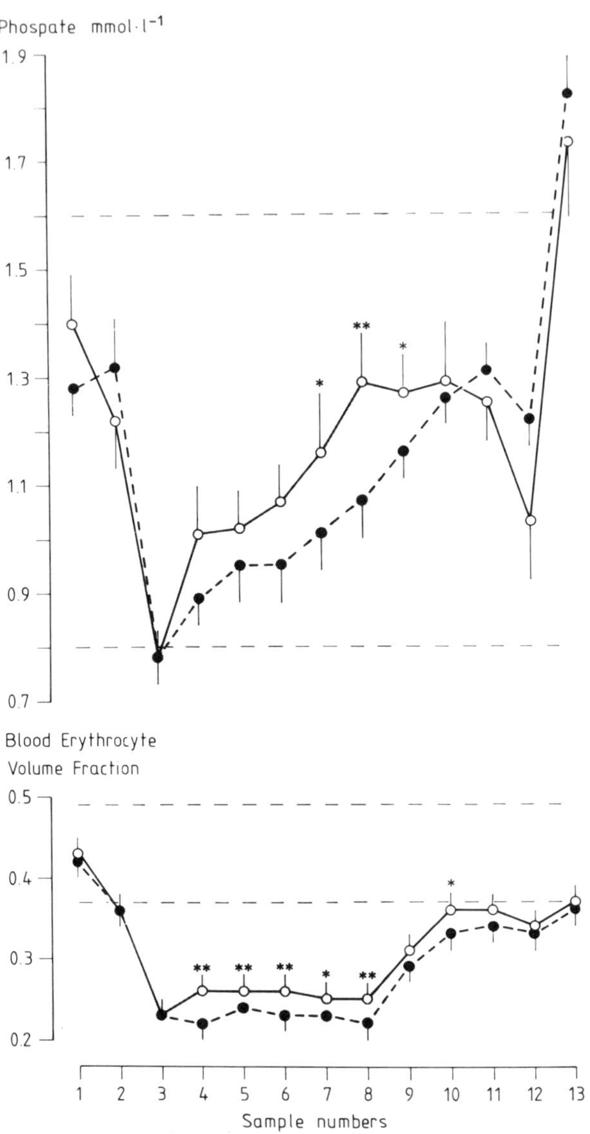

Fig 13–2.—Plasma phosphate and blood erythrocyte volume fraction levels during and after cardiopulmonary bypass in alpha-stat (*filled circles*) and pH-stat (*open circles*) patients. *Vertical line* at each sample represents 90% confidence for the mean. *Area between the horizontal dashed lines* is the reference interval. (* P < .05, ** P < .01, *** P < .001 between the 2 groups.) (Courtesy of Kancir CB, Madsen T: *Scand J Thorac Cardiovasc Surg* 26:151–155, 1992.)

bypass. Different phosphate patterns may relate to the varying effects of adding CO_2 and respiratory acidosis on cellular metabolism.

▶ After reading this paper carefully, I am not so sure whether the phosphate balance that occurred in the pH-stat patients vs. that which occurred in the alpha-stat patients was better or worse; all I can say is that it was different. Although alpha-stat cardiopulmonary bypass management has now mostly supplanted pH-stat, we still are not sure whether that move was clinically important or resulted in clinical improvement. The most recent studies from animal models at hypothermia have not shown that there really is very much difference in terms of cerebral blood flow or metabolism or distribution of cerebral blood flow and metabolism between these 2 methods. However, this study showed at least 1 difference that perhaps will prove interesting: a difference in phosphate metabolism. At the moment, I do not know how to interpret this finding.—J.H. Tinker, M.D.

Barbiturates Impair Cerebral Metabolism During Hypothermic Circulatory Arrest

Siegman MG, Anderson RV, Balaban RS, Ceckler TL, Clark RE, Swain JA (Natl Heart, Lung, and Blood Inst, Bethesda, Md; Allegheny Singer Hosp, Pittsburgh, Pa; Univ of Nevada, Las Vegas)
Ann Thorac Surg 54:1131–1136, 1992   101-94-13–3

Background.—Barbiturate administration can reduce the neuropsychiatric complications of intracardiac surgery. Phosphorus-31 nuclear magnetic resonance (NMR) spectroscopy was used to determine the effects of barbiturates on cerebral tissue energy state during cardiopulmonary bypass, hypothermic circulatory arrest, and reperfusion.

Methods.—A 4.7-T magnet was used to obtain NMR spectra from sheep at 37°C, during bypass before and after drug administration at 37°C and 15°C, throughout 1 hour of hypothermic circulatory arrest, and during 2 hours of reperfusion. Eight animals received a 40-mg bolus of sodium thiopental per kg during bypass at 37°C. Thiopental infusion was continued at a rate of 3.3 $mg/kg^{-1}/min^{-1}$ until the animals went into hypothermic circulatory arrest; another 8 animals received no barbiturate.

Findings.—The barbiturate-treated animals had a lower tissue energy state than the control animals, as reflected by phosphocreatine/adenosine triphosphate ratio, during cardiopulmonary bypass at 15°C. Throughout all periods of arrest and reperfusion, phosphocreatine/ adenosine triphosphate ratios were lower in the barbiturate group. The cerebral energy state typically seen in hypothermia was prevented by thiopental, leading to a decreased energy state during hypothermic arrest and subsequent reperfusion.

Conclusion.—Giving thiopental before inducing hypothermic circulatory arrest is not cerebroprotective and may even have an adverse effect on the energy state of the brain, possibly by inhibition of glycolysis. These results warrant reevaluation of the use of systemic hypothermia for patients undergoing surgical procedures associated with cerebral ischemia.

▶ The authors believe that preservation of the cerebral energy state is crucial to cerebral protection and, because thiopental does not allow the normal increase seen in cerebral energy state during hypothermia, they have somehow concluded that it may therefore not be a cerebral protectant. We have previously operated under the assumption that increasing cerebral energy states simply enabled faster deterioration to occur when there was a limited availability of substrates. At first glance, this article seems to be at variance with much of the previous work of Michenfelder and many others. Although I do not think it is really inconsistent, the article's conclusion, which goes against barbiturates, is not really warranted by the data. Barbiturates prevent the increase in cerebral energy state. Whether that is good or bad is debatable, based on this study, but it is probably good because of the number of previous studies that have shown functional correlations.—J.H. Tinker, M.D.

Hyperbaric Oxygenation for Arterial Air Embolism During Cardiopulmonary Bypass

Kol S, Ammar R, Weisz G, Melamed Y (Carmel Lady Davis Hosp, Haifa, Israel)
Ann Thorac Surg 55:401–403, 1993   101-94-13-4

Introduction.—Arterial air embolisms that occur during cardiopulmonary bypass can lead to serious brain damage and death. Although retrograde perfusion has been proposed as a means of reducing the amount of air obstructing cerebral vessels, only half the gas has been recovered in this way in an animal model.

Series.—The value of hyperbaric oxygenation was examined in 6 patients who were referred with an arterial air embolism that complicated cardiopulmonary bypass. Four of the patients had undergone coronary bypass graft surgery, whereas 1 each had undergone closure of an atrial septal defect and aortic valve replacement. The patients were treated in a large multiplace hyperbaric chamber.

Outcomes.—Both patients who began hyperbaric oxygen therapy within 2–3 hours of the event recovered completely. When treatment was delayed to see how the embolism was influencing recovery, 2 of 4 patients died, and 1 was left with severe neurologic impairment. The remaining patient had a mild motor deficit that affected 1 leg.

Conclusion.—A massive arterial air embolism calls for the immediate institution of hyperbaric oxygen therapy, even before neurologic signs of cerebral ischemia appear.

▶ We also saw such a case recently, and we have a hyperbaric chamber in our institution. The results in terms of decreasing the overall content of cerebral air, as measured by scanning, were truly remarkable. Of course, each of these cases is an "$n = 1$," because there is no control group in which the exact same volume and distribution of air has not been treated by hyperbaric oxygen. However, anecdotal evidence in this paper and others indicates that hyperbaric oxygen therapy for intracerebral air that is created during cardiopulmonary bypass or another procedure is effective.—J.H. Tinker, M.D.

Hydroxyethyl Starch as a Prime for Cardiopulmonary Bypass: Effects of Two Different Solutions on Haemostasis

Kuitunen A, Hynynen M, Salmenperä M, Heinonen J, Vahtera E, Verkkala K, Myllylä G (Helsinki Univ Central Hosp; Finnish Red Cross Transfusion Service, Helsinki)
Acta Anaesthesiol Scand 37:652–658, 1993   101-94-13–5

Introduction.—Hydroxyethyl starch (HES), although it is an effective expander of intravascular volume, may have adverse effects on hemostasis. If large doses of HES solutions are administered rapidly to the patient, as when priming for a cardiopulmonary bypass (CPB), the effect may be clinically significant. Whether a low-molecular-weight (LMW) solution would have less of an effect on coagulation than a high-molecular-weight (HMW) solution was determined in patients undergoing coronary artery bypass grafting (CABG).

Methods.—Eligible patients included those without a history of cardiac surgery and coagulation disorders. Forty-five such patients undergoing CABG were prospectively randomized to receive Ringer's acetate, 2,000 mL; a LMW HES preparation (LMW-HES); or an HMW HES preparation (HMW-HES) as their CPB prime. The final volume of the prime was completed to 2,000 mL with Ringer's acetate in the HES groups. The 3 groups were comparable in preoperative characteristics, operative data, and coagulation parameters at baseline.

Results.—During and after CPB, the hematocrit was slightly lower in both HES groups than in the Ringer's group. Both HES groups had a significantly lower serum total-protein level than the Ringer's group in all samples that were obtained after the start of CPB. One hour after CPB, there was a tendency for plasma fibrinogen level to be lower in the HMW-HES group than in the Ringer's group. Compared with the Ringer's group, plasma levels of von Willebrand's factor antigen and factor VIII procoagulant activity were significantly more depressed after CPB in both HES groups; the activated partial thromboplastin time was more prolonged; and the maximal amplitude of thromboelastographic tracing was more decreased in the HES groups.

Conclusion.—The LMW and HMW HES solutions impaired hemostatic parameters in a similar manner. Because HES can alter platelet function, the platelet defect resulting from CPB itself may be worsened by adding HES to the priming solution of the CPB circuit. Use of the HES solution can also increase the fibrinolysis-induced bleeding tendency in cardiac surgical patients. Use of HES solutions should be avoided in the CPB prime, especially in patients at increased risk for bleeding.

▶ I included this article from 1993 to emphasize that the literature often reviews things we thought we knew. I thought we had pretty well decided that the different HES solutions had various anticoagulant effects. Apparently, their relative inexpensiveness has led the authors to entertain again the possibility that these solutions might be reasonable to use in priming for CPB. However, they once again discovered that at least from the standpoint of bleeding after cardiac operations, these solutions are not ideal.—J.H. Tinker, M.D.

14 Anesthesia for Vascular Procedures

Myocardial Infarction After Reconstruction of the Abdominal Aorta
Kalra M, Charlesworth D, Morris JA, Al-Khaffaf H (Withington Hosp, Manchester, England)
Br J Surg 80:28–31, 1993   101-94-14-1

Background.—Although it is reasonable to screen all patients awaiting for surgery on aortic abdominal aneurysm for ischemic heart disease, it is not clear which measures of myocardial function to use. One approach is to select patients for more advanced tests on the basis of the clinical data and ECG findings, but which clinical factors signify an increased risk of postoperative myocardial infarction must be known.

Objective.—Risk factors that dispose to cardiac complications were sought in 555 patients who had either elective or urgent reconstruction of the abdominal aorta, e.g., symptomatic aneurysm or pregangrenous changes. An attempt was made to maintain the blood pressure throughout surgery; to minimize operating time, particularly clamp time; and to limit the loss of blood.

Results.—Thirty-five patients (6.3%) had perioperative myocardial infarction develop, and 12 of them (2.2%) died. Multiple logistic regression analysis identified 4 preoperative factors that independently predicted postoperative infarction: history of transient ischemic attacks, elevated serum creatinine, age older than 60 years, and angina necessitating regular treatment. A scoring system based on these factors identified 150 patients who were at high risk of perioperative infarction, including 69% of the patients who actually had an infarct and 83% of those who died.

Conclusion.—It is feasible to use a stepped process for selecting patients to undergo aortic aneurysm surgery. Those identified as being at high risk on the basis of the clinical findings can undergo dipyridamole-thallium or gated acquisition scanning preoperatively.

▶ This study, like many others, confirms that clinical criteria can be used to segregate low-risk patients from high-risk patients. If there is a rationale for identifying high-risk patients in whom therapy should be increased either pre-operatively or postoperatively, such patients can be segregated by further

"

tests such as exercise testing, dipyridamole echocardiography, or dipyridamole thallium scintigraphy.

The authors found independent risk factors and their respective relative risk ratios to be age older than 60 years (relative risk ratio, 3); serum creatinine greater than 2.5 mg/dL (3.7); history of transient ischemic attacks (5.1); and history of angina (2.74). This study and many others have demonstrated that knowing the patient's history is very important before prescribing more costly tests before vascular surgery.—M.F. Roizen, M.D.

Relationship Between Postoperative Anemia and Cardiac Morbidity in High-Risk Vascular Patients in the Intensive Care Unit

Nelson AH, Fleisher LA, Rosenbaum SH (Yale Univ, New Haven, Conn)
Crit Care Med 21:860–866, 1993   101-94-14-2

Objective.—The implication of postoperative anemia for the development of myocardial ischemia and morbid cardiac events was examined in a case-control study of 27 consecutive high-risk patients who had infrainguinal arterial bypass surgery on an elective basis. None of the patients had a hematocrit less than 30% preoperatively.

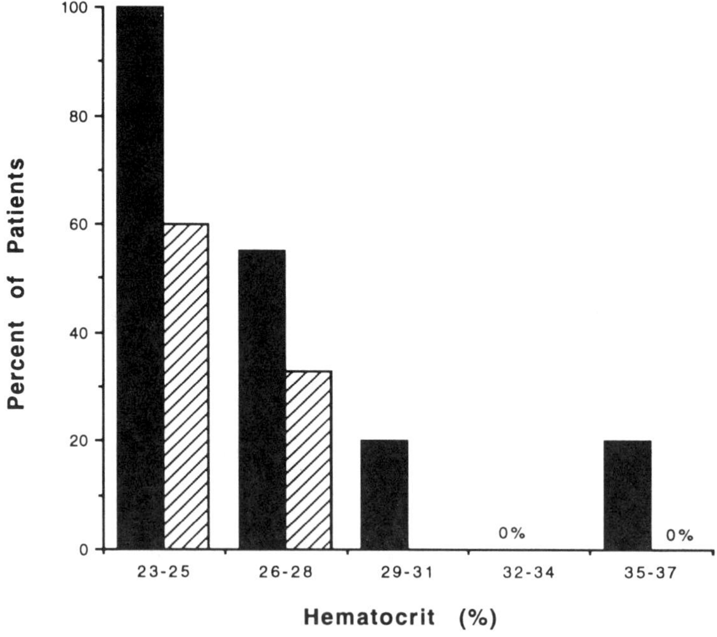

Fig 14–1.—Incidence of postoperative myocardial ischemia and morbid cardiac events as related to hematocrit. *Filled bars* represent myocardial ischemia; *hatched bars* represent morbid cardiac events. (Courtesy of Nelson AH, Fleisher LA, Rosenbaum SH: *Crit Care Med* 21:860–866, 1993.)

Methods.—The patients had continuous ambulatory ECG monitoring that began the evening before surgery and continued for as long as 80 hours postoperatively. Myocardial ischemia was defined as 1 mm or greater of horizontal or downsloping ST-segment depression or 2 mm or greater of ST-segment elevation that lasts 1 minute or longer on the ambulatory ECG.

Results.—Of the 27 patients, 8 received blood transfusions on the first postoperative day. By analysis of the receiver operating characteristic curve, a hematocrit of 28% was deemed to be the best threshold value below which morbid cardiac events (e.g., cardiac death, myocardial infarction, unstable angina, ischemic pulmonary edema) were most likely to occur (Fig 14–1). Of the 13 patients with a hematocrit below 28%, 10 had myocardial ischemia postoperatively, and 6 had morbid cardiac events. Only 2 of 14 patients with higher hematocrit levels had myocardial ischemia, and none had morbid cardiac events. Patients with morbid events also exhibited myocardial ischemia postoperatively.

Conclusion.—Anemia after major surgery may contribute to both postoperative myocardial ischemia and morbid cardiac events in high-risk patients with vascular disease.

▶ This article is extremely important, because it indicates that the transfusion trigger in patients with cardiac disease should be different from that in patients without cardiovascular disease. The authors found that the transfusion trigger should be around 28% to 30% in patients with ischemic heart disease. This agrees with the preconceived theoretical knowledge that oxygen delivery is maximal around a hematocrit of 30%. This figure takes into consideration the decreased resistance to flow, the reduced viscosity, and the lessened carrying capacity of oxygen. Every now and then, experiments such as this prove theoretic considerations to be correct.—M.F. Roizen, M.D.

Ancrod Versus Heparin for Anticoagulation During Vascular Surgical Procedures
Cole CW, Bormanis J, Luna GK, Hajjar G, Barber GG, Harris KA, Brien WF (Univ of Ottawa, Ont, Canada; Univ of Western Ontario, London, Canada)
J Vasc Surg 17:288–293, 1993   101-94-14–3

Background.—Ancrod, a thrombin-like enzyme that is derived from the venom of the Malayan pit viper, depletes the α-fibrinopeptides but not fibrinopeptide-β from fibrinogen. It has been successfully used as an alternative to heparin in patients with venous thrombosis. The effects and early results of ancrod and heparin as anticoagulants in patients undergoing infrainguinal vascular reconstructions were compared.

Methods.—The trial included 28 patients—14 randomized to receive heparin and 14 to ancrod. Those in the heparin group received 100 units of the anticoagulant per kg intravenously after the vessels were dissected and before placement of arterial clamps. Patients in the ancrod group were given 70 units in normal saline during 12 hours, until the serum fibrinogen stabilized between .2 and .5 g/L. When the fibrinogen level had stabilized, ancrod was discontinued and the patient was taken to the operating room. Ancrod was restarted after the operation when fibrinogen levels began to increase again. The dose required was usually 70 units per 24 hours.

Results.—No patient in either group required a blood transfusion because of hemorrhaging during the operation. No instances of clotting of blood within the grafts or native vessels occurred during the surgical procedures. One patient in each group underwent a thrombectomy because of graft occlusion during the first 24 hours after surgery. Those in the ancrod and heparin groups were similar in their rate of complications, hospital course, and patency at 1 month.

Conclusion.—Most alternatives to heparin have been less effective as anticoagulants. Ancrod achieves anticoagulation through a mechanism that does not affect platelets or other coagulation factors, and it may be valuable when heparin cannot be used or is ineffective. Unfortunately, this safe and effective alternative to heparin is only approved for limited use in the United States.

▶ Many people do not believe any anticoagulation is needed for infrainguinal vascular reconstruction, so, if nothing is needed, ancrod is no more dangerous than heparin. This appears to be the first test in which it did not cause adverse events, at least not in the doses used in these few patients. Whether ancrod has value as a replacement for heparin when anticoagulation is really needed remains to be determined.—M.F. Roizen, M.D.

The Importance of Intraoperative Detection of Residual Flow Abnormalities After Carotid Artery Endarterectomy
Kinney EV, Seabrook GR, Kinney LY, Bandyk DF, Towne JB (Med College of Wisconsin, Milwaukee)
J Vasc Surg 17:912–923, 1993   101-94-14-4

Background.—Although the clinical efficacy of carotid endarterectomy has been proven, the procedure is still associated with residual or recurrent stenosis in 9% to 22% of patients. If recurrent carotid stenosis increases the incidence of late ipsilateral stroke, intraoperative inspection and postoperative surveillance are important to detect such lesions. The relationship between residual flow abnormalities and the incidence of subsequent recurrent internal carotid stenosis/occlusion and ipsilateral stroke was investigated.

Methods.—Four hundred thirty patients with 461 carotid endarterectomies were studied prospectively. The adequacy of the repair was assessed by ultrasound assessment alone in 142 cases, by ultrasound and arteriography in 268, and by clinical inspection in 51. Duplex ultrasonography was done to confirm patency and classify the severity of internal carotid artery (ICA) stenosis after surgery. On the basis of intraoperative examinations, 26 carotid endarterectomy sites were revised during surgery.

Findings.—Patients with normal, mildly abnormal, or no ultrasound completion studies had comparable 30-day morbidity rates. Permanent and temporary neurologic deficits occurred in 1.3% and 2.6%, respectively. Six patients died, 4 of strokes and 2 of myocardial infarctions. According to life-table analysis, patients with residual flow abnormality or no study had an increased incidence of more than 50% of diameter-reducing ICA stenosis or occlusion. Patients with normal intraoperative flow assessments had a significantly lower rate of late ipsilateral stroke than the rest of the patients. During a mean 30 months of follow-up, the incidence of late stroke was higher in patients with ICA restenosis or occlusion than in patients without recurrent stenosis.

Summary.—In this series, intraoperative ultrasonography identified severe residual flow abnormalities in 26 of 461 carotid endarterectomies, and immediate revision was done in 25 cases without any adverse events. Confirmation of a normal repair at surgery is the best way to minimize ischemic neurologic events and anatomical restenosis after carotid endarterectomy.

Selective Monitoring in Abdominal Aortic Surgery

Adams JG Jr, Clifford EJ, Henry RS, Poulos E (St Paul Med Ctr, Dallas)
Am Surg 59:559–563, 1993   101-94-14-5

Background.—In patients undergoing abdominal aortic surgery, monitoring by a flow-directed pulmonary artery catheter is considered integral to perioperative management. In fact, several investigators have advocated its routine use. However, catheter insertion and maintenance require extensive time and effort and are not without risk to the patient. A subgroup of patients was identified that could be safely monitored with a central venous catheter during the perioperative period.

Patients and Methods.—A total of 128 patients undergoing elective infrarenal abdominal aortic surgery was prospectively assessed for risk of perioperative myocardial dysfunction, using criteria determined by the history, physical examination, chest radiography, and ECG. Of these, 45 patients with no identifiable cardiac risk factors were subsequently monitored perioperatively with a central venous catheter.

Results.—In all 45 patients who underwent surgery for abdominal aortic aneurysmal disease or aortoiliac disease (66.7% and 33.3%, respectively), no intraoperative complications were noted. Twelve patients experienced 15 postoperative complications, primarily of either a pulmonary (7) or gastrointestinal (3) nature. The cardiac-related morbidity was 4.4%, including congestive heart failure in 1 patient and renal failure in another. No perioperative myocardial infarctions were noted. One postoperative death occurred secondary to aspiration pneumonia.

Conclusion.—Patients with no identifiable coronary artery disease can be managed perioperatively using a central venous catheter, with admissibly low cardiac-related morbidity and mortality.

▶ Confirmation of the efficacy of a single monitor in a complex disease that has many unpredictable variables is probably not realistic. The decision to place a pulmonary artery catheter may be appropriately influenced by the perceived presence or absence of significant ischemic heart disease or impaired myocardial contractility. Nevertheless, to choose to place or avoid use of a pulmonary artery catheter solely on the basis of a single variable (ischemic heart disease) seems to defeat the value of individualizing decisions based on the entire patient and the probable surgical and anesthetic course.—R.K. Stoelting, M.D.

15 Anesthesia for Noncardiac Thoracic Procedures

Prophylactic Digitalization Fails to Control Dysrhythmia in Thoracic Esophageal Operations
Ritchie AJ, Tolan M, Whiteside M, McGuigan JA, Gibbons JRP (Royal Victoria Hosp, Belfast, Northern Ireland)
Ann Thorac Surg 55:86–88, 1993   101-94-15-1

Objective.—The ability of digitalization to prevent atrial fibrillation during thoracic surgery was evaluated in 80 consecutive patients undergoing elective esophageal surgery. Although 10 patients had myocardial disease, none had inadequate respiratory reserve, hypoxemia on breathing room air, or current dysrhythmia.

Methods.—Patients in the prospective, randomized trial received 2 doses of 500 μg of digoxin the day before surgery and 250 μg at the time of premedication. Postoperatively they received 250 μg daily for 9 days, with the dose adjusted to maintain a serum digoxin level of 1–2 μg/mL. Serum digoxin was measured by radioimmunoassay 6 hours after dosing.

Results.—Mortality was 6%; however, no dysrhythmia occurred in any of the 26 patients who were operated on for benign disease, whether or not digoxin was given. Among the 54 patients with malignant disease, 46% of 26 patients who were digitalized and 32% of the 28 who were not digitalized experienced dysrhythmias. All these dysrhythmias would have been expected to have been prevented by digoxin therapy or to have been related to such treatment.

Conclusion.—Preoperative digitalization was of no apparent benefit to patients undergoing elective esophageal surgery. In this setting, older patients with malignant disease are the most likely to have dysrhythmia develop, and it occurs most often on the day of surgery.

▶ Use of prophylactic digoxin before vascular and thoracic surgery has been advocated as a way of improving cardiac performance and decreasing the lethality of arrhythmias and the consequences of dysrhythmias when they occur. Too many things in this article are left unexplained to make it desirable reading, unless you simply want to explore the subject further. For example we do not know whether the dysrhythmias in the digoxin group were less lethal, had less association with myocardial ischemia, had better rate control, or were associated with less hemodynamic disturbance than those in the nondigoxin group, or vice versa. We also do not know about the well-being of the patients or anything about their renal excretion of digoxin or their preexisting potassium levels. Clearly, more data and a more thorough method of reporting by a study of equal quality are needed before prophylactic digitalization is abandoned.—M.F. Roizen, M.D.

Haemodynamic and Metabolic Consequences of Aortic Occlusion During Abdominal Aortic Surgery

Whalley DG, Salevsky FC, Ryckman JV (Cleveland Clinic Found, Ohio; Royal Victoria Hosp, Montreal)
Br J Anaesth 70:96–98, 1993   101-94-15–2

Introduction.—In patients undergoing aortic reconstruction, infrarenal aortic cross-clamping may be associated with significant increases in systemic vascular resistance (SVR), which may further compromise cardiac performance in patients with coronary artery disease. There are conflicting reports regarding whether patients with occlusive disease have smaller increases in SVR at the time of cross-clamping than those with aneurysms. The hemodynamic and metabolic effects of infrarenal aortic cross-clamping in patients undergoing aortic reconstruction for repair of aneurysmal or occlusive disease were examined.

Methods.—Of the 20 patients in the prospective study, 12 had aneurysms and 8 had atherosclerotic occlusive disease. Intravenous, intra-arterial, and thermodilution pulmonary artery catheters were inserted for measurement of hemodynamic variables at baseline, 5 minutes after cross-clamping, and before as well as 15 minutes after removal of the cross-clamp. Metabolic variables were measured at similar intervals.

Findings.—There was a highly significant and positive correlation between the cross-clamp–associated change in SVR and the change in base deficit associated with the removal of the cross-clamp. The aneurysm and occlusion groups showed no differences in regression analysis or in mean change in SVR and base deficit. There was also a positive correlation between the maximum increase in mixed venous serum lactate concentration and the duration of aortic cross-clamping.

Conclusion.—A significant relationship was shown between the change in SVR with aortic cross-clamping and the subsequent increase in base deficit after the cross-clamp is removed. This finding, along with the relationship between increased mixed venous serum lactate concentration and the duration of cross-clamping, suggests the importance of the collateral circulation in the development of metabolic acidoses during aortic surgery. No difference was found in the SVR response for patients with aneurysmal vs. occlusive disease.

▶ This article validates the obvious: Increased SVR on cross-clamp relates to lack of collateral circulation, and longer surgery times are associated with more anerobic metabolism. However, the article does not indicate what the authors did to minimize SVR changes when the cross-clamp was applied. I would like to have such methodologic information and to know whether we could prevent the changes and whether they are important. Nevertheless, this article adds important physiologic data and acid-base data to our already substantial knowledge of what happens with aortic cross-clamping.—M.F. Roizen, M.D.

Paraplegia Following Thoracic Aortic Cross-Clamping in Dogs: No Difference in Neurological Outcome With a Barbiturate Versus Isoflurane
Mutch WAC, Graham MR, Halliday WC, Teskey JM, Thomson IR (Univ of Manitoba, Winnipeg, Canada)
Stroke 24:1554–1560, 1993   101-94-15–3

Background.—Paraplegia is a potential complication of surgery to reconstruct the thoracic aorta. The influence of anesthetic on neurologic outcome after cross-clamping of the aorta has not been well studied. Therefore, 2 anesthetic regimens were compared in a dog model of thoracic aortic cross-clamping: intravenous infusion of the barbiturate methohexital vs. the inhaled agent isoflurane. A better neurologic outcome was expected with methohexital, because of superior neuronal protection and greater spinal cord perfusion pressure with barbiturates.

Methods.—After surgical preparation and 30 minutes of stabilization, 9 dogs were randomized to receive intravenously administered methohexital (group M), and another 9 dogs were randomized to receive isoflurane (group I). The thoracic aorta was occluded for 30 minutes and then released. Hemodynamics and CSF pressure were measured at baseline, 2 minutes after cross-clamping, 20 minutes after cross-clamping, 5 minutes after unclamping, and 30 minutes after resuscitation. Neurologic evaluation was performed at 24 hours. The spinal cord was then studied histopathologically.

Results.—There was no difference in spinal cord perfusion pressure between the 2 groups of dogs at any time during the study. The neurologic outcome was not significantly different between the 2 groups.

Conclusion.—There was no difference in the incidence of paraplegia after thoracic aortic cross-clamping when dogs were anesthetized with either isoflurane or methohexital. There appears to be no advantage to the use of barbiturate anesthesia in this canine model.

▶ Paraplegia or paraparesis after thoracic aneurysm resection is an unavoidable complication that reflects surgical interruption of the blood supply to the spinal cord. Although perfusion pressure and oxygenation are under the anesthesiologist's control, it is incorrect to assume that spinal cord dysfunction is preventable if only higher perfusion pressures had been possible. The patient should be fully advised of the risk of this feared complication before he or she consents to this life-saving surgery.—R.K. Stoelting, M.D.

16 Anesthesia for Outpatient Procedures

Patients' Ratings of Outpatient Visits in Different Practice Settings: Results From the Medical Outcomes Study
Rubin HR, Gandek B, Rogers WH, Kosinski M, McHorney CA, Ware JE Jr
(Johns Hopkins Med Institutions, Baltimore, Md; New England Med Ctr Hosps, Boston; RAND, Santa Monica, Calif)
JAMA 270:835–840, 1993   101-94-16-1

Objective.—Knowledge of how payment strategies affect features of care would enable consumers to make informed choices among alternative systems and clinicians to receive specific feedback about areas to improve. Patients' ratings of specific outpatient visits across 5 practice types were compared.

Methods.—Data were obtained from the Medical Outcomes Study that was conducted in 1986 in Boston, Chicago, and Los Angeles. In each city, physicians in 3 types of practice organizations were sampled: a staff model health maintenance organization (HMO), multispecialty group (MSG) practices, and solo or single-specialty small group (SOLO) practices. Both MSG and SOLO practices included patients who belonged to prepaid health plans or had traditional, fee-for-service (FFS) indemnity insurance. Adult patients were asked by providers to complete a visit rating questionnaire after they had seen a physician and before they left the office. The sample was weighted to represent the population of patients that visited physicians in each of the 5 practice types: HMO prepaid, MSG prepaid, MSG FFS, SOLO prepaid, and SOLO FFS.

Results.—Responses were obtained from 17,671 patients. In overall ratings, 55% rated their visit as excellent, 32% as very good, 11% as good, and 2% as fair or poor. The highest ratings were given to physicians' technical skills and personal manner (64% and 73% excellent, respectively). The worst-rated aspect of the visit was the office wait, which earned an excellent rating from only 32% of subjects. Patients of SOLO FFS practitioners were more likely to give excellent overall and specific visit ratings than those in the other 4 practice types. Physicians whose visit ratings were in the lowest quintile were nearly 4 times as likely to be left by patients within 6 months as were physicians in the highest quintile.

Conclusion.—Many patients see considerable room for improvement in their outpatient visits. Access to service was a significant problem, and it was worse in large organizations, especially HMOs. Providers need to reduce the length of office visit waits and spend more time with patients. From the patients' point of view, small, single-specialty practices provide superior care.

▶ Clearly, reducing waiting time and spending more time answering patients' questions are important elements in patient satisfaction that we should all take into account. Automated histories that can simplify our job so we do not have to interrupt patients 18 seconds into their response can provide us with extra time to focus on delivering the information the patient wants. Such technology may be an important adjunct to our future practice.—M.F. Roizen, M.D.

Assessment and Selection of Patients for Day Surgery in a Public Hospital
Rudkin GE, Osborne GA, Doyle CE (Royal Adelaide Hosp, Australia)
Med J Aust 158:308–312, 1993   101-94-16–2

Introduction.—The practice of day surgery has only recently become widespread in Australia. Because of cost considerations, the assessment of patients before day surgery may be inadequate. Anesthetists can play a key role in implementing an effective system of patient selection. Methods used for adult patient assessment and selection for day case surgery were described.

Methods.—At the study institution, the Day Surgery Unit (DSU) is a functionally separate unit established in 1988. Five thousand patients underwent day surgery between May of 1989 and April of 1992. Patients are selected by surgeons and referred to the DSU no less than 2 days before surgery to allow adequate time for assessment. An anesthetic questionnaire is administered, and the patients are given instructions for the day of surgery. All test results are reviewed by an anesthetist before the day of surgery. Patients are required to have someone escort them home after surgery. Nursing staff members provide telephone follow-up (Fig 16–1).

Results.—The initial screening resulted in 46% of all patients being reviewed by an anesthetist before the day of surgery. More than half the patients underwent general anesthesia. There were 110 patients (2.4%) who were judged to be unsuitable for day surgery; most of these were elderly and had been referred for ophthalmic surgery. The most frequently ordered preoperative investigation (8.5% of patients) was electrocardiography. Postsurgery, the nursing staff was able to contact 87% of all patients by telephone, 99% of whom expressed satisfaction with the day surgery service. There were 64 unanticipated hospital admissions, 1.28% of the total, which was a satisfactory rate. Most admissions were for bleeding or other direct surgical complications.

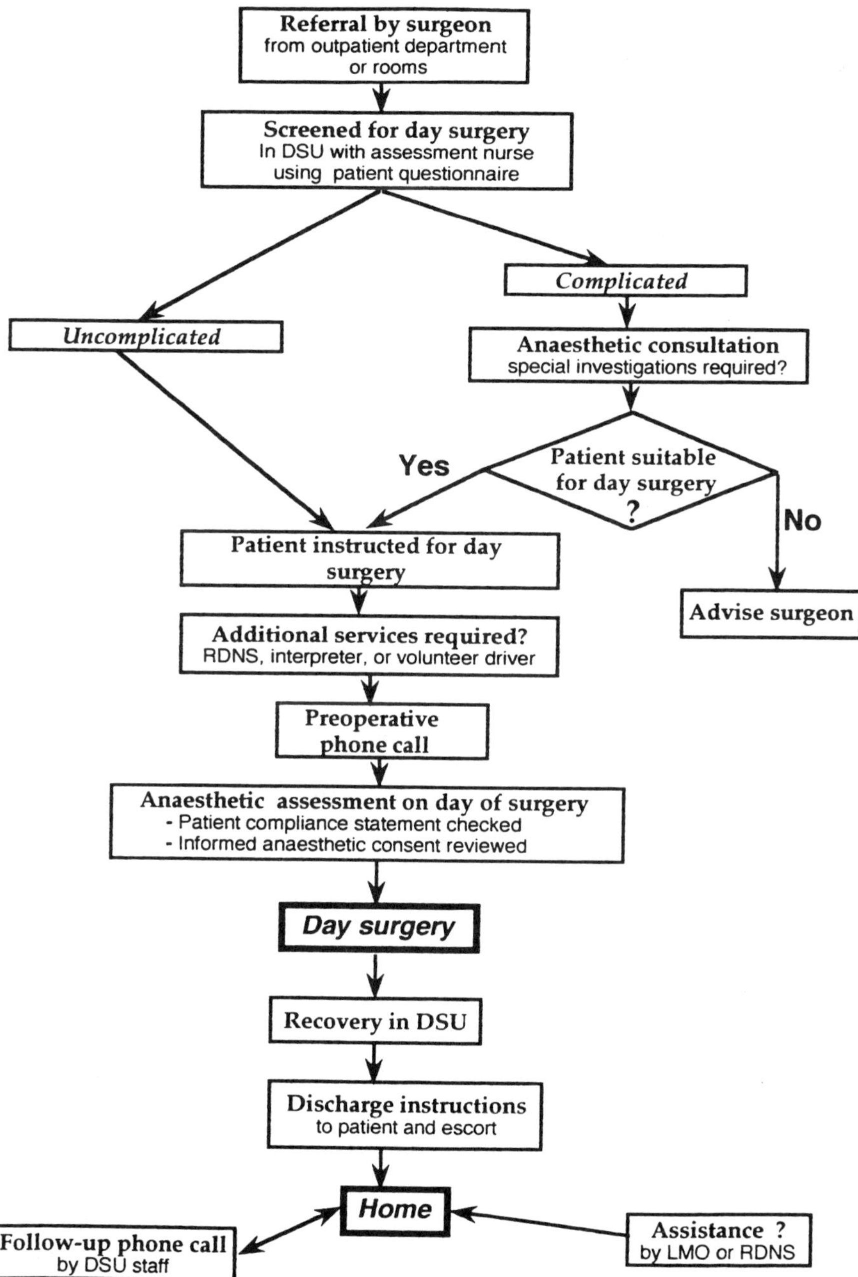

Fig 16–1.—Screening and assessment of day surgery patients. (Courtesy of Rudkin GE, Osborne GA, Doyle CE: *Med J Aust* 158:308–312, 1993.)

Conclusion.—Selection of suitable patients and procedures allows day surgery to be a successful and cost-effective alternative to hospital admission. Contributing to the success of this DSU were a dedicated day surgery area, a skilled nursing staff, use of a comprehensive patient questionnaire, and coordination by anesthetists who were experienced in day surgery.

▶ Two aspects of this article deserve special mention: (1) All patients who were referred to anesthetists for screening were first screened with a patient questionnaire to help the physicians make more efficient use of time. I favor this streamlining of obtaining patient information, and I commend Rudkin and colleagues for doing so. (2) Notably, 2.4% of the patients referred were judged to be unsuitable for day surgery. We do not know whether patients had delays on the day of surgery or how many delays occurred among the other 54% of patients who were not referred by the surgeons to the pre-screening clinic; presumably, they were healthier patients.

In our studies, we now use a questionnaire that the patient completes in the surgeon's office. The physician then faxes or electronically transfers it to us so we can review it and make a decision, based on the assigned risk index and the patient's history, whether we need to see the patient before the morning of surgery. This system has worked so well that many of us will probably start having questionnaires completed in the surgeon's office and electronically transmitted to us. This way, we will see only the sickest patients or those who want consultative questions answered. We can then make the most efficient use of our time and that of the patient. On the other hand, there is an advantage to seeing everyone, because pain relief mechanisms, alleviation of anxiety, and other preoperative suggestions can be made that may reduce the hospital stay for inpatients and facilitate the recovery in all patients as well.—M.F. Roizen, M.D.

Documenting Local Anesthesia Patient Care: Developing the Tool
Kendall F (Parkridge Med Ctr, Chattanooga, Tenn)
AORN J 58:715–719, 1993   101-94-16–3

Background.—The operating room staff at Parkridge Medical Center in Chattanooga, Tennessee, sought to update and improve methods of documenting the evaluation and monitoring of patients who were given local anesthesia.

A New Form.—They created a separate form by modifying existing forms. The new form included patient identification, procedural information, the initials of staff members, the patient's history and physical findings, the results of a postoperative assessment, and transport information. A graph for documenting medications and vital signs was also included. The staff provided input into each section of the new form, and information on patient assessment and the medical history was later excluded as unnecessary; however, a section on patient allergies was retained. Small check-off boxes were used wherever possible.

Conclusion.—When developing new documentation forms, it is advisable to invite the input of staff members who will be using them.

▶ The author has developed something that resembles an anesthetic record to me, but it does contain some nursing items, such as sponge counts and skin conditions. Perhaps we can learn from some of what they have done to improve our forms, but it seems like an awfully long run for a short slide.—M.F. Roizen, M.D.

Inhaled Induction and Emergence From Desflurane Anesthesia in the Ambulatory Surgical Patient: The Effect of Premedication
Kelly RE, Hartman GS, Embree PB, Sharp G, Artusio JF Jr (New York Hosp-Cornell Univ)
Anesth Analg 77:540–543, 1993   101-94-16–4

Purpose.—Desflurane has a low blood-gas coefficient, suggesting that it might be associated with rapid induction of anesthesia; its pungency, however, might be associated with retarded induction. Whether premedication with fentanyl and midazolam could reduce airway irritability on induction without adversely affecting the hemodynamic profile of desflurane was studied.

Methods.—The study sample comprised 18 ambulatory patients, American Society of Anesthesiologists physical status I or II, who were scheduled for elective surgical procedures. The 10 patients in the premedication group received fentanyl, 1 μg/kg, and midazolam, .04 mg/kg, 5 minutes before induction with desflurane, 3.5% in 60% nitrous oxide and oxygen; the 8 controls received no premedication. The study was blinded only during follow-up.

Results.—Premedication had no effect on either induction or emergence, but it did significantly reduce the end-tidal and inspired concentrations of desflurane at loss of consciousness, 10% and 14% vs. 5% and 9%, respectively, in the control group. All patients in the control group had airway irritability, compared with only 30% in the premedication group. None of those in the premedication group had apnea, compared with 38% of the control group. Those in the control group had an increase in mean arterial pressure and heart rate after they lost consciousness. Patients in both groups had a decrease in mean arterial pressure, with no change in heart rate, at the time of incision. All expressed satisfaction with their anesthesia.

Conclusion.—Premedication with fentanyl and midazolam is useful during induction of anesthesia with desflurane. It reduces airway reactivity, decreases anesthetic requirements, and provides hemodynamic stability during induction; however, it does not hasten induction or prolong recovery from anesthesia.

▶ I endorse the timing, route of administration, drug selection, and dose used in this report. Although it was not measured in this study, greater patient relaxation in the postoperative period would be another benefit of this regimen.—R.K. Stoelting, M.D.

Desflurane Versus Propofol Anesthesia: A Comparative Analysis in Outpatients
Lebenbom-Mansour MH, Pandit SK, Kothary SP, Randel GI, Levy L (Univ of Michigan, Ann Arbor)
Anesth Analg 76:936–941, 1993   101-94-16-5

Introduction.—The new inhalational anesthetic desflurane has a relatively low blood-gas solubility coefficient and produces rapid induction and recovery in humans.

Study Plan.—The characteristics of desflurane anesthesia were compared with those of propofol in 60 outpatients who were scheduled for orthopedic surgery. In 2 groups, induction with propofol was followed by either desflurane and nitrous oxide (group 1) or propofol infusion and nitrous oxide (group 2). Other groups received desflurane with nitrous oxide (group 3) or without nitrous oxide (group 4) for both induction and maintenance of anesthesia. Propofol was given in a dose of 2.5 mg per kilogram. Nitrous oxide was used in a 60% concentration with oxygen.

Results.—The quality of infection was inferior when desflurane was used, with patients exhibiting more breath-holding and excitation. Those who were induced and maintained with desflurane emerged more rapidly than patients in any of the other groups, as reflected in their ability to give their names. Intermediate recovery, as demonstrated by psychomotor function tests, was best in patients given propofol and in those given desflurane for induction and maintenance. Postoperative narcotic requirements were comparable in all groups. Vomiting was most frequent among patients who were given desflurane and nitrous oxide. The anesthetics had similar hemodynamic effects.

Conclusion.—Desflurane is a problematic induction agent, but it is suitable for maintaining anesthesia in patients who are having ambulatory surgery.

▶ I am impressed by the enormous difference in the incidence of vomiting. When desflurane was used for both induction and maintenance, as in group 3, a 50% incidence of vomiting occurred, which is clearly unacceptable. A number of groups have referred to the possibility that propofol may have antiemetic properties. It seems apparent that some combination of propofol and desflurane might be much more suitable for outpatient anesthesia. Also, it is clear that desflurane is not simply a "faster" isoflurane. We are going to have a learning curve with it.—J.H. Tinker, M.D.

17 Anesthesia for General Surgery and Orthopedics

Laparoscopic Cholecystectomy During Pregnancy in Symptomatic Patients

Morrell DG, Mullins JR, Harrison PB (Univ of Kansas–Wichita; HCA–Wesley Med Ctr, Wichita, Kan)

Surgery 112:856–859, 1992   101-94-17–1

Introduction.—Most patients with symptomatic biliary tract disease during pregnancy are managed conservatively, with a cholecystectomy recommended after delivery. However, other studies suggest an aggressive surgical approach may be the most appropriate. Although pregnancy has been considered an absolute contraindication to laparoscopic cholecystectomy, several studies have suggested that this applies only to advanced intrauterine pregnancy.

Treatment.—In 1991, 5 women at 13 to 23 weeks' gestation underwent a laparoscopic cholecystectomy for symptomatic cholelithiasis or acute cholecystitis.

Outcome.—Four patients were delivered of healthy newborns, and the fifth was still pregnant and progressing normally at the last report. There was no maternal or fetal morbidity, and the postoperative course of all patients was unremarkable.

Conclusion.—Laparoscopic cholecystectomy can be performed safely in the second trimester of pregnancy, and it appears to be the optimal management for selected patients who have symptomatic biliary tract disease during pregnancy.

▶ The authors performed 5 successful laparoscopic cholecystectomies during the second trimester of pregnancy. Until now, laparoscopic surgery has been limited to the first trimester of pregnancy. To my knowledge, no published study has examined the fetal response to laparoscopic surgery in laboratory animals. Most surgeons are reluctant to perform laparoscopic surgery during the third trimester, because of the risk of injury to the enlarged gravid uterus.—D.H. Chestnut, M.D.

Effectiveness of Perioperative Recombinant Human Erythropoietin in Elective Hip Replacement

Laupacis, A, for the Canadian Orthopedic Perioperative Erythropoietin Study Group (Ottawa Civic Hosp, Ont, Canada)
Lancet 341:1227–1232, 1993   101-94-17–2

Background.—Because of the risk of viral infection transmission, attempts have been made to reduce the transfusion requirements of patients undergoing surgery. Whether recombinant human erythropoietin decreases blood transfusion needs in patients having elective hip arthroplasty was investigated.

Methods.—Two hundred eight patients were enrolled in the multicenter, double-blind, randomized, placebo-controlled trial. All were given daily subcutaneous injections of erythropoietin or placebo beginning 10 days before surgery, at which time the 78 patients in group 1 received placebo for 14 days. The 77 patients in group 2 were given erythropoietin, 300 units per kilogram to a maximum of 30,000 units, for 14 days, and the 53 patients in group 3 were given placebo on days 10–6 before surgery, with erythropoietin being administered for the next 9 days.

Findings.—A primary outcome event, which was defined as any transfusion or a hemoglobin concentration of less than 80 g/L, occurred in 46% of group 1 patients, 23% of group 2 patients, and 32% of group 3 patients. The mean number of transfusions for those in groups 1, 2, and 3 was 1.14, .52, and .7, respectively. Respective mean reticulocyte counts the day before the operation were 72, 327, and 170 $\times$ 10^9/L. Five patients in group 1, 8 in group 2, and 8 in group 3 had deep venous thrombi. Patients with a hemoglobin concentration of less than 135 g/L before randomization benefited most from erythropoietin.

Summary.—In patients undergoing elective hip arthroplasty, when erythropoietin was given for 14 days perioperatively, it reduced the need for blood transfusion; the treatment was well tolerated.

▶ This is the first study of which I am aware that showed that erythropoietin given before elective surgery reduced transfusion requirements. Although this is an important consideration, it did not completely eliminate such requirements, perhaps predeposit in combination with recombinant human erythropoietin administration would do so.—M.F. Roizen, M.D.

Anesthetic Techniques During Surgical Repair of Femoral Neck Fractures: A Meta-Analysis

Sorenson RM, Pace NL (Univ of Utah, Salt Lake City)
Anesthesiology 77:1095–1104, 1992   101-94-17–3

Introduction.—Hip fractures typically occur in older women, who frequently have serious chronic illnesses. It is uncertain whether regional or general anesthetic techniques are preferable for these patients. A meta-analysis compared the survival of patients with traumatic femoral neck fractures who underwent surgical repair during regional or general anesthesia.

Data Analysis.—Thirteen randomized, controlled trials were found in peer reviewed journals. In addition to 30-day mortality, operative blood loss and the occurrence of deep venous thrombosis were reviewed. For dichotomous outcomes, both the difference in probabilities and the odds ratio were calculated. A random-effects bayesian meta-analysis technique was used to combine study data, estimate parameters, and create 95% confidence levels.

Findings.—Older women predominated in the studies reviewed. The great majority underwent open reduction with internal fixation. Both intravenous and inhalational techniques of general anesthesia were used, but isoflurane was not administered. Most patients were operated on within 3 to 4 days after injury. Deep venous thrombosis was 31% more frequent in patients who were given general anesthesia than in those who received regional anesthesia. Odds ratio analysis indicated that deep vein thrombosis was nearly 4 times more likely to occur after general anesthesia. No difference in estimated operative blood loss was apparent. Mortality was 2.7% lower after regional anesthesia, not a significant difference. Death was 1.5 times more likely with general anesthesia, but the lower limit of the 95% confidence interval was close to 1.

Conclusion.—No important difference in mortality was found between hip fracture patients who had repair with general anesthesia and those who were given regional anesthesia.

▶ Such outcome data are crucial in confirming the efficacy or lack thereof of alternative techniques and therapies. Those who insist on a specific technique for hip surgery should take note of the absence of any difference in outcome in this patient population.—R.K. Stoelting, M.D.

18 Anesthesia for Neurosurgery

Monitoring of Brainstem Function During Vertebral Basilar Aneurysm Surgery: The Use of Spontaneous Ventilation
Manninen PH, Cuillerier DJ, Nantau WE, Gelb AW (Univ Hosp, London, Ont, Canada)
Anesthesiology 77:681–685, 1992   101-94-18–1

Objective.—Whether spontaneous ventilation is a useful marker of brain stem function in patients having posterior fossa surgery was determined using retrospective and prospective observations made from 1981 to 1988.

Patients and Methods.—Forty charts were reviewed, and 10 other patients were evaluated prospectively. The respective mean ages were 46 and 57 years. In many patients, a moderate degree of induced hypotension was used when dissecting an aneurysm before spontaneous ventilation began. In addition to routine cardiovascular and respiratory monitoring, brain stem auditory-evoked potentials and somatosensory-evoked potentials were recorded throughout the procedure.

Findings.—In the retrospective series, 9 of 40 patients had respiratory changes, and 4 of them became apneic during temporary occlusion of the vertebral artery. Only 2 of these patients had cardiovascular changes at the same time, and only 2 of 13 who were monitored had changes in evoked potentials. In the prospective series, 4 of 10 patients had respiratory changes. Three patients, 2 of whom were apneic during vertebral artery occlusion, had a simultaneous change in evoked potentials, but none had cardiovascular changes. In 1 patient, all these parameters changed.

Conclusion.—Permitting a patient who is undergoing posterior fossa surgery to breathe spontaneously provides a useful early indicator of brain stem ischemia, especially when the vertebrobasilar system is temporarily occluded. Cardiovascular changes generally occur later than respiratory changes, and evoked potential monitoring is not always available or usable.

▶ The key to analyzing this process is the change that has occurred in providing anesthesia for neurosurgery during the past 20 years. Before electroencephalography and somatosensory-evoked potentials, it was common practice to use spontaneous ventilation during posterior fossa surgery and to examine changes in the ventilatory pattern as indicators of subtle changes in brain stem function. However, controlled ventilation became customary, because spontaneous ventilation often resulted in hypercapnea, which can lead to swelling of the brain, impairment of the surgical view, and the possibility of damage to brain structures. At the same time, many anesthesiologists believed that monitoring cardiovascular variables was as sensitive as monitoring respiration for detecting brain stem ischemia; therefore, many anesthesiologists advocated low ventilation. However, as Manninen and colleagues pointed out, the areas of the brain stem where respiratory and hemodynamic control reside and where conduction of sensory and motor pathways takes place are adjacent but anatomically discrete. From this study, it appears that changes in respiration that can be detected by the use of spontaneous ventilation are in fact *important early warning signs of a decrement in brain stem function.* Although it is unclear whether detecting these changes will lead to changes in patient outcome, studies to determine that presumably will be forthcoming.—M.F. Roizen, M.D.

Protection From Postischemic Spinal Cord Injury by Perfusion Cooling of the Epidural Space

Tabayashi K, Niibori K, Konno H, Mohri H (Tohoku Univ, Miyagi, Japan)
Ann Thorac Surg 56:494–498, 1993   101-94-18-2

Purpose.—A number of techniques have been proposed to prevent the catastrophic complication of spinal cord injury after successful surgery on the thoracic aorta. Hypothermia may protect against spinal cord ischemia, but proposed methods of hypothermia are not appropriate for all patients with an aneurysm of the thoracic aorta. Dogs were used to determine the protective effects of epidural space perfusion cooling during occlusion of the descending thoracic aorta.

Methods.—Sixteen dogs were randomized into 3 groups. Two groups were subjected to 1 hour of aortic occlusion, 1 with and the other without cooling of the spinal cord by perfusion of the epidural space with chilled saline solution. The third group underwent 2 hours of occlusion with perfusion cooling. The effects of the procedure were assessed by noting the development and severity of motor disturbance 1 week after the procedure. The evaluation also included a histologic examination of the spinal cord.

Results.—Of the 5 animals that received no perfusion cooling, 4 had spastic paraplegia with rigidly extended hind limbs develop. Of 6 dogs that received 1 hour of perfusion cooling, 5 were normal; the other dog could not walk, although it could move its hind legs somewhat. All 5 dogs in the 2-hour perfusion group were normal. On histologic examination, paraplegic dogs showed degeneration of the gray matter with macrophage infiltration, whereas the normal dogs had enlargement of the central canal, slight edema, and a few dark neurons.

Conclusion.—This animal study suggests that epidural space perfusion cooling is an effective way to decrease the incidence of spinal cord injury after temporary occlusion of the descending thoracic aorta. This technique might be clinically useful in all patients with thoracic aneurysm, even those who are in shock because of acute dissection or rupture. However, the short- and long-term effects of perfusion cooling on neurologic function will first have to be evaluated in the laboratory.

19 Anesthesia for Obstetrics and Gynecology

Labor Analgesia and Anesthesia

Comparison Among Intrathecal Fentanyl, Meperidine, and Sufentanil for Labor Analgesia

Honet JE, Arkoosh VA, Norris MC, Huffnagle HJ, Silverman NS, Leighton BL
(Thomas Jefferson Univ, Philadelphia)

Anesth Analg 75:734–739, 1992
101-94-19-1

Background.—Small-gauge spinal catheters have been successfully used to provide labor analgesia. These newly developed catheters enable administration of multiple intrathecal doses of a lipid-soluble opioid, such as fentanyl, meperidine, or sufentanil. No study has systematically compared these 3 drugs.

Methods and Findings.—The analgesic efficacy of intermittent injections of intrathecal fentanyl, 10 μg, meperidine, 10 mg, and sufentanil, 5 μg, was compared in 65 parturients in the first stage of labor. Onset and duration of effective analgesia were comparable among the 3 groups. However, women given meperidine had significantly lower pain scores after cervical dilatation exceeded 6 cm. Adverse effects were mild pruritus and nausea. Variable decelerations of the fetal heart rate increased in the groups given fentanyl and meperidine after intrathecal drug injection. In all neonates, 5-minute Apgar scores were 7 or more.

Conclusion.—Intermittent intrathecal injections of fentanyl, meperidine, or sufentanil can produce sufficient analgesia in first-stage labor. Analgesia appears to be more reliable with meperidine as the first stage of labor advances.

▶ Among the opioids used in clinical practice, meperidine is the only 1 that has local anesthetic qualities. As a result, is it not surprising that intrathecal meperidine provided better relief of the somatic pain of advanced labor. In this study, the authors gave intermittent doses of opioid through a 28-gauge spinal catheter. The Food and Drug Administration has withdrawn spinal microcatheters from the market, because of concern about cauda equina syndrome after their use for administration of continuous spinal anesthesia. It is

"

impractical to use a 20-gauge epidural catheter to provide continuous spinal analgesia in healthy parturients, because of the high incidence of postdural puncture headache. Therefore, some anesthesiologists favor intrathecal administration of a single dose of a lipid-soluble opioid as part of a combined spinal-epidural technique.—D.H. Chestnut, M.D.

A Twenty-Year Retrospective Analysis of the Efficacy of Epidural Analgesia-Anesthesia When Administered and/or Managed by Obstetricians

Farabow WS, Roberson VO, Maxey J, Spray BJ (High Point Regional Hosp, NC; Wake Forest Univ, Winston-Salem, NC)
Am J Obstet Gynecol 169:270–278, 1993   101-94-19–2

Purpose.—Epidural anesthesia and analgesia have come into widespread use for women in labor. The recent trend toward specialty care raises the question of whether obstetricians or anesthesiologists should be the ones to administer epidural analgesia-anesthesia. The safety and efficacy of epidural anesthesia that was administered by obstetricians in a community hospital were evaluated retrospectively.

Methods.—The analysis included data on 14,598 epidural procedures performed during 31,818 births in a 20-year period. Spinal anesthesia was administered or supervised by obstetricians with varying levels of

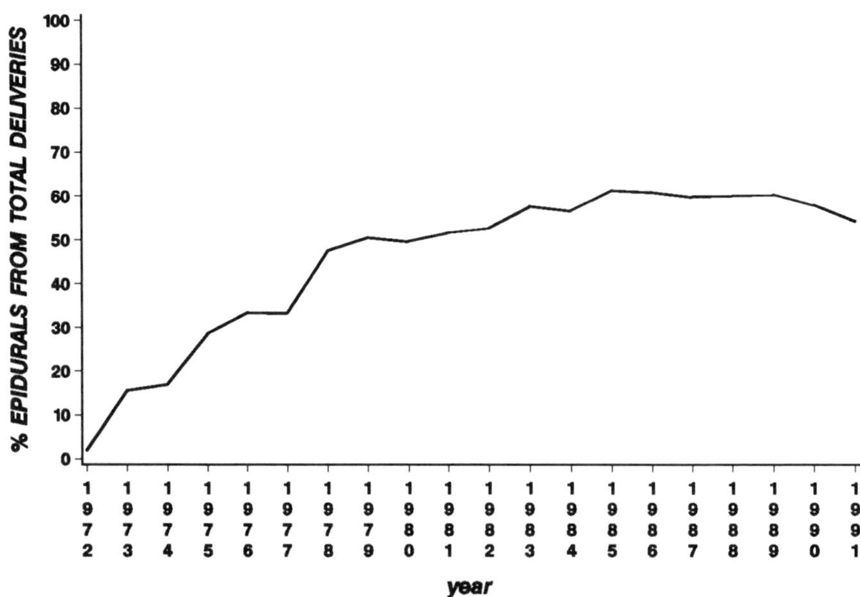

Fig 19–1.—Frequency of epidural anesthesia plotted as percentage of total deliveries for each year from 1972 through 1991. (Courtesy of Farabow WS, Roberson VO, Maxey J, et al: *Am J Obstet Gynecol* 169:270–278, 1993.)

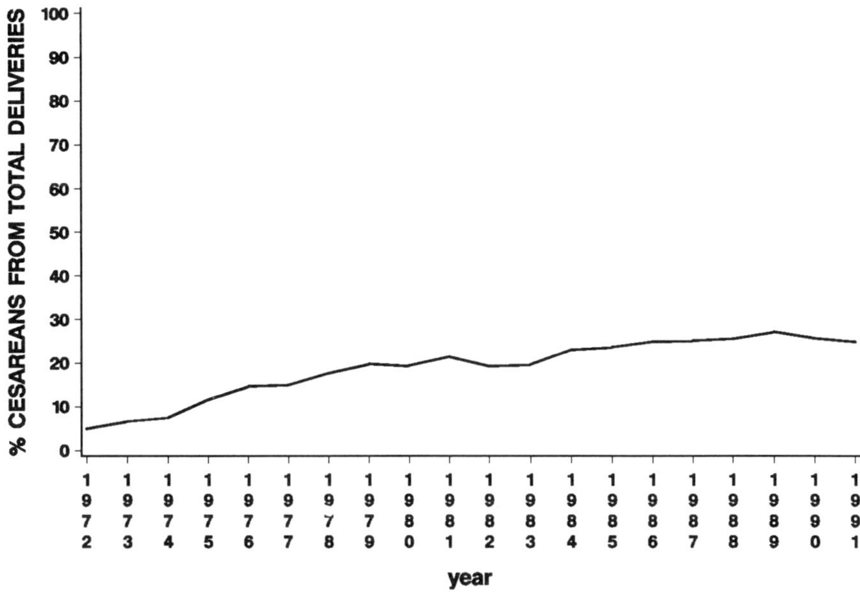

Fig 19–2.—Frequency of cesarean sections plotted as percentage of total deliveries for each year from 1972 through 1991. (Courtesy of Farabow WS, Roberson VO, Maxey J, et al: *Am J Obstet Gynecol* 169:270–278, 1993.)

training and experience. Trends over time were examined, with particular attention paid to any recorded complications during labor or delivery. Odds ratios were calculated to look for associations between epidural anesthesia and oxytocin stimulation, episiotomy, assisted vaginal delivery, and cesarean section.

Results.—No maternal deaths or serious complications were associated with the use of epidural anesthesia. Patient acceptance of the procedure was excellent, and the frequency of its use increased steadily during the years (Fig 19–1). Less than 5% of patients who received epidural anesthesia required additional anesthesia. Use of epidural anesthesia was greater in women who required oxytocin augmentation (odds ratio, 6.4); forceps delivery (4.8); and episiotomy (1.6). The cesarean section rate increased gradually over the years (Fig 19–2), until most patients did not receive epidural anesthesia (.31).

Conclusion.—Epidural anesthesia-analgesia has been shown to be a safe and effective procedure when it is administered or supervised by obstetrician-gynecologists in a community hospital. Its use has been increased in women requiring oxytocin augmentation, episiotomy, and assisted vaginal delivery and reduced in women undergoing cesarean section, mainly because of the high number of repeat and emergency cesarean sections.

▶ The authors claimed that "of the 14,598 epidural procedures, there were no maternal deaths or serious sequelae associated with the use of epidural anesthesia." They obtained their data from the delivery room logs at their hospital. It is unclear whether this method of data retrieval enabled them to ascertain any serious complications that may have resulted from epidural anesthesia. At the University of Iowa, the delivery room logs would not be my choice as a source of information regarding anesthetic complications.

As managed care gains a greater foothold in obstetric practice, some obstetricians may be reluctant to share a piece of the reimbursement pie with anesthesiologists. Unfortunately, it is difficult for obstetricians to maintain competence in the prevention, recognition, and management of the rare but serious complications of regional anesthesia. For years, obstetricians, hospitals, and patients have struggled to increase the involvement of anesthesiologists in obstetric care. I hope that health-care reform will not push anesthesiologists out of the labor and delivery suite.—D.H. Chestnut, M.D.

Does the Choice of Local Anesthetic Affect the Catecholamine Response to Stress During Epidural Anesthesia?

Stevens RA, Beardsley D, White JL, Kao T-C, Teague PJ, Spitzer L (Uniformed Services Univ of the Health Sciences, Bethesda, Md; Georgetown Univ, Washington, DC; Natl Naval Med Ctr, Bethesda, Md)
Anesthesiology 79:1219–1226, 1993   101-94-19-3

Background.—There is evidence that neural blockade by local anesthesia may lessen some of the physiologic sequelae of surgery of the lower abdomen or lower extremity. Blocking segments that subserve the adrenal medulla would be expected to counter the release of catecholamines into the circulation. Nevertheless, epidural anesthesia with 2-chloroprocaine reportedly does not alter the circulating epinephrine level in young, healthy subjects and lowers the norepinephrine level only when there is pinprick analgesia to C8.

Objective and Methods.—Nine healthy men aged 33–43 years received epidural anesthesia on 3 occasions at intervals of at least 48 hours, using .75% bupivacaine, 2% lidocaine, and 3% 2-chloroprocaine (all without epinephrine). Blood was sampled using a central venous catheter 20 minutes after catheter placement and during cold pressor testing before and after epidural analgesia to T1. The test entailed immersing the patient's hand in an ice water bath for 90 seconds.

Results.—No significant changes followed the production of stage 2 epidural block. The mean arterial pressure, heart rate, and cardiac index increased during the first cold pressor test, as did the plasma epinephrine and norepinephrine levels. None of the local anesthetics attenuated the heart rate and cardiac index responses to cold pressor testing, but they all lessened the increase in arterial pressure. Epidural bupivacaine and 2-chloroprocaine limited the increase in plasma catecholamines associated with cold pressor testing, but lidocaine did not.

Conclusion.—Lumbar epidural anesthesia to T1 using plain anesthetic solutions produces only partial sympathetic blockade. When examining patient outcomes after epidural anesthesia, the particular local anesthetic used should be taken into account.

▶ This study clearly indicated that epidural anesthesia is not a generic procedure, even among a large group of patients with a uniform sensory level. Thus, the choice of drug(s) may affect the hemodynamic response to stress during labor and/or surgery.—D.H. Chestnut, M.D.

A Comparison of Intrathecal, Epidural, and Intravenous Sufentanil for Labor Analgesia
Camann WR, Denney RA, Holby ED, Datta S (Harvard Med School, Boston)
Anesthesiology 77:884–887, 1992   101-94-19-4

Background.—Recent research suggests that highly lipid-soluble opioids have similar analgesic effects when given epidurally or intravenously. Whether the lipid-soluble opioid sufentanil is more effective given intrathecally than epidurally or intravenously was determined.

Methods.—Twenty-four women in active labor were included. Sufentanil, 10 μg, was given intrathecally to 9, epidurally to 8, and intravenously to 7, using a combined spinal-epidural method. No concomitant local anesthetics were given.

Findings.—The median durations of analgesia were 84, 30, and 34 minutes, respectively, in the intrathecal, epidural, and intravenous groups. Visual analogue scale scores in the intrathecal group declined rapidly and significantly. In the other 2 groups, these scores were unchanged and remained significantly increased at all observation points compared with those in the intrathecal group. Side effects consisted only of pruritus in 3 patients who were given sufentanil intrathecally; none of the patients had a postdural puncture headache.

Conclusion.—Given intrathecally, sufentanil, 10 μg, provides rapid, effective analgesia for 1–2 hours during labor. When this dose was delivered epidurally or intravenously, it did not provide sufficient analgesia. The increased efficacy associated with intrathecal injection suggests a spinal site of action by this route.

▶ Intrathecal sufentanil is most useful when given as part of a combined spinal-epidural technique. The anesthesiologist first gives intrathecal sufentanil, which provides a rapid onset of effective analgesia that has a duration of 1 to 2 hours. The anesthesiologist then places the epidural catheter. Local anesthetic (with or without opioid) can be injected when pain recurs. This technique may be favored by obstetricians who worry that epidural administration of local anesthetic during early labor may increase the likelihood of fetal head malposition and increase the incidence of cesarean section. Some anesthesiologists allow patients to ambulate after intrathecal administration of opioid.

In this study, no patient developed hypotension, although others have observed it after intrathecal sufentanil administration in a substantial number of laboring women. As a result, the anesthesiologist should determine maternal blood pressure at frequent intervals after intrathecal sufentanil administration. It also seems prudent to exclude orthostatic hypotension before allowing a patient to ambulate with assistance.—D.H. Chestnut, M.D.

Spinal Subdural Haematoma in a Parturient After Attempted Epidural Anaesthesia

Lao TT, Halpern SH, MacDonald D, Huh C (Univ of Toronto)
Can J Anaesth 40:340–345, 1993
101-94-19-5

Introduction.—A rare case of spinal hematoma that occurred after epidural anesthesia was attempted in a parturient with severe preeclampsia was described. The cause of the hematoma was unknown, but it may have been spontaneous.

Case Report.—Woman, 36 (gravida 3, para 2), was seen with severe preeclampsia at 30.5 weeks' gestation. She had no history of bleeding disorder but had recently experienced severe back pain radiating down both legs. The pain was not associated with any neurologic deficit. On admission, the patient's blood pressure remained elevated at 160/100 mm Hg despite treatment with magnesium sulfate and parenteral hydralazine. Her activated partial thromboplastin time (aPTT) was 49 seconds; all other tests of coagulation produced normal results. When a small vaginal bleed occurred, placental abruption was suspected, and the patient was prepared for an emergency cesarean section with epidural anesthesia.

Despite a test dose that produced negative results, injection of local anesthetic resulted in a generalized seizure. Epidural anesthetic was abandoned, and general anesthesia was induced. She delivered an infant weighing 895 g with a 5-minute Apgar score of 8. Seventy-two hours later, the woman had bilateral leg weakness, urinary incontinence, absent rectal sphincter tone, and asymmetric leg reflexes. Magnetic resonance imaging confirmed a diagnosis of spinal hematoma. Within 6 hours, a laminectomy was performed, and a blood clot extending from L3 to S1 was removed from the subdural space. The patient made a full neurologic recovery.

Discussion.—The estimated incidence of spinal hematoma in obstetric patients receiving anesthesia is 1 in 500,000. In this patient, it is possible that elevated venous pressure in combination with blood vessel trauma was responsible for the hematoma. The prolonged aPTT was attributed to lupus anticoagulant, because the patient had previously been treated with trifluoperazine for an unspecified psychiatric illness. Nevertheless, without evidence of a bleeding tendency, it is unlikely that a marginally elevated aPTT was an important etiologic factor.

▶ To my knowledge, this is only the third published case of an intraspinal, i.e., epidural or subdural, hematoma after administration of epidural anesthesia in an obstetric patient. Curiously, the patient had a platelet count of 425,000/mm³, a normal prothrombin time (10.5 seconds), and a normal bleeding time (3 minutes). The modest prolongation of the partial thromboplastin time probably resulted from the presence of lupus anticoagulant, which does not increase the likekihood of abnormal bleeding.

The etiology of this patient's hematoma is unclear, and it may not have been the result of the failed attempt to provide epidural anesthesia. The initial bleed may have occurred at the time the patient complained of severe back pain, *before* the attempt to provide epidural anesthesia. This case illustrates that a negative aspiration test and a negative test dose do not exclude intravenous placement of the epidural catheter.—D.H. Chestnut, M.D.

Continuous Extradural Infusion of Lignocaine 0.75% vs Bupivacaine 0.125% in Primiparae: Quality of Analgesia and Influence on Labour
Milaszkiewicz R, Payne N, Loughnan B, Blackett A, Barber N, Carli F (Northwick Park Hosp, Middlesex, England; School of Pharmacy, London) *Anaesthesia* 47:1042–1046, 1992   101-94-19–6

Introduction.—Continuous extradural infusion of a low concentration of local anesthetic during labor has a number of advantages compared with the intermittent bolus method. In the context of infusion techniques, the use of lidocaine during labor was reevaluated and compared with bupivacaine.

Methods.—Study participants were healthy primiparae who requested extradural analgesia. All were at or near term after an uncomplicated pregnancy, and they had a live singleton fetus in cephalic presentation. The women were randomized to receive an extradural infusion of lidocaine .75% after an initial dose of 10 mL of lidocaine 1.5% (42 women) or an infusion of bupivacaine .125% after an initial dose of 10 mL of bupivacaine .25% (44 women). Labor was actively managed according to the hospital protocol. On the day after delivery, all patients were questioned about the quality of analgesia during the first and second stages of labor by an anesthetist who was unaware of the study.

Results.—The mean duration of the extradural infusion was 3.72 hours for lidocaine and 4.55 hours for bupivacaine. More patients required top-ups in the lidocaine group (78%) than in the bupivacaine group (45%). Many women in the lidocaine group received top-ups almost every hour. The duration of the second stage of labor was significantly longer in the bupivacaine group. According to the women's assessments, bupivacaine produced a significantly better quality of analgesia than lidocaine. The 2 groups did not differ significantly in terms of spontaneous and instrumental delivery, fetal distress, or Apgar scores. One patient had a plasma concentration of lidocaine in the toxic range, but no ill effects were noted in the infant.

Conclusion.—Lidocaine was associated with a low incidence of motor block, a relatively short duration of second-stage labor, and a high incidence of spontaneous vaginal delivery, with no detrimental effect on the neonate. Nevertheless, lidocaine, as it was administered in this study, did not provide adequate analgesia during labor and delivery.

▶ This study confirms our experience at the University of Iowa. The continuous epidural infusion of .75% lidocaine does not consistently provide excellent analgesia during either the first or the second stage of labor. By comparison, the continuous epidural infusion of .125% bupivacaine provides analgesia of excellent quality, but a prolonged infusion results in substantial motor blockade. Maintenance of the epidural infusion of .125% bupivacaine until delivery may result in a prolonged second stage and an increased likelihood of instrumental vaginal delivery.—D.H. Chestnut, M.D.

The Effect of Intrapartum Epidural Analgesia on Nulliparous Labor: A Randomized, Controlled, Prospective Trial

Thorp JA, Hu DH, Albin RM, McNitt J, Meyer BA, Cohen GR, Yeast JD (St Luke's Hosp, Kansas City, Mo; Univ of Missouri, Kansas City)
Am J Obstet Gynecol 169:851–858, 1993   101-94-19–7

Background.—Epidural analgesia provides safe, effective pain relief during labor. However, retrospective studies suggest there is an increased risk of dystocia and subsequent cesarean delivery when it is used in nulliparous women. The effects of epidural analgesia on nulliparous labor and delivery were evaluated in a randomized, controlled, prospective study.

Methods.—Nulliparous women with uncomplicated, term, singleton gestations and a spontaneous onset of labor participated in the study. Forty-five patients were given meperidine, 75 mg, and promethazine hydrochloride, 25 mg, intravenously every 90 minutes as needed during the first stage of labor; 48 patients received an initial bolus of .25% bupivacaine followed by continuous .125% bupivacaine infusion through the second stage of labor. A cesarean section was performed in cases of fetal distress, as indicated by fetal heart rate monitoring or arrested cervical dilatation during active labor or descent during the second stage of labor.

Results.—Compared with narcotic analgesia, epidural analgesia significantly prolonged the first and second stages of labor, doubled the need for oxytocin augmentation, and significantly delayed cervical dilatation. A significant, fourfold increase in malposition was observed with epidural analgesia. Twelve of the 13 cesarean deliveries performed were in the epidural group; 4 of those were performed because of dystocia.

Conclusion.—Epidural analgesia in nulliparous labor significantly prolongs the first and second stages of labor and increases the need for oxytocin. Additional effects are an increased frequency of malposition and cesarean delivery because of dystocia. Nulliparous patients should be advised of the heightened risk of cesarean delivery when they are offered epidural analgesia.

▶ In the past, most studies of epidural analgesia during labor evaluated the quality of pain relief and maternal and neonatal safety. Few prospective studies have evaluated whether epidural analgesia increases the incidence of cesarean section. In this study, the authors noted an unbelievable 12-fold increase in the incidence of cesarean section in the epidural group. Unfortunately, they also assumed responsibility for making decisions regarding the method of delivery. Others have introduced an epidural analgesia service or increased the intrapartum use of epidural analgesia without any increase in the cesarean section rate.

In this study, no patient who received epidural analgesia after a 5-cm cervical dilatation underwent cesarean section. As a result, the authors concluded that the adverse effect of epidural analgesia on labor and delivery could be limited by delaying the epidural placement until a cervical dilatation of 5 cm or more had been reached.

At the University of Iowa, we have performed 2 studies that suggest administration of epidural analgesia between a cervical dilatation of 3 and 5 cm does not prolong labor or increase the incidence of cesarean section in nulliparous women.—D.H. Chestnut, M.D.

Effect of Epidural Opioids on Gastric Emptying in Labour
Ewah B, Yau K, King M, Reynolds F, Carson RJ, Morgan B (Queen Charlotte's Maternity Hosp, London; St Thomas' Hosp, London)
Int J Obstet Anesth 2:125–128, 1993   101-94-19–8

Background.—Administering opioid intramuscularly to a woman in labor markedly delays gastric emptying, but no such effect is seen when local anesthesia is given by the epidural route. It is now common practice to use a combination of opioid and local anesthetic in the epidural space. One of the opioids used, fentanyl, delays gastric emptying during labor and after cesarean section.

Objective.—The effects of both fentanyl and diamorphine on gastric emptying were examined in women who received bupivacaine epidurally during labor.

Study Plan.—The 36 participants all had pregnancies greater than 36 weeks' gestation and a cervical dilatation of less than 7 cm when they were given the initial dose of epidural bupivacaine. They then were randomized to receive 10 mL of .25% bupivacaine alone or combined with fentanyl, 50 μg, or diamorphine, 2.5 mg, or 10 mL of .125% bupivacaine alone or combined with fentanyl, 100 μg, or diamorphine, 5 mg, when they first asked for a top-up. The groups were demographically and clinically comparable. Gastric emptying was estimated by measuring the absorption of paracetamol after an oral dose of 1.5 g, which was given 30 minutes after the top-up.

Results.—Peak plasma paracetamol levels were significantly lower in women who were given diamorphine, 5 mg, than in those given bupivacaine alone. Both fentanyl and diamorphine in the larger dose prolonged the time to peak paracetamol level. Adding 100 μg of fentanyl to bupivacaine doubled the duration of analgesia, whereas diamorphine, 5 mg, increased it 80%. The lower doses of each drug did not significantly prolong analgesia. No significant group differences in Apgar scores were noted.

Conclusion.—Epidurally administered opioids may significantly delay gastric emptying. Therefore, a cesarean section delivery, if required, should be done under regional rather than general anesthesia. Women who are given epidural opioids when they are in labor should receive an H_2-antagonist prophylactically.

▶ Obstetricians and anesthesiologists have long known that systemic opioids delay gastric emptying during labor. In the past, an argument in favor of intrapartum epidural analgesia was that it allowed physicians to avoid the adverse effects of systemic opioids on gastric emptying. It is not surprising that epidural fentanyl delays gastric emptying, because its epidural route of administration results in blood levels of drug similar to those that occur after intravenous administration.

The authors acknowledged that the delayed gastric emptying may also have resulted from a direct spinal effect. Although I agree that it is preferable that such patients receive regional anesthesia for emergency cesarean section, I do not agree that epidural opioid administration mandates the prophylactic administration of an H_2-antagonist during labor.—D.H. Chestnut, M.D.

Epidural Anesthesia During Labor and Stress Incontinence After Delivery
Viktrup L, Lose G (Univ of Copenhagen)
Obstet Gynecol 82:984–986, 1993   101-94-19-9

Objective.—Because experience has suggested that a number of obstetric factors may play a role in the development of stress incontinence after vaginal delivery, the preventive value of epidural anesthesia was examined in 208 primiparae seen in a 6-month period; none were incontinent before or during pregnancy. The women, whose median age was 26 years, were asked about stress incontinence 3 months postpartum.

Findings.—Of the 208 women, 45 received epidural anesthesia during labor. The first stage of labor had lasted significantly longer in these women, and vacuum extraction was more frequently used. Twelve of the women who were given epidural anesthesia (27%) and 13% of the others experienced stress incontinence, a marginally significant difference. Incontinence was significantly associated with the length of the second stage of labor but not with the duration of the first stage or the use of vacuum extraction. Episiotomy did not predispose the women to stress incontinence, and epidural anesthesia was unrelated to the presence of stress incontinence 1 year postpartum.

Conclusion.—That epidural anesthesia for labor protects against the occurrence of stress incontinence in the postpartum period was not confirmed. In fact, incontinence was more frequent in women who were given epidural anesthesia than in those who received other forms of analgesia.

▶ The authors performed this study in response to a letter to the editor that suggested that intrapartum epidural anesthesia may prevent the subsequent development of stress urinary incontinence (SUI) (1). The authors of this study did not confirm that epidural anesthesia protects against the subsequent development of SUI. Rather, they indicated there was an increased incidence of transient SUI in women who had received epidural anesthesia (P = .05). Most cases of SUI had resolved by 1 year postpartum in both groups of patients. The authors noted that their findings were compatible with "electrophysiologic studies showing that the pudendal nerve function postpartum is similar in women who receive epidural anesthesia and in those who do not" (2).—D.H. Chestnut, M.D.

References

1. Schuessler B, et al: *Lancet* ii: 762, 1988.
2. Snooks SJ, et al: *Int J Colorectal Dis* 1:20, 1986.

Epidural Anesthesia Complicated by Fluid Collection Within the Spinal Cord
Katz N, Hurley R (Brigham & Women's Hosp, Boston)
Anesth Analg 77:1064–1065, 1993   101-94-19–10

Introduction.—Spinal cord injury is a rare complication of epidural anesthesia that can result from needle injury, epidural hematoma formation, cord ischemia secondary to arterial spasm or injury, or an epidural abscess. In other cases, a neurologic abnormality may develop after epidural anesthesia as a result of existing medical problems, patient positioning, or surgery itself.

Case Report.—Woman, 32 years, was seen for elective section delivery at 39 weeks' gestation who had an epidural catheter placed uneventfully in the L3–4 interspace and advanced 4 cm. However, as soon as an injection of 2% lidocaine was attempted, there were painful paresthesias in the lower back, buttocks, posterior thighs and calves, and feet. Six top-up doses totaling 44 mL were required for anesthesia at the chest level, and each injection produced the same symptoms. A cesarean section was done, and sensation returned fully 6 hours after catheter placement. However, severe back pain continued, and there was urinary retention. Radiating back pain was described on day 3 when examination revealed tenderness in the L2–4 region, mild weakness of the left leg, and areas of hypesthesia in both legs. The patient's reflexes were reported to be normal, but a week later they were impaired despite normal sensation and less pain. An expansile syrinx involving the conus medullaris from T11–12 to the L1 level was shown by MRI. At 3 months, the patient reported mild-to-moderate radiating back pain; repeat MRI revealed no change.

Discussion.—In this case, the catheter tip may have been against or, more likely, within the spinal cord, but a preexisting syrinx also is a possibility. Even at the L3–4 level, the conus medullaris is within range of a rostrally directed epidural catheter. It is critical not to inject when the patient describes paresthesia.

▶ Serious neurologic complications of epidural anesthesia are rare. The authors indicated that they might have avoided the complication described in this report if they had followed an old rule: Never continue to inject when the patient experiences a paresthesia.—D.H. Chestnut, M.D.

Double-Blind Evaluation of Patient-Controlled Epidural Analgesia During Labor
Fontenot RJ, Price RL, Henry A, Reisner LS, Weinger MB (Univ of California, San Diego)
Int J Obstet Anesth 2:73–77, 1993   101-94-19–11

Background.—Many patients in labor prefer to control the level of analgesia, but neither parenteral administration nor a constant epidural infusion of local anesthetic is a practical means of doing this. Recent research suggests that patient-controlled epidural analgesia (PCEA) is a safe means of providing consistent and adequate analgesia during labor.

Study Design.—A randomized, double-blind study was planned to compare PCEA with continuous epidural analgesia (CEA) in 39 American Society of Anesthesiologists physical status I or II women in active

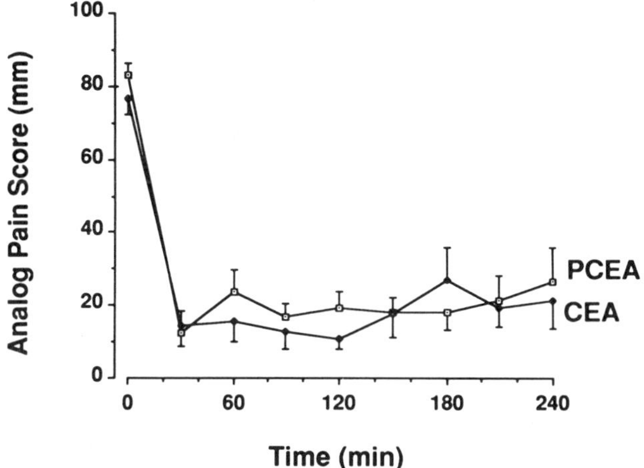

Fig 19–3.—Visual analogue pain scores for patients receiving CEA vs. PCEA. A score of 0 equated with no pain whereas a score of 100 equated with the worse pain imaginable. There were no significant differences in the pain scores during the 4-hour study. (Courtesy of Fontenot RJ, Price RL, Henry A, et al: *Int J Obstet Anesth* 2:73–77, 1993.)

labor who had already received 8 mL of .25% bupivacaine for epidural analgesia. The patients were randomized to receive either a continuous infusion of .125% bupivacaine at a rate of 12 mL/hr or a background infusion of 4 mL/hr. The latter patients were allowed to self-administer

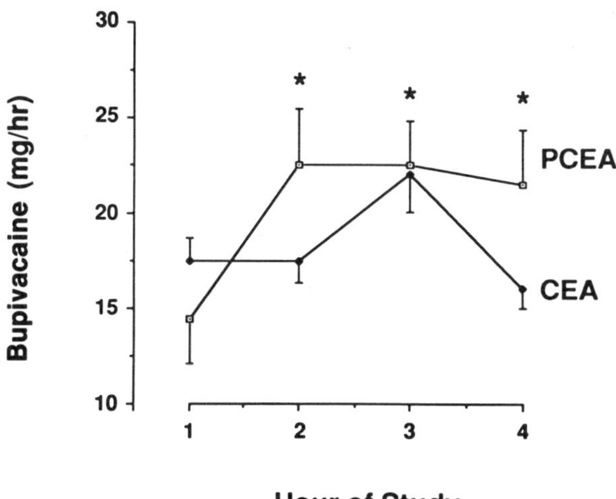

Fig 19–4.—Hourly drug usage for patients receiving CEA vs. PCEA. There was a statistically significant increase in drug use with time only in the PCEA (* = $P < .05$; subsequent hours compared with first hour). The total dose of bupivacaine administered in the CEA and PCEA groups did not differ significantly at any time point. (Courtesy of Fontenot RJ, Price RL, Henry A, et al: *Int J Obstet Anesth* 2:73–77, 1993.)

boluses of 3 mL at 10-minute intervals up to 15 mL/hr. Patients in both groups received supplemental doses of 5 mL of .25% bupivacaine when they reported inadequate analgesia. The 2 groups were similar in body size, gravidity, duration of labor, and motor and sensory blockade.

Results.—There were no significant differences between the PCEA and CEA groups in the frequency of hypotension or in the infants' Apgar scores. Patients in the 2 groups were equally satisfied with their analgesia, and no significant differences in pain scores were noted (Fig 19–3). The total amounts of anesthetic delivered were comparable in the 2 groups, but the PCEA patients used significantly more per hour after the first hour (Fig 19-4). Forty percent of patients in the CEA group and only 15% of those in the PCEA group required supplemental doses of bupivacaine.

Conclusion.—Patient-controlled epidural anesthesia is an effective and safe means of administering analgesia during labor. It may provide more consistent analgesia than CEA and require less staff time.

▶ During labor, PCEA is a double-edged sword. On the 1 hand, it may decrease manpower requirements for the provision of intrapartum analgesia. On the other hand, it may decrease the personal involvement of the anesthesiologist in patient care. I hope that the anesthesiologist's role will not be reduced to that of a technician who places a needle and catheter in the epidural or subarachnoid space.—D.H. Chestnut, M.D.

Intrathecal Sufentanil for Labor Analgesia: Sensory Changes, Side Effects, and Fetal Heart Rate Changes

Cohen SE, Cherry CM, Holbrook RH Jr, El-Sayed YY, Gibson RN, Jaffe RA (Stanford Univ, Calif)
Anesth Analg 77:1155–1160, 1993   101-94-19–12

Background.—Intrathecal sufentanil reportedly provides good relief of labor pain for as long as 4 hours. However, experience with a combined spinal-epidural technique suggests that most patients have sensory changes in their legs and that hypotension and fetal heart rate abnormalities are occasional problems.

Study Plan.—The duration of analgesia and the attendant hemodynamic changes were studied in a retrospective series of 90 patients who received sufentanil, 10 μg, in 1 mL of saline intrathecally during active labor. A combined spinal-epidural technique was used in these cases. Eighteen similarly managed parturients were studied prospectively.

Observations.—One fifth of the women in the retrospective series required no further analgesia. The mean duration of pain relief exceeded 2 hours. Patients frequently described feelings of warmth, tingling, and, occasionally, numbness in their legs in addition to pruritus. One patient transiently had trouble breathing deeply and swallowing. Five patients

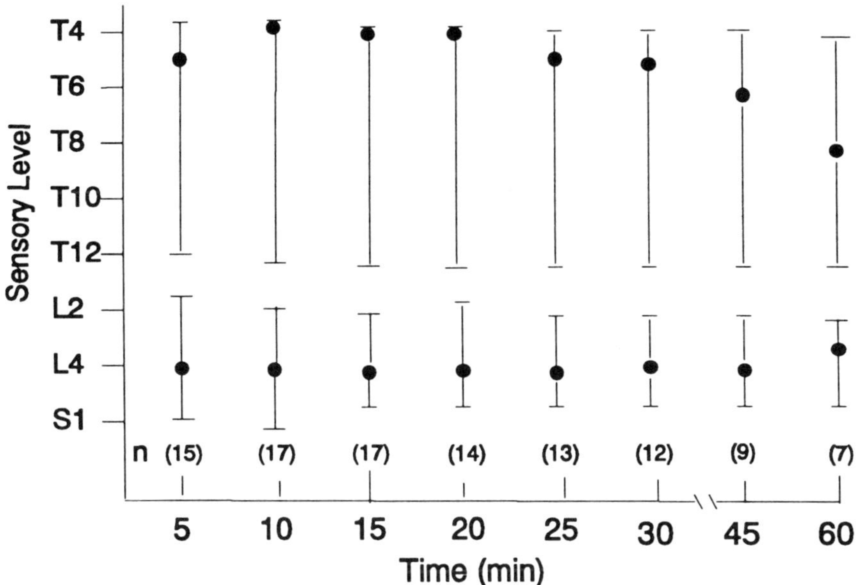

Fig 19–5.—Median (*circles*) upper and lower levels of decreased sensation to pinprick. *Vertical bars* represent the range. *Values in parentheses* refer to number of patients exhibiting sensory changes at each observation time. (Courtesy of Cohen SE, Cherry CM, Holbrook RH Jr, et al: *Anesth Analg* 77:1155–1160, 1993.)

required a small dose of ephedrine because of hypotension. Only 1 infant had a low Apgar score. In the prospective series, profound analgesia developed rapidly in all but 1 patient. Significant sensory changes lasted about 1 hour (Fig 19–5). All the patients requested more analgesia; 11% became hypotensive (Fig 19–6), but none required ephedrine. The patients were mildly sedated. Significant fetal heart rate changes were seen in 15% of evaluable records, but they were not considered to be clinically meaningful.

Conclusion.—Intrathecal sufentanil appears to be ideal for the woman whose labor is progressing rapidly and for those who ask for analgesia at an advanced stage of labor. However, it should be used cautiously if hemodynamic stability is a critical concern.

▶ The authors observed maternal hypotension in a sizeable number of women who received intrathecal sufentanil, 10 μg. Furthermore, they also observed evidence of definite sensory changes in most patients. The etiology of the hypotension is unclear, but the authors speculated that "at least in part, these effects result from a local anesthetic action of the opioid." Patients who receive intrathecal opioids during labor should be given at least the same level of surveillance that is provided for patients who receive epidural local anesthetics. In addition, ambulation should be avoided in patients with evidence of orthostatic hypotension. The potential for extensive sensory

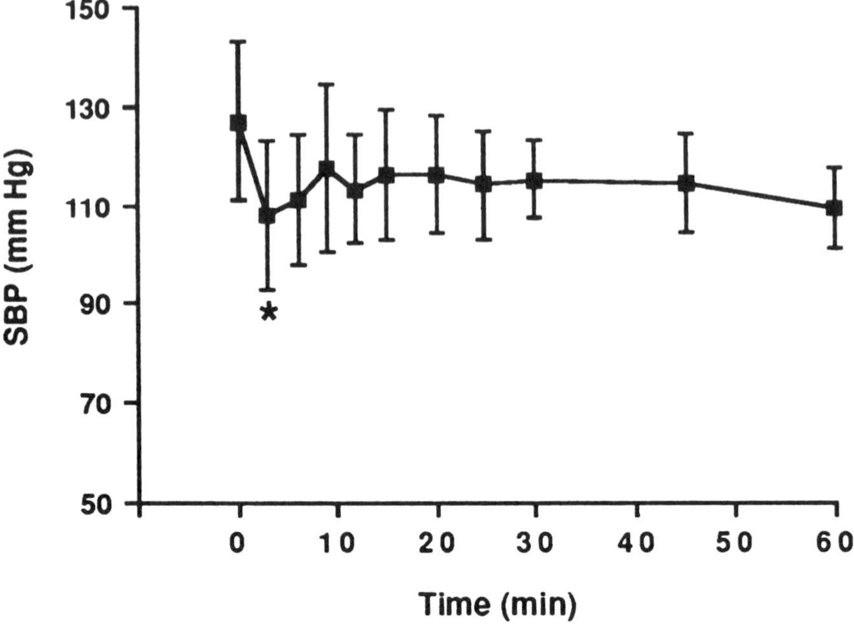

Fig 19–6.—Systolic blood pressure (mean ± standard deviation) after intrathecal injection of sufentanil. *P < .05 vs. control. (Courtesy of Cohen SE, Cherry CM, Holbrook RH Jr: *Anesth Analg* 77:1155–1160, 1993.)

changes mandates the constant attendance of a support person during attempted ambulation after intrathecal opioid administration.—D.H. Chestnut, M.D.

Intrathecal Sufentanil Labor Analgesia: The Effects of Adding Morphine or Epinephrine

Grieco WM, Norris MC, Leighton BL, Arkoosh VA, Huffnagle HJ, Honet JE, Costello D (Thomas Jefferson Univ, Philadelphia)
Anesth Analg 77:1149–1154, 1993   101-94-19–13

Objective.—Intrathecal opioids can provide profound labor analgesia. An attempt was made to prolong analgesia induced by intrathecal sufentanil by adding morphine or epinephrine.

Study Design.—Forty-one healthy nulliparous women at term who were having regular, painful uterine contractions had a lumbar epidural catheter placed and received sufentanil, 10 µg. In addition, 13 women received 200 µg of epinephrine and 15 received 250 µg of morphine. Patients requesting further analgesia received 10 mL of .25% bupivacaine epidurally. A blinded observer recorded blood pressure and changes in cervical dilatation.

Results.—There were no significant group differences in time to delivery, the method of delivery, pruritus, or infant Apgar scores. Analgesia developed rapidly in all cases, with no significant group differences. The addition of epinephrine tended to prolong analgesia, and the addition of morphine significantly increased its duration. Patients who were given morphine in addition to sufentanil remained comfortable for longer than those in the other groups after the initial dose of epidural bupivacaine. Pruritus and nausea were most evident in patients treated with morphine, but there were no significant group differences in blood pressure.

Conclusion.—Both epinephrine and morphine prolong analgesia when added to intrathecal sufentanil. However, the use of morphine may lead to pruritus and nausea, and for this reason it should not be given routinely to produce analgesia during labor.

▶ The addition of morphine, .25 μg, to sufentanil, 10 μg, resulted in only a modest prolongation of analgesia during labor. However, women who received both sufentanil and morphine experienced significantly more nausea and pruritus than women in the other 2 groups. I agree with the authors that the modest prolongation of analgesia does not justify the increase in side effects associated with the addition of morphine, .25 μg. A larger dose, e.g., .4 mg of morphine, should be given to obtain satisfactory intrathecal analgesia for most of the first stage of labor in the majority of laboring women. Unfortunately, this dose of intrathecal morphine results in a high incidence of pruritus and nausea.—D.H. Chestnut, M.D.

Epidural Anesthesia for Labor in an Ambulatory Patient
Breen TW, Shapiro T, Glass B, Foster-Payne D, Oriol NE (Harvard Med School, Boston)
Anesth Analg 77:919–924, 1993   101-94-19–14

Background.—Although it is generally accepted as the most effective method for pain relief, epidural anesthesia during labor has disadvantages for some patients, including a possible prolongation of the second stage of labor, a possible increase in the incidence of assisted deliveries, and confinement to bed. Epidural fentanyl alone or an ultra–low-dose bupivacaine-epinephrine-fentanyl regimen may provide satisfactory analgesia for labor and delivery as it enables the patient to ambulate safely.

Methods.—The effect of these 2 epidural analgesic regimens on the ability to ambulate was compared in a prospective, randomized, double-blind study. Fifty-three patients received epidural fentanyl in a 75-μg bolus and an infusion of fentanyl, 2.5 μg/mL, at 15 mL/hr. Another 77 patients received ultra–low-dose bupivacaine (.04%), epinephrine (1.7 μg/mL), and fentanyl (1.7 μg/mL) in a 15-mL bolus followed by an infusion at 15 mL/hr. Data collected for each patient included an evaluation of the intensity of the motor block (table).

Modified Bromage Score (Intensity of Motor Block)

1 = Complete block (unable to move feet or knees)
2 = Almost complete block (able to move feet only)
3 = Partial block (just able to move knees)
4 = Detectable weakness of hip flexion (between scores 3 and 5)
5 = No detectable weakness of hip flexion while supine (full flexion of knees)
6 = Able to perform partial knee bend

(Courtesy of Breen TW, Shapiro T, Glass B, et al: *Anesth Analg* 77:919–924, 1993.)

Findings.—Adequate analgesia was obtained rapidly in 90.6% of the patients in the first group and in 92.2% of the patients in the second group. About 70% of the patients in both groups were able to ambulate. The second regimen provided a longer duration of analgesia. Hip flexion weakness that precluded ambulation occurred in 17% of the patients in the second group; orthostatic hypotension occurred in 9% of this group. Neonatal outcomes for the 2 groups were comparable.

Conclusion.—Many patients who are given epidural analgesia for pain relief during labor obtain satisfactory analgesia with fentanyl alone or with a low-dose mixture of bupivacaine, fentanyl, and epinephrine. About 70% of these patients are able to ambulate. Patients who want to ambulate should have no obstetric or anesthetic contraindications to walking, normal leg strength, no orthostatic hypotension, and the ability to satisfactorily perform a partial knee bend from a standing position before they are allowed to walk.

▶ Some physicians and nurses contend that ambulation hastens labor and decreases the likelihood of a malpositioned fetal head. In the past, early administration of epidural analgesia necessitated early confinement to bed. Use of intraspinal (epidural or intrathecal) *opioid* techniques may enable the anesthesiologist to provide effective analgesia during early labor, because it preserves the patient's ability to ambulate. However, I have some reservations about the wisdom of attempted ambulation in patients who have received an epidural injection of local anesthetic (as did the patients in the second group in this study). Anesthesiologists who allow ambulation after administration of an intraspinal analgesia should pay attention to the 4 requirements outlined by the authors of this study. I also agree with the authors that no patient should ambulate unaccompanied.—D.H. Chestnut, M.D.

Posture and the Spread of Hyperbaric Bupivacaine in Parturients Using the Combined Spinal Epidural Technique

Patel M, Samsoon G, Swami A, Morgan B (Queen Charlotte's and Chelsea Hosp, London)
Can J Anaesth 40:943–946, 1993

100-94-19–15

Background.—Spinal anesthesia is becoming more frequently used in obstetric practice. Previous studies have examined the effect of posture on the spread of isobaric bupivacaine in pregnant women, but no similar studies of hyperbaric bupivacaine have been reported.

Methods.—This randomized study had a twofold objective: to compare the effects of a sitting position vs. a left lateral position on the spread of hyperbaric bupivacaine, as given by the combined spinal extradural technique, and to evaluate the quality of analgesia provided by 10 mg of bupivacaine given in this manner. The subjects were 50 healthy patients scheduled for elective cesarean section under regional anesthesia. Both groups received .5% hyperbaric bupivacaine, 2 mL, while in a sitting or a left lateral position. All injections were given with a 27-gauge, 120-mm long spinal needle using a single-space combined spinal extradural technique.

Results.—Analgesia at T4 was achieved in 7.7 minutes in the lateral group and in 10.8 minutes in the sitting group. A grade 3 motor block was achieved in 6.9 and 9.4 minutes, respectively. Epidural supplementation was required by 9 women in the sitting group, compared with just 1 in the lateral group. Hypotension occurred in 48% of patients in the lateral group, compared with 13% in the sitting group. The rate of nausea was 61% and 22%, respectively. There was no difference in neonatal outcome between the 2 groups.

Conclusion.—Analgesia for cesarean section is more rapidly and effectively achieved if the injection is given with the patient in the lateral rather than the sitting position. If the induction is performed by the single-space combined extradural technique with the patient in a sitting position, more than 10 mg of hyperbaric bupivacaine should be used if rapid analgesia to T4 is required.

▶ Others have observed that the lateral position is preferable to the sitting position during the administration of hyperbaric spinal anesthesia for cesarean section. During performance of single-shot spinal anesthesia, use of the sitting position may result in an inadequate cephalad sensory level. With the combined spinal-epidural technique, use of the sitting position increases the likelihood that epidural supplementation will be required. Use of the sitting position also entails the risk of hypotension, if a long time is required to insert and secure the epidural catheter. I am biased in favor of the lateral position for most spinal and epidural procedures in obstetric patients, unless maternal obesity mandates the use of the sitting position.—D.H. Chestnut, M.D.

Aortocaval Compression in the Sitting and Lateral Decubitus Positions During Extradural Catheter Placement in the Parturient

Andrews PJD, Ackerman WE III, Juneja MM (Univ of Louisville, Ky; Norton Hosp, Louisville, Ky)
Can J Anaesth 40:320–324, 1993   101-94-19–16

Background.—Hypotension from aortocaval compression has been reported in the supine recumbent and lateral decubitus positions. The incidence of concealed aortocaval compression in the 2 positions most often used during epidural space identification has not been established. The incidence of concealed aortocaval compression in the left lateral decubitus and sitting positions in the parturient at term was determined.

Methods.—Forty American Society of Anesthesiologists physical status I or II parturients at term and in active labor were studied. All had required epidural analgesia. By random assignment, 22 women were placed in group 1, positioned in the left lateral decubitus position, and 18 were placed in group 2, in the sitting position. Cardiac output (CO) was recorded every 1 minute for 5 minutes before, during, and for 5 minutes after epidural catheter insertion using the BoMED NCCOM3-R7 thoracic electrical bioimpedance (TEB) monitor.

Findings.—Of the 22 patients in the left lateral decubitus position, 17 had a greater than 25% decrease in CO_{TEB}, compared with 5 of the 18 patients in the sitting position. Patients in the lateral decubitus position had a greater percentage change in CO_{TEB} than those in the sitting position. Compared with the left lateral decubitus position, there was a reduced incidence of aortocaval compression during identification of the epidural space in the sitting position.

Conclusion.—Concealed aortocaval compression is common during epidural space identification. It appears to occur more frequently in the left lateral decubitus position than in the sitting position, with marked flexion of the spine. Identification of the epidural space should therefore be done in the sitting position and when compromise of the uteroplacental unit is suspected.

▶ For years I have preferred to ask pregnant women to assume the lateral decubitus position during identification of the epidural space. In an earlier study, we observed that leaner patients tend to prefer the lateral decubitus position, whereas heavier patients tend to favor the sitting position (1). It seems intuitive that the lateral decubitus position should result in better uteroplacental perfusion than the sitting position. Suonio and colleagues (2) noted that mean placental blood flow in 10 pregnant women decreased 23% when they moved from the left lateral recumbent to the sitting position. Anecdotally, I have observed several cases of unexplained fetal bradycardia during identification of the epidural space in the sitting position. Because it is often difficult to use Doppler ultrasound to monitor the fetal heart rate in patients who are sitting, I ask the obstetrician to place a fetal scalp electrode before the patient assumes the sitting position for identification of the epidural space.

This study challenges my long-held bias against use of the sitting position. I wonder whether acute dorsiflexion in the lateral decubitus position affects venous return differently than acute dorsiflexion in the sitting position. It would be interesting to compare fetal heart rate (and perhaps fetal oxygenation) during identification of the epidural space using either of these 2 positions. Until someone documents improved outcome with the sitting position, I intend to continue to use the lateral decubitus position, except in morbidly obese patients.—D.H. Chestnut, M.D.

References

1. Vincent RD, Chestnut DH: *Int J Obstet Anesth* 1:9, 1991.
2. Suonio S, et al: *Ann Clin Res* 8:22, 1976.

When to Remove an Epidural Catheter in a Parturient With Disseminated Intravascular Coagulation

Sprung J, Cheng EY, Patel S (Med College of Wisconsin, Milwaukee)
Reg Anesth 17:351–354, 1992   101-94-19–17

Background.—Intraspinal hematoma can complicate indwelling epidural catheterization for anesthesia during labor. In this case report, acute coagulopathy developed in a parturient with an epidural catheter inserted for cesarean delivery.

Case Report.—Woman, 27, was hospitalized for induction of labor that was indicated by postmaturity with intrauterine growth retardation. Labor induction was unsuccessful, and a cesarean section was planned. Through an epidural catheter, 15 mL of 2% lidocaine with 1:200,000 epinephrine was titrated over 10 minutes. A T3 sensory block was obtained with no evidence of hypotension. A healthy baby was delivered. An oxytocin infusion was begun while the surgeon was manually delivering the placenta. The patient suddenly became confused, showing only a pain withdrawal response. Her respiration became labored. Perioral cyanosis developed, and pulse oximetry readings failed. Tonic-clonic seizures then occurred, followed by a loss of measurable blood pressure. Oxygen was administered, and the patient was intubated under direct laryngoscopy. Mechanical ventilation was begun. A normal saline fluid challenge and a 100-μg phenylephrine intravenous bolus produced a return of palpable pulses. After hemodynamic stabilization, the surgery was completed, and the patient was sent to the intensive care unit. The epidural catheter was still in place. Within 2 hours, the patient sustained several more seizures and episodes of bleeding around vascular catheter sites and from the incision site and the vagina. After she was stabilized again, the epidural insertion site was examined. There were no signs of bleeding, the patient was able to move both lower extremities spontaneously, and there were no focal neurologic deficits. The catheter was then carefully removed. The patient was closely observed for signs of lower extremity neurologic deficits for the next 24 hours. She had no further episodes of hemodynamic instability. Her oxygenation improved with diuretic therapy over 48 hours. Positive end-expiratory pressure and forced inspiratory oxygen were reduced gradually. The disseminated intravascular coagulation resolved within 24 hours. Three days after the cesarean section, the patient regained consciousness. She was weaned from mechanical ventilation and extubated. Ten days after admission, she was discharged home.

Conclusion.—Severe secondary coagulopathy can occur in parturients with indwelling epidural catheters. Because these catheters can migrate and bleeding can begin, they should be removed as early as possible. However, when bleeding around the epidural catheter site or intraspinal bleeding is evident, the catheter should be left in place because of the possible tamponading effect. In either case, frequent neurologic assessment is needed to detect the early signs of intraspinal bleeding. The clinician should try to correct the coagulopathy until the underlying disorders that caused the bleeding can be treated.

▶ There is still controversy regarding when to remove an epidural catheter in patients with evidence of coagulopathy. Some physicians worry that removal of the catheter may precipitate bleeding; this seems unlikely. The catheter should be removed as soon as possible. An indwelling catheter can migrate and cause trauma to an epidural vein, which can increase the likelihood of an epidural hematoma. I question the authors' recommendation of leaving the catheter in place in patients who have evidence of bleeding around the epidural catheter site. If the catheter can be removed easily, it should be removed as soon as possible. Of course, an effort should be made to correct the coagulopathy.—D.H. Chestnut, M.D.

Epidural Infusions for Nulliparous Women in Labour
A Randomised Double-Blind Comparison of Fentanyl/Bupivacaine and Sufentanil/Bupivacaine (St Thomas' Hosp, London)
Anaesthesia 48:856–861, 1993   101-94-19–18

Background.—For women in labor who are receiving epidural analgesia, it is preferable to minimize motor block for a number of reasons. Epidural opioids can permit administration of a decreased dose of local anesthetic and thereby reduce motor blockade. In a randomized, double-blind trial, systemically equivalent doses of fentanyl and sufentanil, both given with low-dose bupivacaine, were compared for quality of analgesia and the occurrence of side effects, particularly motor blockade.

Methods.—The study sample comprised 60 nulliparous women who requested epidural analgesia during labor. The women were randomly assigned to receive epidural infusions of .0625% bupivacaine containing either fentanyl, 2.5 μg/mL^{-1}, or sufentanil, .25 μg/mL^{-1}, both beginning at 12 mL/hr. The women were assessed hourly for the extent of the block, pain, and the degree of motor blockade.

Results.—The 2 groups did not differ in the duration of each stage of labor or in the mode of delivery. They had a similar quality of analgesia in the first and second stages of labor and at delivery. There was no difference in their dose requirements for bupivacaine. Of the women who received fentanyl, 90% required no or only 1 top-up, as did 87% of those receiving sufentanil. Motor blockade, which was limited to hip movement, developed in 5 of the fentanyl group and 4 of the sufentanil group. Pruritus occurred in 6 women in each group. Neonatal parameters did not differ between groups, and both groups reported a high rate of satisfaction with their first- and second-stage analgesia. There were also no any differences in the occurrence of postnatal symptoms, including perineal pain and localized backache.

Conclusion.—There were no significant differences in effectiveness between fentanyl and sufentanil when they were given with low-dose bupivacaine in an epidural infusion during labor. Both regimens provided excellent analgesia with a low incidence of side effects. The mothers reported a high level of satisfaction with their pain relief, and there were no apparent adverse effects on the baby.

▶ Several years ago, we published 2 studies (1, 2) of the epidural administration of .0625% bupivacaine with fentanyl, 2 μg/mL. We also demonstrated that this regimen provides effective intrapartum analgesia with very little motor block. Subsequently, we largely abandoned it in favor of .125% bupivacaine *without* fentanyl for 3 reasons. First, the .0625% bupivacaine/.0002% fentanyl technique was labor intensive. Second, some inexperienced residents used the fentanyl, which always provides at least partial analgesia through a systemic effect, to conceal a malpositioned epidural catheter. Third, we observed 2 cases of neonatal respiratory depression after epidural administration of a large dose of fentanyl. Soon, the pediatric residents were blaming all incidences of neonatal respiratory depression on epidural fentanyl.

Now we only add fentanyl to the solution of bupivacaine when a patient continues to complain of pain, despite a symmetric sensory level of at least T10. Then we add fentanyl rather than giving additional bupivacaine, which would increase the risk of significant motor blockade. We also arbitrarily limit the total intrapartum dose of fentanyl to 150 μg.—D.H. Chestnut, M.D.

References

1. Chestnut DH, et al: *Anesthesiology* 68:754, 1988.
2. Chestnut DH, et al: *Anesthesiology* 72:613, 1990.

Anesthetic and Obstetric Outcome in Morbidly Obese Parturients

Hood DD, Dewan DM (Wake Forest Univ, Winston-Salem, NC)
Anesthesiology 79:1210–1218, 1993   101-94-19–19

Introduction.—Morbid obesity increases the risks of surgery in non-pregnant patients for many reasons. In pregnant women, obesity is associated with an increased rates of diabetes, hypertension, preeclampsia, and primary operative delivery. In addition, obese women are more likely to deliver large infants but less likely to deliver prematurely.

Study Population.—Anesthesia records were collected prospectively for 117 parturients who delivered infants in 1978–1989 and who weighed more than 300 lb at the time of delivery. Each was matched with the first patient weighing less than 300 lb who was attended by the same obstetrician and delivered in the same month. Gravidity and parity were similar in the 2 groups, but the obese women were significantly older than the control group and had more advanced gestational ages.

Observations.—Sixty-two percent of the morbidly obese women and 24% of control women had cesarean section deliveries. Nearly half of all obese women in labor required an emergency section, compared with 9% of the corresponding control women. Epidural analgesia was used during labor and vaginal delivery in comparable percentages of the 2 groups, but the obese women required more catheter changes. The frequency of regional anesthesia for section delivery also was similar. The obese women remained in the hospital longer after either an operative or vaginal delivery. Premature births were substantially less frequent in the obese group; only 9% of singleton infants weighed less than 2,500 g at birth, compared with 24% of the control women's infants.

Conclusion.—The need for operative delivery is much increased in morbidly obese women, usually because of a failure to progress. Although placement of an epidural catheter early in labor is a reasonable step, provision for emergency airway management is mandatory.

▶ This is a very helpful clinical study from 2 anesthesiologists with a long-standing history in the anesthetic management of morbidly obese parturients. The authors made 2 striking observations. First, 62% of the morbidly obese women underwent a cesarean section. Second, epidural anesthesia was used successfully for labor and cesarean section in 74 of 79 morbidly obese women. Only 3 women had failed epidural anesthesia for cesarean section, and only 1 morbidly obese patient required intraoperative induction of general anesthesia. Although these results are exemplary, they illustrate that the anesthesiologist must be prepared to administer general anesthesia—*and manage the airway*—in a morbidly obese patient who receives regional anesthesia for cesarean section.—D.H. Chestnut, M.D.

Isoflurane in Labour
Wee MYK, Hasan MA, Thomas TA (St Michael's Hosp, Bristol, England)
Anaesthesia 48:369–372, 1993   101-94-19–20

Objective.—Whether adding .2% isoflurane to self-administered Entonox (50% nitrous oxide in nitrogen) in the first stage of labor provides better pain relief than Entonox alone without making parturients much drowsier was investigated.

Study Design.—Seventeen American Society of Anesthesiologists physical status I parturients aged 16–38 years who requested inhalational analgesia during normal labor participated in the study. They inhaled Entonox alone and Entonox with .2% isoflurane added for alternating 1-hour periods in random order during a 3-hour study period. The gases were self-administered using a standard Entonox demand-valve and breathing system.

Results.—Linear analogue scores for pain were significantly lower when women used the Entonox-isoflurane combination than when they used Entonox alone. Improved scores correlated closely with the mothers' subjective evaluation of pain relief. The use of isoflurane was associated with higher scores for drowsiness, but none of the mothers appeared to be drowsy or disoriented, and good verbal contact was maintained at all times. Nausea was not a major problem. All women progressed to spontaneous vaginal delivery, and the Apgar score of all infants were normal.

Conclusion.—Supplementation of Entonox with .2% isoflurane provides superior analgesia during labor without causing undue drowsiness.

▶ Few hospitals in the United States use inhalation analgesia during the first stage of labor, and I have no enthusiasm for the administration of a potent halogenated agent during the first stage of labor. In this study, it is not clear who supervised the self-administration of the inhalation agents. I agree with the authors that we need to identify alternative methods of effective analgesia for patients when regional anesthesia is unavailable or contraindicated.—D.H. Chestnut, M.D.

Severe Bronchospasm During Epidural Anaesthesia
Wang CY, Ong GSY (Univ Malaya, Kuala Lumpur, Malaysia)
Anaesthesia 48:514–515, 1993   101-94-19–21

Introduction.—Bronchospasm that occurs during anesthesia can potentially impair oxygenation and even cause death. With 1 exception, all reported cases have occurred during general anesthesia.

Case Report.—Woman, 38, had had asthma for 10 years when she was scheduled for an elective cesarean section. Two previous operative deliveries using general and epidural anesthesia had been uncomplicated. The asthma was well controlled by salbutamol tablets. Mild expiratory rhonchi were noted at the time of delivery. A test dose of .5% bupivacaine was delivered uneventfully by an epidural catheter, and further anesthetic mixed with fentanyl produced a sensory block at T4. Systolic hypotension was treated with intravenous ephedrine. Respiratory distress began shortly after total sensory block. The patient was tachypneic, and marked expiratory rhonchi were noted bilaterally. Bronchospasm was resolved by nebulized salbutamol, and a healthy infant was subsequently delivered.

Conclusion.—Anaphylaxis was not a probable cause of bronchospasm in this patient. Blockade of the sympathetic nerve supply to the lung, with a concomitant decline in circulating adrenaline, probably was responsible.

▶ Some anesthesiologists have long speculated that a high regional block, with its attendant sympathetic blockade, might cause bronchoconstriction as a result of unopposed vagal activity in asthmatic patients. This case report suggests that such a phenomenon may occur, although clinical experience suggests that it is *very rare.* Endotracheal intubation is a known trigger for the development of bronchospasm in asthmatic patients. Regional anesthesia continues to be the preferred anesthetic technique for most asthmatic patients who require a cesarean section.—D.H. Chestnut, M.D.

Aortic Stenosis, Cesarean Delivery, and Epidural Anesthesia

Brian JE Jr, Seifen AB, Clark RB, Robertson DM, Quirk JG (Univ of Arkansas, Little Rock)
J Clin Anesth 5:154–157, 1993   101-94-19–22

Introduction.—The stenotic aortic valve limits cardiac output and, under the increased cardiovascular demands of pregnancy, may lead to exertional dyspnea, angina, and syncope. Maternal mortality of 17% has been reported, with a rate of 40% when pregnancy is terminated electively. Epidural anesthesia has been recommended for use in these patients, but its hemodynamic effects in this setting are uncertain.

Case Report.—Woman, 23, was seen at 32 weeks' gestation who gave a history of congenital subvalvular aortic stenois. Valve replacement had been done at age 9 years, and at age 13 the prosthesis was replaced because of aortic insufficiency. A St Jude's prosthesis had been placed at age 15 years, and the patient had done well until age 18, when congestive failure developed. The valve gradient at that time was 80 mm Hg. Subsequently, the patient had stopped using diuretic and anticoagulant therapy against medical advice. The patient was admitted for elective section delivery and tubal ligation at 36 weeks' gestation. A lumbar epidural catheter was placed, and fractional doses of 1.5% lidocaine with 1:200,000 epinephrine were administered in 5-mL increments. Ringer's lactate solution was infused to maintain cardiac filling pressures. Hemodynamic values remained relatively stable, although the cardiac output declined 19%. Oxytocin was discontinued when the pulmonary artery pressure and pulmonary vascular resistance increased and the systemic vascular resistance declined. Epidural analgesia was maintained for 24 hours with .125% bupivacaine.

Discussion.—The use of ephedrine to treat declining blood pressure in patients with aortic stenosis may have detrimental hemodynamic consequences. This patient had some degree of cardiac reserve before pregnancy, but it was not clear whether she had enough added reserve to tolerate labor and delivery. Oxytocin, which is reported to be a peripheral vasodilator, had adverse effects on peripheral and pulmonary resistances in this patient.

▶ Historically, many anesthesiologists have considered aortic stenosis a relative contraindication to the administration of regional anesthesia. In recent years, others have reported the safe administration of epidural anesthesia in a small number of pregnant women with severe aortic stenosis (1). Slow induction of epidural anesthesia (as was done in this case) and adequate left uterine displacement are essential. Some anesthesiologists have stated that epidural anesthesia can be given to almost anyone, if it is given slowly. I continue to prefer an opioid-based general anesthetic technique for most patients with severe aortic stenosis who require cesarean section. The risks of maternal aspiration and neonatal respiratory depression are overstated in these patients. With careful planning, these risks can be anticipated and managed successfully.

As an aside, it appears that this patient's aortic stenosis was the sole indication for her cesarean section. At the University of Iowa, we reserve cesarean section for obstetric indications, even in patients with valvular heart disease. It is not clear why some physicians believe that elective cesarean section results in less maternal stress than labor and vaginal delivery.—D.H. Chestnut, M.D.

Reference

1. Easterling TR, et al: *Obstet Gynecol* 72:113, 1988.

Cesarean Section (Including Postoperative Analgesia)

A Comparative Study of Patient-Controlled Epidural Fentanyl and Single Dose Epidural Morphine for Post-Caesarean Analgesia

Yu PYH, Gambling DR (Grace Hosp, Vancouver, BC, Canada; Univ of British Columbia, Vancouver, Canada)
Can J Anaesth 40:416–420, 1993   101-94-19–23

Introduction.—Epidural morphine is effective for post-cesarean analgesia, but the opioid is associated with a number of adverse side effects. Epidural fentanyl, which is more lipophilic than morphine, is reported to provide reliable analgesia with fewer undesirable side effects. In this prospective, randomized, double-blind study, the effectiveness of patient-controlled epidural analgesia using fentanyl was compared with a single dose of epidural morphine.

Methods.—Study subjects were 22 women who were seen for elective lower segment cesarean delivery with epidural anesthesia. Half received fentanyl (100 μg) 20 minutes after delivery. Using a patient-controlled analgesic device, they self-administered a maximum of 2 epidural fentanyl boluses 50 μg with a lockout period of 5 minutes for a maximum of 2 doses per hour. The remaining patients received a single 3-mg bolus of epidural morphine intraoperatively. Their patient-controlled analgesic devices were filled with .9% sodium chloride. At 2, 4, 8, and 24 hours after administration of the initial dose of study drugs, the patients were evaluated for pain, satisfaction with pain relief, nausea, and pruritus. Data were also collected on the number of patient demands for epidural analgesia; the number of treatments for pain, itching, or nausea; and the time to independent ambulation.

Results.—The mean time to first ambulation was shorter for patients who received fentanyl than for those who were given morphine (18 vs. 22 hours). The fentanyl and morphine groups reported similar pain relief, satisfaction with pain relief, and use of supplemental analgesics. The 2 groups also had the same degree of nausea and clinically unimportant respiratory depression. Pruritus was less common in the fentanyl group at 8 and 24 hours. The mean 24-hour dose of epidural fentanyl used was 680 μg.

Conclusion.—The analgesia provided by patient-controlled epidural analgesia with fentanyl to patients who underwent cesarean delivery was equal to that offered by a single dose of epidural morphine. Fentanyl is less likely to cause pruritus and permits patients to titrate their own analgesia.

► In this study, the primary advantage of patient-controlled epidural fentanyl analgesia was a decrease in the incidence and severity of pruritus. The authors acknowledged 2 problems with patient-controlled epidural fentanyl: (1) the potential for migration or dislodgment of the catheter; and (2) the increased cost, when compared with that of a single dose of epidural morphine. I commend the authors for their levelheaded conclusion that "this method of analgesia may be suitable for the motivated patient with a history of severe pruritus after epidural morphine administration."—D.H. Chestnut, M.D.

Electrocardiographic Changes During Cesarean Section: A Cause for Concern?

Zakowski MI, Ramanathan S, Baratta JB, Cziner D, Goldstein MJ, Kronzon I, Turndorf H (New York Univ)
Anesth Analg 76:162–167, 1993   101-94-19–24

Introduction.—As many as 60% of women who undergo cesarean section under regional anesthesia have electrocardiographic ST-segment changes consistent with myocardial ischemia. Continuous Holter monitoring was used to determine whether these changes were associated with permanent myocardial damage, specific symptoms, intraoperative events, or hemodynamic changes.

Methods.—One hundred seventy consecutive healthy parturients were studied. Their ST-segment changes were recorded from 2 hours before to 3 hours after surgery. One hundred twenty women had lumbar epidural anesthesia (LEA), and 50 had subarachnoid anesthesia (SA). Transthoracic two-dimensional echocardiograms were obtained in 30 women having LEA.

Findings.—The ST segment was depressed or increased 160 times in 44 patients in both groups. Ninety-eight percent of the changes were noted between anesthesia induction and the end of surgery. Seventy-eight percent of the episodes registered −1 mV. Although the number of episodes tended to increase after delivery in the LEA group, the frequency remained constant in the SA group. ST-segment depression occurred in 38% of the women given LEA and in 14% of those given SA. There was no wall motion abnormality in the echocardiogram during ST-segment depression. The 12-lead electrocardiogram and plasma myocardial specific creatine kinase did not suggest myocardial injury. Operative events did not predict ST-segment changes. In 10% of time epochs, tachycardia was related to ST-segment changes.

Conclusion.—Although the incidence of ST-segment changes in these subjects was 25%, there was no evidence of myocardial ischemia or infarction. The group undergoing spinal anesthesia had a significantly lower incidence of heart rate and ST-segment changes than those who underwent epidural anesthesia.

▶ The etiology of electrocardiographic ST-segment changes in healthy patients undergoing cesarean section is unclear. However, this and other studies suggest that myocardial ischemia is not responsible for these changes in most parturients. In this study, it is curious that there was a lower incidence of ST-segment changes in patients who received epidural anesthesia when compared with those who received spinal anesthesia. This may, in part, reflect the slightly slower heart rate in patients who received spinal anesthesia.—D.H. Chestnut, M.D.

Prophylactic Intramuscular Ephedrine Prior to Caesarean Section

Rout CC, Rocke DA, Brijball R, Koovarjee RV (Univ of Natal, Durban, South Africa)
Anaesth Intensive Care 20:448–452, 1992   101-94-19-25

Introduction.—The incidence of hypotension in women undergoing spinal anesthesia for cesarean section is unacceptably high, despite the use of crystalloid preload and uterine displacement. Some authorities have suggested the prespinal administration of prophylactic vasopressor agents. The timing and extent of maternal hemodynamic changes after intramuscular ephedrine injection were documented.

Methods.—Thirty healthy parturients agreed to participate in the randomized, double-blind trial. Women received an intramuscular injection of .9% sodium chloride, 25 mg of ephedrine, or 50 mg of ephedrine 30 minutes before general anesthesia was induced for cesarean section.

Findings.—Ninety percent of the women who received ephedrine, 50 mg, and 50% who received 25 mg had reactive hypertension of 20% or more compared with control values. Women in the 50-mg group had a mean maximum increase of 28.2%. Maternal pH was significantly reduced in women who were given ephedrine, 50 mg. Neonatal acid-base status was significantly impaired in the 50-mg group. Umbilical venous and arterial pH were significantly lower in this group than in the control group.

Conclusion.—The prophylactic administration of intramuscular ephedrine before spinal anesthesia is not recommended, because it is associated with an unacceptably high incidence of maternal hypertension. Also, if general anesthesia becomes necessary, prophylactic intramuscular ephedrine may also result in adverse neonatal biochemical changes.

▶ The authors concluded that "prophylactic administration of intramuscular ephedrine prior to spinal anesthesia is associated with an unacceptably high incidence of maternal hypertension. . . ." This study does not justify that conclusion, because all patients subsequently received general anesthesia. Nonetheless, it is unclear why ephedrine would be given intramuscularly rather than intravenously before administration of spinal anesthesia for cesarean section. After intramuscular administration, the absorption of ephedrine is unpredictable. Hypertension may occur in the occasional case of failed spinal anesthesia. I prefer to wait and give both a bolus and infusion of ephedrine *intravenously* immediately *after* the intrathecal injection of local anesthetic.—D.H. Chestnut, M.D.

Effects of Propofol and Thiopental on Maternal and Fetal Cardiovascular and Acid-Base Variables in the Pregnant Ewe

Alon E, Ball RH, Gillie MH, Parer JT, Rosen MA, Shnider SM (Univ of Califor-

nia, San Francisco)
Anesthesiology 78:562–576, 1993   101-94-19–26

Background.—Propofol, a relatively new agent, is being used increasingly for nonobstetric surgical procedures. However, its effects on uterine blood flow are not well documented.

Methods.—A chronically instrumented pregnant sheep model was used to determine the effects of induction and maintenance of propofol-induced anesthesia on maternal and fetal cardiovascular and acid-base variables. A 2-mg bolus of propofol per kg was used for induction. For maintenance, 1 of 3 continuous infusions was used: 150, 300, or 450 $\mu g/kg^{-1}/min^{-1}$. Animals in a control group were given thiopental for anesthesia induction and isoflurane for maintenance.

Findings.—No adverse effects on maternal or fetal mean arterial pressure, heart rate, base excess, fetal heart rate variability, or uterine blood flow were associated with propofol. Uterine blood flow declined temporarily during induction and intubation with thiopental, but it was stable during propofol induction. However, succinylcholine administration for intubation in animals that were given propofol resulted in a severe, transient maternal bradycardia. The anesthesia provided by continuous infusion of 300 $\mu g/kg^{-1}/min^{-1}$ of propofol appeared to be satisfactory.

Conclusion.—If these findings can be applied to humans, they suggest that anesthesia induction and maintenance with propofol and 50% nitrous oxide in oxygen do not adversely affect the fetus. However, there may be a risk of severe maternal bradycardia during anesthesia induction when propofol and succinylcholine are used.

▶ Others have observed that concurrent administration of both propofol and succinylcholine entails a risk of bradycardia. At the University of Iowa, we have observed at least 1 case of asystole in a young, healthy, nonpregnant patient who received both propofol and succinylcholine for rapid-sequence induction of general anesthesia. Because succinylcholine remains the preferred muscle relaxant during rapid-sequence induction in most pregnant patients, I avoid using propofol during administration of anesthesia for cesarean section.—D.H. Chestnut, M.D.

Spinal Anaesthesia for Caesarean Section: Comparison of 22-Gauge and 25-Gauge Whitacre Needles With 26-Gauge Quincke Needles
Shutt LE, Valentine SJ, Wee MYK, Page RJ, Prosser A, Thomas TA (St Michael's Hosp, Bristol, England; Queen Alexandra Hosp, Portsmouth, England)
Br J Anaesth 69:589–594, 1992   101-94-19–27

Introduction.—The renewed interest in spinal anesthesia, especially for lower-segment cesarean section, has spawned new refinements in spinal needle design. The performance of the 26-gauge Quincke needle was compared with that of the 22- and 25-gauge Whitacre needles.

Methods.—One hundred fifty women undergoing elective cesarean section with spinal anesthesia were randomly assigned to 1 of 3 groups, each of which received the anesthetic with a different needle. The ease of insertion, the number of attempted needle insertions before identification of CSF, the quality of subsequent analgesia, and the incidence of postoperative complications were compared.

Findings.—Although there were differences between groups, they were not significant. Postdural puncture headache occurred in 1 woman in the 22-gauge Whitacre group, none in the 25-gauge Whitacre group, and 5 in the 26-gauge Quincke group. Of these 6 cases of headache, 5 occurred after a single successful needle insertion. In 15 women, more than 2 needle insertions were needed; 7 patients in this group experienced backache. Only 12 of the 129 women who needed 1 or 2 insertions had backache.

Conclusion.—A low incidence of postdural puncture headache was associated with the use of 22- and 25-gauge Whitacre needles in women undergoing elective cesarean section. Postoperative backache was more likely to occur when more than 2 attempts were made to insert the needle.

The Sprotte Needle and Post Dural Puncture Headache Following Caesarean Section

Ross AW, Greenhalgh C, McGlade DP, Balson IG, Chester SC, Hutchinson RC, Ashley JE (Royal Women's Hosp, Carlton, Victoria, Australia)
Anaesth Intensive Care 21:280–283, 1993   101-94-19–28

Introduction.—The problem of postdural puncture headache (PDPH) in patients undergoing cesarean section has been difficult to resolve. Some studies in which the Sprotte needle was used found no headaches or only slight headaches in obstetric patients, but the results have been variable. The rate of PDPH was prospectively studied in patients who had a cesarean section and were given anesthesia by Sprotte and Quincke needles.

Methods.—During an 18-month period, 104 patients underwent cesarean section with spinal anesthesia using the 24-gauge Sprotte needle. Patients with a known history of recurrent headache were excluded. The women were followed postoperatively for a minimum of 5 days and questioned regarding symptoms consistent with PDPH. A comparison group consisted of 40 women undergoing cesarean section who had spinal anesthesia administered using 26-gauge Quincke needles.

Results.—Anesthesia was successful in 103 patients with the Sprotte needle and in 38 patients with the Quincke needle. Ten patients (9.6%)

in the Sprotte needle group had PDPH; 2 cases were severe. There were 8 (20%) cases, 3 of which were severe, in the Quincke needle group.

Conclusion.—The high incidence of headache associated with the Quincke needle occurred despite orientation of the needle bevel parallel to the longitudinal direction of the dural fibers. This technique has been reported to reduce the incidence of PDPH. Because of the uneven sizes of the Sprotte and Quincke groups, the difference between the 2 needles with regard to PDPH was not statistically significant. Clinically relevant headaches continue to occur with the Sprotte needles. Despite the various advantages of spinal anesthesia, the epidural technique has a far lower incidence of headache that requires blood patching.

▶ During the last decade, few innovations have affected my practice more than the introduction of the noncutting (pencil point) spinal needles (Abstract 101-94-19–27). A decade ago, some of our residents completed their training without having given a single spinal anesthetic for a cesarean section. We now give spinal anesthesia to approximately 40% of our patients who require cesarean section. The article by Ross et al. (Abstract 101-94-19–28) illustrates that the use of a Sprotte or Whitacre needle does not result in a *zero* incidence of PDPH. However, use of a Sprotte or a Whitacre needle results in severe PDPH in less than 1% of our patients. During attempted epidural anesthesia, the incidence of unintentional dural puncture is approximately 2%, and approximately 75% of those patients will experience severe PDPH. Thus, use of a Sprotte or Whitacre needle may result in a lower incidence of severe PDPH than what occurs with planned epidural anesthesia for cesarean section. Currently, we use a 25-gauge Whitacre needle for most patients who receive spinal anesthesia for cesarean section. The Whitacre needle is not as expensive as the Sprotte needle. It is also easier for inexperienced residents to use a 25-gauge needle than a 27-gauge needle. I use a 120-mm 24-gauge Sprotte needle when performing a needle-through-needle combined spinal-epidural technique.—D.H. Chestnut, M.D.

A Two-Dose Epidural Morphine Regimen for Cesarean Section Patients: Therapeutic Efficacy

Zakowski MI, Ramanathan S, Turndorf H (New York Univ)
Acta Anaesthesiol Scand 36:698–701, 1992   101-94-19–29

Introduction.—Because epidural morphine does not offer pain relief to most patients who have cesarean section after the first 24 hours, supplemental analgesics are routinely required beyond this period. The efficacy of a second dose of epidural morphine, 5 mg, administered 24 hours after the first dose was evaluated.

Methods.—The study group consisted of 104 consecutive American Society of Anesthesiologists physical status I patients who were scheduled for elective cesarean section. They were alternately assigned to receive a single 5-mg dose of epidural morphine (group 1) or 2 doses (group 2). The patients did not know whether the second epidural dose was morphine or saline. Using a visual analogue scale, an independent observer asked the patients to rate their nausea, itching, and analgesia 24 hours after each injection. Patients received supplemental analgesic tablets and medications for nausea and itching if they requested them.

Results.—Fifty patients from each group were available for analysis. Fewer patients in group 1 complained of nausea and itching, but more group 1 patients complained of postoperative pain on the second day, despite the use of oral analgesics. In group 2, the second dose of morphine produced a significantly lower incidence and severity of nausea and itching than did the first dose. Supplementary analgesics beyond 48 hours were required by significantly more patients in group 1 (76%) than in group 2 (36%). No patient from either group required treatement for nausea and itching after the second injection. No serious complications occurred in either group.

Conclusion.—The administration of a second epidural morphine dose reduces or eliminates the need for supplemental narcotics in patients who have undergone cesarean section. This finding suggests that morphine has a residual effect at the spinal opioid receptors. Development of acute tolerance to morphine may explain the absence of increased nausea and itching with the second dose. The authors have used this 2-dose regimen with success in more than 1,800 patients.

▶ At the University of Iowa, we offer a single dose of intraspinal morphine for postcesarean analgesia. We give 3.5 mg to women who receive epidural anesthesia and .2 mg to patients who receive spinal anesthesia. Most patients experience satisfactory analgesia for approximately 24 hours. Subsequently, most require oral analgesics only. Few of our patients require a parenteral injection of an opioid. I am not convinced that the risk-benefit ratio justifies the 2-dose regimen described in this study. Furthermore, how many third-party payers reimburse the anesthesiologist for administering a second dose of epidural morphine?—D.H. Chestnut, M.D.

Postcesarean Delivery Epidural Patient-Controlled Analgesia: Fentanyl or Sufentanil?
Cohen S, Amar D, Pantuck CB, Pantuck EJ, Goodman EJ, Widroff JS, Kanas RJ, Brady JA (Albert Einstein College of Medicine, Bronx, NY; Cornell Univ, New York; Columbia Univ, New York)
Anesthesiology 78:486–491, 1993   101-94-19–30

Background.—Both fentanyl and sufentanil cause a lower incidence of opioid-induced side effects than morphine when they are administered epidurally for postcesarean delivery analgesia. Bupivacaine and epinephrine are often added to fentanyl and sufentanil to reduce opioid requirements. The incidence of side effects and patient satisfaction during prolonged epidural patient-controlled analgesia (PCA) infusions of these combinations of analgesic agents were compared.

Methods.—The study group consisted of 250 patients who were scheduled for elective cesarean delivery. They were randomized into 2 epidural PCA infusion groups, with half receiving fentanyl, 2 μg/mL, and half receiving sufentanil, .8 μg/mL. Both infusions also contained .01% bupivacaine and epinephrine, .5 μg/mL. The initial infusion rate was 16 mL/hr; self-administered 3-mL boluses were available every 15 minutes by PCA. Plasma samples were obtained at various periods to determine opioid concentrations.

Results.—The 2 groups had similar pain scores and similar pain relief. The infusion durations, 50.4 hours with fentanyl and 53.5 hours with sufentanil, did not differ significantly. The total number of times PCA requests were made was greater with fentanyl (106.7) than with sufentanil (70.8). Vomiting occurred more frequently with sufentanil; pruritus, nausea, and sedation occurred at similar rates for the 2 groups. Lightheadedness and dizziness occurred in 42 patients approximately 1–2 hours after the sufentanil infusion was discontinued; this side effect was reported by only 1 patient in the fentanyl group.

Conclusion.—Both fentanyl and sufentanil administered by epidural PCA succeeded in providing pain relief to postcesarean patients. There were fewer PCA requests for sufentanil, but this opioid was associated with a greater incidence of vomiting during infusion and dizziness after infusion. Sufentanil is significantly more costly and offers no advantages over fentanyl.

▶ This study suggested that epidural sufentanil provides no advantages over epidural fentanyl when it is combined with bupivacaine and epinephrine for postcesarean analgesia. I am not convinced that epidural PCA offers substantial advantages over intravenous PCA after cesarean section. The future of epidural PCA is in doubt. It is unclear whether third-party payers will continue to reimburse anesthesiologists for providing this service. In our hospital, we offer patients a single dose of either epidural or intrathecal morphine for postcesarean analgesia. Patients who reject this option receive intravenous PCA.—D.H. Chestnut, M.D.

Adequacy of General Anesthesia for Cesarean Section
King H-K, Ashley S, Brathwaite D, Decayette J, Wooten DJ (Charles R Drew Univ, Los Angeles)
Anesth Analg 77:84–88, 1993   101-94-19–31

Background.—In patients undergoing general anesthesia during cesarean section, the time from induction of anesthesia to birth is directly related to depression of the newborn after delivery. Therefore, to minimize anesthesia duration, the rapid-sequence induction of anesthesia is delayed until immediately before surgical incision. However, the lack of wash-in and anesthetic transfer times may impair the quality of anesthesia during the initial incision. The adequacy of commonly used general anesthesia for cesarean section was evaluated.

Patients and Methods.—The isolated forearm technique was used in 30 patients aged 17 to 35 years. All patients were scheduled for nonemergent abdominal delivery, and all were American Society of Anesthesiologists physical status I and II. Intravenous thiopental, 3 mg/kg, 250 mg maximum, and succinylcholine, 1.5 mg/kg, were used to induce anesthesia, followed by a mixture of 50% nitrous oxide, 50% oxygen, and .5% halothane at a flow of 5 L/min, as well as end-tidal carbon dioxide at 40 mm Hg. A .1% succinylcholine infusion was used to maintain paralysis. After the eyelash reflex was no longer noted, patients received taped instruction through headphones at 1-minute intervals for 10 minutes. They were advised to flex their fingers if they could hear, to make a fist or squeeze the investigator's hand if pain was felt, to remember 5 target words, and to respond with specific physical signals during subsequent interviews. Three sets of randomly assigned tapes were used. Other variables, including eye centering, pupil size, sweating, and lacrimation, were simultaneously monitored during induction, laryngoscopy/intubation, and skin incision, followed by 1-minute intervals for 10 minutes. Brain activity was also monitored by a computerized aperiodic analysis of an electroencephalogram (Lifescan). Postanesthesia interviews were conducted during recovery and 24 hours later.

Results.—At the time of skin incision, 29 patients signaled awareness by flexing their fingers, 26 had lacrimation, and 24 made a fist or squeezed the investigator's hand, indicating the perception of pain. At 1 minute after skin incision, 23 signaled awareness, and 19 signaled pain. At 2 minutes, 6 signaled awareness, 2 signaled pain, and 1 demonstrated signs of awareness for an additional minute. During postoperative interviews, no patients remembered intraoperative activities, target words, or responded to the physical signals requested in the taped instructions. A significant shift of the activity edge to the left was noted during brain activity monitoring, with a decreased frequency after induction and during endotracheal intubation in all patients. An abrupt, marked increase in frequency during skin incision was also revealed in 25 patients, followed by a marked slowing after narcotic administration.

Conclusion.—Adequate anesthesia is not provided at the time of skin incision when surgery is begun immediately after endotracheal intubation.

▶ The authors gave an inadequate dose of thiopental, i.e., 3 mg/kg, with a maximum dose of 250 mg. I typically give at least 4 mg of thiopental per kg during induction of general anesthesia for cesarean section. I also give a preinduction dose of opioid to patients in whom I want to blunt the hypertensive response to laryngoscopy and intubation. Nonetheless, it is time to reevaluate the practice of allowing the obstetrician to make the skin incision immediately after rapid-sequence induction and endotracheal intubation. Perhaps this practice is appropriate in cases of severe fetal distress, but it is of dubious value in patients who are receiving general anesthesia for a nonemergent cesarean section.—D.H. Chestnut, M.D.

Plasma Catecholamines and Neonatal Condition After Induction of Anaesthesia With Propofol or Thiopentone at Caesarean Section
Gin T, O'Meara ME, Kan AF, Leung RKW, Tan P, Yau G (Chinese Univ of Hong Kong, Shatin)
Br J Anaesth 70:311–316, 1993   101-94-19–32

Background.—Increased maternal sympathetic nervous system activity may decrease placental perfusion, resulting in an unfavorable neonatal outcome. Catecholamine response and neonatal effects in Chinese patients with uncomplicated, singleton pregnancies who were undergoing cesarean deliveries were investigated.

Patients and Methods.—Sixty-one patients were included in this study. Thirty-one patients were randomly assigned to receive thiopental, 4 mg/kg^{-1}, whereas the remaining 30 patients received propofol, 2 mg/kg^{-1}. Preoxygenation was performed in all patients for 3 minutes before a rapid-sequence induction of anesthesia, followed by suxamethonium, 1.5 mg/kg^{-1}. After 1 minute, a laryngoscopy was performed, and tracheal intubation was completed by 2 minutes. Atracurium, nitrous oxide, and isoflurane were used to continue anesthesia. Catecholamine assays were performed using maternal venous blood samples taken at 0, 1, 2, 3, 4 minutes and at delivery.

Results.—After tracheal intubation, patients in the thiopental group had a greater increase in mean arterial pressure from baseline values, at 29 $\pm$ 15 mm Hg, compared with 18 $\pm$ 14 mm Hg in the propofol group. Both groups experienced increased concentrations of norepinephrine and epinephrine after tracheal intubation. Patients in the thiopental group had greater maximum norepinephrine concentrations at 413 $\pm$ 177 pg/mL^{-1} compared with 333 $\pm$ 108 pg/mL^{-1} in the propofol group. However, no between-group differences were noted for epinephrine concentrations. Comparable between-group results were noted for neonatal Apgar scores, neurobehavioral testing and umbilical catecholamine, blood-gas tension, and oxygen content analysis.

Conclusion.—Propofol decreased the hypertensive and catecholamine response associated with laryngoscopy and tracheal intubation. However, no improvements in neonatal outcome were demonstrated.

▶ The authors observed a small difference between groups in the hypertensive response to laryngoscopy and intubation. In my judgment, the difference was clinically insignificant and not sufficient to justify the use of propofol during rapid-sequence induction of general anesthesia for cesarean section.

There is a small group of pregnant women who are at risk for severe hypertension and adverse sequelae during laryngoscopy and intubation. In those patients, I prefer to take other precautions, e.g., administration of an antihypertensive agent and/or an opioid, to attenuate the hypertensive response. In my practice, I can think of no reason to give propofol during rapid-sequence induction of general anesthesia for cesarean section.—D.H. Chestnut, M.D.

Complications During Spinal Anesthesia for Cesarean Delivery: A Clinical Report of One Year's Experience
Juhani TP, Hannele H (Tampere Univ, Finland)
Reg Anesth 18:128–131, 1993   101-94-19–33

Background.—Spinal anesthesia has many advantages for patients undergoing cesarean delivery. It is easy to perform, has a rapid onset of action, and requires only a small amount of anesthetic agent. In addition, it enables early breast-feeding. However, spinal anesthesia for cesarean delivery is also associated with many complications. The complication rate and factors that correlate with complications during spinal anesthesia for cesarean delivery in a single institution were determined.

Patients and Methods.—A total of 284 patients who were scheduled for cesarean delivery with hyperbaric .5% bupivacaine spinal anesthesia during a 1-year period was enrolled. Of these, 160 had elective and 124 had nonelective cesarean deliveries. Complications that occurred during the observation period were analyzed.

Results.—Hyperbaric .5% bupivacaine provided reliable anesthesia, with a failure rate of only 2.8%. Hypotension and nausea were the most frequent complications and were noted in 42% and 14% of the patients, respectively. Hypotensive periods occurred before delivery in 81% of the patients, although no correlations with low Apgar scores or low pH in the umbilical artery of the infant were noted. Elective procedures and operations without prophylactic ephedrine infusion were identified as risk factors for hypotension. Nausea occurred significantly more often when a lower interspace was used for administration of the subarachnoid block.

Conclusion.—Spinal anesthesia is a safe, effective, and fast-acting method of anesthesia for cesarean delivery. However, because of the high incidence of minor complications, patients must be carefully monitored during spinal anesthesia to ensure optimal outcomes for both mother and fetus.

▶ I give prophylactic ephedrine to most patients who receive spinal anesthesia for cesarean section. I also typically give approximately 1,500 mL of Ringer's lactate before administration of spinal bupivacaine. I then give an intravenous 5- to 10-mg bolus of ephedrine immediately *after* the injection of local anesthetic and add ephedrine, 25 mg, to the remaining 500 mL of fluid in the second bag of Ringer's lactate. Although this regimen does not prevent all cases of hypotension, mild and transient hypotension does not adversely affect the condition of the newborn.—D.H. Chestnut, M.D.

Comparison of the 25-Gauge Whitacre With the 24-Gauge Sprotte Spinal Needle for Elective Caesarean Section: Cost Implications

Campbell DC, Douglas MJ, Pavy TJG, Merrick P, Flanagan ML, McMorland GH (Univ of British Columbia, Vancouver, Canada)
Can J Anaesth 40:1131–1135, 1993   101-94-19–34

Objective.—Both the Sprotte and Whitacre pencil-point spinal needles, which are used to provide spinal anesthesia for surgical delivery, reportedly carry a low risk of postdural puncture headache (PDPH). Because the 25-gauge Whitacre needle is less costly than the 24-gauge Sprotte needle, their relative safety and ease of use were determined in a prospective, double-blind, comparative study.

Study Design.—A total of 304 American Society of Anesthesiologists physical status I and II women who were having an elective cesarean section with spinal anesthesia were included in the study. The patients were monitored daily for 5 days by an investigator who did not know which needle had been used. The needle was introduced in the midline in the L2–3 or the L3–4 interspace to administer hyperbaric .75% bupivacaine solution, preservative-free morphine, and fentanyl. The 2 groups were comparable both demographically and with respect to the number and ease of needle insertions.

Results.—In 2 patients in each group, it was not possible to identify the subarachnoid space. After successful dural puncture, subarachnoid block failed in 2% of the Sprotte group and in 1.3% of the Whitacre group. About one fifth of the patients had a nonspinal headache in the postpartum period. The incidence of PDPH was 4% in the Sprotte

			Documented Incidence of PDPH With the 24-Gauge Sprotte	
Author	*Year*	*Study type*	*Incidence of PDPH*	
Sprotte *et al.*[2]	1987	Prospective	(0.02%)	
Cesarini *et al.*[5]	1990	Prospective	0/55	(0%)
Mayer *et al.*[19]	1991	Prospective	0/23	(0%)
Leeman *et al.*[3]	1991	Prospective	2/55	(3.6%)
Ross *et al.*[17]	1992	Retrospective	2/132	(1.5%)
Devcic *et al.*[4]	1992	Prospective	4/71	(5.6%)

(Courtesy of Campbell DC, Douglas MJ, Pavy TJG, et al: *Can J Anaesth* 40:1131–1135, 1993.)

group and .66% in the Whitacre group. One patient in each group required a blood patch. The occurrence of PDPH was not related to the difficulty of needle placement. Significantly fewer patients in the Whitacre group than in the Sprotte group required supplemental analgesia (3.3% vs. 17.3%).

Discussion.—The reported frequency of PDPH has increased as spinal anesthesia has been used more often in parturients (table). Both the 24-gauge Sprotte and the 25-gauge Whitacre spinal needles reliably deliver effective spinal anesthesia with a low risk of PDPH. The Whitacre needle is a reasonable choice, because it is less expensive.

▶ Some anesthesiologists have expressed concern that the large size of the hole at the distal end of the Sprotte needle might increase the likelihood of injecting some of the local anesthetic outside the subarachnoid space, i.e., within the subdural and/or the epidural space. In this study, there was no difference between groups in the incidence of failed block, but more women in the Sprotte group required supplemental analgesia during surgery. The results would have been more convincing had the anesthetists been blinded to the group assignment. Nevertheless, the 25-gauge Whitacre needle is less expensive than the 24-gauge Sprotte needle, so it seems logical to choose the former for administration of single-shot spinal anesthesia for cesarean section.—D.H. Chestnut, M.D.

Venous Air Embolism During Cesarean Section: More Common Than Previously Thought
Lew TWK, Tay DHB, Thomas E (Kandang Kebau Hosp, Singapore)
Anesth Analg 77:448–452, 1993   101-94-19–35

Background.—The reported incidence of venous air embolism (VAE) in cesarean delivery ranges from 11% to 52%. These variations are the result, in part, of differing study designs and definitions of positive Doppler events. Monitoring increased expired nitrogen concentration (FEN_2) is a specific diagnostic method that is commonly used in other surgical procedures to detect air embolism. The current study monitored FEN_2 and precordial Doppler imaging to determine the incidence of VAE during cesarean delivery with general anesthesia. The effect of a 10-degree reverse Trendelenburg tilt in preventing VAE was also evaluated.

Methods.—Thirty women undergoing cesarean delivery with general anesthesia were randomized into 2 groups: Women in group A were placed in the horizontal position with a left lateral tilt, and those in group B were placed in a 10-degree reverse Trendelenburg/left lateral tilt. Inspired and expired nitrogen concentration, obtained by a side stream sampling catheter, was measured with a Raman scattering analyzer. An ultrasonic Doppler transducer that was placed parasternally over the fourth intercostal space was monitored through headphones by a single listener. Air embolism was diagnosed if FEN_2 increased .1 vol%

from baseline or if the Doppler signal changed to chirping or broken-up roaring.

Results.—Expired nitrogen concentration monitoring demonstrated a similar incidence of VAE in the 2 groups: 93.3% in group A and 100% in group B; 23 episodes in group A and 19 in group B. Fifty-six Doppler changes were detected; however, 45% of Doppler events in group A and 35% of those in group B did not correspond with FEN_2 increases.

Conclusion.—Cesarean section conducted with general anesthesia has a very high incidence of VAE, which is not lowered by the use of the reverse Trendelenburg position. Because Doppler monitoring has limited sensitivity for true VAE, FEN_2 should be monitored routinely in cesarean delivery with general anesthesia.

▶ Venous air embolism occurs during cesarean section in a substantial number of parturients. Most air emboli are small, and morbidity and mortality are rare. I am not aware of a single published case of maternal mortality secondary to VAE during cesarean section. However, not all adverse outcomes are published, and I suspect that some maternal deaths have resulted from VAE during cesarean section. However, no study has demonstrated the need to make major changes in anesthetic management to decrease the risk of VAE during cesarean section. The authors noted that "whether the results of this study indicate a need for routine placement of central venous pressure catheters in all parturients undergoing operative delivery remains debatable." There is no need for debate; neither this study nor any other published study justifies the risk or the cost of placing a central venous pressure catheter in healthy pregnant women who are undergoing cesarean section.—D.H. Chestnut, M.D.

An Ethical Justification for Emergency, Coerced Cesarean Delivery
Chervenak FA, McCullough LB, Skupski DW (New York Hosp/Cornell Med Ctr, New York; Baylor College of Medicine, Houston)
Obstet Gynecol 82:1029–1035, 1993   101-94-19–36

Background.—When a woman refuses a cesarean section delivery that has been advised for the benefit of the fetus, 1 response is to seek a court order. However there are emergency cases where a court-ordered intervention has been clinically irrelevant, because there is not enough time to obtain judicial review much less a court order. Whether it sometimes is ethically justified to resist a woman's refusal of an emergency section delivery and coerce her into undergoing the procedure was considered.

Existing Arguments.—Most legal opinions, as well as the American Medical Association Board of Trustees, have opposed court-ordered cesarean delivery in all cases, although the board has acknowledged that there may be instances in which it is acceptable. Many think that the maternal right to refuse the procedure is an absolute, but this argument is inconsistent with the obligation not to unnecessarily cause harm to the term fetal patient. Of course, this assumes that the term fetus without a lethal anomaly is, in fact, a patient. Some who would allow a coerced, court-ordered cesarean delivery have failed to address the emergency situation.

Ethically Inadequate Arguments.—It may be claimed that in the emergency setting, the mother is not truly able to give informed consent, but this is not the case. The act of simply coming to the hospital and accepting preliminary treatment does not constitute consent to operative delivery. Attempts to establish fetal rights are problematic, because it is not possible to show conclusively that the fetus possesses an independent moral status.

A *Justification.*—Coerced emergency cesarean section must rest on the established beneficence-based obligations of the pregnant woman and her obstetrician to the term fetal patient and future child. A highly reliable judgment is required that on balance, operative delivery will prevent serious infant morbidity or death. The woman must not be resisting in a manner that will significantly increase the chances of her being harmed. In addition, there must be insufficient time to consider obtaining a court order. It is appropriate for physicians to take a preventive approach toward refusal of operative delivery, particularly when the patient does not speak English as her first language.

▶ Several years ago, I received a *stat* page to administer anesthesia for emergency cesarean section in a patient with persistent fetal bradycardia. I met the patient in the operating room, where she stated that she did not want to undergo a cesarean section. Both the husband and the obstetrician were at her side, and they urged me to anesthetize her as soon as possible. The patient offered no resistance, but she clearly stated that she did not want to undergo a cesarean section. Meanwhile, the fetal monitor demonstrated a persistent fetal heart rate of 60 beats per minute. There was little doubt in my mind that this baby would soon die if it remained in utero. I administered general anesthesia, and a depressed, acidotic infant was promptly delivered. The infant responded to resuscitative measures, and both the infant and the mother had an uneventful hospital course. After surgery, the mother thanked me for the care I had provided, specifically for proceeding with anesthesia despite her refusal. Our hospital attorney informed me that I did the wrong thing and that I was vulnerable to a charge of battery. I think that this case satisfied the 3 requirements for an "emergency, coerced cesarean delivery," as outlined in this article. Medicine is a challenging profession, and we are well paid, in part, because we must make tough decisions. I encourage all anesthesiologists who provide care for obstetric patients to read this article in its entirety.—D.H. Chestnut, M.D.

Comparison of Two Fentanyl Doses to Improve Epidural Anaesthesia With 0.5% Bupivacaine for Caesarean Section

Halonen PM, Paatero H, Hovorka J, Haasio J, Korttila K (Helsinki Univ Central Hosp)
Acta Anaesthesiol Scand 37:774–779, 1993   101-94-19-37

Background.—Spinal opioids appear to be useful in epidural anesthesia for cesarean section. One report has recommended that fentanyl, 100 µg, be added to .5% bupivacaine to improve the quality of epidural blockade. However, the same report warns against administering the opioid near delivery to mothers with premature labor or an acidotic fetus, or both. Whether a smaller dose of fentanyl, 50 µg, would improve the quality of epidural blockade sufficiently was investigated in a double-blind study.

Methods.—Ninety women having elective cesarean section with epidural anesthesia were randomly assigned to receive saline, 2 mL, or fentanyl, 50 or 100 µg, in 2-mL volume added to .5% bupivacaine. The women in the groups were similar with respect to weight, height, parity, and number of previous cesarean sections.

Findings.—Both doses of fentanyl improved anesthesia and reduced discomfort during surgery. In both fentanyl groups, the epidural blockade more often reached the fifth thoracic segment. The patients had significantly less pain and required less intravenous diazepam during surgery. The operating conditions also were better than those in the control

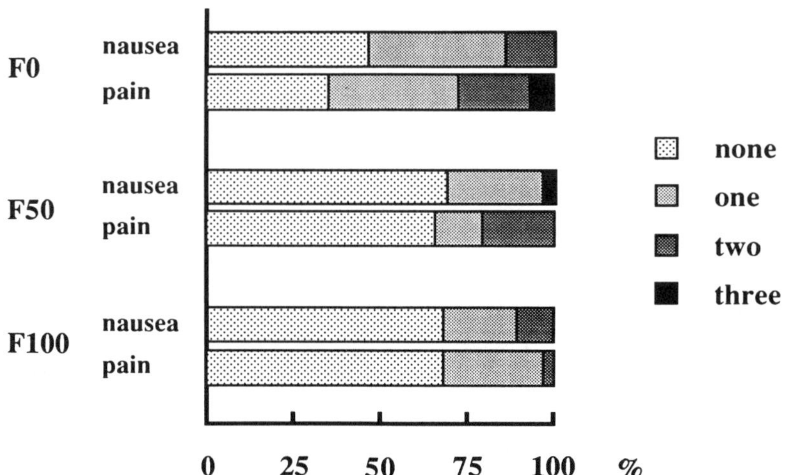

Fig 19–7.—Number of episodes of pain and nausea during cesarean section conducted under epidural anesthesia with .5% bupivacaine. Adjucnt to .5% bupivacaine: FO, saline; F50, fentanyl 50 µg; F100, fentanyl 100 µg. Contingency table analysis for pain $P = .0236$ between groups, and for nausea $P = .1835$, not significant. (Courtesy of Halonen PM, Paatero H, Hovorka J, et al: *Acta Anaesthesiol Scand* 37:774–779, 1993.)

group. Neonatal Apgar scores and cord blood pH were comparable in all groups. After surgery, the time to treatment for pain requested by the patient was more than 1 hour longer in the fentanyl groups. However, the total amount of postoperative analgesics needed in the first 24 hours did not differ among groups. Mild pruritus, which did not require treatment, occurred more often in patients who were given fentanyl than in those given saline. The frequency of nausea and pain was significantly lower in the fentanyl groups (Fig 19–7).

Conclusion.—A dose of fentanyl, 50 μg, added to .5% bupivacaine increases patient comfort and improves the quality of epidural anesthesia for patients undergoing cesarean section. The addition of fentanyl, 100 μg, does not provide any further advantage.

▶ The results of this study differ from those of Helbo-Hansen and colleagues (1). In this study, Halonen and associates observed that the addition of 50 μg of fentanyl to .5% bupivacaine improved the quality of epidural anesthesia for cesarean section and that administration of 100 μg did not provide any additional advantage. In contrast, the authors observed that the addition of 50 μg of fentanyl to .5% bupivacaine did not improve analgesia and that it was necessary to add either 75 μg or 100 μg of fentanyl to yield a demonstrable benefit. Why not use 2% lidocaine with 1:200,000 epinephrine rather than .5% bupivacaine? Fentanyl rarely needs to be added to the solution of lidocaine, and lidocaine is probably safer for the mother than bupivacaine.—D.H. Chestnut, M.D.

Reference

1. Helbo-Hansen HS, et al: *Int J Obstet Anesth* 2:21, 1993.

Evaluation of Prognostic Factors for Vaginal Delivery After Cesarean Section

Jakobi P, Weissman A, Peretz BA, Hocherman I (Technion-Israel Inst of Technology, Haifa)
J Reprod Med 38:729–733, 1993   101-94-19–38

Introduction.—Vaginal birth after cesarean section (VBAC) is a widely accepted and safe procedure, with a success rate of more than 60% in selected patients. However, 90% of pregnant American women who underwent a previous cesarean section choose a repeat cesarean section, largely because of pessimism regarding their chances for a successful vaginal delivery. The predictive value and relative importance of various prognostic factors and their usefulness in selecting patients for VBAC were evaluated.

Methods.—Univariate and multivariate analyses were used to evaluate 15 prognostic factors related to past and present pregnancies in 261 women with 1 previous cesarean section. All women were undergoing a trial of spontaneous labor. Those with other than a low transverse incision, as well as those with a nonvertex presentation, multiple gestation, or prolonged or delayed labor, were excluded.

Results.—The final predictive model identified 6 significant prognostic factors: previous breech, previous successful VBAC, station at admission, admission without rupture of membranes, dilatation at admission, and previous failure to progress. The overall predictive value was 68%, but the predictive value for successful vaginal delivery was excellent, with 95% of women who were predicted to deliver vaginally actually doing so. Predictive value for failed vaginal delivery was lower; two thirds of women in whom vaginal delivery was predicted to fail delivered vaginally.

Conclusion.—The chances for successful VBAC are good, even in women with a less favorable prognosis, suggesting that a liberal approach to VBAC should be adopted. However, many women and their physicians consider a 60% chance too low. With the ability to predict successful VBAC accurately, more women may be encouraged to elect a trial of labor.

▶ Other studies have confirmed that a trial of labor results in vaginal delivery in most women with a history of cesarean section, even when the indication for the previous cesarean section was failure to progress or cephalopelvic disproportion. At the University of Iowa Hospitals and Clinics, we require a trial of labor in almost all patients with a history of low transverse cesarean section. We do not perform an elective repeat cesarean section unless there is an obstetric indication for cesarean section or there is a specific contraindication to a trial of labor, e.g., classic uterine scar. Some obstetricians consider a history of 2 low transverse uterine incisions to be a contraindication to a trial of labor.—D.H. Chestnut, M.D.

Maternal Effects of Adding Epidural Fentanyl to 0.5% Bupivacaine for Caesarean Section

Helbo-Hansen HS, Bang U, Lindholm P, Klitgaard NA (Odense Univ Hosp, Denmark)
Int J Obstet Anesth 2:21–26, 1993   101-94-19–39

Introduction.—Bupivacaine .5% is frequently used for epidural anesthesia in women undergoing operative delivery, but its onset of action is relatively slow and several patients have described nausea or pain during surgery. Fentanyl has significantly improved the quality of analgesia when added to plain .5% bupivacaine and has also reduced the time to onset of analgesia.

Study Design.—The minimal dose of fentanyl that enhances epidural bupivacaine analgesia was determined in a prospective, randomized trial undertaken in 80 healthy women scheduled for elective section delivery at term. The patients had fentanyl, 50, 75, or 100 μg, added to 20 mL of .5% bupivacaine, and a control group received bupivacaine alone. Additional bupivacaine was given as needed at 30 minutes and thereafter to achieve a bilateral block to the T4 level.

Results.—The weight-related dose of fentanyl did not correlate with the time to loss of pinpick sensation at T4, and there were no significant group differences in the degree of motor block during or after surgery. Patients given fentanyl, 75 or 100 μg, required supplemental anesthetic less often than control patients, and fewer of them required intravenous opiate for pain relief during surgery. Pain scores were less in patients treated with fentanyl, but not significantly so. Hypotension was no more frequent in patients treated with opiates, but more of these patients had mild-to-moderate pruritus. No patient had clinically evident respiratory depression.

Conclusion.—Adding fentanyl, 75 or 100 μg, to .5% bupivacaine enhances epidural anesthesia in women undergoing cesarean section without producing serious side effects.

Neonatal Effects of Adding Epidural Fentanyl to 0.5% Bupivacaine for Caesarean Section

Helbo-Hansen HS, Bang U, Lindholm P, Klitgaard NA (Odense Univ Hosp, Denmark)
Int J Obstet Anesth 2:27–33, 1993   101-94-19–40

Background.—An epidural injection of opioid was introduced to improve analgesia for pregnant women during labor and cesarean section, and the placental transfer of fentanyl was quantified. The neonatal effects of adding fentanyl to .5% bupivacaine for epidural anesthesia also were assessed in women undergoing elective cesarean section at full term.

Methods.—Eighty women were randomly assigned to 1 of 4 groups. Saline or fentanyl, 50, 75, or 100 μg, was added to 20 mL of .5% bupivacaine.

Findings.—All groups had comparable Apgar scores, time to sustained respiration, and umbilical acid-base values. When data from all fentanyl groups were analyzed together, the median umbilical artery to maternal vein fentanyl concentration ratio was .34. In the assessment of neurologic and adaptive capacity, neonates of mothers who were given fentanyl had lower supporting reaction scores at 2 hours and active tone at 24 hours compared with control group neonates. However, there were no differences among groups in other neurobehavioral test criteria (Fig 19–8).

Conclusion.—Epidural administration of fentanyl, 50–100 μg, added to .5% bupivacaine at elective cesarean delivery did not depress full-term neonates. However, the umbilical plasma levels of fentanyl indicate that

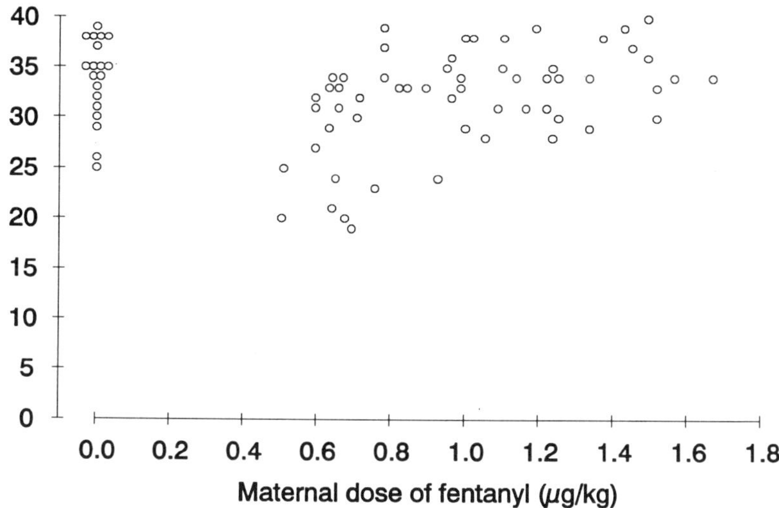

Fig 19–8.—Total Neurologic and Adaptive Capacity Scoring System (NACS) score and epidural dose of fentanyl per kg of maternal body weight at 15 minutes after delivery. There was no correlation (correlation coefficient with 95% confidence limits .12 [⁻.11 to .34, *P* value is .3]) between dose of fentanyl and the total NACS score. (Courtesy of Helbo-Hansen HS, Bank U, Lindholm P, et al: *Int J Obstet Anesth* 2:27–33, 1993.)

the safety margin is small, suggesting that it is important to select the lowest effective dose of fentanyl to improve epidural anesthesia before delivery.

▶ When I was a resident at Duke, I asked a professor why we used .75% rather than .5% bupivacaine. (This was before we learned that bupivacaine was more cardiotoxic than lidocaine and also before the Food and Drug Administration had withdrawn its approval for the use of .75% bupivacaine in obstetric patients.) He replied, "If you use .5% bupivacaine in 1 patient, you will understand why we do not use it." I tried it, and I understood. Epidural administration of .5% bupivacaine does not consistently provide satisfactory anesthesia for cesarean section. It can be made to work, provided there is enough time to wait and give a reinforcing dose to "repaint the fence." Unfortunately, this requires time and patience, which often are in short supply on a busy obstetric service. Therefore, it is not surprising that anesthesiologists have sought ways to improve the efficacy of .5% bupivacaine. Maternal epidural administration of 50 to 100 µg of fentanyl improves the efficacy of .5% bupivacaine and does not result in clinically significant neonatal respiratory depression (Abstract 101-94-19–39). The neurobehavioral effects are subtle. However, Helbo-Hansen et al. (Abstract 101-94-19–40) acknowledged that the safety margin was small.

In contrast, inadequate anesthesia is rarely a problem when epidural anesthesia is given using 2% lidocaine with 1:200,000 epinephrine. Lidocaine has several advantages over bupivacaine. It has a faster onset and is less cardiotoxic than bupivacaine. It is not necessary to add fentanyl to lidocaine before delivery in most patients. Why give an opioid before delivery unless it is necessary? I cannot remember the last time that I used .5% bupivacaine during administration of epidural anesthesia for cesarean section.—D.H. Chestnut, M.D.

Prevention of Aspiration in Obstetrics

Intravenous Ranitidine Reduces the Risk of Acid Aspiration of Gastric Contents at Emergency Cesarean Section

Rout CC, Rocke DA, Gouws E (Univ of Natal, Durban, South Africa; Med Research Council, Durban, South Africa)
Anesth Analg 76:156–161, 1993   101-94-19–41

Introduction.—The most common cause of anesthesia-related maternal death is aspiration of gastric contents. Combinations of H_2-receptor antagonists and a nonparticulate antacid are increasingly being used before elective cesarean, but the best combination of agents for women undergoing emergency surgery has not been established. Gastric pH and volume, as well as number of patients at risk of acid aspiration of gastric contents, were determined in a group of women undergoing emergency cesarean section with general anesthesia.

Methods.—Data on 595 women were analyzed. Patients were randomized to receive ranitidine, 50 mg intravenously, or placebo at the time the decision was made to do a cesarean section. All patients also received 30 mL of .3 M sodium citrate on entry to the operating room. Aspiration of gastric contents was done immediately after endotracheal intubation (PI) and before tracheal extubation. Patients with pH values less than 3.5 and volumes exceeding 25 mL were considered at risk of acid aspiration if regurgitation were to occur.

Findings.—After intubation, 4% of the patients in the citrate-only group and 2.3% in the ranitidine-citrate group were considered to be at risk. Before extubation, 5.6% and .3% in the citrate-only and combination groups, respectively, were at risk. After endotracheal intubation, the pH in patients given the combination treatment was significantly higher than in patients given citrate only. If the study drug was given more than 30 minutes before the PI sample, none of the patients given ranitidine were at risk compared with 3.2% in the citrate-only group.

Conclusion.—Regional anesthesia for cesarean section may not always be possible, particularly in emergency cases. In such cases, use of the most effective prophylactic regimen against acid aspiration is required. The current findings show that intravenous ranitidine, 50 mg, given at the time it is decided to do a cesarean section reduces the risk of acid aspiration, as long as at least 30 minutes have passed between injection and induction of anesthesia.

▶ Most anesthesiologists agree that pregnant women should receive pharmacologic aspiration prophylaxis before emergency cesarean section, but there is no consensus as to the ideal regimen. To my knowledge, no study has demonstrated that any regimen reduces maternal morbidity or mortality. I do not know whether it is cost-effective, but I give both ranitidine and metoclopramide intravenously, and sodium citrate orally, to most patients who require an emergency cesarean section. I omit the ranitidine and metoclopramide in those patients who require general anesthesia for *stat* cesarean section. There is little efficacy in giving an H_2-receptor antagonist and metoclopramide immediately before induction of general anesthesia.—D.H. Chestnut, M.D.

An Evaluation of Gastric Emptying Times in Pregnancy and the Puerperium
Whitehead EM, Smith M, Dean Y, O'Sullivan G (London Chest Hosp; Natl Hosp for Neurology and Neurosurgery, London; St Thomas' Hosp, London)
Anaesthesia 48:53–57, 1993   101-94-19–42

Background.—Pulmonary acid aspiration syndrome still contributes to maternal morbidity and mortality. The effect of pregnancy on gastric emptying is not well understood. Gastric emptying times through pregnancy and the postpartum period were investigated.

Methods.—Five groups of women were included: nonpregnant controls of reproductive age, women who were 8–10 weeks pregnant who were scheduled for vaginal termination, women who were 16–24 weeks pregnant, women at 34 weeks' gestation or more in whom vaginal delivery was expected, and women in the postpartum period after a normal vaginal delivery. All the participants were healthy, with no history of gastrointestinal disease or drug ingestion that could affect gastric motility. An indirect paracetamol absorption technique was used to measure gastric emptying.

Findings.—Gastric emptying times did not differ significantly between nonpregnant women and pregnant women or mothers 18 hours after delivery or more. However, 2 hours after delivery, gastric emptying was significantly delayed. In this group, the median values of the peak paracetamol concentration were 12.5 mg/L^{-1}; the time to reach the peak, 120 min; and the area under the paracetamol concentration-time curve, 3.8 mg/L^{-1}/hr. For the nonpregnant women, these values were 20.8 mg/L^{-1}, 40 minutes, and 13.5 mg/L^{-1}/hr, respectively.

Conclusion.—From the second day postpartum, healthy mothers appear to be at no greater risk of pulmonary acid aspiration than nonpregnant women. However, the pattern of gastric emptying between 2 hours and 18 hours after delivery has yet to be determined.

▶ The authors confirmed that gastric emptying is delayed during the first 2 hours after vaginal delivery but that it is normal between 18 and 48 hours after delivery; they did not assess gastric emptying between 2 and 18 hours after delivery. This is problematic for anesthesiologists who are asked to provide anesthesia for postpartum tubal ligation. I provide anesthesia for postpartum tubal ligation immediately after vaginal delivery *only* if the patient received satisfactory epidural anesthesia for labor and delivery and *only* if I can extend the block satisfactorily. Otherwise, I delay administration of anesthesia for postpartum tubal ligation until at least 8 hours after vaginal delivery.—D.H. Chestnut, M.D.

Acute Myocardial Infarction in Parturient

Anaesthetic Management of a Parturient With Myocardial Infarction Related to Cocaine Use
Liu SS, Forrester RM, Murphy GS, Chen K, Glassenberg R (Northwestern Univ, Chicago)
Can J Anaesth 39:858–861, 1992   101-94-19-43

Introduction.—The incidence of cocaine use in parturients is estimated to be from 11.8% to 20%. Numerous maternal and fetal complications are associated with the use of the drug. A case of myocardial infarction (MI) related to cocaine abuse was studied. Peripartum MI has a high mortality rate and has been considered a rare event.

Case Report.—Woman, 33, was seen at 36 weeks' gestation in severe respiratory distress. She had smoked crack cocaine within the past hour and had a history of hypertension. The patient's initial blood pressure was 240/130 mm Hg, and she required immediate tracheal intubation. A precordial ECG demonstrated left ventricular hypertrophy with 4 mm of ST elevation in leads V2 and V3. Her cervix was 3–4 cm dilated, and the uterus was contracting every 3–5 minutes. When fetal heart tracing revealed a tachycardia at 180 beats per minute with poor variability, labor was induced with oxytocin (Pitocin). Midazolam and fentanyl were used for sedation. Vecuronium, 10 mg, was given, and controlled ventilation was instituted with a 10-cm positive and expiratory pressure at 100% inspired oxygen. After 4 hours, a 2,185-g female infant was delivered with outlet forceps. The woman recovered from the non–Q-wave MI and was discharged receiving metoprolol, diltiazem, and enalapril.

Discussion.—To date, only 82 cases of peripartum MI have been reported. Atherosclerotic disease is the most common cause. Third-trimester MI carries a higher mortality rate (45%) than first- and second-trimester MI (23%). The fetal outcome generally correlates with the maternal outcome. Since 1982, there have been 58 reports of MI temporally related to cocaine use. Most cases have involved young men. Cocaine can compromise the cardiovascular system both through sympathomimetic effects and vasoconstrictive effects on coronary arteries. The normal cardiovascular changes that occur during pregnancy may add to the stress on the maternal heart. Cases such as this may become more common as the incidence of cocaine abuse grows.

▶ The epidemic of cocaine abuse has been among the great tragedies of the last decade. A substantial number of women continue to abuse cocaine during pregnancy. Cocaine use is more common in women who live in the inner city, but it is also a problem in suburbia. Perinatal complications of cocaine abuse include congenital anomalies, intrauterine growth restriction, preterm labor, abruptio placentae, and fetal distress. Physicians should consider the diagnosis of cocaine toxicity in patients who are seen with unexplained, severe hypertension during pregnancy. Likewise, physicians should suspect cocaine toxicity in otherwise healthy women who are seen with evidence of myocardial ischemia. In this case, I commend the obstetricians for not performing a knee-jerk cesarean section. Among pregnant patients who suffer a myocardial infarction, cesarean section should be reserved for *obstetric* indications.—D.H. Chestnut, M.D.

Mortality and Outcomes

Vaginal Birth After Cesarean Section: Acceptance and Outcome at a Rural Hospital
Walton DL, Ludlow D, Willis DC (432 Med Group, Misawa Air Base, Japan; Univ of Miami, Fla)
J Reprod Med 38:716–718, 1993   101-94-19-44

Objective.—Although there is convincing evidence concerning the success rate of vaginal birth after cesarean section (VBAC) at tertiary care centers, there are few data concerning the experience with VBAC in other settings. Any effect of VBAC on the increasing national cesarean section rate will require its adoption by patients and physicians in rural and community hospitals.

Patients.—Sixty-two patients were considered possible candidates for an attempted VBAC in a 2-year period at the obstetric clinic of a 24-bed United States Air Force hospital in an isolated area of Japan. Vaginal birth after cesarean section was encouraged, beginning at the first prenatal visit. Seventy-nine percent of the patients requested a trial of labor; 24% of them were excluded from consideration, usually because of an estimated fetal weight greater than 4,000 g. In 3 cases, patients changed their minds late in the pregnancy.

Results.—Vaginal delivery was successful in 88% of women who had a trial of labor, including 3 patients with numerous previous cesarean sections. There were 4 failures of VBAC, all of which occurred in patients with a history of cephalopelvic disproportion. Another 2 patients with this history successfully delivered vaginally. The only perinatal morbidity was 1 fetus who died in utero at 40 weeks. One woman had postcesarean endometritis, and another sustained a vaginal sidewall laceration after an outlet forceps delivery.

Conclusion.—Good acceptance and outcome of VBAC have been reported at an isolated military hospital. Hesitance on the part of physicians, rather than patients, may explain the less frequent use of VBAC at community hospitals. Although further study is needed, rural hospitals should be encouraged to offer VBAC.

▶ Others have confirmed that VBAC can be performed safely in small community hospitals. In fact, the American College of Obstetricians and Gynecologists does not require a faster response time for emergency cesarean section in patients who attempt a VBAC than in patients with no history of a cesarean section. One major limitation to attempted VBAC in rural hospitals is the shortage of anesthesia personnel. The authors of this study obtained admirable results, despite the fact that epidural analgesia often was not available.

Many women refuse VBAC because they fear that they will again experience a long, painful labor, which will again result in cesarean section. In this study, the authors acknowledged that 3 women reversed their original decision to attempt VBAC because of their fear of pain and the authors' inability to guarantee the availability of epidural analgesia. In my judgment, the availability of effective intrapartum analgesia is a necessary component of a successful VBAC program.—D.H. Chestnut, M.D.

Maternal Mortality in New Zealand
Aickin DR (Christchurch School of Medicine, New Zealand)
N Z Med J 106:375–376, 1993   101-94-19–45

Background.—Pregnancy- and puerperium-related deaths in New Zealand have been reported since 1969. Maternal mortality in New Zealand from 1986 to 1988 was analyzed and compared with rates from Australia and the United Kingdom during the period from 1985 to 1987.

Methods and Findings.—All women who die while pregnant or who were pregnant within 3 months of their death are reported under the provisions of the Maternal Morality Research Act. The causes and circumstances of the death are then assessed. The rate of obstetric deaths to total births in New Zealand was 9.6 per 100,000 in the period studied. The rates in the United Kingdom and Australia were 6.2 and 4.4 per 100,000, respectively. Of the 16 deaths that occurred in New Zealand in the study period, 6 were caused by sepsis. There were 5 cases of puerperal infection with group A β-hemolytic streptococci (table).

Conclusion.—There is a continuing need for careful analysis of obstetric outcomes. Health-care providers must report maternal deaths and

| Cause of Direct Obstetric Deaths 1969–1988 | | | | | | | | |
1969-71	72-4	75-7	78-80	81-3	84-5	86-8	Total	% of 155
Thromboembolic disease								
12	7	2	6	1	2	0	30	19.4
Anaesthetic 7	6	5	1	5	0	1	25	16.7
Eclampsia, pre-eclampsia/ chronic reneal disease								
10	3	4	3	1	0	3	24	15.5
Intrapartum/ postpartum haemorrhage								
1	4	3	2	1	2	2	15	9.7
Ruptured uterus 1	6	2	0	1	0	1	11	7.1
Septicaemia (inc. puerperal sepsis)								
1	2	5	1	1	0	6 (5)	16	10.3
Ectopic 5	1	2	0	2	0	1	11	7.1
Abortion (inc. septicaemia and haemorrhage)								
3	1	2	0	0	1	0	7	4.5
Amniotic fluid embolism								
3	1	1	0	0	2	2	9	5.8
Transfusion hepatitis								
1	0	2	0	0	0	0	3	1.9
Others 0	0	3	0	1	0	0	4	2.6
Total 44	31	31	13	13	7	16	155	

(Courtesy of Aickin DR: *N Z Med J* 106:375–376, 1993.)

provide information when appropriate so that trends in maternal mortality can be followed.

▶ Anesthesia was the second leading cause of maternal death in New Zealand between 1969 and 1988. Only 1 of the 25 maternal deaths that resulted from anesthesia occurred after 1983. Other studies have noted that failed intubation and pulmonary aspiration of gastric contents are the 2 leading causes of anesthesia-related maternal death. It is tempting to speculate that the apparent decline in the number of anesthesia-related maternal deaths in New Zealand may have resulted, in part, from an increased use of regional anesthesia.—D.H. Chestnut, M.D.

Cognitive Deficits in Women After Childbirth

Eidelman AI, Hoffmann NW, Kaitz M (Hebrew Univ, Jerusalem)
Obstet Gynecol 81:764–767, 1993   101-94-19–46

Introduction.—Many new mothers describe feelings of confusion and forgetfulness immediately after delivery, but studies of cognitive function have given contradictory results.

Study Design.—One hundred women with a mean age of 27 years, who had uncomplicated pregnancies and delivered normal infants at term, were given standardized neuropsychological tests. All participants had completed at least 12 years of education. Twenty childless women and 15 high-risk pregnant women in the third-trimester were also studied, along with 39 men whose wives had recently delivered a normal infant. Cognitive function was measured using the Wechsler Logical Memory Test of verbal recall and the Wechsler Visual Reproduction Test of visual-spatial perception and memory.

Results.—The parturients had significantly lower cognitive test scores on the first postpartum day than did nonpregnant control women. Those who were not given intrapartum analgesia had particularly low scores. The parturients had scores on days 2 and 3 that did not differ significantly from those of nonpregnant women. The women with high-risk pregnancies had lower Logical Memory Test scores than nonpregnant women on the first day; the same was true for the fathers.

Conclusion.—Parturients should not be instructed in child care until at least the second postpartum day, and it may be wise to provide written instructions. Fathers also exhibit defective memory function in the early postpartum period. Early discharge may be dangerous for high-risk women.

▶ Labor and delivery results in both physical and mental stress. This study provided objective evidence that supports anecdotal reports of confusion and forgetfulness after childbirth. Of interest to anesthesiologists, the administration of intrapartum analgesia, i.e., meperidine and promethazine, did not exacerbate the maternal cognitive deficit after delivery. In fact, the authors noted that "women who did not receive any medication had a more global deficit on the first postpartum day than did the mothers who received medication." As a result, the authors concluded that the observed cognitive effect was not a side effect of intrapartum narcotic medication but was the result of the stress of labor and delivery. It seems reasonable to speculate that epidural analgesia, which attenuates the intrapartum stress response more effectively than systemic opioids, would protect cognitive function at least as well as systemic opioid administration. I hope that these authors perform a second study in which patients receive epidural analgesia rather than systemic meperidine.—D.H. Chestnut, M.D.

Other Medical Conditions and Pregnancy

Asthma in Pregnancy

Clark SL, Natl Asthma Education Program Working Group on Asthma and

Pregnancy, NIH, Natl Heart, Lung, and Blood Inst (NIH, Bethesda, Md; Univ of Utah, Salt Lake City)
Obstet Gynecol 82:1036–1040, 1993   101-94-19–47

Background.—The NIH recently issued a comprehensive report on asthma and pregnancy developed by a panel of obstetricians, pharmacologists, internists, allergists, and pulmonologists.

Asthma in Pregnancy.—Asthma is a lung disease characterized by airway obstruction that at least partially resolves spontaneously or after treatment. It is characterized by airway inflammation and airway responsiveness to various stimuli, including environmental irritants, viral respiratory infections, cold air, or exercise. The various mechanisms that are hypothesized to explain airway hyperresponsiveness in asthma include airway inflammation, abnormalities in bronchial epithelial integrity, changes in autonomic neural control of airways, changes in intrinsic bronchial smooth-muscle function, alterations in the volume and composition of the airway liquid lining layer, defects in control of bronchial blood flow, and abnormal airway geometry.

Discussion.—Asthma in pregnant women tends to be undertreated in the United States, partly because of an unfounded fear that the drug treatment will adversely affect the fetus. The 4 key components of treatment of asthma in pregnancy are objective evaluation of maternal lung function and fetal well-being, avoidance or control of precipitating environmental factors, drug therapy (table), and patient education.

Conclusion.—The undertreatment of pregnant women with asthma is a major problem in asthma management in the United States. Fears that pharmacologic therapy will harm the fetus are unfounded. Pharmacologic therapy, along with an objective assessment of maternal lung function and fetal well-being, avoidance or control of precipitating factors in the environment, and patient education are the keys to successfully managing asthma in pregnancy.

▶ Epidemiologic studies suggest that there is an increased incidence of mortality secondary to asthma in the United States. The reasons are unclear, but undertreatment is probably responsible for a substantial number of deaths. I have provided care for several asthmatic pregnant women who required intubation and mechanical ventilation during pregnancy. In each case, there was evidence of undertreatment of patient's disease. All obstetricians and anesthesiologists who provide care for obstetric patients should read this article in its entirety.—D.H. Chestnut, M.D.

Drugs and Dosages Preferred for Use for Asthma and Associated Conditions
During Pregnancy

Drug class	Specific drug	Dosage
Anti-inflammatory	Cromolyn sodium	Two puffs four times a day (inhalation); two sprays in each nostril two to four times a day (intranasal for nasal symptoms)
	Beclomethasone	Two to five puffs two to four times a day (inhalation); two sprays in each nostril twice a day (intranasal for allergic rhinitis)
	Prednisone	Burst for active symptoms: 40 mg/day, single or divided dose for 1 week, then taper for 1 week. If prolonged course is required, single AM dose on alternate days may minimize adverse effects.
Bronchodilator	Inhaled beta$_2$-agonist	Two puffs every 4 hours as needed
	Theophylline	Oral: Dose to reach serum concentration of 8-12 μg/mL.
Antihistamine	Chlorpheniramine	4 mg by mouth up to four times per day, 8-12 mg sustained-release twice a day
	Tripelennamine	25-50 mg by mouth up to four times a day, 100 mg sustained-release twice a day
Decongestant	Pseudoephedrine	60 mg by mouth up to four times a day, 120 mg sustained-release twice a day
	Oxymetazoline	Intranasal spray or drops up to 5 days for rhinosinusitis
Cough	Guaifenesin	2 tsp by mouth four times a day
	Dextromethorphan	As above
Antibiotics	Amoxicillin	3 weeks' therapy for sinusitis

Note: This table presents drugs and suggested dosages for home management of asthma and associated conditions. These examples do not imply that other, similar agents in each category are not equally appropriate.

(Courtesy of Clark SL, National Asthma Education Program Working Group on Asthma and Pregnancy, NIH, et al: *Obstet Gynecol* 82:1036–1040, 1993.)

Interactions of Human Immunodeficiency Virus Infection and Pregnancy

Alger LS, Farley JJ, Robinson BA, Hines SE, Berchin JM, Johnson JP (Univ of Maryland, Baltimore)

Obstet Gynecol 82:787–796, 1993   101-94-19–48

Introduction.—Antenatal screening programs for HIV infection are increasing the number of seropositive women who are seen by obstetricians. Both HIV infection and pregnancy itself exert independent immunosuppressive effects. How HIV infection interacts with pregnancy in a relatively representative population of American women seeking prenatal care was determined in a group of largely asymptomatic women whose risk factors were not limited to drug use.

Study Population.—Groups of 101 HIV-seropositive and 97 seronegative women were closely matched for age, parity, marital status, and risk factors. Those in both groups were older than the general population, were less often married, and had had more deliveries and abortions. Most women were black, unemployed, and receiving Medicaid. The women were evaluated at the time of enrollment, at delivery, and 6–8 weeks postpartum.

Findings.—The seropositive women were more often black than those who were seronegative, but they were more likely to have private insurance. Infected women had sought prenatal care later in pregnancy, although those in both groups delayed the start of prenatal care longer than the general population. Intravenous drug use was the most common risk factor in both seropositive and seronegative women. Reported risk behaviors declined significantly during pregnancy in both groups. Seropositive women were relatively likely to have condylomata and to have a higher body temperature when admitted in labor, but they were not at increased risk of antepartum medical problems. Only 1 woman had an AIDS-defining opportunistic infection during the evaluation period. Serologic status did not influence either the obstetric outcome or the status of the newborn infant. Hematologic indices were initially abnormal in the seropositive women, but they did not become worse during the course of pregnancy.

Implications.—Pregnancy apparently does not significantly alter the early course of HIV-related disease in women who are asymptomatic when they first seek prenatal care. In addition, seropositivity for HIV does not appear to compromise either the maternal or neonatal outcome. These conclusions apply only to women in developed countries where nutrition and health care are adequate.

▶ Other studies have suggested that pregnancy does not affect the early course of HIV in asymptomatic women. Conversely, HIV infection does not affect perinatal outcome. However, the authors acknowledged that vertical transmission seemed to be the greatest threat associated with pregnancy.—D.H. Chestnut, M.D.

Anesthetic Management of the Pregnant Patient With Marfan Syndrome

Gordon CF III, Johnson MD (Harvard Med School, Boston)
J Clin Anesth 5:248–251, 1993
101-94-19–49

Introduction.—Classic Marfan syndrome occurs in 4–6 of every 100,000 births. The mean age at death is 32 years; 95% of deaths are attributable to cardiovascular complications.

Case 1.—Woman, 38, with Marfan syndrome, mitral valve prolapse, and aortic root enlargement was seen at 38 weeks' gestation for controlled induction of labor. Aortic and mitral regurgitant flow was insignificant. Atenolol was given orally, and the patient was closely monitored. Epidural analgesia was given with .25% bupivacaine to obtain sensory block at T8, and fentanyl was added. Hypotension responded to intravenous phenylephrine, 40 μg. A low forceps delivery was performed, and analgesia was maintained with oral opioid analgesics.

Case 2.—Woman, 25, was seen at 35 weeks' gestation and was scheduled for induction at 38 weeks. She had Marfan syndrome with mitral valve prolapse and an enlarged aortic root but no cardiac symptoms. Maintenance therapy consisted of oral atenolol. Tachycardia developed during labor after induction of epidural analgesia. Labetalol was given intravenously, and fentanyl was given epidurally after an outlet forceps delivery.

Recommendations.—In women with preexisting cardiovascular disease, it is desirable to minimize increases in contractility and sudden changes in blood pressure during labor. Beta-blockade should be continued or initiated. Direct and indirect beta-agonists, vagolytic drugs, and potentially hypertensive agents should be avoided. Vaginal delivery is possible, with cesarean delivery reserved for obstetric indications and impending aortic rupture. Dense conduction block and oxytocin augmentation will facilitate labor. If pushing is minimal, low forceps delivery should be considered. Parturients should be monitored in an intensive care setting for at least 6 hours after an uncomplicated delivery.

▶ I agree with the authors that in pregnant women with Marfan syndrome, a cesarean section should be reserved for obstetric indications and that epidural anesthesia is the analgesic technique of choice during labor. Patients with a dilatated aortic root are at risk for acute aortic dissection. After delivery, these patients should continue to be cared for in an intensive care setting.—D.H. Chestnut, M.D.

Preeclampsia

Coagulation Studies in the Preeclamptic Parturient: A Survey

Voulgaropoulos DS, Palmer CM (Univ of Arizona, Tucson)
J Clin Anesth 5:99–104, 1993   101-94-19–50

Introduction.—Although 5% of all pregnancies are complicated by preeclampsia, which may be associated with clotting factor and platelet deficiencies, little is known about the morbidity from coagulopathy that may occur in parturients.

Objective.—Current practice in evaluating coagulation status before inducing regional anesthesia in preeclamptic parturients was examined by sending a questionnaire to the chairmen of all 113 registered anesthesiology residency training programs in the United States. Usable responses were obtained from 74 programs.

Findings.—Regional anesthesia was used in most operative deliveries and in just more than half of vaginal deliveries. The number of tests requested increased with the severity of preeclampsia, but most programs required fewer tests in the urgent than in the elective setting. One fifth of the respondents favored using spinal rather than epidural anesthesia in patients with mild coagulopathy. Most anesthesiologists preferred not to use regional anesthesia when documented coagulopathy was present, even with a difficult airway. Several respondents believed that thromboelastography may be the best way of defining the risk of regional anesthesia in a patient at increased risk of coagulopathy.

Conclusion.—In general, no coagulation tests are considered to be necessary before undertaking regional anesthesia in mildly preeclamptic parturients. Only in severe cases is a platelet count required.

▶ At the University of Iowa, we rarely obtain a bleeding time measurement before administration of epidural anesthesia in preeclamptic patients. There is no evidence that the bleeding time correctly predicts the risk of epidural hematoma in a preeclamptic patient. Furthermore, there is a very low incidence of epidural hematoma after administration of epidural anesthesia in pregnant patients. To my knowledge, there are only 3 published cases of intraspinal, i.e., epidural or subdural, hematoma after administration of epidural anesthesia in pregnant patients. Only 1 of those 3 patients was preeclamptic, and she had a *normal* bleeding time (1). I assess the platelet count before administration of epidural anesthesia in preeclamptic patients, but I do not require other assessments of coagulation unless the patient has thrombocytopenia, abnormal liver function tests, or clinical evidence of coagulopathy.—D.H. Chestnut, M.D.

Reference

1. Lao TT, et al: *Can J Anaesth* 40:340, 1993.

Fetal Pulse Oximetry

Preliminary Experience With Intrapartum Fetal Pulse Oximetry in Humans

Dildy GA, Clark SL, Loucks CA (Univ of Utah, Salt Lake City; Intermountain Health Care Perinatal Ctrs, Salt Lake City, and Provo, Utah)
Obstet Gynecol 81:630–635, 1993
101-94-19–51

Background.—Fetal heart rate monitoring is highly specific in detecting fetal well-being, but such specificity is lacking when fetal compromise is suggested. Theoretically, fetal pulse oximetry offers several advantages over fetal heart rate monitoring by enabling direct assessment of arterial oxygen saturation and tissue perfusion in addition to fetal pulse rate. A preliminary experience with intrapartum fetal pulse oximetry was reported.

Study Design.—Oxygen saturation and pulse rate data were recorded in 73 women during active labor, using the Nellcor N-400 Fetal Oxygen Saturation Monitor and the FS-10 Oxisensor. The Oxisensor was designed to operate in a reflectance mode against the surface of the fetal head. The preferred site of placement was on the fetal temple or cheek, and the sensor was held in place by the static forces of the lateral uterine wall.

Findings.—The mean duration of monitoring was 161.4 minutes, and sensor contact was achieved 67.3% of the time during labor. Oxygen saturation and pulse rate data were recorded successfully in all patients. A reliable signal was achieved 50.1% of the time during labor. The average fetal oxygen saturation was 57.9%. There were no complications.

Discussion.—The potential for research and clinical applications of intrapartum fetal pulse oximetry are promising. Clearly, there are technical obstacles that must be overcome, including reliable continuous readings throughout labor, calibration of monitors using normal fetal oxygen saturations, false or loss of signals, and optical interference from meconium, fetal anemia, and caput. Clinical studies are also warranted to define the correlation between monitor and actual arterial oxygen saturation in the fetus as well as its correlation with newborn outcome.

▶ Electronic fetal heart rate (FHR) is a relatively sensitive method for the detection of intrapartum fetal hypoxemia. Unfortunately, FHR monitoring is not very specific for the diagnosis of intrapartum fetal distress, that is, it is associated with a large number of false-positives. This results in part because electronic FHR monitoring is an *indirect* method of fetal assessment. Fetal pulse oximetry holds the promise of providing a direct assessment of fetal oxygenation. However, technical problems must be overcome, and outcome studies should be used to determine whether the use of fetal pulse oximetry improves perinatal outcome.—D.H. Chestnut, M.D.

Gynecologic Procedures (Including In Vitro Fertilization)

Anesthesia for In Vitro Fertilization: A Comparison of 1.5% and 5% Spinal Lidocaine for Ultrasonically Guided Oocyte Retrieval

Manica VS, Bader AM, Fragneto R, Gilbertson L, Datta S (Harvard Med School, Boston)
Anesth Analg 77:453–456, 1993   101-94-19–52

Background.—In in vitro fertilization procedures, ultrasonically guided oocyte retrieval is a relatively short procedure that is performed on an outpatient basis. Spinal block appears to be the optimal choice for anesthesia, and the optimal technique should permit good surgical anesthesia with a short recovery time. The relative regression of equal doses of different concentrations of hyperbaric spinal lidocaine during transvaginal ultrasound-guided oocyte retrieval was compared.

Methods.—In a double-blind, randomized fashion, 56 American Society of Anesthesiologists physical status I and II patients received spinal anesthesia with either 60 mg of hyperbaric 1.5% lidocaine (4 mL) or 60 mg of hyperbaric 5% lidocaine (1.2 mL) in combination with fentanyl, 10 μg.

Outcome.—Both groups had excellent analgesia, as evidenced by a score of 0 on the visual analogue scale throughout the procedures. Sensory level, maximum motor block, intravenous sedation requirements, time to 2-segment regression, and time to full sensory recovery did not differ between groups. However, those in the group receiving 1.5% lidocaine had significantly shorter times to ambulation, voiding, full motor recovery, and discharge. There were no adverse effects.

Conclusion.—The use of 1.5% hyperbaric lidocaine (60 mg) provides an equally excellent analgesia but with a significantly shorter recovery time than 5% hyperbaric lidocaine. The use of 1.5% hyperbaric lidocaine is a good choice for spinal anesthesia for transvaginal oocyte procedures.

▶ At the University of Iowa Hospitals and Clinics, we use modest doses of intravenous alfentanil and midazolam to provide satisfactory analgesia to most patients who undergo transvaginal oocyte retrieval. We reserve spinal anesthesia for those few patients who desire a totally painless procedure or who were dissatisfied with the analgesia that was provided during a previous procedure. In practice, this means that we give spinal anesthesia to no more than 3% of our patients who undergo transvaginal oocyte retrieval. When given a choice, most patients prefer a little intraoperative discomfort to a needle in the back.—D.H. Chestnut, M.D.

Minimum Effective Combination Dose of Epidural Morphine and Fentanyl for Posthysterectomy Analgesia: A Randomized, Prospective, Double-Blind Study

Tanaka M, Watanabe S, Ashimura H, Akiyoshi Y, Nishijima Y, Sato S, Naito H
(Univ of Tsukuba, Ibaraki, Japan; Mito Saiseikai Gen Hosp, Ibaraki, Japan)
Anesth Analg 77:942–946, 1993

101-94-19–53

Background.—Concomitant use of epidural fentanyl and epidural morphine (EPM) overcomes the analgesic latency associated with EPM. Nevertheless, clinical studies of epidural fentanyl as an adjunct to EPM have produced equivocal results because of differences in surgical procedure, sequence of narcotic administration, and drug dose. The dose-response relationship of post-EPM administration of fentanyl for posthysterectomy analgesia was examined to determine the minimum effective combination dose.

Methods.—In this randomized, double-blind, prospective study, radical abdominal hysterectomy was performed in 120 patients using a standardized anesthesia protocol. Patients received 1 of 6 postsurgical anesthesia regimens: epidural morphine (2 mg or 4 mg) administered 60 minutes before the end of surgery alone, or followed by epidural fentanyl (50 μg or 100 μg) 15 minutes before the end of surgery. Pain was assessed immediately after surgery and within the subsequent 2, 3, 6, 12, 18, and 24 hours using a 10-cm visual analogue scale (VAS).

Results.—The VAS scores were significantly lower with combination regimens than with morphine monotherapy through the first 6 postoperative hours, but they became similiar therafter. All morphine/fentanyl combinations provided a significantly longer duration of analgesia than either morphine monotherapy dose. Supplemental analgesia requirements were significantly lower with all combinations compared with morphine, 2 mg, and with all but the morphine, 2 mg/fentanyl, 50 μg, compared with morphine, 4 mg.

Conclusion.—Administration of epidural fentanyl after EPM improves and prolongs early postoperative analgesia. The minimum combination dose for posthysterectomy analgesia is morphine, 2 mg/fentanyl, 50 μg. Neither the quality nor the duration of analgesia is improved by larger doses.

► We routinely offer either epidural or intrathecal morphine to almost all patients who receive either epidural or spinal anesthesia for cesarean section at the University of Iowa Hospitals and Clinics. We have had great success with epidural and intrathecal morphine in this patient population. By contrast, I have had little success with epidural and intrathecal morphine in *nonpregnant* patients who have undergone hysterectomy. In my experience, it is difficult to predict an individual patient's dose requirement. My only experience with clinically significant respiratory depression (and near respiratory arrest) occurred in a healthy, young woman who received epidural anesthesia for a vaginal hysterectomy. Epidural administration of 3.5 mg of morphine did not result in satisfactory postoperative analgesia. Three hours after epidural administration of an additional 1.5 mg of morphine, the patient had a respiratory rate of 4 breaths per minute and was almost unresponsive.

Epidural administration of 3.5 mg of morphine (or intrathecal administration of .2 mg) consistently provides excellent postcesearean analgesia in our patient population. However, I prefer to use intravenous patient-controlled analgesia in nonpregnant patients who have undergone a hysterectomy.—D.H. Chestnut, M.D.

20 Pediatric Anesthesia

Induction

The Effect of Cricoid Pressure on Preventing Gastric Insufflation in Infants and Children

Moynihan RJ, Brock-Utne JG, Archer JH, Feld LH, Kreitzman TR (Stanford Univ, Calif)

Anesthesiology 78:652–656, 1993					101-94-20-1

Background.—The routine use of ventilation by mask in pediatric anesthetic practice as well as in critical care and resuscitation is not without risk. Forcing gas into the stomach can lead to regurgitation and pulmonary aspiration of gastric contents. Distention of the stomach can also provide an extrathoracic competitor to ventilation, and obstruction of central venous return can result. The use of cricoid pressure to prevent gastric gas insufflation has been studied in adults and to some extent in children. The airway pressures at which gastric inflation occurs in paralyzed and nonparalyzed anesthetized children, with and without cricoid pressure, were determined.

Method.—Fifty-nine children aged 2 weeks to 8 years who were scheduled for elective surgery received an inhalational induction of anesthesia with holothane, nitrous oxide, and oxygen. A single observer monitored the upper abdomen for air entry. In the first study, which was carried out without paralysis, the proximal airway pressure was slowly increased by gradually closing the pop-off valve on the anesthesia machine until gas could be heard entering the stomach, the pop-off point, or until the peak inspiratory pressure (PIP) reached 40 cm of water. The pressurization procedure was then repeated 3 times as the application and removal of cricoid pressure were varied. The children were then paralyzed (study 2), and the experiment was repeated by testing the effects with and without cricoid pressure.

Results.—When appropriately applied, cricoid pressure was 100% effective in preventing gas insufflation into the stomach in children up to 40 cm of water PIP, both with and without paralysis. Moreover, paralysis significantly decreased the median pop-off point in any given patient.

Conclusion.—Appropriate application of cricoid pressure is a potentially valuable technique during airway management by mask of children undergoing surgery. However, care should be taken to apply the appropriate pressure, particularly in young infants who are at risk of airway obstruction.

▶ I remain skeptical about the value of routine use of cricoid pressure. Properly performed, this maneuver makes visualization of the glottic opening impossible during direct laryngoscopy. Aspiration, although it is a rare complication, still occurs despite the alleged application of cricoid pressure. More important than cricoid pressure is attention to maintaining a patent upper airway—a skill inherent in the practice of anesthesiology.—R.K. Stoelting, M.D.

Cardiovascular Effects of I.V. Induction in Children: Comparison Between Propofol and Thiopentone

Aun CST, Sung RYT, O'Meara ME, Short TG, Oh TE (Chinese Univ of Hong Kong, Shatin)

Br J Anaesth 70:647–653, 1993

101-94-20-2

Introduction.—A major criticism of propofol is its effect on arterial pressure. In both adults and children, induction of anesthesia with

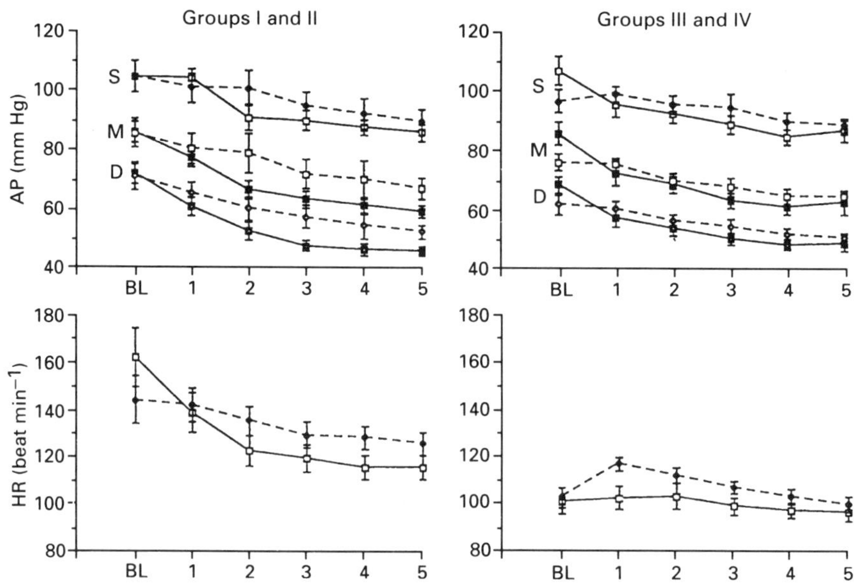

Fig 20–1.—*Abbreviations: HR,* heart rate; *AP,* arterial pressure; *BL,* baseline (before induction); *1–5,* time after induction; *S,* systolic pressure; *M,* mean arterial pressure; *D,* diastolic pressure. Cardiovascular responses during induction of anesthesia in the children younger than 2 years of age (groups I and II) and children aged 2–12 years (groups III and IV). Propofol (*solid line*); thiopentone (*dashed line*). (Courtesy of Aun CST, Sung RYT, O'Meara ME, et al: *Br J Anaesth* 70:647–653, 1993.)

propofol is associated with a significantly greater reduction in arterial pressure than occurs with thiopental. Pulsed Doppler echocardiography was used to compare the cardiovascular effects of the 2 agents when used for intravenous induction of anesthesia in children.

Patients and Methods.—Forty-five healthy Chinese children who were scheduled for elective surgery were randomly allocated in a double-blind manner to receive either propofol, 2.5 mg/kg^{-1}, or thiopental, 5 mg/kg^{-1}. The children ranged in age from 8 months to 12 years and were grouped according to age: younger than 2 years and 2–12 years. Anesthesia was maintained by spontaneous ventilation with 70% nitrous oxide and .5% halothane in oxygen. Measurements of arterial pressure, heart rate, and stroke volume were made before induction and at 1-minute intervals for 5 minutes after induction.

Results.—Four patients had inadequate Doppler recordings and were excluded from analysis. At baseline, mean heart rates and systemic vascular resistance values were greater in toddlers than in older children. Both age groups and anesthetic agent groups showed a significant decrease in systolic, mean, and diastolic arterial pressures after induction. For both age groups, the differences were significantly greater after propofol than after thiopental (Fig 20–1). The heart rate was stable in older children, but it decreased significantly in toddlers; the decrease was significantly greater with propofol (24%) than with thiopental (11%). Changes in stroke volume and systemic vascular resistance were similar for the age and anesthetic agent groups.

Conclusion.—Intravenous induction of anesthesia with propofol in children was associated with more cardiovascular depression than an equipotent dose of thiopental. The greater decrease in heart rate after propofol suggests that it causes more baroreflex depression than thiopental. A similar finding was reported in studies of adult patients.

▶ I selected this paper so I could complain about it. The authors picked 1 dose of propofol, 2.5 mg/kg, and 1 dose of thiopental, 5 mg/kg. Because there was no dose-response curve here, I do not know how the authors can conclude much of anything. Their suggestion that propofol causes more baroreflex depression than thiopental may be true at these single doses of each. Pharmacologic studies of anesthetic drugs must move toward legitimate pharmacology, which means dose-response curves.—J.H. Tinker, M.D.

Emesis and Voiding Postoperatively

Propofol Anesthesia Reduces Emesis and Airway Obstruction in Pediatric Outpatients
Martin TM, Nicolson SC, Bargas MS (Children's Hosp, Philadelphia; Univ of Pennsylvania, Philadelphia)
Anesth Analg 76:144–148, 1993   101-94-20-3

Background.—Children's resistance to placement of an intravenous cannula often results in induction with an inhalation agent, usually halothane. However, in children, propofol appears to be associated with faster recovery and less vomiting than halothane.

Methods.—The effects of and recovery from anesthesia in healthy, premedicated children receiving inhaled anesthetics or propofol were studied. The 68 children in the former group, group 1, had a mean age of 3.8 years and a mean weight of 17.7 kg. The 75 children in group 2 had a mean age and weight of 3.3 years and 16.3 kg, respectively.

Findings.—The incidence of vomiting was lower in the children who received propofol than in those who received volatile agents. Children who received an inhaled agent had a higher incidence of airway obstruction during induction of anesthesia. Nineteen percent of the children had withdrawal of the extremity with propofol injection. In group 2, the arterial blood pressure was higher at loss of consciousness, laryngoscopy, and tracheal intubation. The 2 groups were comparable in the length of time from the end of surgery to extubation of the trachea, recovery scores, and length of time spent in the postanesthetic care unit (PACU) and the day surgery unit. Pain scores recorded in the PACU also did not differ between the 2 groups.

Conclusion.—Propofol can be safely used to induce and maintain anesthesia in healthy children undergoing outpatient procedures. This, along with the low incidence of vomiting and airway obstruction in the group given propofol, supports the use of this drug in this patient population.

▶ The antiemetic effect of propofol by unknown mechanisms is a commonly described attribute of this drug. A lower incidence of airway obstruction during induction of anesthesia compared with an inhaled anesthetic is not likely to be a unique characteristic of propofol.—R.K. Stoelting, M.D.

Postoperative Voiding Interval and Duration of Analgesia Following Peripheral or Caudal Nerve Blocks in Children

Fisher QA, McComiskey CM, Hill JL, Spurrier EA, Voigt RE, Savarese AM, Beaver BL, Boltz MG (Univ of Maryland, Baltimore)
Anesth Analg 75:173–177, 1993   101-94-20–4

Introduction.—For children undergoing orchiopexy or herniorrhaphy, it is not clear whether caudal anesthesia prolongs the interval before voiding after surgery or whether the addition of epinephrine to caudal nerve block prolongs postoperative analgesia. Postoperative micturition and duration of analgesia were studied in 82 children aged 6 months to 10 years who had a herniorrhaphy or orchiopexy.

Setting.—Surgery was performed with general anesthesia with nitrous oxide and halothane, and all patients received D_5 lactated Ringer's solution equivalent to 6 hours, maintenance during surgery. At the end of surgery, patients were randomly assigned to receive 1 of 3 regional anesthetic injections of .25% bupivacaine; 1 group received caudal injections, .75 mL/kg; another received caudal injections with epinephrine 1:200,000, .75 mL/kg; and the third received ilioinguinal-iliohypogastric nerve block with epinephrine 1:200,000, .4 mL/kg per side, through the wound edges by the surgeon. All patients received oral fluids ad libitum after surgery.

Outcome.—Seventy-four patients had successful blocks. The time to first postoperative micturition varied widely from 25 to 630 minutes, but it did not differ significantly among the 3 groups. Seven children took more than 8 hours to void, but none required further intervention. More than 60% of patients had sustained pain relief for at least 4 hours, and there were no significant differences among the groups. By 24 hours, 66% of all patients required analgesics.

Conclusion.—In children undergoing inguinal-scrotal surgery, the time to postoperative voiding is variable and not prolonged by caudal analgesia. The addition of epinephrine does not measurably prolong analgesia or delay voiding. Ilioinguinal-iliohypogastric nerve block and caudal bupivacaine with or without epinephrine are equally effective in providing postoperative analgesia.

▶ The lack of a demonstrable prolongation of time to voiding in patients receiving caudal analgesia has obvious implications in outpatient surgery.—S.E. Abram, M.D.

Ventilation and Postanesthetic Apnea

Are All Preterm Infants Younger Than 60 Weeks Postconceptual Age at Risk for Postanesthetic Apnea?
Malviya S, Swartz J, Lerman J (Univ of Toronto)
Anesthesiology 78:1076–1081, 1993   101-94-20-5

Background.—Several reports suggest that preterm and ex-preterm infants are at risk of life-threatening apnea after general anesthesia. However, there is agreement on the likelihood of postanesthetic apnea occurring in infants between 44 and 60 weeks of postconceptual age.

Study Population.—Ninety-one consecutive preterm infants who were less than 37 weeks' gestational age at birth and less than 60 weeks' postconceptual age at the time of surgery were studied prospectively. They received a total of 101 general anesthetics. Infants scheduled for postoperative ventilatory support were not included. Cardiorespiratory monitoring was done overnight. Anesthetic management was individualized.

Observations.—Ten infants had numerous episodes of apnea and bradycardia after 12 procedures; all but 1 of them were less than 44 weeks' postconceptual age (Fig 20–2). The infants with postanesthetic apnea were significantly younger (in terms of postconceptual age) and

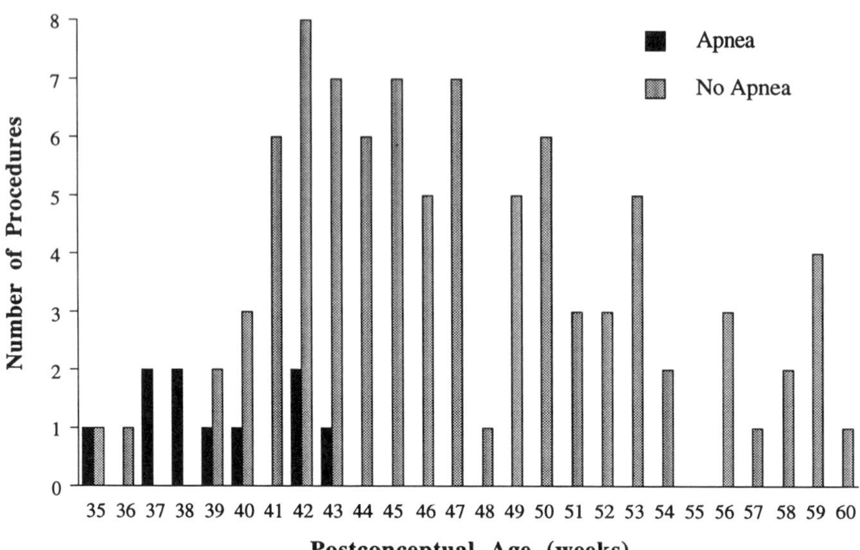

Fig 20–2.—Incidence of postanesthetic apnea with respect to postconceptual age. All episodes of postanesthetic apnea occurred in infants younger than 44 weeks' postconceptual age with the exception of 1 who was excluded from the study. (Courtesy of Malviya S, Swartz J, Lerman J: *Anesthesiology* 78:1076–1081, 1993.)

smaller at the time of surgery than those without apneic episodes. Of the 9 affected infants, 6 had a history of neonatal apnea. Four infants required repeated tactile stimulation, and 4 required 100% oxygen by continuous positive airway pressure. No infant had to be intubated. Seven other infants, all more than 44 weeks' postconceptual age, had episodes of bradycardia that lasted 3 to 5 seconds.

Conclusion.—Ex-preterm infants of less than 44 weeks' postconceptual age should be managed where intensive respiratory care is available. Infants of less than 50 weeks' postconceptual age should be monitored overnight in a hospital, even after minor surgery. Older infants should be closely watched in the postanesthetic recovery unit for 2 hours after anesthesia is discontinued.

▶ In this study, 12 apnea-free hours identified an infant who did not have postanesthetic apnea. The problem is that age-old question, namely, When does the postanesthetic period end? Infants are subjected to the risk of sudden infant death syndrome. Can we infer from this study that if an apneic period occurs more than 12 hours postanesthesia, it should be referred to as something other than postanesthetic apnea? Despite this, it makes sense that preterm infants might have a greater likelihood of postanesthesia apnea than full-term infants. Although this finding is not surprising, it is better documented in this paper than in any other article I have seen.—J.H. Tinker, M.D.

Ventilation and Thoracoabdominal Asynchrony During Halothane Anesthesia in Infants

Benameur M, Goldman MD, Ecoffey C, Gaultier C (Hôpital Antoine Beclere, Clamart, France; Hôpital Bicetre, France)
J Appl Physiol 74:1591–1596, 1993   101-94-20-6

Purpose.—Although it is the most commonly used anesthetic in children, there are relatively few studies of the action of halothane in infants. Because chest wall compliance is higher in infants than in older children, it is logical that halothane's effects on rib cage behavior—and therefore on decreases in ventilation—would be more important in early infancy. The effects of various concentrations of halothane in infants and children were examined to evaluate the ventilatory consequences of high chest wall compliance during anesthesia.

Methods.—Three different fractions of minimal alveolar concentration were studied at .75, 1, and 1.5 minimal alveolar concentration (MAC). The subjects were 10 infants younger than 1 year of age and 11 children 1 year of age or older. All were studied before undergoing elective abdominal surgery under anesthesia. Measurements were made after each of 3 equilibration periods, at the end of which the patients had identical inspired and expired concentrations of halothane.

Results.—Although minute ventilation decreased by 21% at .75 to 1 MAC in the infants, the children showed no significant change. The tidal volume decreased with the halothane level, with a decrease of 33% in the infants vs. 23% in the children. The ratio of inspiratory to total time (T_I/T_T) increased with the halothane level in the children but not in the infants; the latter had a decrease in T_I at higher halothane levels. Although the infants had increasing thoracic paradox at greater halothane levels, the children did not. The infants had a greater increase in thoracic paradox in association with the decrease in tidal volume between .75 and 1.5 MAC.

Conclusion.—Smaller infants rely more on inspiratory intercostal muscle activity to stabilize the thorax. This results in greater ventilatory depression during halothane-induced depression of inspiratory intercostal muscle activity. Therefore, infants younger than 1 year of age are at risk of significant hypoventilation during spontaneous breathing under halothane anesthesia of 1 MAC or greater.

▶ The authors found that smaller infants depend more on intercostal activity and less on other so-called secondary muscles of respiration. Pediatric anesthetists have long contended that if possible, infants should be anesthetized before intubating the trachea or undertaking other painful procedures. This study confirms our clinical impression that this is not easily done.—J.H. Tinker, M.D.

Minute Ventilation During Mask Halothane Anaesthesia in Infants and Children

Brown KA, Bissonnette B, Holtby H, Ein S, Shandling B (Univ of Toronto)
Can J Anaesth 40:112–118, 1993   101-94-20-7

Background.—There are few data on minute ventilation (MV) values in spontaneously breathing anesthetized infants. This is partly because most studies have grouped infants with children and normalized their ventilation data on a per-kilogram basis.

Methods.—Minute ventiltation was examined during elective mask halothane anesthesia (HA) ventilation in 12 pediatric surgical patients. The patients were all undergoing herniorrhaphy; 7 were infants (mean age, 3 months) and 5 were children (mean age, 3 years). Pneumotachography was used to measure airflow. During the operation, analogue signals of pressure and flow were recorded for later playback, when the flow signal was mathematically integrated to volume for breath-by-breath analysis.

Results.—Minute ventilation was no different between the 2 groups. Both groups demonstrated rapid, shallow breathing during HA, when the tidal volume was 2.9 mL/kg^{-1} in the infants vs. 3.7 mL/kg^{-1} in the children. Both groups had lower values for tidal volume during HA than during emergence (Fig 20–3). No between-group differences were noted

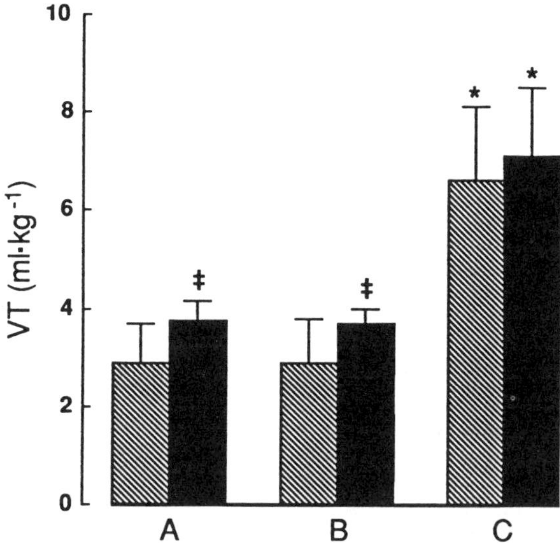

Fig 20–3.—Histogram (mean ± 1 SD) summarizing group values for tidal (VT$_x$) during HA and recovery in both groups. During HA, VT$_A$ and VT$_B$ were lower than VT$_C$ in both groups (P < .05). During HA, VT$_A$ and VT$_B$ were lower in group I (*hatched*) than in group II (*solid*) (P < .05). There was no difference in VT$_C$ between groups. *, intragroup statistical differences from stage A (P < .05); ‡, intergroup statistical difference from group I (P < .05). (Courtesy of Brown KA, Bissonnette B, Holtby H, et al: *Can J Anaesth* 40:112–118, 1993.)

in the mean inspiratory flow. The infants had a lower mean inspiratory flow during HS than during emergence but the children did not. No differences between or within groups were noted for the inspiratory duty cycle.

Conclusion.—Infants appear to have greater reductions in tidal volume during HA than older children. As a result, infants may be predisposed to hypercarbia during HA. Both infants and children have reduced MV values during HA.

▶ I selected this paper because it seemed to be high-quality science but also because I wanted to alert readers that these authors are competent in administering halothane anesthesia by mask to spontaneously breathing small infants. Many anesthesiologists intubate such infants when they are awake, with nothing to blunt the noxious stimulation. Many pediatric anesthesiologists recommend some form of anesthesia for such infants. This article confirms that it can be done.—J.H. Tinker, M.D.

Air Embolus During Caudal

Probable Venous Air Embolism During Caudal Anesthesia in a Child
Guinard J-P, Borboen M (Centre Hospitalier Universitaire Vaudois, Lausanne, Switzerland)
Anesth Analg 76:1134–1135, 1993   101-4-20–8

Background.—Caudal anesthesia is often given to children because it is safe, effective, and easy to use. A small amount of air is often injected through the needle or catheter to exclude the possibility of subcutaneous injection. A complication resulting from this maneuver was studied.

Case Report.—Boy, 26 months, was undergoing surgery for repair of a scrotal hypospadias. General anesthesia was induced, and the child was prepared for caudal anesthesia. A 22-gauge, 2.9-cm-long needle was inserted into the hiatus between the sacral cornua, at 60 degrees with the bevel maintained in a ventral position. At the first attempt, there was a distinct pop, indicating sacrococcygeal membrane puncture. The angle of the needle was flattened, and the catheter was pushed 5 mm further into the caudal epidural space. There was no particular resistance. After negative blood and fluid aspiration, 2.5 mL of air was injected through the catheter. No subcutaneous emphysema was evident. Within 10–15 seconds, however, the boy's heart rate decreased from 130 to 95 beats per minute. Pulse oximetry decreased from 99% to 85%, and end-tidal carbon dioxide decreased from 35 to 20 mm Hg. A whirring noise, which had been previously unheard, was auscultated simultaneously over the left precordium. The patient was immediately placed head down, and the rate of lactated Ringer's solution was increased. When the caudal catheter was withdrawn, its end was partially covered with blood. Within 45 seconds, the boy's heart rate increased again and the murmur disappeared. The end-tidal carbon dioxide and pulse oximetry normalized gradually after 5 minutes. During the next 10 minutes of observation, no other adverse events occurred, and the surgeons decided to proceed. A similar catheter was inserted for caudal anesthesia by the same technique, except for air injection, without complication. After surgery, the child had bilateral motor weakness for 2 hours; otherwise, his recovery was uneventful. He was discharged from the hospital after 8 days with no sequelae.

Conclusion.—A venous air embolism apparently resulted when air was used to identify the caudal space in inducing a central block. The catheter had been placed without difficulty using a standard technique.

▶ We have been placing sharpened hollow needles near (or in) nerve structures since the 1880s. We still do not have a way of verifying an extravascular location of the tip of the needle, despite the fact that we can drive a missle 7,000 miles and put it inside a 55-gallon drum (almost).

Although we make a big deal about regional anesthesia, it actually is merely 1 of several drug delivery systems that are available to the anesthesiologist. I know this will get me in trouble, but I think regional anesthesia is the least accurate and the most difficult to control of all the anesthesia drug delivery systems. This case report did not indicate that we should avoid caudal anesthesia in anesthetized children. However, it does remind us that we cannot tell for certain exactly where the tip of that needle might be located. A whole generation of young anesthesiologists has, I think, been "brainwashed" into believing that anesthesia is extraordinarily safe, and the government has been brainwashed into believing the same thing. Cases like this should bring us back to reality.—J.H. Tinker, M.D.

Hemodynamic Responses

Halothane Concentrations Required to Block the Cardiovascular Responses to Incision (MAC CVR) in Infants and Children
Ishizawa Y, Dohi S (Univ of Tsukuba, Ibaraki, Japan; Univ of Gifu, Japan)
Can J Anaesth 40:18–23, 1993   101-94-20–9

Introduction.—There are insufficient data on the age-related changes in automatic activity that occur in children under anesthesia. Among the suggested means of studying these changes is the concept of MAC BAR, the concentration needed to block adrenergic responses to incision in half the subjects. The concentration of halothane in nitrous oxide necessary to block cardiovascular responses (MAC CVRs) in skin incisions in infants and children was investigated.

Methods.—The halothane-nitrous oxide MAC CVR in 64 unpremedicated infants and children was examined. The children ranged in age from 1 month to 7 years, and all were American Society of Anesthesiologists physical status I and II. Halothane-nitrous oxide anesthesia was induced slowly in each patient, and an endotracheal tube was placed. The steady-state end-tidal halothane concentration was established for 10 minutes, after which Dixon's "up-and-down" technique

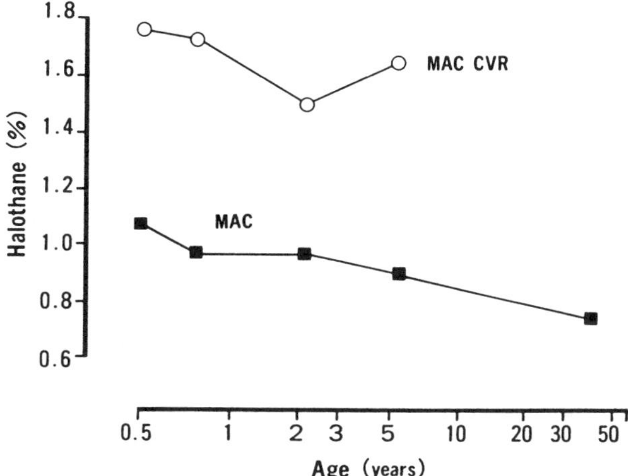

Fig 20–4.—Values of MAC CVR50 are calculated as concentrations of halothane. Age adjustments of MAC value for halothane are based on data from Gregory et al. (Courtesy of Ishizawa Y, Dohi S: *Can J Anaesth* 40:18–23, 1993.)

was used to assess MAC CVR. An increase of more than 10% in the mean arterial pressure or heart rate was interpreted as a positive cardiovascular response.

Results.—With 60% nitrous oxide, the mean MAC CVR values for halothane were 1.16% for infants as old as 6 months, 1.17% for those age 7–12 months, .95% for those age 1–3 years, and 1.12% for those age 4–7 years (Fig 20–4). The value for children age 1–3 years was lower than that for the other age groups. Correlations were noted between changes in mean arterial pressure, heart rate, and pupillary diameter in younger infants and children.

Conclusion.—The values of MAC CVR50 of halothane in infants and children are higher than those required to block motor responses. Children aged 1–3 years appear to have the lowest MAC CVR values. Further studies of the anesthetic requirement, as related to postoperative outcome are needed.

▶ These authors referred to a variant of the term MAC BAR, which was coined by Roizen and associates (1). I cannot understand why these authors are calling it MAC CVR. It seems to me that MAC CVR, as identified by these authors, is exactly the same as the old term MAC BAR. Why do we need more jargon?—J.H. Tinker, M.D.

Reference

1. Roizen MF, et al: *Anesthesiology* 54:390, 1981.

Neonatal Surgery

Neonatal Surgery: Intensive Care Unit Versus Operating Room
Finer NN, Woo B-C, Hayashi A, Hayes B (Royal Alexandra Hosp, Edmonton, Alta, Canada; Univ of Alberta Hosp, Edmonton, Alta, Canada)
J Pediatr Surg 28:645–649, 1993   101-94-20–10

Introduction.—To avoid the morbidity associated with transferring a critically ill neonate to an operating room, such infants now undergo surgery in a designated area of the neonatal intensive care unit (NICU). The infant is transferred to this area on the overhead radiant warmer, using a portable gas source to power the ventilator.

Study Population.—Eighty-one procedures were carried out in the NICU in the past 4 years, and 112 were performed in the operating room. The respective mean birth weights were 1,758 and 2,457 g, and the respective gestational ages were 31.3 and 35.8 weeks. The infants in the NICU weighed less at the time of surgery. More than three fourths of these infants required mechanical ventilation compared with one fourth of those who had surgery in the operating room.

Results.—Mortality was significantly higher in the NICU group (table), but this was ascribed to the greater degree of prematurity and more associated illness in this group. Surgery was thought to be the major factor contributing to death in the NICU group in only 1 instance. Two wound

| | Procedures and Mortalities | | | |
| | NICU | | OR | |
Procedure	No	Deaths	No	Deaths
Bowel surgery and ostomies	40	7	56	1
Repair of oomphalocele	1	0	1	0
Repair of gastroschisis	1	0	1	0
Repair of inguinal hernia	2	0	12	0
Repair of CDH	10	2	3	0
Ligation of PDA	3	1	0	0
Repair of TEF	1	0	2	0
Bilateral cryopexy	10	0	0	0
Urological	5	1	20	0
Miscellaneous	8	1	17	1
Total	81	12	112	2

Abbreviations: CDH, congenital diaphragmatic hernia; *PDA,* patent ductus arteriosus; *TEF,* tracheoesophageal fistula.
(Courtesy of Finer NN, Woo B-C, Hayashi A, et al: *J Pediatr Surg* 28:645–649, 1993.)

infections were documented in the operating room group, and 1 was documented in the NICU group.

Conclusion.—The unstable newborn infant can have surgery in the NICU with no greater risk of morbidity or mortality than accrues to surgery performed in an operating room.

▶ The authors were the first to admit that this report was simply the result of observations of 2 very different and highly selected populations. Despite the limitations of this study, many critically ill patients underwent successful surgery and were spared the potential complications of transportation to a distant operating room, at what might be assumed to be a considerable economic savings. However, I would be interested in how our Canadian colleagues in anesthesiology viewed these complex pediatric surgeries being performed using high-dose fentanyl and pancuronium without the supervision of an anesthesiologist.—D.M. Rothenberg, M.D.

21 Transfusion, Fluids, and Electrolytes

Informed Consent for Blood Transfusion: A Regional Hospital Survey
Eisenstaedt RS, Glanz K, Smith DG, Derstine T (Temple Univ, Philadelphia)
Transfusion 33:558–561, 1993   101-94-21–1

Introduction.—Shifting social attitudes have expanded the circumstances in which written documentation of informed consent may be desirable. The American Association of Blood Banks endorses the concept of seeking informed consent from transfusion recipients. To determine the types of policies regarding informed consent for transfusion that are now in place, a survey of hospitals in 3 mid-Atlantic states was conducted.

Methods.—The 92 hospitals were located in New Jersey, Pennsylvania, and Delaware. The 21-item survey included general sections about the size and location of the hospital and specific questions on the design and content of their informed consent form, if such a form was used. Eighty-one (88%) of the hospitals contacted responded to the survey.

Results.—Approximately half (46%) of responding institutions had 200–400 beds. Fourteen percent were affiliated with a major medical school, and 21% were community hospitals with a medical school affiliation. Fifty-three percent of the surveys were completed by medical directors, 37% by blood bank supervisors, and 10% by hospital or nursing administrators. Fifty (62%) hospitals required written informed consent before blood transfusion; 39 had a document that was specifically used for this purpose. Most forms mentioned the possibility of complications, although few estimated the frequency of adverse reactions or described alternatives to allogeneic transfusion. The attending physician was responsible for obtaining consent in only 28 of 49 institutions. The reading level of 34 informed consent documents was rated as difficult or very difficult.

Conclusion.—Although most hospitals responding to the survey require written informed consent for blood transfusion, an analysis of these forms suggests that most do not fulfill the fundamental tenets of informed consent: benefits, risks, and the availability of alternatives. Verbal explanations by the patient's attending physician are likely to provide more information than many of these forms. Informed consent for transfusion should be inititiated well in advance of the procedure, presented in a document that uses easily understood language and offers the options of allogeneic blood and designated donations from freinds or relatives.

▶ Once again we find a rationale for a preoperative clinic, that is, to give appropriate and informed consent for transfusion. Many of us do not give such informed consent, and many surgeons give it woefully inadequately, but perhaps as we move into a managed care world and insurers want to discourage patients from having expensive, extensive surgery, informed consent for transfusion will be 1 of the ways of discouraging patients from having marginally beneficial surgery.

We should remember the tenents of informed consent—discussion of benefits, risks, and the availability of alternatives—given long enough in advance so the patient can consider it. This study does not answer who will pay for informed consent. However, it does reveal that most institutions do not give it appropriately, and the cost of such consent is not a minor issue. The attending physician did not obtain informed consent for blood transfusion in 64 of the 92 hospitals that responded to the survey.—M.F. Roizen, M.D.

Subcutaneous Recombinant Human Erythropoietin and Autologous Blood Donation Before Coronary Artery Bypass Surgery

Kulier AH, Gombotz H, Fuchs G, Vuckovic U, Metzler H (Univ of Graz, Austria)
Anesth Analg 76:102–106, 1993   101-94-21–2

Background.—The time required for accumulation of sufficient blood and the power of the erythropoietic response may limit the success of autologous blood donation before elective surgery, especially for patients with coronary artery disease. Recombinant human erythropoietin (rHuEPO) can improve preoperative autologous blood donation, but reported regimens use high doses at frequent intervals. A more practical regimen of rHuEPO for patients who donate autologous blood before primary elective coronary artery bypass grafting (CABG) was evaluated.

Methods.—The regimen evaluated consisted of a single weekly subcutaneous dose of 400 IU/kg, plus 270 mg of oral iron sulfate and .35 mg of folate. Twenty-four men who were awaiting CABG were randomized to receive either this regimen or oral iron only. Both groups were seen weekly. If their hemoglobin level was more than 12 g/dL, as many as 4 units of autologous blood was taken at these visits. The operation was performed without knowledge of whether the patients had received rHuEPO.

Results.—The rHuEPO group had consistently higher hemoglobin values than the iron-only group, permitting the collection of greater red cell volumes—775 vs. 682 mL, respectively. Homologous blood was needed at surgery in 8 of 12 of the iron-only group vs. just 1 of 12 of the rHuEPO group.

Conclusion.—The practical rHuEPO regimen reported effectively stimulates erythropoiesis and compensates for the hemoglobin decrease in patients donating autologous blood before elective CABG. Further research is needed to optimize rHuEPO dosage for patients awaiting various surgical procedures and to address the postoperative period.

▶ This article presented a more economical regimen in an attempt to increase the hemoglobin concentration of surgery patients with combinant erythropoietin, using a lower-cost dosing regimen than has been used in the past. It appears that this regimen was effective. I suppose much more information will be needed before we can finally evaluate the appropriate therapeutic dose and the timing of the predeposit to be supplemented with recombinant erythropoietin.—M.F. Roizen, M.D.

The Cost-Effectiveness of Preoperative Autologous Blood Donation for Total Hip and Knee Replacement

Birkmeyer JD, Goodnough LT, AuBuchon JP, Noordsij PG, Littenberg B (Dartmouth-Hitchcock Med Ctr, Lebanon, NH; Washington Univ, St Louis, Mo)
Transfusion 33:544–551, 1993   101-94-21–3

Background.—The frequency of preoperative autologous blood donation is increasing dramatically. However, the cost-effectiveness of this procedure has not been fully explored. A decision analysis was done to determine the cost-effectiveness of autologous blood donation for hip and knee replacement.

Methods.—Data on red cell use in 629 patients who had surgery at 2 tertiary care centers were used in the analysis. Cost-effectiveness was expressed as cost per quality-adjusted year of life saved.

Findings.—At centers 1 and 2, autologous blood donation for bilateral and revision joint replacement costs $40,000 and $241,000, respectively, per quality-adjusted year of life saved. For primary unilateral hip replacement, autologous blood donation costs $373,000 and $740,000 per quality-adjusted year of life saved at centers 1 and 2, respectively. The procedure was least cost-effective for primary unilateral knee replacement. Variations among procedures in the cost-effectiveness of autologous blood donation resulted from the differences between autologous blood collections and transfusion requirements. The reduced cost-effectiveness documented at center 2 resulted from higher transfusion rates in autologous blood donors than in nondonors.

Conclusion.—Autologous blood donation is not as cost-effective as other accepted medical procedures. Avoiding overcollection and overtransfusion of autologous blood may greatly improve its cost-effectiveness.

▶ The cost analysis is contingent on acceptance of the assumptions and ranges for the diseases prevented. Something gnawing in their analysis of this study is that the range for a post-transfusion hepatitis of 3 per 100 of 1% is 30 to 120 times less than 1% to 4% in the published data that I have seen. The published data in this study are for conversion to hepatitis C antigen/antibody positivity, not the occurrence of post-transfusion hepatitis, which is perhaps an important difference. This discrepancy would completely change the value and make this preoperative donation a very cost-effective practice.

The authors also did not take into account the anxiety caused in patients who have received homologous rather than autologous units. Such anxiety is obviously substantial and would again change the analysis in favor of autologous units. This article shows the problem of a cost-benefit analysis performed by prominent people who use unvalidated assumptions as well as my analysis, which is based on incorrect data.—M.F. Roizen, M.D.

Intratracheal Perfluorocarbon Administration Combined With Mechanical Ventilation in Experimental Respiratory Distress Syndrome: Dose-Dependent Improvement of Gas Exchange

Tütüncü AS, Faithfull NS, Lachmann B (Erasmus Univ, Rotterdam, The Netherlands; Univ of Istanbul, Turkey; Alliance Pharmaceutical Corp, San Diego, Calif)

Crit Care Med 21:962–969, 1993   101-94-21–4

Introduction.—Advances in conventional mechanical ventilation have improved survival in respiratory distress syndrome, but this complex syndrome remains a major problem in the intensive care unit. In surfactant-deficient lungs, oxygenated perfluorocarbon liquids have been used as an alternative respiratory medium because of their low surface tension and their ability to dissolve large amounts of respiratory gases. Rabbits were used to determine the efficacy of intratracheal perfluorocarbon plus conventional mechanical ventilation in acute respiratory failure.

Fig 21–1.—**Top left,** arterial blood partial pressure of oxygen (Pao_2) before lavage (*BL*), after lavage (*0*), and after treatment with perfluorocarbon or saline. The *bar* represents the lavage procedure (*L*). After the lung lavage, Pao_2 shows significant ($P < .05$, Wilcoxon signed-rank test) decrease in both groups. **Top right,** changes in arterial blood partial pressure of carbon dioxide ($Paco_2$) after intratracheal instillation of perfluorocarbon or saline in combination with mechanical ventilation for 15 minutes. **Bottom right,** arterial pH (mean $\pm$ standard deviation; 8 torr = 1 kPa) is seen to decrease in both groups subsequent to lung lavage (*L*). **Bottom left,** peak airway pressures ($Peak_{awp}$) before lavage, after lavage (*0*), and in response to perflourocarbon or saline administration. Mean data are significantly ($P < .005$, Mann-Whitney U test) different from the saline group at all treatment doses. (Courtesy of Tütüncü AS, Faithfull NS, Lachmann B: *Crit Care Med* 21:962–969, 1993.)

(continued)

Fig 21–1 (cont).

Pao₂ (torr)
600
500
400
300
200
100
0
Perflubron
Saline
Paco₂ (torr)
70
60
50
40
30
Saline
Perflubron
Peak_awp (cm H₂O)
35
30
25
20
15
10
Saline
Perflubron
pH
7.60
7.50
7.40
7.30
7.20
7.10
Perflubron
Saline
BL
L
0
3
6
9
12
15
mL/kg

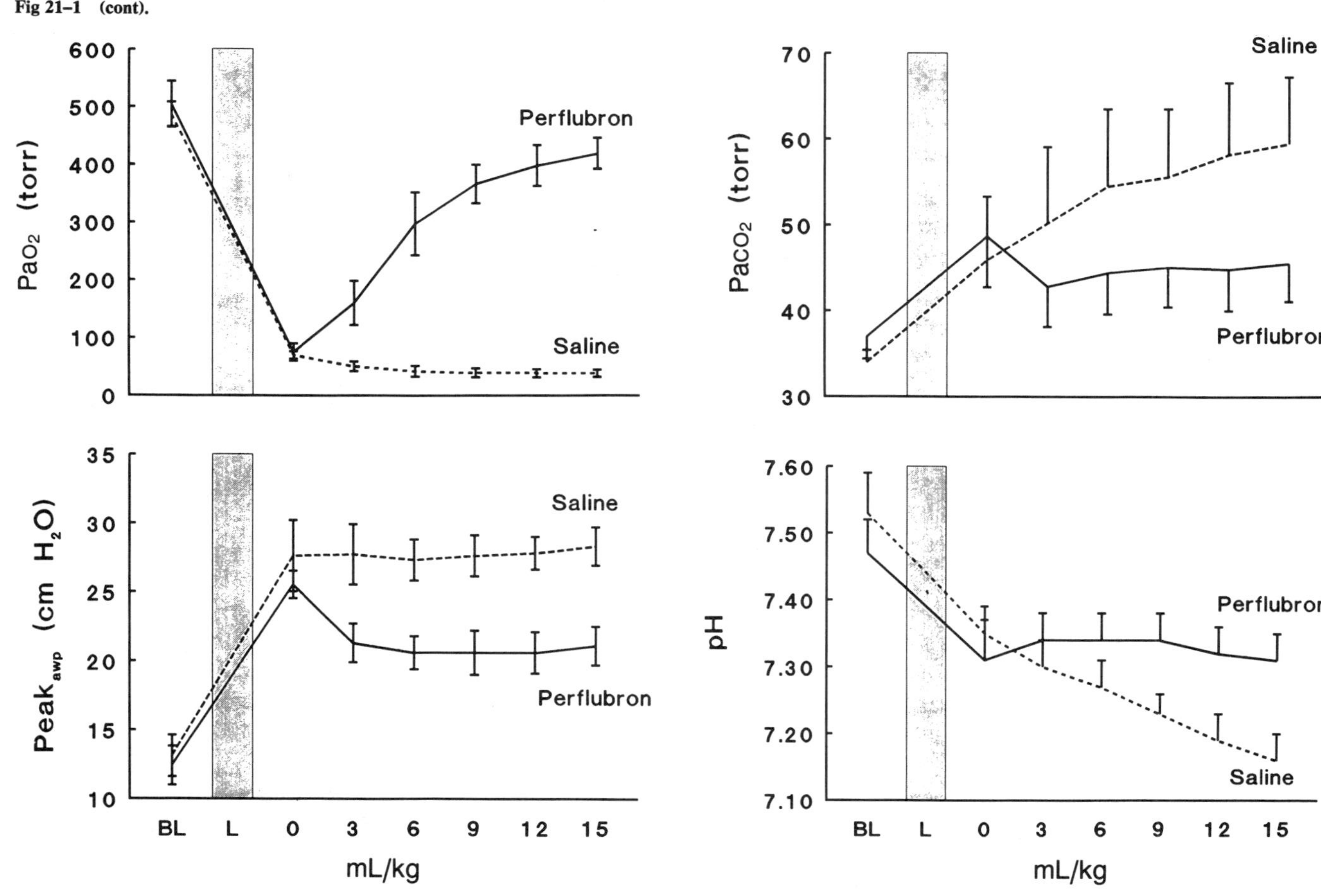

Methods.—In the prospective study, adult male New Zealand rabbits underwent repeated lung lavage with saline to induce respiratory failure. One group of animals was randomized to perfluorocarbon treatment, consisting of intratracheal instillation of incremental doses of 3 mL/kg of each liquid, for a total volume of 15 mL/kg, whereas the other group received placebo treatment. The animals were studied after 15 minutes of volume-controlled ventilation at a tidal volume of 12 mL/kg, a frequency of 30 breaths per minute, fraction of inspired oxygen of 1, and a positive end-expiratory pressure of 6 cm of water.

Results.—After the first dose of perfluorocarbon, the arterial blood partial pressure of oxygen increased from 75 to 420 torr and the arterial blood partial pressure of carbon dioxide decreased from 49 to 43 torr (Fig 21–1). Both values remained stable thereafter. Perfluorocarbon treatment also induced significant declines in airway pressures. The alveolar ventilation was well preserved, whereas alveolar dead space decreased and remained stable. Perfluorocarbon treatment was well tolerated.

Conclusion.—Dramatic improvements in pulmonary parameters were seen in perfluorocarbon-treated rabbits in acute respiratory failure. The type of ventilatory support used in this study may represent an effective and simple technique of clinical perfluorocarbon application.

▶ Although it is too early to speculate on the clinical efficacy of perfluorocarbon therapy for acute lung injury, this fascinating and elegant study represents an exciting area of research.—D.M. Rothenberg, M.D.

Effects of Buffering in Hypercapnia and Hypercapnic Hypoxemia

Wetterberg T, Sjöberg T, Steen S (Univ of Lund, Sweden)
Acta Anaesthesiol Scand 37:343–349, 1993   101-94-21–5

Objective.—Buffer therapy appears to be ineffective in clinical lactic acidosis and harmful in experimental models. However, its effects in hypercapnic acidosis are unknown. The effects of buffering in extreme hypercapnia and hypercapnic hypoxemia were determined.

Methods.—Twelve mechanically ventilated pigs were exposed to extreme hypercapnia, at a partial pressure of carbon dioxide in arterial blood ($PaCO_2$) of 20 kilopascal and a fractional concentration of oxygen in inspired gas (FIO_2) of .4 for 8 hours. Half of the animals received a continuous infusion of isotonic buffers—sodium bicarbonate and trometamol—whereas the other half did not. The mean rate of buffer infusion was 13.6 mL/kg/hr^{-1}. After 8 hours, both groups were exposed to hypercapnic hypoxemia in the form of stepwise increases in FIO_2, with the fractional concentration of carbon dioxide in inspired gas ($FICO_2$) kept at .2.

Results.—Buffered animals had an arterial pH of 7.21, compared with 7.01 for controls. There were no differences in serum osmolality or $PaCO_2$. The buffered group had an attenuation of the hemodynamic response to hypercapnia compared with controls; they also had a lower heart rate, mean arterial pressure, mean pulmonary arterial pressure, and pulmonary vascular resistance. During hypercapnic hypoxemia, both groups had increased pulmonary vascular resistance, and the hemodynamic differences disappeared, except for the difference in heart rate. The arterial oxygen saturation was higher at a FIO_2 of .15 in the buffered group than in the controls. At a FIO_2 of .10, the control animals died in a mean of 14 minutes, whereas the buffered group survived with a stable mean arterial pressure.

Conclusion.—The results in pigs suggest that buffering to a pH of 7.21 attenuates the hemodynamic response in extreme hypercapnia and improves survival in hypercapnic hypoxemia. The physiologic mechanisms of these benefits remain to be established. These findings differ significantly from those reported in metabolic acidosis.

▶ Theoretically, permissive hypercapnia minimizes barotrauma and mitigates the degree of lung damage imposed by positive-pressure mechanical ventilation. The use of bicarbonate or nonbicarbonate buffers in this setting appears to offset the deleterious effects of extreme respiratory acidosis.—D.M. Rothenberg, M.D.

Carbicarb, Sodium Bicarbonate, and Sodium Chloride in Hypoxic Lactic Acidosis: Effect on Arterial Blood Gases, Lactate Concentrations, Hemodynamic Variables, and Myocardial Intracellular pH

Rhee KH, Toro LO, McDonald GG, Nunnally RL, Levin DL (Univ of Arizona, Tucson; Univ of Texas, Dallas)
Chest 104:913–918, 1993   101-94-21–6

Introduction.—Carbicarb is a new agent that buffers in a manner similar to sodium bicarbonate without the net generation of carbon dioxide. It is a 1:1 mixture of disodium carbonate and sodium bicarbonate with a much lower partial pressure of carbon dioxide (PCO_2), a higher pH, and less osmolality than sodium bicarbonate. The carbonate ion, a strong base in Carbicarb, abstracts hydrogen ions from buffer acid and from dissolved carbon dioxide to produce the bicarbonate ion. Because these 2 major sources of proton supply are in blood and in tissues perfused by capillaries, the buffer acids and PCO_2 do not increase with Carbicarb administration. It was hypothesized that Carbicarb would correct hypoxic lactic acidosis more effectively than sodium bicarbonate.

Methods.—In 21 young mongrel dogs, hypoxic lactic acidosis was induced with a fractional concentration of oxygen in inspired gas (FIO_2) of .09 and stabilized with serial measurements of arterial blood gases and pH during 2–3 hours, resulting in an arterial pH of 7.2 with a partial

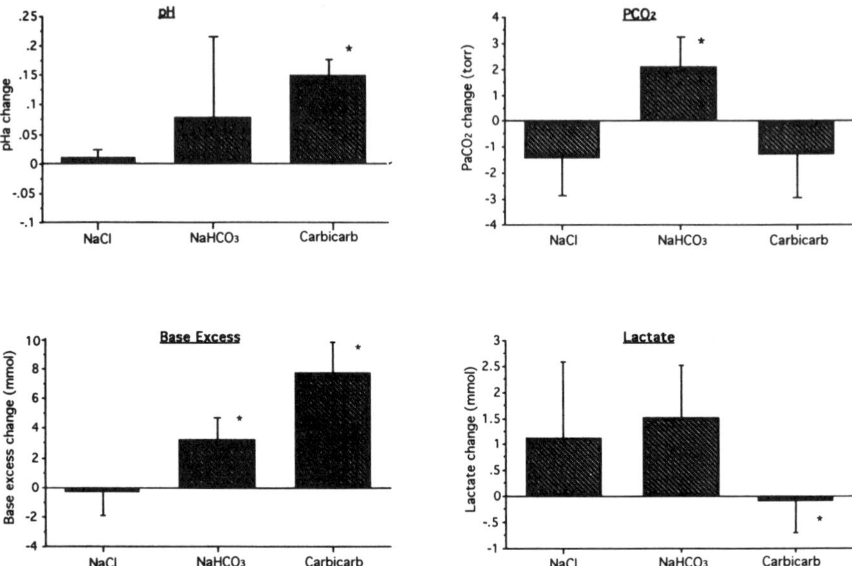

Fig 21–2.—*Abbreviations: NaCl,* sodium chloride; *NAHCO₃,* sodium bicarbonate; *pHa,* arterial pH. Changes of values in pH, P_{CO_2}, base excess, and lactate concentration in arterial blood before and after infusion of each agent. *Columns* indicate mean values of each agent, and *vertical bars* indicate 1 SD error of each value. *Asterisk* indicates $P < .05$. (Courtesy of Rhee KH, Toro LO, McDonald GG, et al: *Chest* 104:913–918, 1993.)

pressure of oxygen (PO_2) of 28 mm Hg. The animals were then randomly assigned to Carbicarb, sodium bicarbonate, or sodium chloride infusion for 30 minutes. Arterial blood gases, pH, lactate concentrations, and hemodynamic variables were measured before and 30 minutes after completion of the infusion.

Results.—Sodium bicarbonate infusion was associated with a significant increase in arterial PCO_2, compared with Carbicarb or sodium chloride. With the Carbicarb infusion, arterial pH, base excess, and cardiac index increased significantly without a significant increase in arterial serum lactate concentration (Fig 21-2). In addition, the stroke volume index increased significantly and heart rate decreased with the Carbicarb infusion (Fig 21-3). Systemic vascular resistance and pulmonary vascular resistance indices decreased similarly in the 3 groups. The arterial pH correlated well with myocardial intracellular pH, as determined by simultaneous nuclear magnetic spectroscopy. In contrast with previous studies, no detrimental hemodynamic effect or paradoxical intracellular acidosis was noted with sodium bicarbonate administration.

Discussion.—Carbicarb administration in hypoxic lactic acidosis improves hemodynamics compared with sodium bicarbonate and sodium chloride. The increased stroke volume with Carbicarb administration is not the result of decreased vascular resistances but rather of improved arterial pH and myocardial intracellular pH. Because Carbicarb does not

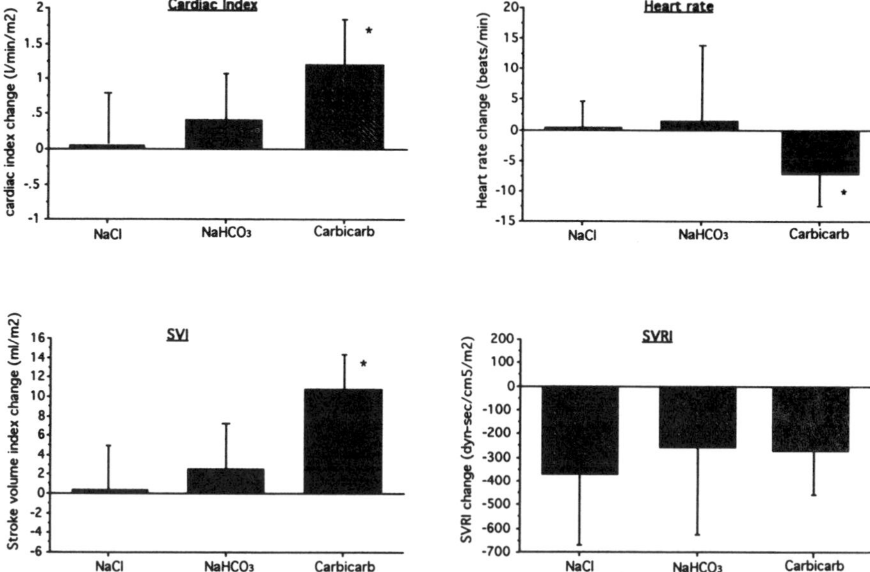

Fig 21–3.—*Abbreviations: NaCl,* sodium chloride; $NAHCO_3$, sodium bicarbonate; *SVI,* stroke volume index; *SVRI,* systemic vascular resistance index. Changes of values in cardiac index, heart rate, stroke volume index, and systemic vascular resistance index before and after infusion of each agent. *Columns* indicate mean values of each agent, and *vertical bars* indicate 1 SD error of each value. *Asterisk* indicates $P < .05$. (Courtesy of Rhee KH, Toro LO, McDonald GG, et al: *Chest* 104:913-918, 1993.)

increase carbon dioxide levels, it would be more effective than sodium bicarbonate in treating hypoxic lactic acidosis with decreased myocardial function and may facilitate the treatment of combined metabolic and respiratory acidosis with adequate ventilation.

▶ Carbicarb appears to have many beneficial effects with none of the concerns of hypertonicity and CO_2 generation that are seen with sodium bicarbonate administration. This agent may also prove to be useful in regulating pH in patients who are undergoing permissive hypercapnia.—D.M. Rothenberg, M.D.

22 Coagulation/Anticoagulation

Identification of Patients at Risk for Excessive Blood Loss During Coronary Artery Bypass Surgery: Thromboelastograph Versus Coagulation Screen
Dorman BH, Spinale FG, Bailey MK, Kratz JM, Roy RC (Med Univ of South Carolina, Charleston)
Anesth Analg 76:694–700, 1993   101-94-22–1

Introduction.—In an effort to devise a reliable preoperative screening test to identify patients undergoing cardiothoracic surgery who are at risk of increased operative bleeding, a study was designed to evaluate a range of coagulation tests in 60 patients who were scheduled to have coronary artery bypass surgery.

Methods.—A complete coagulation screen was performed as well as activated clotting time estimates and a thromboelastograph. Blood loss was determined by weighing sponges and measuring blood in suction canisters.

Observations.—The mean duration of cardiopulmonary bypass was 100 minutes and for surgery it was 5 hours. Total crystalloid and colloid

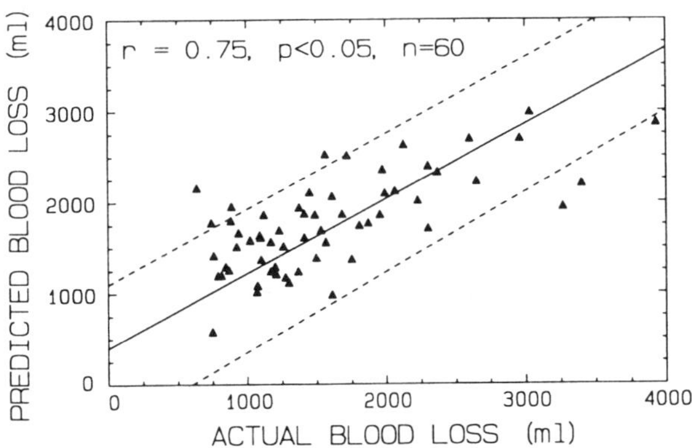

Fig 22–1.—Scatter plot of predicted vs. actual blood loss for 60 patients undergoing coronary artery bypass surgery. Predicted blood loss was modeled using platelet count, bleeding time, and prothrombin time as coagulation screening parameters. The *solid line* represents the regression line, and the *dashed lines* are the 95% confidence interval. (Courtesy of Dorman BH, Spinale FG, Bailey MK, et al: *Anesth Analg* 76:694–700, 1993.)

requirements averaged 5.5 and 1.4 L, respectively. Forty-eight percent of the patients required an average of 2.5 units of blood, and the total intraoperative blood loss averaged 1,590 mL. Components of the thromboelastograph totally failed to predict blood loss. However, it was possible to predict perioperative blood loss using the bleeding and prothrombin times and the platelet count (Fig 22–1).

Conclusion.—Elements of the routine preoperative coagulation profile can help identify patients who are at increased risk of losing excessive blood during coronary artery bypass surgery.

▶ The thromboelastograph (TEG) has been shown to be quite useful clinically in terms of understanding the pathophysiology of excessive bleeding after cardiopulmonary bypass. This study sought to discover whether preoperative TEG could be used to predict postcardiopulmonary bypass coagulopathies. It did not prove to be as useful as a predictor of trouble as the routine preoperative coagulation screen. However, this does not seem to in any way diminish the postoperative usefulness of TEG in the treatment of these problems.—J.H. Tinker, M.D.

Preparation of Autologous Fibrin Glue From Pericardial Blood

Kjaergard HK, Weis-Fogh US, Thiis JJ (Univ of Copenhagen)
Ann Thorac Surg 55:543–544, 1993
101-94-22–2

Background.—Autologous fibrin glue is a hemostatic agent that can be prepared using ethanol. The possible preparation of autologous fibrin glue from pericardial and mediastinal blood was tested to determine its usefulness in hemostasis and blood salvaging during cardiac operations.

Patients and Methods.—Twenty-eight patients aged 30–71 years were scheduled for elective coronary artery bypass grafting. After sternotomy, 44 mL of pericardial and mediastinal blood was drawn into a syringe containing 6 mL of heparin and citrate as anticoagulant. After separation of plasma from the blood cells by centrifugation, the fibrinogen was precipitated with 99% ethanol by incubation at 0°C for 30 minutes. To ensure sterility, the preparation was completed in a closed system. The second component of the glue contained 1,200 IU/mL of thrombin, 100 mmol/L of calcium chloride, and 6,000 kallikrein inactivation units per milliliter of aprotinin.

Results.—The mean volume of fibrinogen concentrate was 2.1 ± .7 mL, with a concentration of 25.1 ± 7.5 mg/mL. After .3 parts of thrombin solution was added, the total volume of the two-component fibrin glue was 2.7 mL. The glue was sterile and prepared in less than 90 minutes.

Conclusion.—The advantages of this glue include protection from transmission of viral diseases and immunologic reactions. It is suitable for use as a hemostatic agent and as a sealant for pulmonary air leak and high-porosity vascular prostheses. A new device that allows glue to be prepared in less than 30 minutes is currently being tested.

Inhibition of Platelet Function by Heparin: An Etiologic Factor in Post-bypass Hemorrhage

John LCH, Rees GM, Kovacs IB (St Bartholomew's Hosp, London)
J Thorac Cardiovasc Surg 105:816–822, 1993   101-94-22-3

Objective.—Heparin-related bleeding in noncardiac surgery patients may be related to impaired platelet function. The effects of heparin on platelet function were explored in 290 patients undergoing cardiac surgery.

Management.—Platelet function was evaluated using the hemostatometer. The extracorporeal circuit was primed with Hartmann solution that contained 10,000 units of heparin, and patients received 300 units per kilogram of heparin intravenously before the start of cardiopulmonary bypass. More heparin was given as needed to maintain an activated clotting time above 500 seconds throughout the bypass period.

Findings.—In vitro studies demonstrated a proaggregatory effect of heparin at 5 units/mL in 8.6% of patients, mild-to-moderate inhibition of platelet function in 58.6%, and severely inhibited platelet function in 32.8%. These groups exhibited no substantial clinical differences and no differences in antiplatelet medication. The in vitro findings correlated well with ex vivo measurements made in blood taken after heparinization. In 111 patients, preoperative measurements of platelet function after exposure of blood to heparin correlated significantly with postoperative blood loss after 4, 12, and 18 hours. The mean blood loss at 18 hours was 713 mL in patients with in vitro findings of mildly to moderately inhibited platelet function and 1,172 mL in those with severe platelet dysfunction.

Conclusion.—Heparin alters platelet function in patients who have cardiac surgery. This may contribute to bleeding after cardiopulmonary bypass. It may be possible to preoperatively identify patients who are at the greatest risk of excessive postoperative bleeding.

▶ Heparin is a biological product with a variety of interactions. The authors found a wide variation of inhibition of platelet function preoperatively and a severe inhibition of platelet function postoperatively in patients after cardiopulmonary bypass. It is well known that heparin interferes with platelet function, among its many other effects. I cannot understand why the authors believe this well-known effect "appears to be a previously unrecognized etiologic factor in bleeding after cardiopulmonary bypass." If heparin is a known inhibitor of platelet function, which it is, I do not understand what is really new in this paper. In their discussion, the authors cited at least 10 studies that clearly showed various types of modification of platelet function by heparin.

Admittedly, I selected this paper to criticize it, but I also chose it to point out to readers that there are some new developments in anticoagulation for cardiopulmonary bypass. For instance, there is a substance called ancrod (see Abstract 101-94-14–3), which is an enzymatic defibrinogenator, and another called hirudin, which is a competitive inhibitor of thrombin. Ancrod is derived from pit viper toxin, and hirudin is derived from the leech. What goes around comes around. Just thought you would like to know.—J.H. Tinker, M.D.

Abnormal Peri-Operative Haemorrhage in Asymptomatic Patients Is Not Predicted by Laboratory Testing

MacPherson CR, Jacobs P, Dent DM (Univ of Cape Town, South Africa; Univ of Cincinnati, Ohio)
S Afr Med J 83:106–108, 1993
101-94-22–4

Background.—Failure to detect bleeding disorders can lead to the unexpected loss of excessive blood during major elective surgery. However, extensive hemostatic screening is costly and may not be appropriate for low-risk patients.

Study Design.—The prothrombin time, activated partial thromboplastin time, bleeding time, and platelet count were estimated in 111 asymptomatic patients who were scheduled for elective major thoracic or general surgery. None of the patients had a positive bleeding history or had ingested aspirin. In a second phase, disordered hemostasis was sought in 49 patients who had required more blood perioperatively than expected among 1,872 who were operated on.

Findings.—Of the 111 patients screened, 8 had a prolonged partial thromboplastin time and 1 had mild thrombocytopenia; none of these patients bled excessively. Technical problems related to vascular surgery or malignant disease may have accounted for excessive blood loss in 23 of the 49 patients reviewed. In 9 other patients, extensive granulation tissue was present in relation to tuberculosis or irradiation. Eight technical errors were made. In 4 patients, a postoperative hemoglobin estimate prompted transfusion. In 5 patients, there was no apparent indication for transfusion.

Conclusion.—Screening for coagulation function preoperatively is not cost-effective for asymptomatic patients who are at low risk. Such testing is not likely to predict abnormal bleeding.

▶ This article adds data on a few more than 100 patients to the already extant data on 30,000 patients that show there is no benefit to asymptomatic patients being screened for coagulation abnormalities. Not only is there no benefit, such screening may actually be hazardous. As a result, the risk-benefit ratio of screening for clotting abnormalities in otherwise asymptomatic patients is not cost-effective or risk-effective. For a review of the subject, see Chapter 25 on preoperative evaluation of the asymptomatic patient in Miller's 1994 edition (1).—M.F. Roizen, M.D.

Reference

1. Roizen MF: Preoperative evaluation, in Miller RD (ed): *Anesthesia*, 4th ed. New York, Churchill-Livingstone, 1994.

23 Critical Care Medicine

Outcome Studies

▶↓ The next 2 articles represent major contributions to the critical care literature and are essential reading for all physicians routinely involved in the management of an intensive care unit.—D.M. Rothenberg, M.D.

Improving Intensive Care: Observations Based on Organizational Case Studies in Nine Intensive Care Units: A Prospective, Multicenter Study

Zimmerman JE, Shortell SM, Rousseau DM, Duffy J, Gillies RR, Knaus WA, Devers K, Wagner DP, Draper EA (George Washington Univ, Washington, DC; JL Kellogg Graduate School of Management, Evanston, Ill; Northwestern Univ, Evanston, Ill; et al)
Crit Care Med 21:1443–1451, 1993　　　　　　　　　　　　101-94-23–1

Background.—Expenditures for intensive care services now exceed $40 billion per year in the United States. Previous research suggests there are wide variations in the appropriateness and efficiency of use of the intensive care unit (ICU) for patient care. Factors related to superior ICU effectiveness were assessed in this prospective multicenter study.

Methods.—Included were 9 ICUs at 5 teaching and 4 nonteaching hospitals from different areas of the country. A detailed on-site analysis was based on each unit's Acute Physiology and Chronic Health Evaluation (APACHE) II risk-adjusted mortality rates. Three of the 9 ICUs were predicted to have better, 3 worse, and 3 average risk-adjusted hospital survival. A team of clinical and organizational researchers interviewed nurses and physicians and observed care and communication practices in the units. The effectiveness of the ICU was measured by the ratio of the actual to the predicted hospital death rate; efficiency was measured by the ratio of the actual to the predicted length of ICU stay.

Results.—Among the 9 hospitals selected for in-depth analysis, the mean number of hospital beds was 455 and the mean hospital occupancy rate was 69.5%. The average number of ICU beds was 11.8 and the mean ICU occupancy rate was 78.9%. Those ICUs with higher performance frequently evidenced a team satisfaction–oriented culture characterized by commitment to excellence in patient care and empowerment of nurses. Higher performing units had patient-centered cultures. The medical directors and nurse managers of these units were dedicated

---

Examples of Best Practices for Coordinating Care Within the ICU and
With Other Areas of the Hospital

Within ICU
 Specific guidelines and protocols for medical and nursing care
 Physician credentialing for selected procedures, e.g., intubation,
  invasive monitoring
 Updated protocols for limiting life-supporting therapy
 Physician rounds made early, facilitating communication and
  planning by nurses
 Orientation, written guidelines, and close supervision for residents
 Rounds and conferences with pharmacist, dietition, radiologist
 Emphasis on decentralized services (satellite pharmacy, labo-
  ratory, and radiograph viewing) in or close to ICU
 Guidelines for nursing change of shift report
Between ICU and Other Areas
 New nurses oriented to emergency, recovery, step-down units
 Standardized nursing reports for patients transferred from ICU;
  interunit conferences for long-term, complex cases
 Floor care for hopelessly ill or chronically ventilated patients with
  a do-not-resuscitate order and other treatment limits
 Direct phone line from visiting area to unit clerk
 Administrative and support services emphasize importance of
  satisfying "internal customers"

(Courtesy of Zimmerman JE, Shortell SM, Rousseau DM, et al: *Crit Care Med* 21:1443–1451, 1993.)

---

to continuous learning and improvement. There were specific, written guidelines and protocols for medical and nursing care. Communication was frequent and open, enhancing coordination among physicians, nurses, pharmacists, and other staff members (table).

Conclusion.—All ICUs offered examples of practices to avoid and practices to emulate. The units with superior risk-adjusted survival could not be distinguished by structural and organizational questionnaires or global judgments of on-site investigators. Although professional skill and technologic capabilities are vital to superior performance, these qualities need to be rooted in a patient-centered, problem-solving culture.

▶ This article confirms what those who practice critical care medicine have intuitively known for some time, namely, that excellence in an ICU is based on goal-oriented problem solving, strong nursing, medical leadership, and communication among all services.—D.M. Rothenberg, M.D.

Eliminating Needless Testing in Intensive Care: An Information-Based Team Management Approach

Roberts DE, Bell DD, Ostryzniuk T, Dobson K, Oppenheimer L, Martens D, Honcharik N, Cramp H, Loewen E, Bodnar S, Guenther A, Pronger L, Roberts E, McEwen TA (Univ of Manitoba, Winnipeg, Canada)

Crit Care Med 21:1452–1458, 1993   101-94-23–2

Introduction.—Providing intensive care is comparatively expensive and often futile, but the demand will continue as new treatment modalities are developed. Rationing critical care services has been mentioned as a way to control the cost of intensive care. A cost-effective, practical management approach may produce sustained reductions in the use of laboratory resources and costs.

Methods.—An interventional study with prospective data collection was conducted in a 10-bed adult surgical intensive care unit (ICU) and an 8-bed adult medical ICU in a tertiary care hospital. Data were obtained from 647 consecutive patients admitted during a 7-month baseline period, 1,236 patients admitted during a 1-year intervention period, and 2,349 patients admitted during a 2-year follow-up.

Interventions.—A management data base was used to track the use of 123 laboratory investigations during the baseline period. Nine tests that accounted for 57.7% of all tests were targeted for reduction, including determinations of blood gases, glucose, potassium, ECG, chest radiograph, sodium, chloride, complete blood count with differential, and serum osmolality. A multidisciplinary committee within the ICU developed specific policies to reduce the use of these tests. These policies were applied to all patients admitted during the 1-year intervention and 2-year follow-up periods.

Outcome.—During the intervention period, there was an overall reduction of 25% in tests per admission. The most dramatic reductions occurred in the 9 targeted tests, ranging from 19% to 46%. In contrast, significant reductions occurred in only 13 of the 114 untargeted investigations. Based on actual hospital costs, the potential annual cost savings was more than $150,000 Canadian. Reduced laboratory use was not associated with increased ICU mortality rate, prolonged ICU lengths of stay, or increased drug costs. Furthermore, the reductions in the frequency of targeted tests were maintained during the 2-year follow-up.

Conclusion.—Application of an information-based multidisciplinary management system in the ICU results in a marked and sustained reduction in unnecessary testing in a cost-effective manner. Rationing of intensive care services may eventually be necessary, but identification and reduction of needless testing can be a safe and effective cost-containment strategy in the ICU.

▶ I suggest that all of us who insist on or expect a "fresh set" of data for ICU rounds every morning reevaluate this rubber-stamp policy in the name of both cost containment and teaching.—D.M. Rothenberg, M.D.

Intensive Care Unit Outcome in the Very Elderly

Kass JE, Castriotta RJ, Malakoff F (Univ of Connecticut, Hartford)
Crit Care Med 20:1666–1671, 1992   101-94-23-3

Introduction.—The population of the very elderly—persons aged 85 years and older—is projected to increase in the United States to 4.6 million by the year 2000. Allocation of intensive care resources to this age group is expected to have a significant impact on health-care costs. The effects of age, previous functional status, and severity of illness on acute and long-term mortality rates and functional status of the very elderly after an intensive care unit (ICU) admission were examined.

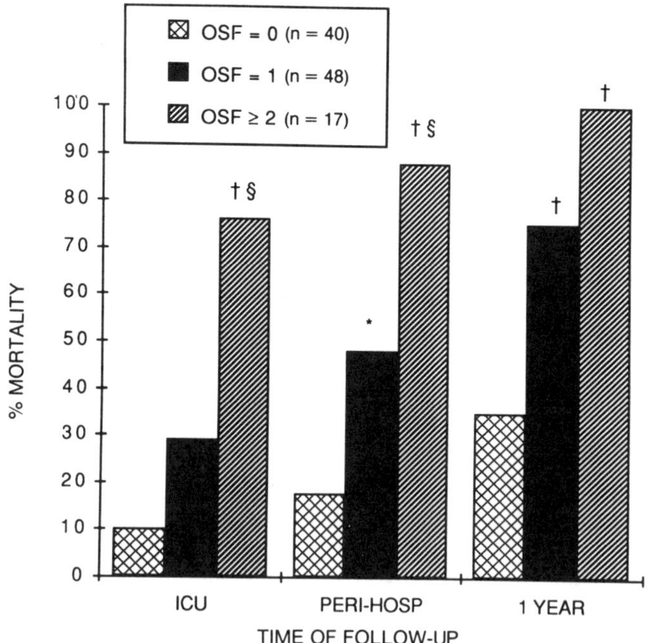

Fig 23–1.—Mortality rate vs. time of follow-up and number of organ system failures (OSF). * $P <$ .01 when compared with OSF = 0, † $P <$ .001 when compared with OSF = 0, § $P <$ .01 when compared with OSF = 1. (Courtesy of Kass JE, Castriotta RJ, Malakoff F: *Crit Care Med* 20:1666–1671, 1992.)

Methods.—Study subjects were all patients, aged 85 years or older, admitted to an ICU during a 2-year period. Cardiac patients were admitted to a separate coronary care unit. Patients were retrospectively entered in the first year of the study and prospectively entered thereafter. Outcome measures were mortality (in the ICU, at 30 days after hospital discharge, and at 1 year), activity of daily living scores, and organ system failure score at the time of the ICU admission.

Results.—The study group of 62 women and 43 men had a mean age of 89.4 years. Their mean length of stay was 5 days in the ICU and 16.1 days in the hospital. The ICU, 30-day posthospital discharge, and 1-year mortality rates were 30%, 43%, and 64%, respectively. At each period, mortality was significantly increased for patients with 2 or more organ system failures (Fig 23–1). Most (86%) patients who survived up to 6 months after hospital discharge survived to 1 year with little change from baseline in activities of daily living scores. The severity of illness was associated with higher ICU and 1-year mortality rates. Age and functional status before admission were not predictive of mortality.

Conclusion.—Acute severity of illness is the most important predictor of mortality after an ICU admission in patients aged 85 years and older. Most very elderly patients who survive to 1 year do not have deterioration in functional status. Few of the very elderly survive after admission to the ICU with 2 or more organ system failures.

Long-Term Outcome of Critically Ill Elderly Patients Requiring Intensive Care

Chelluri L, Pinsky MR, Donahoe MP, Grenvik A (Univ of Pittsburgh, Pa)
JAMA 269:3119–3123, 1993   101-94-23–4

Introduction.—Individuals aged 65 years and older make up about 13% of the United States population but use nearly one third of all health-care resources. Given the steep increases in health-care expenditures, some have suggested that age be used as a criterion for the cost-effective allocation of resources. Whether severity of illness, rather than age, determines long-term survival and quality of life in these patients was determined.

Methods.—Patients aged 65 years and older requiring admission to an intensive care unit (ICU) during a 3-month period were enrolled in the study. Organ transplant patients, those with a poor prognosis secondary to cancer, and patients who had uncomplicated elective surgery were excluded. The patients were divided into 2 groups: aged 65–74 years and aged 75 years and older. Those who survived hospitalization were evaluated for mortality and quality of life at 1, 6, and 12 months after discharge.

Results.—The younger group included 43 patients (mean age, 69 years); the older group included 54 patients (mean age, 81 years). The

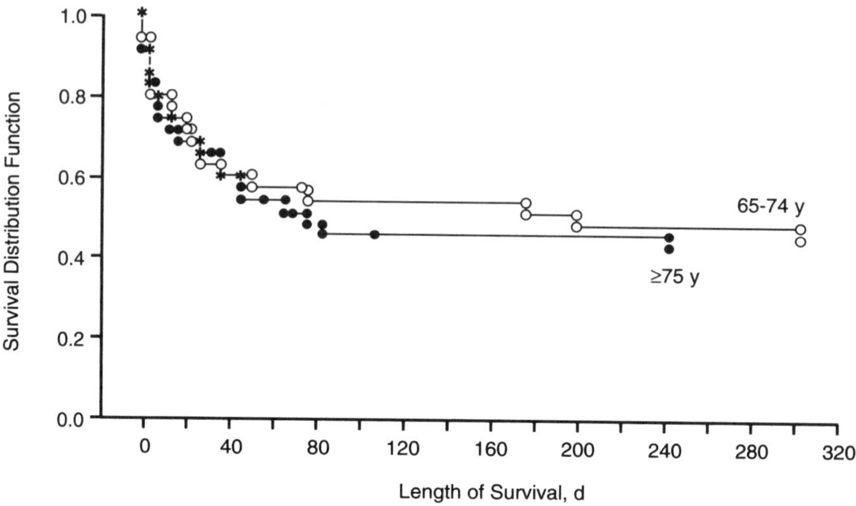

Fig 23–2.—Kaplan-Meier survival analysis based on age. Length of survival: 65–74 years of age, 166 ± 21 days; 75 years of age or older, 123 ± 15 days (mean ± SE) ($P = .5$). *Asterisk* indicates similar rates of survival at this point in time. (Courtesy of Chelluri L, Pinsky MR, Donahoe MP, et al: *JAMA* 269:3119–3123, 1993.)

groups did not differ significantly in length of hospital stay, hospital charges, or mortality at 1 year (Fig 23-2). The severity of illness, however, was related to mortality. Patients readmitted to an ICU during the same hospitalization were more likely to die in the hospital than those

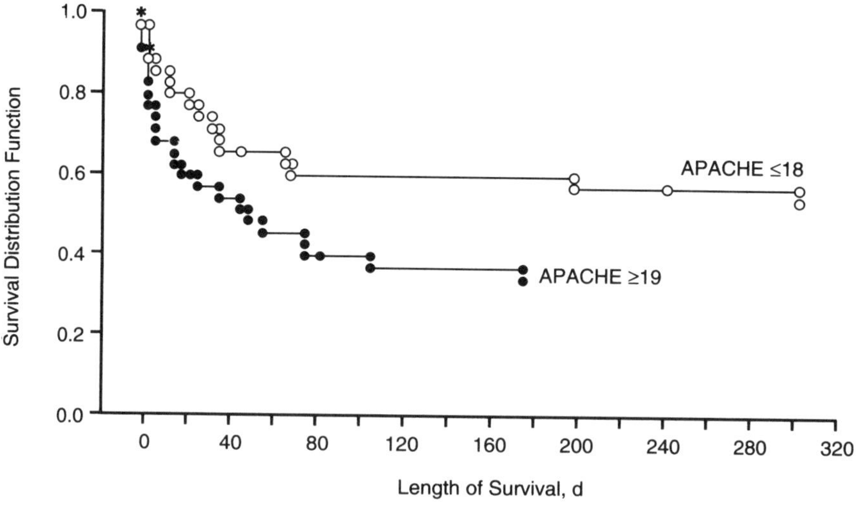

Fig 23–3.—Kaplan-Meier survival analysis based on APACHE II score. Length of survival: APACHE II score 18 or less, 188 ± 20 days; 19 or higher, 82 ± 11 days (mean ± SE) ($P = .04$). *Asterisk* indicates similar rates of survival at this point in time. (Courtesy of Chelluri L, Pinsky MR, Donahoe MP, et al: *JAMA* 269:3119–3123, 1993.)

	%	
One-Year Follow-up of Hospital Survivors		
	65-74 y (n = 18)	75-94 y (n = 20)
Residence		
Home	100	80
Nursing home/other	0	20
Rehospitalization		
Yes	33	30
No	56	50
Unknown	11	20
Willing to receive ICU care again*		
Yes	72	70
No	6	10
Unknown	22	20
Perception of ICU care		
Positive	66	60
Negative	0	5
Neutral/don't remember	6	15
Unknown	28	20

(Courtesy of Chelluri L, Pinsky MR, Donahoe MP, et al: JAMA 269:3119–3123, 1993.)

who did not require readmission (73% vs. 33%, respectively). None of the patients admitted to the hospital after cardiac arrest survived 1 year. Patients with an Acute Physiology and Chronic Health Evaluation (APACHE) II score of 18 or less survived longer than those with an APACHE II score of 19 or more, irrespective of age (Fig 23–3). At each of the 3 follow-up periods, the 2 age groups did not differ significantly in quality of life. Most of the 38 long-term survivors were living at home and would be willing, if necessary, to receive intensive care again (table).

Conclusion.—The decision to use intensive care should consider long-term outcome and quality of life. In patients aged 65 years and older, increased age alone was not a reliable predictor of outcome. The cost of each year of life saved, not including physician fees and expenditures after hospital discharge, was $21,768.

▶ These 2 studies (Abstracts 101-94-23-3 and 101-94-23-4) failed to identify age as an independent risk factor of ICU mortality. For the elderly and the very elderly, only severity of illness scores and the number of organs involved in organ system failure predicted early and late mortality. A 36% and 39% 1-year survival rate was seen in the first and second of these 2 studies, respectively, with both studies showing an adequate quality of life. These results suggest that if rationing of ICU care becomes necessary, age alone should not be a determinant of ICU admission.—D.M. Rothenberg, M.D.

Cardiogenic Shock Complicating Acute Myocardial Infarction in Patients Without Heart Failure on Admission: Incidence, Risk Factors, and Outcome

Leor J, Goldbourt U, Reicher-Reiss H, Kaplinsky E, Behar S, SPRINT Study Group (Sheba Med Ctr, Tel Hashomer, Israel)
Am J Med 94:265–273, 1993   101-94-23-5

Background.—Individuals with a large myocardial infarction (MI) and with clinical signs of heart failure seeking medical attention are at a higher risk of the subsequent development of cardiogenic shock and of

Independent Predictors for Cardiogenic Shock by
Multivariate Analysis

Variable	Relative Odds*	90% CI
Age, by 10-year increments	2.45	1.50–4.02
Female gender	1.51	0.91–2.50
History of angina	2.64	1.36–3.76
History of stroke	2.12	1.26–6.35
Peripheral vascular disease	1.99	0.95–4.18
LDH >4 times the normal	3.16	1.79–5.57
Increased serum glucose on admission by increments of 40 mg/dL	3.52	2.13–5.84

Abbreviations: CI, confidence interval; *LDH*, lactate dehydrogenase.
* Odds are for presence vs. absence of attributes and for increments as described of continuous variables (age, serum glucose).
(Courtesy of Leor J, Goldbourt U, Reicher-Reiss H, et al: *Am J Med* 94:265–273, 1993.)

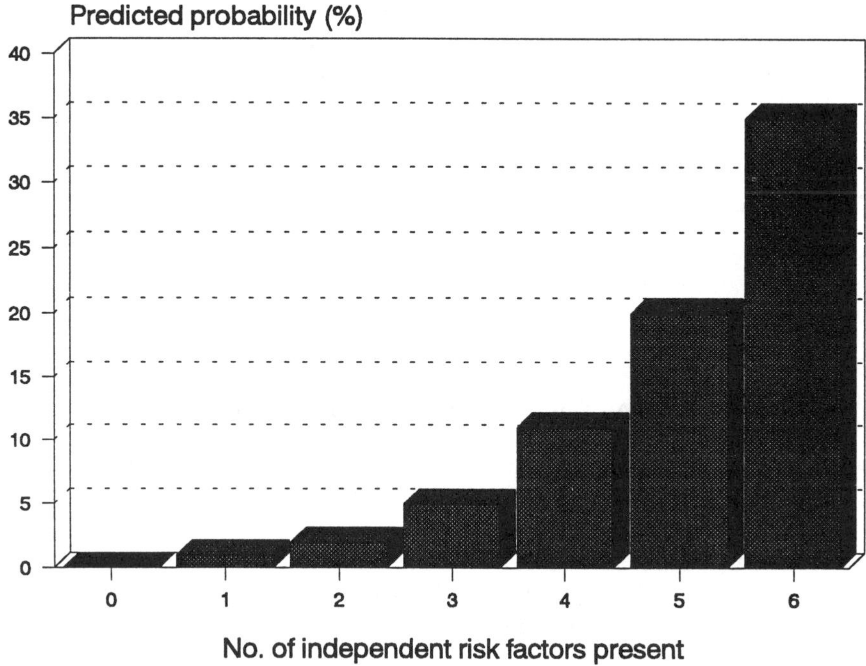

Fig 23–4.—Predicted probability for the in-hospital development of cardiogenic shock according to the number of independent risk factors present. (Courtesy of Leor J, Goldbourt U, Reicher-Reiss H, et al: *Am J Med* 94:265–273, 1993.)

dying. However, little is known about the development of cardiogenic shock in patients with acute MI seen without clinical signs of heart failure.

Methods and Findings.—Clinical data on 5,839 consecutive patients admitted with acute MI were analyzed to determine the incidence, predictors for occurrence, and outcome of in-hospital development of cardiogenic shock in patients seen without heart failure. Of the total group, 3,465 patients (59%) did not have heart failure on admission. In 3% of these patients cardiogenic shock developed during hospitalization. This represented 24% of all cases of in-hospital cardiogenic shock. In 66%, cardiogenic shock developed more than 24 hours after admission. All but 3 patients with cardiogenic shock died. The in-hospital mortality rate among patients without cardiogenic shock was 5%. Independent predictors for the development of shock in the hospital were age, female gender, history of angina, history of stroke, peripheral vascular disease, peak lactate dehydrogenase levels exceeding 4 times the norm, and hyperglycemia on admission. Patients with 6 risk factors, excluding lactate dehydrogenase values, had an estimated probability of 35% for the development of in-hospital cardiogenic shock (table; Fig 23–4).

Conclusion.—A significant percentage of patients with MI in whom cardiogenic shock developed after admission were free of heart failure at the time of admission. Several risk factors were determined to facilitate early identification of subgroups at risk for cardiogenic shock in otherwise low-risk patients.

▶ By identifying this subgroup of patients, it is possible that early attempts to improve myocardial perfusion (e.g., angioplasty and coronary artery bypass grafting) may decrease mortality. Studies randomizing high-risk patients to medical and surgical management seem warranted.—D.M. Rothenberg, M.D.

The Utility of Routine Daily Chest Radiography in the Surgical Intensive Care Unit
Silverstein DS, Livingston DH, Elcavage J, Kovar L, Kelly KM (UMD-New Jersey Med School, Newark)
J Trauma 35:643–646, 1993   101-94-23-6

Introduction.—Although daily chest x-ray films (CXRs) are routinely obtained from patients in surgical intensive care units (ICUs), the necessity for this practice has not been demonstrated. To assess the value of routine chest radiography, the morning CXRs of patients admitted to 2 surgical ICUs during a 1-month period were prospectively evaluated.

Methods.—One surgical ICU was in a level I trauma center and the other was in a large affiliated community hospital. Only the routine morning CXRs were evaluated. The radiographic findings were divided into 2 categories: the location of medical devices (correct, minor incorrect, or major incorrect position) and cardiopulmonary pathologic states. The cardiopulmonary pathologic processes seen on CXRs were examined as to presence and type and whether the process was improved, worsened, without change, or a new finding.

Results.—A total of 525 consecutive CXRs from 112 patients were evaluated. Patients at the community hospital were predominantly undergoing elective procedures; injuries were more common in trauma center patients. Of 1,028 tubes and catheters examined, 55 were in a minor incorrect position and 13 were in a major incorrect position requiring adjustment; 78 CXRs were read as normal. A total of 775 cardiopulmonary pathologic processes was noted in the remaining 477 films. Most of these (65%) showed no change from the previous CXR. Of the 89 new findings noted in all the films, only 3 required immediate action (2 pneumothoraces and 1 large pleural effusion).

Conclusion.—In this broad cross section of surgical patients admitted to the surgical ICU, routine daily CXRs revealed few new findings regarding either medical device placement or cardiopulmonary pathologic processes. Clinical necessity should determine the directive for a morning CXR. Total charges accrued during the 1-month study for routine CXRs and radiologic interpretation were $54,125. Thus, a more selective approach to this type of monitoring could significantly reduce health-care expenditures and free staff for other duties.

▶ Economic constraints are a major incentive to get the doctor back to the bedside to examine the patient!—D.M. Rothenberg, M.D.

Monitoring Gastric Tonometry

Assessment of Splanchnic Oxygenation by Gastric Tonometry in Patients With Acute Circulatory Failure

Maynard N, Bihari D, Beale R, Smithies M, Baldock G, Mason R, McColl I
(Guy's Hosp, London; Lewisham Hosp, London)
JAMA 270:1203–1210, 1993   101-94-23-7

Introduction.—Up to 85% of deaths that occur in surgical intensive care units (ICUs) are associated with acute circulatory failure and progression to multiple-organ failure. The clinical condition resulting from these events is described as the sepsis syndrome or a state of nonbacterial clinical sepsis. Splanchnic ischemia may play a role in such cases, leading to a reduction in gut barrier function. The importance of splanchnic ischemia with acute circulatory failure was investigated by the use of gastric tonometry.

Methods.—Study subjects were 83 consecutive patients in 2 general ICUs in London. The patients had a mean age of 60.7 years and a mean 24-hour Acute Physiology and Chronic Health Evaluation (APACHE) II

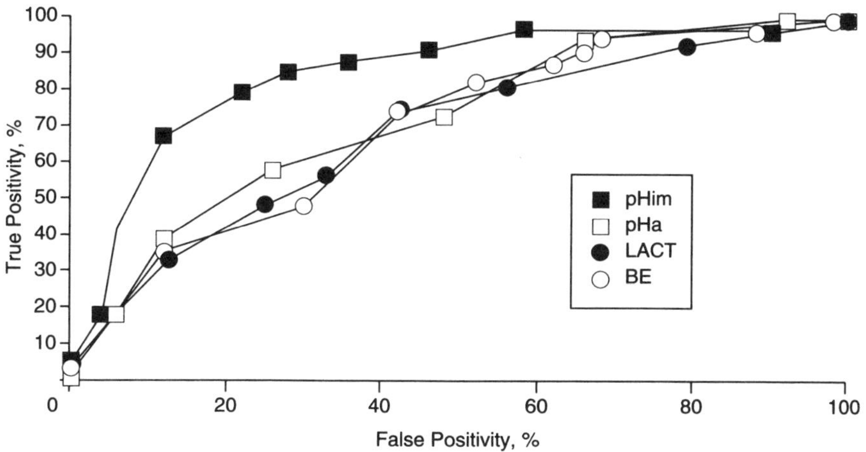

Fig 23–5.—*Abbreviations: pHim,* intramucosal pH; *pHa,* arterial pH; *LACT,* mixed venous lactate concentration; *BE,* standard base excess. Receiver operating characteristic curves for intramucosal pH and metabolic parameters. (Courtesy of Maynard N, Bihari D, Beale R, et al: *JAMA* 270:1203–1210, 1993.)

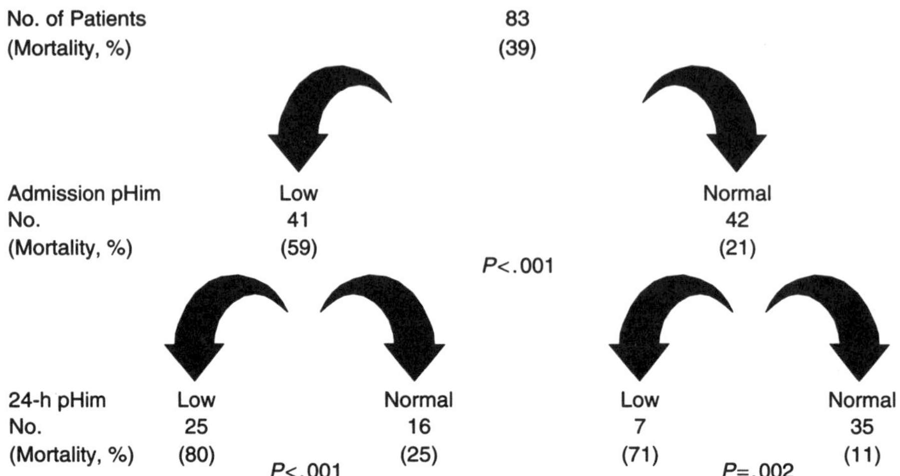

Fig 23–6.—Mortality according to intramucosal pH (*pHim*) on admission and at 24 hours. (Courtesy of Maynard N, Bihari D, Beale R, et al: *JAMA* 270:1203–1210, 1993.)

score of 20.3 All had acute circulatory failure in the first 24 hours after admission to the ICU and were receiving mechanical ventilation at the time of the study. Gastric intramucosal pH and hemodynamics, oxygen transport, and metabolic variables were measured at admission and at 12 and 24 hours after admission.

Results.—The ICU mortality rate of the patients studied was 39.7%; the hospital mortality rate was 41%. The receiver operating characteristic curve for intramucosal pH and metabolic parameters is shown in Figure 23-5. Compared with survivors, nonsurvivors had a significantly higher heart rate and a significantly lower mean arterial pressure. Survivors and nonsurvivors had no consistent differences in cardiac index, oxygen delivery, and oxygen uptake. The mean gastric intramucosal pH was 7.4 on admission and at 24 hours in survivors; corresponding findings for nonsurvivors—7.28 and 7.24, respectively—differed significantly from that of survivors (Fig 23-6). Admission arterial pH was significantly lower in nonsurvivors, base excess was more negative, and lactate concentration was higher. Of the variables studied, gastric intramucosal pH had a very high sensitivity (88%) for the prediction of an ICU death. The likelihood ratio for gastric intramucosal pH was 2.32, higher than any other variable.

Conclusion.—Gastric intramucosal pH as measured by tonometry was the most reliable indicator of adequacy of tissue oxygenation in these patients. Inadequate oxygenation of the gut is associated with a poor outcome, and attempts to improve splanchnic blood flow and gastric intramucosal pH may help to increase survival in patients with multiple-organ failure.

▶ This article adds to the growing literature supporting the use of gastric intraluminal pH (pHi) as a sensitive indicator of gastrointestinal hypoperfusion. If a dysfunctional gastrointestinal tract may predispose to bacterial translocation and the development of a sepsis syndrome and multiple-organ failure, this parameter may be an early indicator of such changes. Utilizing these data by directing therapy to improve pHi may be more useful than the more commonly used parameters of oxygen delivery.—D.M. Rothenberg, M.D.

Comparison of Clinical Information Gained From Routine Blood-Gas Analysis and From Gastric Tonometry for Intramural pH
Boyd O, Mackay CJ, Lamb G, Bland JM, Grounds RM, Bennett ED (St George's Hosp, London)
Lancet 341:142–146, 1993   101-94-23-8

Introduction.—Measurements of gastric intramucosal pH (pH_i) can yield valuable clinical information in a wide range of patients who are critically ill. One study reported that the mortality rate was lower among patients monitored and treated for decreases in pH_i than among patients monitored for blood pressure and urine output. Whether information gained from the measurement of pH_i could be obtained from other measurements of metabolic acidosis was investigated.

Methods.—The study group consisted of 20 consecutive patients admitted to an intensive care unit. Collection of measurement sets was started as soon as correct placement of a pulmonary artery catheter and tonometer was confirmed by radiography. A mean of 8 data sets per patient was obtained. Variables examined were arterial pH, partial pressure of oxygen, partial pressure of carbon dioxide (pCO_2), oxygen saturation, tonometer balloon fluid pCO_2, arterial pressures, and cardiac output. Results were used to calculate bicarbonate concentration, base deficit or excess in blood and extracellular fluid, and pH_i. Relationships between the variables and pH_i were assessed by within-subject comparisons.

Results.—The markers of metabolic acidosis—base deficit in blood and extracellular fluid and bicarbonate concentration—were significantly correlated with pH_i (Fig 23–7). Taking a pH_i less than 7.32 as a clinically important lower limit of the normal range, the lower limits of normal ranges for other variables can be calculated from the regression equations when pH_i is 7.32. A blood base deficit of -4.65 or less and an extracellular fluid base deficit of -6.13 or less could estimate pH_i below 7.32 with a sensitivity of at least 77% and a specificity of at least 96%.

Conclusion.—Gastric tonometry is more expensive and time-consuming than routine blood gas analysis. Information obtained by gastric to-

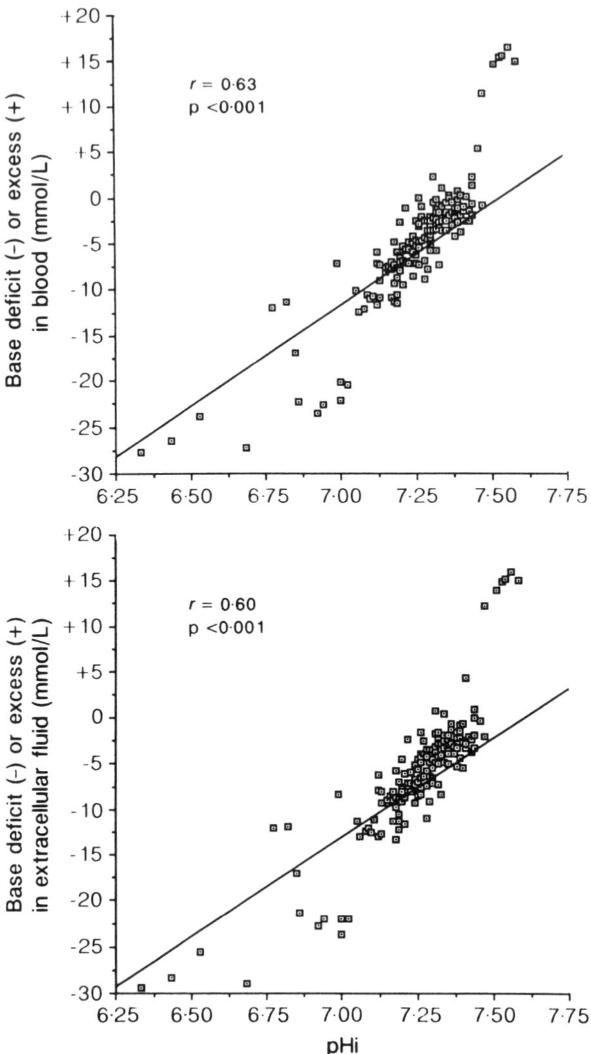

Fig 23–7.—Scatter grams and within-subject correlations of blood and extracellular base deficits/excesses with pH$_i$. (Courtesy of Boyd O, Mackay CJ, Lamb G, et al: *Lancet* 341:142–146, 1993.)

nometry for measurement of pH$_i$ can be calculated from routine analysis of base deficit in blood or extracellular fluid.

▶ It seems only fair to report that others have not found pHi to be any better an indicator of critical illness than a routine arterial blood gas analysis. As exciting as this field of monitoring is, I would not discard arterial lines and pulmonary artery catheters just yet!—D.M. Rothenberg, M.D.

Gastric Intramural pH as a Predictor of Success or Failure in Weaning Patients From Mechanical Ventilation

Mohsenifar Z, Hay A, Hay J, Lewis MI, Koerner SK (Univ of California, Los Angeles)

Ann Intern Med 119:794–798, 1993

101-94-23-9

Background.—Various criteria have been used in the past to predict the outcome of trials weaning patients from mechanical ventilation. Most have good sensitivity and negative predictive value (they predict successful extubation), but none reliably predict weaning failure. Recent evidence indicates that gastric intramural pH (pHi) predicts the risk for massive gastrointestinal bleeding, sepsis, and multiple-organ failure, along with prediction of outcome in patients who are critically ill. Whether gastric pHi can be used to predict the success of weaning was investigated.

Methods.—Twenty-nine patients receiving assisted mechanical ventilation for respiratory failure, and who were considered ready to be weaned, participated. Simultaneous samples of arterial blood and gastric juices were taken during assisted mechanical ventilation and during weaning trials. The predictor variable was calculated according to the following equation: $6.1 + \log$ bicarbonate/(gastric carbon dioxide pressure $[P_{CO_2}] \times .0307$). Patients were considered to be successfully weaned if they supported spontaneous ventilation for more than 24 hours after extubation.

Results.—The patients who could not be weaned had significantly reduced gastric pHi (7.36 during mechanical ventilation compared with 7.46 during weaning). Patients who were successfully weaned did not experience a change in pHi. Through discriminant analysis, gastric pHi during weaning was shown to be the best single predictor of weaning outcome. A diminution of pHi of more than .09 would have correctly

Threshold Values During Weaning to Predict Outcome

Variable	Weaning Successful ($n = 18$)	Weaning Failed ($n = 11$)
	n/n	
pHi >7.30 or a change of <0.09	18/18	0/11
Tidal volume ≥325 mL	18/18	9/11
Respiratory frequency ≤38	18/18	8/11
Negative inspiratory pressure ≤20 cm H$_2$O	18/18	10/11
Frequency/tidal volume ≤105	18/18	8/11

(Courtesy of Mohsenifar Z, Hay A, Hay J, et al: *Ann Intern Med* 119:794–798, 1993.)

classified 9 of 11 unsuccessful cases, and all 18 successful cases. The next best prediction was an increase in gastric PCO_2 of 10 mm Hg or more (table). The following prediction rule was 100% successful: If the initial gastric pH is less than 7.3, or if it decreases by .09 or more during the weaning attempt, classify the patient as a potential failure.

Conclusion.—Clearly, patients who fail to be weaned experience a significant decrease in gastric pHi within 20–30 minutes. Patients who are successfully extubated, on the other hand, have no change in pHi. Apparently, commonly used weaning indices, such as respiratory rate, tidal volume, maximum negative inspiratory pressure, and the ratio of frequency to tidal volume, may not be as good predictors of weaning failure as gastric tonometry.

▶ This paper nicely demonstrated the potential utility of gastric pHi outside of the realm of multiorgan failure. In this study, pHi was calculated using gastric juice CO_2 obtained from a standard nasogastric tube. This was done to avoid a prolonged equilibration phase as is necessary with a gastric tonometer. The predictive value of this measurement appears to be related to blood being diverted from the splanchnic bed to the respiratory muscles, thus signifying an inability to increase oxygen delivery. Larger studies verifying this finding may prove this technique to be a simple and accurate method of avoiding premature extubation.—D.M. Rothenberg, M.D.

Blood Conservation

Evaluation of a New Blood-Conserving Arterial Line System for Patients in Intensive Care Units
Silver MJ, Jubran H, Stein S, McSweeney T, Jubran F (Cleveland Clinic Found, Ohio; Ohio State Univ Hosp, Columbus)
Crit Care Med 21:507–511, 1993   101-94-23–10

Background.—Conventional arterial line systems require considerable initial blood samples to "flush out" resident heparin. A new blood-conserving arterial line system was evaluated and compared with the conventional system.

Methods.—Paired blood samples were taken from both conventional arterial line systems and the new blood-conserving model. Hematocrit and partial thromboplastin time measurements were obtained, and the samples were compared for the presence of hemodilution or heparin contamination

Results.—A Bland-Altman bias analysis of the 2 blood drawing methods indicated that a randomly determined partial thromboplastin time obtained from the blood-conserving arterial line would lie between 3.32 and −5.11 of the partial thromboplastin time taken from the conventional line. A randomly determined hemotocrit value taken from the new model would lie between 1.97 and −1.85 of that of the conventional line.

Conclusion.—The blood-conserving arterial line exhibits no hemodilution or heparin contamination and does not require the initial discharge of large samples of blood. It provides a welcome means of conserving blood in intensive care.

A Clinical Evaluation of a Blood Conservation Device in Medical Intensive Care Unit Patients

Peruzzi WT, Parker MA, Lichtenthal PR, Cochran-Zull C, Toth B, Blake M (Northwestern Univ Med School, Chicago; Northwestern Mem Hosp, Chicago)
Crit Care Med 21:501–506, 1993   101-94-23-11

Purpose.—Blood conservation in critically ill patients is of utmost concern for all health-care personnel. The efficacy of a blood conservation device used in critically ill patients, the effect of blood conservation on hemoglobin concentration and the need for blood transfusions, whether the blood conservation device led to interference with artificial pressure waveforms, and whether use of this device would result in fewer accidental needle punctures experienced by health-care personnel were examined.

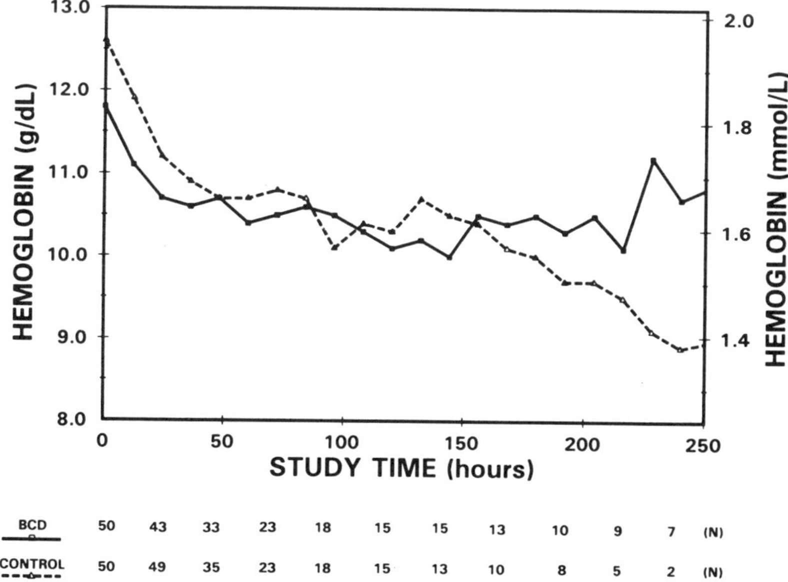

Fig 23–8.—*Abbreviation:* BCD, blood conservation device. Mean hemoglobin concentration of the control vs. the blood conservation group at 12-hour intervals during the study. Differences became statistically significant at 228 hours. (Courtesy of Peruzzi WT, Parker MA, Lichtenthal PR, et al: *Crit Care Med* 21:501–506, 1993.)

Patients and Methods.—A total of 100 consecutive patients admitted to the medical intensive care unit (ICU) were included in this prospective study. All patients required arterial line monitoring for clinical purposes, and they were randomly assigned to either an experimental or a control group. The 50 patients in the experimental group had a blood conservation device incorporated into the arterial pressure monitoring system. The remaining 50 patients (the controls) were monitored by a standard system only. Demographic and clinical traits did not significantly differ between groups.

Results.—Patients in the experimental group had a significantly lower blood volume drawn and discarded from the arterial catheters than did those in the control group. In addition, the total volume of discarded blood was significantly less for patients in the experimental group. On admission, average hemoglobin concentrations were comparable between groups. Concentration levels declined most rapidly during the first 24 hours of admission for both groups and declined more slowly thereafter. In the blood conservation group, the mean hemoglobin concentration was higher after 6 days. However, statistical significance was not reached until 9.5 days after admission (Fig 23–8).

The overall mean change in hemoglobin concentration was 1.2 g/dL during the study, a statistically significant decrease of 9.7%. Concentration levels decreased by 1.4 ± 2.2 g/dL and 1 ± 2.3 g/dL in the control and experimental groups, respectively. Blood volume was a significant and independent predictor of reductions in hemoglobin concentrations. Both groups had similar transfusion requirements. Pressure waveforms were not altered or disrupted by the blood conservation device. Finally, no accidental needle injuries were noted.

Conclusion.—The blood conservation device eliminated a significant factor in the decline of hemoglobin concentrations. With such devices available, the practice of wasting the blood of critically ill patients to prevent preanalytic error should be discontinued.

▶ These articles (Abstracts 101-94-23–10 and 101-94-23–11) reviewed the efficacy of 2 different blood-conservation devices, neither of which interferes with pressure recording, accuracy of hemocrit measurement, or coagulation function. Justifying the use of such devices lies in the elimination of excessive blood discard, as well as in minimizing exposure of health-care workers to blood. Preliminary data here suggest that the use of heterologous blood transfusions may be minimized, and for these reasons, I find these devices to be extremely useful for patients in whom multiple blood sampling is expected. These are now routinely used in our ICU and also in the operating room for such cases as liver transplantation. These devices are ideal in caring for the Jehovah's Witness patient as a method to further minimize blood loss. Finally, these devices would be an initial step in blood conservation at a time when utilization of microchemical analyzers is not yet standard (1).—D.M. Rothenberg, M.D.

Reference

1. Chernow B, et al: *Crit Care Med* 19:313, 1991.

Extrapulmonary Gas Exchange

The Intravascular Oxygenator (IVOX): Preliminary Results of a New Means of Performing Extrapulmonary Gas Exchange

Gentilello LM, Jurkovich GJ, Gubler KD, Anardi DM, Heiskell R (Univ of Washington, Seattle)
J Trauma 35:399–404, 1993

101-94-23-12

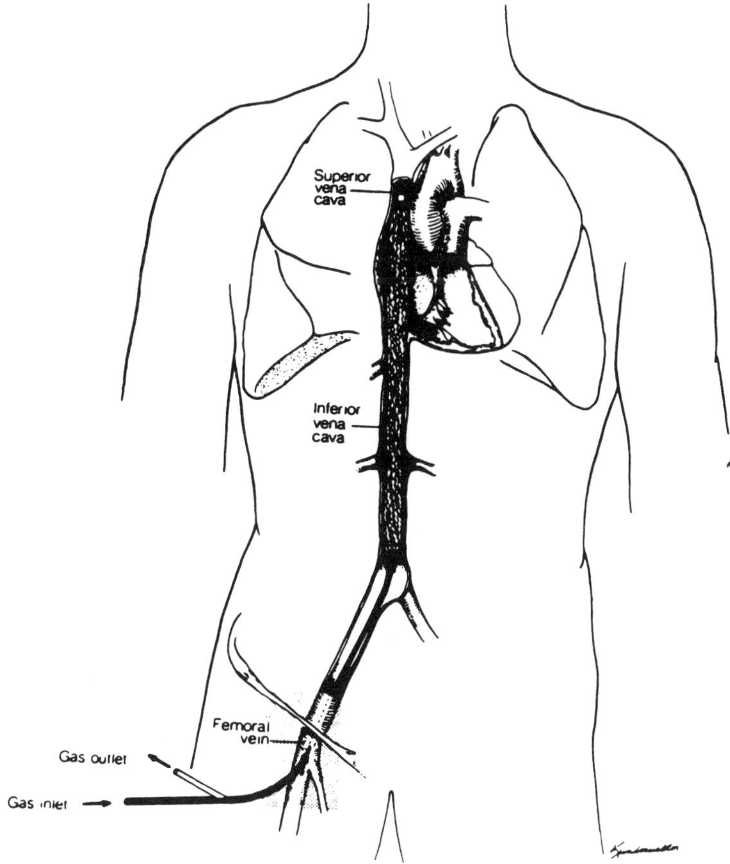

Fig 23–9.—Schematic depiction of the IVOX device. (Courtesy of Gentilello LM, Jurkovich GJ, Gubler KD, et al: *J Trauma* 35:399–404, 1993.)

Background.—Current therapy for adult respiratory distress syndrome (ARDS) with high-minute ventilation, positive end-expiratory pressure, and increased fractional inspired oxygen concentrations is thought to cause increased damage to the lungs. The intravascular oxygenator (IVOX) is a new, temporary, implantable membrane oxygenator designed to transfer gas intravenously. As a pulmonary assist device, it has been reported to transfer enough oxygen and carbon dioxide to justify a clinical trial. Whether IVOX could reduce the level of mechanical ventilatory support in patients with ARDS was determined.

Methods.—The IVOX was inserted in 9 patients who met the diagnostic criteria for ARDS. The device consists of several hundred gas-permeable hollow fibers that are inserted into the vena cava by femoral venous cutdown (Fig 23–9). The flow of gas through the fibers adds oxygen and removes carbon dioxide from the bloodstream. The mean duration of IVOX use was 5.6 ± 4.4 days. Measurements were taken 6, 24, and 48 hours after gas transfer initiation.

Results.—The mean intraoperative blood loss during insertion was 433 ± 240 mL. On average it took 103 ± 23 minutes to insert the device. Of 10 patients, 9 successfully received the IVOX; 1 patient went into cardiac arrest through excessive blood loss. A significant decrease in arterial carbon dioxide pressure (PCO_2) was seen on initiation of gas transfer, but there was little improvement in the alveolar oxygen pressure (PaO_2) or in the arterial oxygen pressure (PaO_2) to fractional concentration of oxygen in inspired gas ratio. Insertion of the IVOX also brought a 35% decrease in the oxygen delivery index (649 ± 155 vs. 422 ± 111 mL O_2/min/m²). Throughout the 48-hour trial period, the oxygen delivery index remained below preinsertion levels, despite efforts to maximize intravascular volume, inotropic support, and hemoglobin levels. Only 2 of the 10 initial patients survived, yet the autopsies revealed no evidence of IVOX-related pathologic damage to the lungs, right heart chamber, valves, or vena cava.

Conclusion.—Past research has revealed that patients with ARDS are more likely to die of sepsis syndrome with multiple-organ failure than lung injury. Therefore, it is unlikely that new supportive therapies, such as IVOX, will greatly influence mortality, particularly if they carry a high complication rate. The decrease in cardiac index and oxygen delivery seen here implies that venous return was impaired, despite vigorous fluid administration. Moreover, none of the ventilator variables measured during minute ventilation (positive end-expiratory pressure and increased fractional inspired oxygen) were significantly reduced by insertion of the device. Further advances in membrane technology are required to improve the gas transfer efficiency of this device and to reduce the adverse effects it has on cardiac output and oxygen delivery.

Clinical Trials of an Intravenous Oxygenator in Patients With Adult Respiratory Distress Syndrome

High KM, Snider MT, Richard R, Russell GB, Stene JK, Campbell DB, Aufiero TX, Thieme GA (Pennsylvania State Univ, Hershey)
Anesthesiology 77:856–863, 1992   101-94-23–13

Background.—Conventional mechanical ventilation may fail to ensure adequate gas exchange in patients with severe adult respiratory distress syndrome (ARDS). Extracorporeal membrane oxygenation may enhance

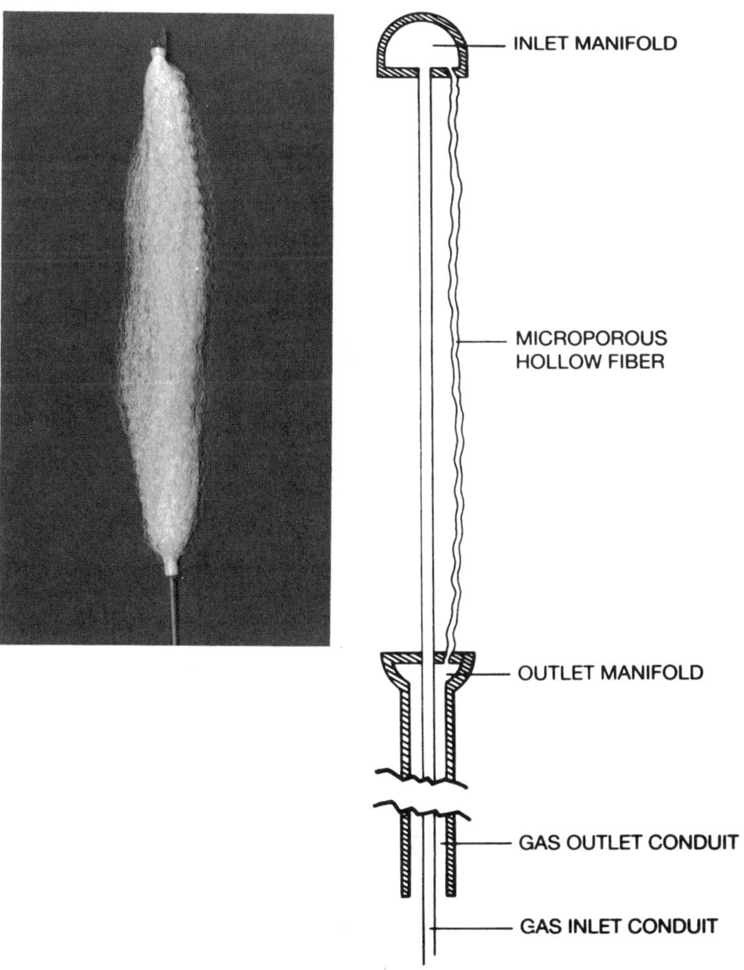

Fig 23–10.—The intravenous oxygenator **(left)** and a schematic diagram **(right).** To clarify gas flow pathways, the schematic diagram shows a single microporous fiber, inlet and outlet manifold, and inlet and outlet conduits. The schematic diagram is not drawn to scale. (Courtesy of High KM, Snider MT, Richard R, et al: *Anesthesiology* 77:856–863, 1992.)

survival, but varying results have been reported, and the approach is costly and labor-intensive. An alternative approach is to use an intravenous oxygenator (IVOX) to provide supplemental transfer of oxygen and carbon dioxide (CO_2), thereby reducing oxygen toxicity and the risk of barotrauma.

Patients and Methods.—Five patients with severe ARDS resulting from aspiration, fat embolism, or pneumonia were treated with an IVOX. The patients underwent tracheal intubation and were sedated and chemically paralyzed. In all cases, the arterial oxygen pressure was less than 60 mm Hg with an inspired oxygen fraction of 1 and a positive end-expiratory pressure of at least 5 cm water.

The IVOX is a cigar-shaped bundle of hollow microporous polypropylene fibers coated with silicone (Fig 23–10). Devices 7–10 mm in diameter, with surface areas of .2–.5 m², are available. An introducer is available to insert the IVOX into the common femoral vein. The furled device is passed into the inferior vena cava and advanced until its tip is in the lower part of the superior vena cava. The IVOX was used for periods of 2 hours to 4 days.

Results.—The extent of gas exchange ranged from 21 to 87 mL/min of CO_2 and from 28 to 85 mL/min of oxygen. The IVOX fulfilled as much as 28% of the requirements for metabolic gas exchange. One patient with a small vena cava had signs of caval obstruction. Three patients had signs of sepsis after insertion of the IVOX. One of the 5 patients survived and was discharged, but the IVOX did not appear to have a significant role in this outcome. Two device removals and 3 autopsies failed to show evidence of acute thromboembolism.

Discussion.—Theoretically, the IVOX can limit the need for mechanical ventilation in patients with severe ARDS. At present, this approach is considered only when the intrapulmonary shunt fraction is less than 35% but greater than 25%; when an inspired oxygen fraction of at least .8 and a positive end-expiratory pressure of 15 cm water or more are needed; when blood cultures are negative for at least 48 hours; and when the common femoral vein and inferior vena cava are large enough to accommodate a size 9 or size 10 IVOX.

▶ In an effort to develop a device that would temporarily relieve the lungs of the constant pressure injury induced by mechanical ventilation and high positive end-expiratory pressures—as well as to improve CO_2 exchange and oxygen delivery—the IVOX failed miserably in these preliminary studies (Abstracts 101-94-23-12 and 101-94-23-13). In its present state, this device appears more cumbersome and potentially more deleterious than adult extracorporeal membrane oxygenation.—D.M. Rothenberg, M.D.

Intensive Care Unit Sedation/Paralysis

Propofol vs Midazolam in Short-, Medium-, and Long-Term Sedation of Critically Ill Patients: A Cost-Benefit Analysis

Carrasco G, Molina R, Costa J, Soler J-M, Cabré L (SCIAS-Hosp de Barcelona)

Chest 103:557–564, 1993   101-94-23–14

Introduction.—Propofol and midazolam are both used for providing continuous sedation in mechanically ventilated critically ill patients in the intensive care unit (ICU). Whereas propofol is much more expensive than midazolam, its use reduces the time needed for recovery of spontaneous respiration. The safety, clinical efficacy, and economic cost of propofol and midazolam were compared when the agents were used to sedate critically ill patients.

Patients.—Eighty-eight patients were entered in the study. Of 46 patients randomized to propofol sedation, 20 were continuously sedated for less than 24 hours, 16 were sedated for 24 hours to 7 days, and 10 were sedated for more than 7 days. Of 42 patients randomized to midazolam, 20 were sedated for less than 24 hours, 12 were sedated for 24 hours to 7 days, and 10 were sedated for more than 7 days. Hours of sedation at the desired level, extubation, and total recuperation times were tabulated for short-term, medium-term, and long-term sedation with either drug, and the costs for each drug were then calculated and compared.

Results.—The mean percentages of hours of adequate sedation were 93% in the propofol group and 82% in the midazolam group. The difference was statistically significant. Recovery after interruption of sedation was significantly faster in propofol-treated patients than in midazolam-treated patients. The correlation between time of propofol administration, time required until extubation, and total recovery was highly significant for short-, medium-, and long-term users. In contrast, neither time required until extubation nor time to total recovery could be predicted when midazolam was used for sedation. The cost of long-term sedation with propofol was 4 times higher than that of long-term sedation with midazolam, but the cost of postsedation care after midazolam was almost 3 times that after propofol. The total long-term sedation cost for propofol was slightly higher than that for midazolam, but the difference did not reach statistical significance.

Conclusion.—In critically ill patients undergoing mechanical ventilation in the ICU, propofol for continuous sedation is as safe as, and clinically more effective than, midazolam. Furthermore, propofol provides a more favorable cost-benefit ratio than does midazolam.

▶ In United States dollars, short-term sedation with propofol saved only $18 per patient. What is more interesting is that patients receiving propofol for more than 7 days were extubated within 48 minutes and discharged to a step-down unit or general ward 108 minutes after discontinuing the drug! This compares with more than 36 *hours* and 54 *hours,* respectively, for midazolam. Given the inherent bias of this understandably unblinded study (I assume it would be difficult to blind the observers from propofol), I would await similar results before accepting these findings as evidence of a tangible cost-benefit ratio.—D.M. Rothenberg, M.D.

Prolonged Administration of Isoflurane to Pediatric Patients During Mechanical Ventilation

Arnold JH, Truog RD, Rice SA (Harvard Med School, Boston; Failure Analysis Associates Inc, Menlo Park, Calif; Stanford Univ, Calif)
Anesth Analg 76:520–526, 1993   101-94-23–15

Background.—Isoflurance is an attractive alternative to intravenously administered drugs for prolonged use during mechanical ventilation. It undergoes limited metabolism and has a relatively low blood-to-gas partition coefficient. The efficacy and toxicities of isoflurane sedation in mechanically ventilated children were examined in a prospective study.

Methods and Findings.—Ten patients, aged 3 weeks to 19 years, were given continuous isoflurane sedation for a mean of 131 minimum alveolar concentration (MAC) hours. All patients were receiving mechanical ventilation and needed large doses of opioids for sedation. The mean peak inorganic fluoride (F−) concentration was 11 μM. The highest F− concentration was 26.1 μM after 441 MAC hours. The F− concentration exceeded 20 μM in only 1 patient. There were no abnormalities in the serum creatinine level or osmolality. Data on creatinine clearance were available for 5 patients receiving a mean 193 MAC hours of sedation. Only 1 patient had a persistent reduction from baseline of more than 20%. Five patients had an abstinence syndrome, consisting of unintentional movements and extreme agitation. All of these children had been given 70 MAC hours or more of isoflurane.

Conclusion.—Isoflurane can be used to sedate mechanically ventilated children for prolonged periods without harming cardiovascular, hepatic, or renal function. Prolonged administration of isoflurane to adults has been reported to significantly increase inorganic fluoride levels.

▶ Prolonged ventilation with anesthetic agents is not new, having been tried many years ago with nitrous oxide, for example. In that trial, effects of nitrous oxide not previously known were soon discovered, including a foul-up of the folic acid system that is so important in blood synthesis. This is why it is a little scary to me to be advocating long-term anesthesia with a drug like isoflurane. Nonetheless, there is always a risk-benefit ratio, and perhaps the alternatives are not as good.—J.H. Tinker, M.D.

Ventilation Management

Prediction of Minimal Pressure Support During Weaning From Mechanical Ventilation

Nathan SD, Ishaaya AM, Koerner SK, Belman MJ (Cedars-Sinai Med Ctr, Los Angeles)
Chest 103:1215–1219, 1993   101-94-23–16

Background.—Pressure support (PS) ventilation, often used to aid weaning from mechanical ventilation, permits a stepwise reduction in ventilatory support and a gradually increasing ventilatory load on the patient. Some investigators have proposed that low levels of PS ventilation can simulate spontaneous breathing, with the PS from the ventilator barely overcoming the resistance of the endotracheal tube and ventilator circuit.

Objective and Methods.—The ability of minimal PS to simulate spontaneous breathing was studied in 7 patients with a mean age of 71 years who had been intubated for a mean of 7½ days and were considered to be weanable by their primary physicians. Minimal PS was calculated as the product of the peak spontaneous inspiratory flow rate and the total airway resistance. The work of breathing was calculated after the patient breathed for 2 minutes at minimal PS or at minimal PS ± 25%.

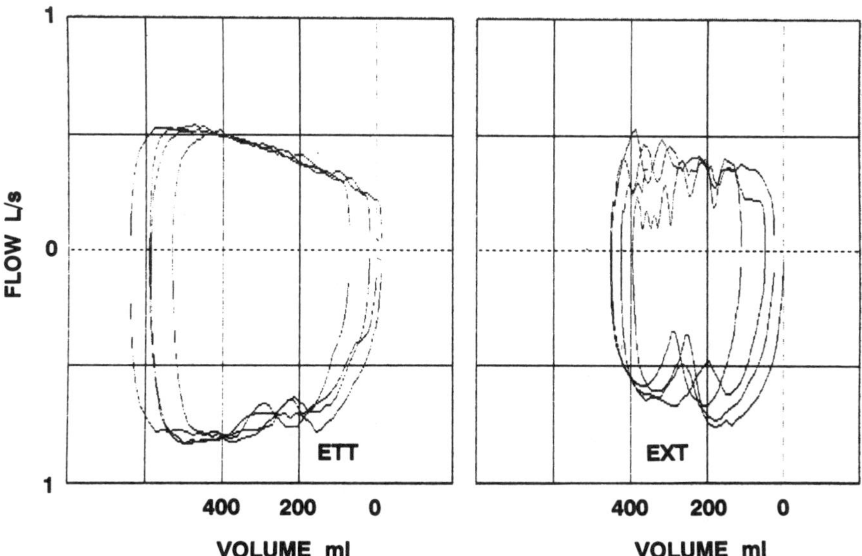

Fig 23–11.—Tidal flow volume loop of patient while breathing with the endotracheal tube (*ETT*) in position and immediately postextubation (*EXT*). Inspiration is below baseline and expiration is above. (Courtesy of Nathan SD, Ishaaya AM, Koerner SK, et al: *Chest* 103:1215–1219, 1993.)

Results.—The mean minimal PS was 7 cm of water, with a range of 4–10 cm of water. The work of breathing increased as the level of pressure support declined. Progressively increasing work of breathing was noted during flow by ventilation and during continuous positive airway pressure ventilation. The change in tidal flow volume after extubation is illustrated in Figure 23–11.

Discussion.—The increased work of breathing associated with decreased PS probably reflects altered airway resistance. The patients were intubated for about a week on average, which was more than enough time for the upper airway to be damaged. Upper airway dysfunction may go unrecognized when inspiratory stridor is not obvious.

▶ The use of PS during mechanical ventilation is an effective method for minimizing the work of breathing. This study attempted to quantify the minimal amount of PS required to overcome system resistance. Whether these calculations are any more effective than bedside observation of the patient after PS application is unanswered by this study, but I suspect it is no different. Finally, the most remarkable finding noted in this study is the degree of silent, postextubation upper airway obstruction. These data should heighten one's awareness in suspecting upper airway obstruction as a cause of acute respiratory failure after extubation.—D.M. Rothenberg, M.D.

Decreasing Imposed Work of the Breathing Apparatus to Zero Using Pressure-Support Ventilation

Banner MJ, Kirby RR, Blanch PB, Layon AJ (Univ of Florida, Gainesville; Shands Hosp, Gainesville, Fla)
Crit Care Med 21:1333–1338, 1993   101-94-23–17

Objective.—Pressure-support ventilation was applied to patients receiving mechanical ventilatory support in an attempt to lower the imposed work of breathing to zero. Eleven adult patients and 4 children with acute respiratory failure from various causes participated in the prospective study. The patients were intubated and were studied while breathing spontaneously and when receiving continuous positive airway pressure ventilation and pressure-support ventilation.

Methods.—The imposed work of the breathing apparatus (the endotracheal tube, breathing circuit tubing, and demand-flow system) was estimated by integrating the pressure measured at the tracheal end of the endotracheal tube from a narrow air-filled catheter and the change in volume from a pneumotachographic flow sensor located between the endotracheal tube and the Y-piece of the breathing circuit (Fig 23–12). The pressure and volume signals were directed to a computerized, portable respiratory monitor that provided a real-time display of the pressure-volume (work) loops. Pressure-support ventilation was applied incrementally until imposed work declined to zero.

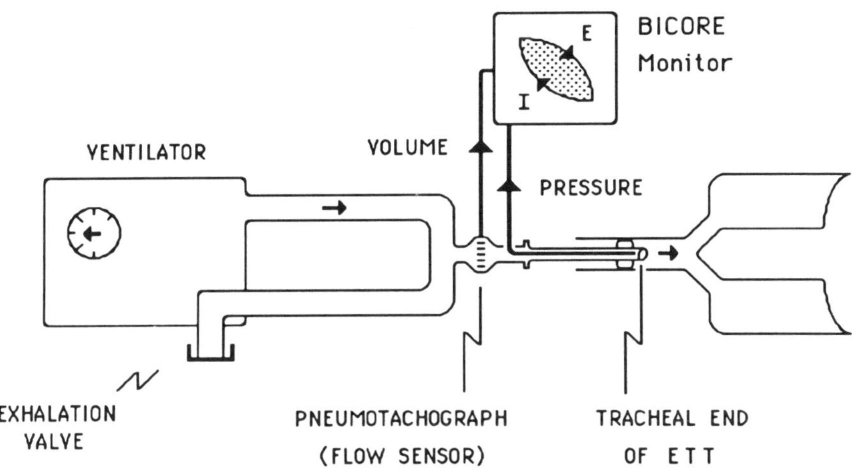

Fig 23–12.—Imposed work of breathing apparatus during spontaneous breathing is determined by measuring pressure with a narrow catheter at the tracheal or carinal end of endotracheal tube (P_{ETT}) and change in volume (dV) with a miniature pneumotachograph positioned between the "Y" piece of ventilatory breathing circuit and the endotracheal tube. Both P_{ETT} and dV are directed to a portable, computerized, bedside monitor (CP-100, Biocore Monitoring Systems) and are integrated to display a pressure-volume (work) loop and calculate imposed work, i.e., the area circumscribed within the loop during inhalation (I) and exhalation (E). (Courtesy of Banner MJ, Kirby RR, Blanch PB, et al: *Crit Care Med* 21:1333–1338, 1993.)

Observations.—Imposed work decreased quadratically when incremental levels of pressure-support ventilation were applied. The imposed mean work was .6 J/L at baseline, without pressure-support ventilation, and decreased to zero at a mean pressure-support ventilation level of 13.5 cm of water.

Discussion.—This is a practical way of measuring imposed work by using a portable bedside monitor. All patients with respiratory failure whose pulmonary mechanics are compromised and who are intubated but breathing spontaneously should receive at least a minimal level of pressure-support ventilation to reduce the work of breathing imposed by the breathing apparatus.

▶ This study nicely described the use of a portable bedside respiratory monitor useful in measuring the work of breathing by real-time assessment of pressure-volume (work) loops. Pressure support was thus accurately instituted to minimize the work of breathing.—D.M. Rothenberg, M.D.

Could the Oxygen Cost of Breathing Be Used to Optimize the Application of Pressure Support Ventilation?

Shikora SA, MacDonald GF, Bistrian BR, Kenney PR, Benotti PN (Harvard Med School, Boston)
J Trauma 33:521–527, 1992

101-94-23–18

Background.—Current techniques for mechanical ventilation have improved outcome in critically ill or injured patients with respiratory failure. However, some of these patients will remain dependent on the ventilator after recovery. A new ventilator modality, pressure support ventilation (PSV), augments spontaneous inspiratory pressure with selected levels of positive airway pressure. Whether bedside measurements of the oxygen cost of breathing (OCOB) would be useful for titrating the optimal level of pressure support was determined.

Methods.—The OCOB, a clinically applicable technique for quantitating the work of breathing, has been shown to be an accurate tool for predicting the potential for weaning a patient from mechanical ventilation. The OCOB is the calculated difference in oxygen consumption between total ventilator support and spontaneous respiration. Nine studies were performed in 8 patients who were ventilator dependent for longer than 12 days because of an inability to sustain respiratory work. The OCOB and other bedside variables of pulmonary function were measured at various levels of PSV.

Oxygen Cost of Breathing, Tidal Volume (Estimated and Actual), and Respiratory Rate After the Application of Pressure Support

Patient Number	$V_{T_{est}}$ (mL)	$OCOB_{cpap}$ (%$\Delta_v\dot{V}O_2$)	$OCOB_{psv}$ (%$\Delta\dot{V}O_2$)	RR (bpm)	$V_{T_{meas}}$ (mL)	PSV (cm H_2O)
1	600–900	30	15	14	800	20
2*	800–1200	24	13	15	760	25
3*	800–1200	42	8	10	800	20
4	900–1350	17	11	15	800	30
5	700–1050	19	2	8	1200	25
6	900–1350	15	9	10	1200	20
7	700–1050	19	7	11	1050	25
8	900–1350	14	−8	11	900	25
9	700–1050	21	13	10	1200	25
Mean ± SD		22 ± 9†	8 ± 7†	12 ± 3	968 ± 194	

Abbreviations: $V_{T_{est}}$, estimated tidal volume; $V_{T_{meas}}$, measured tidal volume; *RR*, respiratory rate.

* Two studies performed on the same patient.

† $P < .001$.

(Courtesy of Shikora SA, MacDonald GF, Bistrian BR, et al: *J Trauma* 33:521–527, 1992.)

Results.—Patients had a mean age of 66 years; all had undergone major surgery. With increasing levels of PSV, the OCOB decreased steadily from 22% to 8% (table). The tidal volume improved with increases in pressure, a statistically significant relationship seen in every study. At the maximum PSV, no patient had a tidal volume less than 700 mL. The respiratory rate decreased significantly and consistently with increasing pressure support. Minute ventilation appeared to be less influenced by PSV. Patients were observed to be more comfortable with PSV than with continuous positive airway pressure.

Conclusion.—Pressure support ventilation delivers a predetermined, regulated amount of positive pressure with each patient-triggered breath. Bedside measurement of OCOB may be a simple and accurate tool for titrating the level of applied pressure support to optimize respiratory work.

▶ This study estimated the work of breathing indirectly by measuring the oxygen cost of breathing via a metabolic cart. Although consistent improvement in respiratory parameters was noted, this technique appears to be somewhat cumbersome. What needs to be determined from the 3 previous studies (101-94-23–16 through 101-94-23–18) is the optimal work of breathing, i.e., where respiratory muscles exercise without fatigue.—D.M. Rothenberg, M.D.

Verbal Communication of Ventilator-Dependent Patients

Manzano JL, Lubillo S, Henríquez D, Martín JC, Pérez MC, Wilson, DJ (Hosp Nuestra Señora del Pino, Las Palmas de Gran Canaria, Canary Islands, Spain)
Crit Care Med 21:512–517, 1993   101-94-23–19

Introduction.—The cuffed tracheostomy speaking tube allows patients receiving mechanical ventilation to speak, but the results have not been satisfactory regarding phonation and communication. The usefulness, advantages, and disadvantages of the Passy-Muir tracheostomy speaking valve were evaluated in a prospective study.

Procedure.—The Passy-Muir unidirectional valve allows air to flow into the lungs during inspiration but closes during expiration to force the expired air to pass around the tracheostomy tube to the glottis, mouth, and nose, allowing the patient to speak. The valve is placed between the tracheostomy tube and the Y-shaped piece of the ventilator's circuit. The following procedures are performed before attaching the Passy-Muir valve to the ventilator-dependent patients: (1) suctioning of tracheal and pharyngeal secretions, (2) deflation of the tracheostomy tube cuff, (3) increasing the tidal volume of the ventilator to maintain the inspiratory pressure before the cuff's deflation, and (4) setting the peak inspiratory pressure alarm and disconnecting the expiratory volume alarm.

Patients.—The efficacy of the valve was evaluated in 10 chronic ventilator-dependent patients who had undergone tracheostomy. All patients had the ability to eliminate tracheobronchial secretions to maintain a patent and unobstructed airway, had adequate gas exchange while ventilated with a fraction of inspired oxygen of $\leq$ .4 (partial pressure of oxygen in the alveoli > 60 torr [8 kPa], arterial blood partial pressure of carbon dioxide < 55 torr [7.3 kPa]), had normal hemodynamics without the need for administration of vasodepressors, and had a normal mental state. Eight patients had pulmonary disease and 2 had neuromuscular disease.

Outcome.—The Passy-Muir tracheostomy speaking tube improved communication in 8 patients, allowing pronounciation of complete sentences with an adequate and intelligible tone during the entire respiratory cycle. Other advantages of the tracheostomy speaking valve were decreased tracheobronchial secretions, improved cough effectiveness, reestablishment of the sense of smell, and considerable improvement in well-being. In all patients, tidal volume was increased > 50% to maintain the previous peak inflation pressure; other cardiorespiratory variables did not change significantly. The use of the tracheostomy speaking valve was impossible in 2 patients: one with severe pulmonary disease in whom cuff deflation prevented adequate ventilation and the other with neuromuscular disease and laryngopharyngeal dysfunction.

Conclusion.—The use of the Passy-Muir tracheostomy speaking tube during mechanical ventilation facilitates patients' verbal communication, allowing a sense of independence and dignity for their care. It is safe and effective for patients with normal upper airway function, but it is extremely important to remember to deflate the tracheostomy tube cuff to avoid severe hyperinflation, barotrauma, and possibly death. In view of these problems, a cuffless tracheostomy tube, which decreases the resistance to the exhaled flow around the tracheostomy tube toward the larynx and avoids the high expiratory pressure that may be generated during coughing, may be used.

► Provided that care is afforded in placing this device, this unidirectional valve may offer a patient a measure of restored dignity in what is often a dehumanizing situation.—D.M. Rothenberg, M.D.

Mechanical Ventilation for the Elderly Patient in Intensive Care: Incremental Charges and Benefits

Cohen IL, Lambrinos J, Fein IA (Albany Med College, NY; Union College, Schenectady, NY)
JAMA 269:1025–1029, 1993   101-94-23–20

Background.—There are concerns regarding the use of critical care resources in individuals who will derive little or no benefit, as measured by cost-effectiveness analysis. Prolonged mechanical ventilation in patients aged 80 years and older may indicate an unfavorable outcome and may be an important variable in assessing the "appropriateness" of intensive care unit resource use.

Study Design.—In a retrospective fashion, all patients in an intensive care unit, aged 80 years and older who required mechanical ventilation for 3 days or more between April of 1985 and October of 1987 in a single, tertiary-care teaching community-hospital were studied. Of the 59 candidates, 45 had complete billing records. For cost-effectiveness analysis, incremental hospital charges from hospital billing records were related to years of life saved. Hospital survivors were followed up for at least 4 years after discharge by means of a telephone survey.

Results.—Ten patients survived the hospitalization; 2 were alive and 1 could not be located at follow-up. Using 1985–1987 dollars, the estimated charge per year of life saved ranged from $51,854 to $75,090. A simple index of age and duration of mechanical ventilation was used to identify a subgroup of patients whose mortality rate approached 100%. Twenty-two patients whose age in years plus duration of mechanical ventilation in days totaled 100 or greater were identified, and only 2 survived hospitalization. For this subgroup of patients, the cost per year of life saved was $181,308. Neither of these patients was alive at follow-up: 1 died 2 months after hospital discharge and the other was discharged to a nursing home and died 4.5 years later.

Conclusion.—In elderly patients who require prolonged mechanical ventilation, each additional year of life is associated with very high charges among those whose sum of age and days of mechanical ventilation is 100 or greater. The cost-effectiveness of prolonged mechanical ventilation in this subgroup is poor. Incremental cost or charge analysis may prove valuable in both clinical and administrative decision-making processes.

▶ This study used age and days of mechanical ventilation to derive a medical and economic "futility" index. Although this work is noteworthy, it was a relatively small, retrospective study and should, therefore, not be applied as a predictive index to any individual patient.—D.M. Rothenberg, M.D.

Infection Therapy

Impact of Previous Antimicrobial Therapy on the Etiology and Outcome of Ventilator-Associated Pneumonia
Rello J, Ausina V, Ricart M, Castella J, Prats G (Universitat Autonoma de Barcelona)
Chest 104:1230–1235, 1993   101-94-23–21

Introduction.—Nosocomial pneumonia is the leading cause of death from nosocomial infection; at particular risk are intubated patients receiving mechanical ventilation. Because ventilator-associated pneumonia (VAP) has a high rate of morbidity and mortality, prophylactic antibiotics have been recommended for intubated patients. The influence of prior antibiotic use on the etiology and mortality of VAP was investigated in a prospective study.

Methods.—Eligible patients were all those in whom pneumonia developed in the study institution's intensive care unit during a 35-month period. Pneumonia was considered to be ventilator associated when its onset occurred after 48 hours of mechanical ventilation. All antimicrobials administered for more than 48 hours during the 10 days preceding the episode of VAP were recorded.

Results.—Of the 150 episodes of nosocomial pneumonia identified in the intensive care unit, 129 met the criteria of VAP. Antibiotics were used for more than 48 hours preceding the onset of VAP in 54 episodes. The mean age of the patients with VAP was 49.5 years. One third (34.1%) of the patients died. Of the 18 patients whose death was directly related to the pulmonary infection, 9 had *Pseudomonas aeruginosa* isolated from culture specimens. Patients who had received prior antimicrobial therapy had a higher mortality rate (27.7%) than patients who did not receive this therapy (4%). Logistic regression analysis identified prior antibiotic use as the only variable significantly influencing the risk of death from VAP. When the etiologic agent was included in the regression equation, however, prior antibiotic use was replaced as a significant risk factor by high-risk pathogens.

Conclusion.—A clear and strong relationship between the use of antibiotics prior to the onset of VAP and the etiologic agent was shown. Thus, the increased mortality associated with prior antibiotic use is caused by the selection of more lethal organisms, such as *P. aeruginosa*. The prognosis was benign when VAP was caused by gram-positive cocci or by *Haemophilus influenzae*. A restrictive antibiotic policy for mechanically ventilated patients to reduce deaths from VAP is suggested.

Ventilator-Associated Pneumonia: A Multivariate Analysis
Kollef MH (Washington Univ, St Louis, Mo)
JAMA 270:1965–1970, 1993   101-94-23–22

Introduction.—Pneumonia is the major cause of death from nosocomial infection. A number of preventive measures have been studied in recent years. A prospective study was designed to identify factors contributing to ventilator-associated pneumonia (VAP) so that effective ways can be found to reduce its frequency.

Study Design.—Data were collected from 277 consecutive patients who required mechanical ventilation for longer than 24 hours. Seventy-five patients were cared for in a medical intensive care unit, 100 in a surgical intensive care unit, and 102 in a cardiothoracic unit. Ventilator-associated pneumonia was defined as a new, persisting infiltrate accompanied by a pleural or blood culture positive for the same organism as the

TABLE 1.—Variables Independently Associated With Intensive Care Unit Mortality by Univariate Analysis

Variable	Nonsurvivors (n=36)	Survivors (n=241)	OR	P
OSFI				
≥3	30 (83.3)	45 (18.7)	21.78	<.001
<3	6 (16.7)	196 (81.3)		
Renal failure				
Yes	26 (72.2)	53 (22.0)	9.22	<.001
No	10 (27.8)	188 (78.0)		
Dialysis				
Yes	10 (27.8)	10 (4.2)	8.88	<.001
No	26 (72.2)	231 (95.8)		
VAP				
Yes	16 (44.4)	27 (10.4)	6.34	<.001
No	20 (55.6)	214 (89.6)		
APS				
≥10	25 (69.4)	65 (26.9)	6.15	<.001
<10	11 (30.6)	176 (73.1)		
Chemical paralysis				
Yes	7 (19.4)	10 (4.2)	5.58	<.001
No	29 (80.6)	231 (95.8)		
APACHE II				
≥15	29 (80.6)	106 (44.0)	5.28	<.001
<15	7 (19.4)	135 (56.0)		
Head elevated				
No	16 (44.4)	37 (15.0)	4.41	<.001
Yes	20 (55.6)	204 (85.0)		
Bilirubin >34.2 μmol/L (2 mg/dL)				
Yes	7 (19.4)	13 (5.4)	4.23	.002
No	29 (80.6)	228 (94.6)		
Duration of MV, d				
≥5	24 (66.7)	88 (36.5)	3.48	.001
<5	12 (33.3)	153 (63.5)		
Lifestyle score				
≥2	20 (55.6)	69 (28.6)	3.12	.001
<2	16 (44.4)	172 (71.4)		
Iatrogenic event				
Yes	13 (36.1)	40 (16.6)	2.84	.005
No	23 (63.9)	201 (83.4)		
IABP				
Yes	6 (16.7)	16 (6.6)	2.81	.038
No	30 (83.3)	225 (93.4)		
Albumin, units				
<3	17 (47.2)	62 (28.8)	2.53	.009
≥3	19 (52.8)	153 (71.2)		
Nutritional support				
Yes	25 (69.4)	114 (47.3)	2.53	.013
No	11 (30.6)	127 (52.7)		
Use of H_2 antagonists				
Yes	24 (68.6)	121 (50.2)	2.16	.042
No	11 (31.4)	120 (49.8)		

(continued)

Table 1 *(continued)*

Emergency surgery				
Yes	11 (30.6)	41 (17.0)	2.15	.052
No	25 (69.4)	200 (83.0)		
Underlying malignancy				
Yes	13 (36.1)	51 (21.2)	2.11	.047
No	23 (63.9)	190 (78.8)		
Immunosuppression				
Yes	17 (47.2)	74 (30.7)	2.02	.049
No	19 (52.8)	167 (69.3)		

Abbreviations: ICU, intensive care unit; *APS,* acute physiology score; *OSFI,* organ system failure index; *MV,* mechanical ventilation; H_2, histamine type 2 receptor; *APACHE,* Acute Physiology and Chronic Health Evaluation; *IABP,* intra-aortic balloon pump; *OR,* odds ratio.
(Courtesy of Kollef MH: *JAMA* 270:1965–1970, 1993.)

tracheal aspirate; cavitation; histologic evidence of pneumonia; or new-onset fever and leukocytosis accompanied by a purulent tracheal aspirate.

Data Analysis.—Both univariate and multivariate analyses were performed on a wide range of variables, including life-style, preadmission status, immunosuppression, malignant disease, and the acute physiology score. In addition, process of care variables were examined, including previous mechanical ventilation, antibiotic treatment, head positioning, and nutritional support. Antiulcer medication, the organ system failure index, and the serum bilirubin value were also taken into account.

Findings.—Ventilator-associated pneumonia developed in 43 patients, 15.5% of the total. The results are summarized in Tables 1 and 2. On stepwise logistic regression analysis, factors independently associated with VAP included an age of 60 years or older, an elevated organ system failure index, previous antibiotic treatment, and supine head positioning early in the course of ventilation. Ventilator-associated pneumonia was more frequent in the cardiothoracic intensive care unit than in the medical unit. The mortality rate was 37% in patients with VAP and 8.5% in the other patients.

TABLE 2.—Variables Independently Associated With
Mortality by Logistic Regression Analysis

Variable	Adjusted OR	95% CI	*P*
OSFI ≥3	16.1	6.1-42.0	<.001
Lifestyle score ≥2	3.1	1.3-7.3	.012
Head not elevated	3.1	1.2-7.8	.016

Abbreviations: OR, odds ratio; *CI,* confidence interval; *OSFI,* organ system failure index.
(Courtesy of Kollef MH: *JAMA* 270:1965–1970, 1993.)

Discussion.—Different intensive care unit populations may be at varying risk for the development of VAP. It is to be hoped that studies such as this one will suggest effective interventions.

Selective Decontamination of the Digestive Tract in Neurosurgical Intensive Care Unit Patients: A Double-Blind, Randomized, Placebo-Controlled Study

Korinek AM, Laisne MJ, Nicolas MH, Raskine L, Deroin V, Sanson-Lepors MJ (Pitié-Salpétrière Hosp, Paris; Lariboisière Hosp, Paris)
Crit Care Med 21:1466–1473, 1993   101-94-23–23

Introduction.—Lower airway infection may occur in more than half of all ventilated neurosurgery patients. Parenteral antibiotic prophylaxis may not prevent bronchopulmonary infection caused by *Staphylococcus aureus* in head-injured patients. There is evidence that selective decontamination of the digestive tract may prevent nosocomial infection in victims of trauma.

Objective.—The efficacy of digestive decontamination was examined in a double-blind, randomized trial in comatose neurosurgery patients who remained in a neurosurgical intensive care unit (ICU) for longer than 5 days and were intubated within 24 hours of admission.

Treatment.—Treated patients received a suspension of 100 mg of polymyxin E, 80 mg of tobramycin, and 500 mg of amphotericin B, instilled 4 times a day through the nasogastric tube. In addition, a carboxymethylcellulose paste containing the same antibiotics in 2% concentra-

Morbidity and Mortality

	SDD (n = 63)		Placebo (n = 60)		*p* Value
No. of infected patients	29	(46 %)	49	(81.6 %)	<.001
No. of infectious episodes	36		71[a]		<.01
Bronchopneumonia	15		25		<.04
Urinary tract infections	12		24		<.01
Sinusitis	2		9		<.02
Bacteremia	2		6		NS
Meningitis/ventriculitis	5		5		NS
Other	0		2		NS
ICU mortality	3		7		NS
Hospital mortality	5		4		NS

Abbreviation: SDD, selective digestive decontamination.
[a] Several patients had more than 1 infection.
(Courtesy of Korinek AM, Laisne MJ, Nicolas MH, et al: *Crit Care Med* 21:1466–1473, 1993.)

tion plus 4% vancomycin was applied to the oral cavity. Control patients received 2 placebo treatments. The study lasted 15 days.

Results.—Evaluable data were obtained from 63 antibiotic-treated patients and 60 placebo recipients. Associated therapies were similar in the 2 groups and both were fed parenterally. The baseline colonization rates were identical, but decontamination significantly reduced colonization of the oropharynx, trachea, and stomach from day 3 to day 12. Bronchopulmonary infection was less frequent in antibiotic-treated patients (table), particularly in trauma victims. Three treated patients and 7 placebo patients died during the study period, all of neurologic deterioration; the difference was not significant.

Costs.—Nearly twice as much was spent on parenteral antibiotics to treat acquired infection in the placebo group. The cost of antimicrobials for treated patients who had infection was nearly threefold greater than that for infected placebo patients.

Discussion.—Selective digestive decontamination nearly halved the infection rate in these comatose neurosurgery patients. Nosocomial infections were significantly less frequent in treated patients. Effective decontamination of the trachea appears to be related to the occurrence of bronchopneumonia.

▶ Prior antibiotic therapy influences the development and outcome of VAP by selecting more virulent pathogens, and by potentially inhibiting additional antibiotic therapy by creating drug-resistant organisms. Although studies utilizing selective decontamination, such as the one presented here (Abstract 101-94-23–23), suggest a lower incidence of VAP, outcome is no different. This may imply that selective decontamination merely prevents less virulent forms of pneumonia (e.g., pseudomonas). Although I assume the debate about selective decontamination will continue, it is clear from these 2 independent studies (Abstracts 101-94-23–21 and 101-94-23–22) that the risk of VAP can at least be minimized by simply avoiding inappropriate antibiotic prophylaxis and by elevating the head of the bed.—D.M. Rothenberg, M.D.

Plasma Cytokine and Endotoxin Levels Correlate With Survival in Patients With the Sepsis Syndrome

Casey LC, Balk RA, Bone RC (Rush-Presbyterian-St Luke's Med Ctr, Chicago)
Ann Intern Med 119:771–778, 1993   101-94-23–24

Background.—The mortality rate from sepsis syndrome remains as high as 60% despite modern antibiotics and supportive measures. It is now recognized that lipopolysaccharide is not directly responsible for the sequelae of sepsis. Instead, it stimulates the production and release of a number of endogenous mediators that themselves produce pathophysiologic changes and sepsis-related death. Identified mediators of

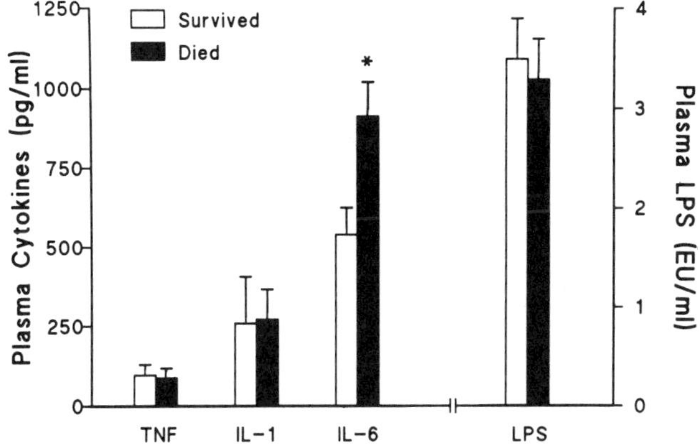

Fig 23–13.—Plasma TNF-α, IL-1β, IL-6, and lipopolysaccharide (*LPS*) levels in patients with sepsis syndrome who survived or died. Plasma IL-6 level was elevated in patients who died (*P* < .01). (Courtesy of Casey LC, Balk RA, Bone RC: *Ann Intern Med* 119:771–778, 1993.)

sepsis include tumor necrosis factor-alpha (TNF-α), interleukin-1β (IL-1β), and IL-6.

Objective.—The relationship between plasma levels of these mediators and lipopolysaccharide and the outcome of sepsis syndrome was examined in 97 patients. Twenty critically ill but nonseptic patients and 20 healthy persons were also studied.

Criteria.—Sepsis syndrome was diagnosed from a temperature above 38.3°C (or below 35.5°C); tachycardia exceeding 90 beats/min; tachy-

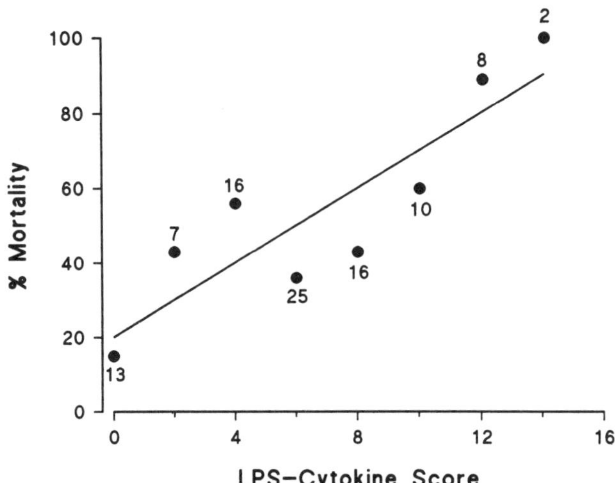

Fig 23–14.—Relation between lipopolysaccharide (*LPS*)-cytokine score and mortality from sepsis syndrome. A unit increase in the LPS-cytokine score was associated with a 5% increase in mortality (*P* < .001) *Numbers under points* represent number of patients with that score. (Courtesy of Casey LC, Balk RA, Bone RC: *Ann Intern Med* 119:771–778, 1993.)

pnea of more than 20 breaths/min; a clinical suspicion of infection; and at least 1 of the following: the presence of hypoxemia, oliguria, unexplained metabolic acidosis, or a recent change in mental status.

Findings.—Tumor necrosis factor-alpha was detected in 54% of the patients with sepsis syndrome (median level, 26 pg/mL); IL-1 was detected in 37% (median level, 20 pg/mL); and IL-6 was detected in 80% (median level, 415 pg/mL). Lipopolysaccharide was present in 89% of this group (median level, 2.6 endotoxin units/mL). All values were higher in septic patients than in the critically ill control patients or healthy subjects. Levels of all mediators were independent of the patient's culture status. Levels of IL-6 were 69% higher in patients who died than in survivors (Fig 23–13). When scores for individual mediator levels and lipopolysaccharide were summed to form a total lipopolysaccharide-cytokine score, mortality increased with the score (Fig 23–14).

Discussion.—Patients with sepsis often had detectable plasma levels of TNF-α and IL-1 and IL-6. Combinations of cytokines with lipopolysaccharide may, even at low levels, be as significant a risk factor as a large increase in any individual factor. Levels of IL-6 correlated most closely with mortality in this study.

Serum Cytokine Levels in Human Septic Shock: Relation to Multiple-System Organ Failure and Mortality
Pinsky MR, Vincent J-L, Deviere J, Alegre M, Kahn RJ, Dupont E (Univ of Pittsburgh, Pa; Free Univ of Brussels, Belgium)
Chest 103:565–575, 1993
101-94-23–25

Introduction.—Despite aggressive therapy, patients with septic shock have a high rate of mortality. The development of multiple-system organ failure (MSOF) appears to contribute to many of these deaths. A common pathogenic link between the initial insult and MSOF in septic shock may be cytokine-related systemic intravascular inflammation. It was hypothesized that levels of inflammatory cytokines, such as tumor necrosis factor (TNF) and interleukin-6 (IL-6), would be elevated in patients with septic shock and predictive of poor outcome.

Methods.—During a 6-month period, 53 episodes of shock (35 septic and 18 nonseptic) were recorded in 52 patients in an intensive care unit. Serum levels of TNF, IL-1, IL-2, IL-6, and interferon-γ were measured serially for the first 48 hours after the onset of hypotension thought to be caused by sepsis in all patients seen in the intensive care unit. Serum cytokine levels were subsequently correlated with clinical status, organ system function, and survival.

Results.—Septic patients, compared with nonseptic patients, had higher mortality rates (41% vs. 17%), an increased likelihood of development of MSOF (29% vs. 6%), and a greater incidence of cirrhosis (21% vs. 0%). During the study period, patients with septic shock had higher

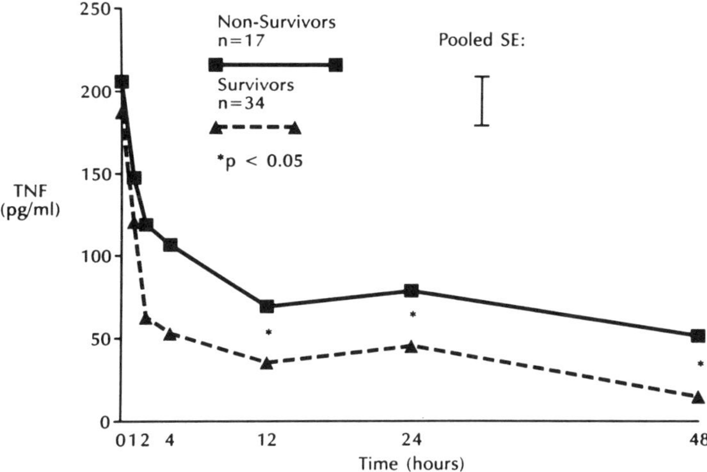

Fig 23–15.—Mean serum TNF levels in survivors and nonsurvivors of shock over time. Note persistent elevation of TNF levels at 12, 24, and 48 hours in nonsurvivors. (Courtesy of Pinsky MR, Vincent J-L, Deviere J, et al: *Chest* 103:565–575, 1993.)

levels of TNF, but there was no relationship between peak TNF level and outcome (Fig 23–15). Cirrhotic patients were more likely than non-cirrhotic patients to acquire MSOF and die (67% vs. 30%). The TNF and IL-6 levels in patients who had MSOF or who died were both elevated and did not decrease with time, whether or not the patient had sepsis (Fig 23–16). No elevations in IL-1, IL-2, or interferon-γ were noted.

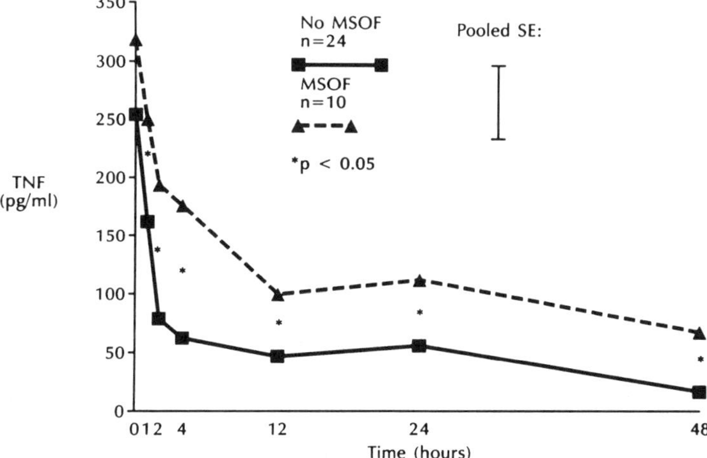

Fig 23–16.—Mean TNF levels in patients with septic shock with subsequent or no MSOF. Note the persistent elevation in TNF levels in patients with septic shock and MSOF. (Courtesy of Pinsky MR, Vincent J-L, Deviere J, et al: *Chest* 103:565–575, 1993.)

Conclusion.—Serum levels of both TNF and IL-6 are higher in septic than in nonseptic shock. The persistence of these cytokines, however, rather than peak levels, predicts poor outcome in patients with shock. This finding suggests a relationship between processes that maintain elevated serum TNF levels and remote organ dysfunction in critically ill patients.

▶ The value of measuring circulatory cytokines may be to identify which patients with the sepsis syndrome would benefit from specific monoclonal antibody therapy. If these studies (Abstracts 101-94-23–24 and 101-94-23–25) are to have routine clinical applicability, standardized assays that yield rapid results will be necessary to direct anticytokine therapy early in the course of sepsis.—D.M. Rothenberg, M.D.

Renal Function

Predictability of Creatinine Clearance Estimates in Critically Ill Patients
Robert S, Zarowitz BJ, Peterson EL, Dumler F (Université Laval, Quebec, Canada; Henry Ford Hosp, Detroit)
Crit Care Med 21:1487–1495, 1993   101-94-23–26

Background.—Accurate measurements of renal function are desirable in critically ill patients to determine the appropriate dosages of medications whose elimination depends on renal function. However, most measurements provide reasonable clinical indication of renal function in the general medical population, but not in critically ill persons. A prospective study in a medical intensive care unit was conducted to evaluate the predictive ability of different creatinine clearance methods as compared with the criterion standard, inulin clearance, and to determine which predictive method yields the most accurate estimation of creatinine clearance.

Methods.—The glomerular filtration rate was measured by the inulin clearance using a standard protocol in 20 critically ill patients in the intensive care unit. The results were compared with 30-minute creatinine clearance, 24-hour creatinine clearance, and creatinine clearance estimates by the Cockcroft-Gault equation. In the Cockcroft-Gault equations, 6 different estimates of creatinine clearance were computed using the patient's ideal body weight, total body weight, or lean body mass with the actual serum creatinine level or a serum creatinine level corrected to 1 mg/dL when the actual value was less than 1 mg/dL. A seventh estimate in the Cockcroft-Gault equation used the lower of ideal body weight or total body weight.

Results.—Linear regression analysis showed a strong correlation between the inulin clearance and the Cockcroft-Gault equation using ideal body weight and corrected serum creatinine level. There was also a good correlation between inulin clearance and the Cockcroft-Gault equation using ideal body weight and the corrected serum creatinine level, as well as between inulin clearance and the Cockcroft-Gault equation using the lower of ideal or total body weight and the higher of the actual or corrected serum creatinine level. The 30-minute and the 24-hour creatinine clearances had poorer agreement with inulin clearance. The Cockcroft-Gault equation using the actual serum creatinine level also performed poorly. Better predictions and higher correlations were achieved when the corrected serum creatinine value was incorporated into the Cockcroft-Gault equation.

Conclusion.—The Cockcroft-Gault equation provides a more accurate prediction of the glomerular filtration rate in the critically ill patient than do urine creatinine clearance measures. The lower of ideal or total body weight should be used, along with the higher of actual serum creatinine or corrected serum creatinine concentration to 1 mg/dL.

▶ Most anesthesiologists probably assess a patient's degree of renal impairment by noting whether the serum creatinine value falls between the laboratories' "asterisks." Estimating creatinine clearance via the Cockcroft-Gault equation, however, points out how often perioperative renal insufficiency is underestimated. Utilizing this simple formula can provide more accurate information in guiding drug dosages and in assessing perioperative renal risk.—D.M. Rothenberg, M.D.

24 Pain and Its Management

Pain Mechanisms

Low Levels of Somatomedin C in Patients With the Fibromyalgia Syndrome: A Possible Link Between Sleep and Muscle Pain
Bennett RM, Clark SR, Campbell SM, Burckhardt CS (Oregon Health Sciences Univ, Portland)
Arthritis Rheum 35:1113–1116, 1992   101-94-24-1

Introduction.—Fibromyalgia is an increasingly recognized syndrome of diffuse musculoskeletal pain and fatigue in the absence of distinctive laboratory or tissue correlations. Fibromyalgia was initially seen as a form of psychogenic rheumatism, but consistent findings of tender areas in specific locations and not in others led to the development of guidelines for the diagnosis of fibromyalgia. Patients with fibromyalgia often have a distinctive stage 4 sleep disturbance characterized by alpha-wave intrusion into the normal delta rhythm. Because growth hormone is critical to muscle homeostasis and repair, the theory that this stage 4 sleep anomaly disrupts the secretion of growth hormone in fibromyalgia patients was investigated.

Methods.—Seventy female patients with fibromyalgia with a mean age of 47.6 years and 55 age-matched female controls with a mean age of 45.6 years participated in the study. Blood samples were obtained from each participant for the measurement of serum somatomedin C, a growth hormone–related peptide, using a peptide-specific radioimmunoassay.

Results.—The mean somatomedin C concentrations were 124.7 ng/mL in patients with fibromyalgia and 175.2 ng/mL in healthy controls. The difference was statistically highly significant. The mean somatomedin C concentration was 129.4 ng/mL in the 27 patients with fibromyalgia who were taking low-dose tricyclic antidepressants to improve sleep and 120.1 ng/mL in the remaining 43 patients who were not taking tricyclic antidepressants. The difference was statistically not significant. No significant correlation was found between somatomedin C levels and body weight, depression or anxiety scores, fatigue, impaired sleep, stiffness, pain, number of tender points, or total myalgic scores.

Discussion.—The low somatomedin C levels found in patients with fibromyalgia support the hypothesis that the stage 4 sleep anomaly present in approximately 60% of patients with the fibromyalgia syndrome disrupts the nocturnal secretion of growth hormone. A lack of regular exercise may be a contributing factor to low somatomedin C levels. The persistent disruption of growth hormone secretion may well predispose fibromyalgia patients to muscle microtrauma and may impair the normal healing of muscle microtrauma, or both.

▶ Fibromayalgia patients have often been labeled as having a psychosomatic or factitious disorder, because routine laboratory studies are often normal. As consistencies in the clinical presentation have become apparent, more physicians are convinced that fibromyalgia is a real clinical entity. Now some new studies are revealing differences in certain hormonal values among these patients. It is not clear whether the somatomedin C deficiencies in these patients is a cause or an effect. It would be of interest to determine whether levels are reduced in patients with other chronic pain syndromes who have associated sleep disruption.—S.E. Abram, M.D.

Alterations in Pain Threshold and Psychomotor Response Associated With Subanaesthetic Concentrations of Inhalation Anaesthetics in Humans
Tomi K, Mashimo T, Tashiro C, Yagi M, Pak M, Nishimura S, Nishimura M, Yoshiya I (Osaka Univ, Japan)
Br J Anaesth 70:684–686, 1993   101-94-24-2

Background.—Some anesthetic agents cause an increase in the pain threshold in subanesthetic concentrations. However, there has been no study of both analgesic and hypnotic actions of inhalation anesthetics. Six currently available inhalation anesthetics were assessed at subanesthetic levels.

Methods.—Six healthy men, aged 29–51 years, volunteered for the study. The effects of 6 agents at subanesthetic levels of .2 minimum alveolar concentration on pain threshold and psychomotor function were determined.

Findings.—Compared with 100% oxygen inhalation, nitrous oxide and methyoxyflurane significantly increased the pain threshold and prolonged the response time to auditory stimuli. By contrast, halothane, enflurane, isoflurane, and sevoflurane prolonged response time to auditory stimuli but did not affect pain perception. With nitrous oxide, the pain threshold remained significantly increased 30 minutes after the anesthetic was stopped, and the response time returned to preinhalation values.

Conclusion.—Nitrous oxide and methoxyflurane apparently possess both analgesic and hypnotic actions at subanesthetic concentrations, whereas halothane, enflurane, isoflurane, and sevoflurane apparently do not. The analgesic action of nitrous oxide persists after it is eliminated.

▶ This paper is included in the YEAR BOOK OF ANESTHESIOLOGY AND PAIN MANAGEMENT because it is an example of several recent studies of effects on psychomotor responses in patients who have residual subanesthetic concentrations of agents "on board." In the United States, over 40% of surgery is now being done on an outpatient basis. These kinds of studies are important as we send more and more patients home (or somewhere outside our hospitals) after general anesthesia.—J.H. Tinker, M.D.

Sex Differences in Responsiveness to Painful and Non-Painful Stimuli Are Dependent Upon the Stimulation Method

Lautenbacher S, Rollman GB (Univ of Western Ontario, London, Canada; Max Planck Inst for Psychiatry, Munich)
Pain 53:255–264, 1993   101-94-24-3

Background.—Although many advances have been made in stimulation techniques and psychophysical evaluation methods, the issue of gender difference in response to experimental pain has not been resolved. One assumption, found in a number of experimental studies of gender differences and deserving further investigation, is that the method of pain induction—thermal, electrical, or mechanical—is not particularly relevant. Previous study results have therefore been interpreted as being dependent on the pain dimension (threshold or tolerance, sensory or affective component) and on higher-order variables, including anxiety, sex role, and hormonal influences. Gender differences in thermocutane-

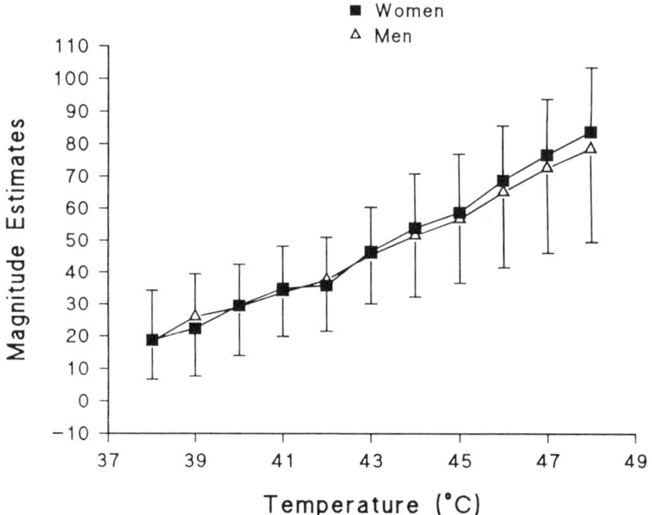

Fig 24–1.—Magnitude estimates of temperature stimuli applied to the forearm ranging from 39°C to 48°C in women and men; mean and 1 SD are given; $n = 14$ for women and $n = 20$ for men. (Courtesy of Lautenbacher S, Rollman GB: *Pain* 53:255–264, 1993.)

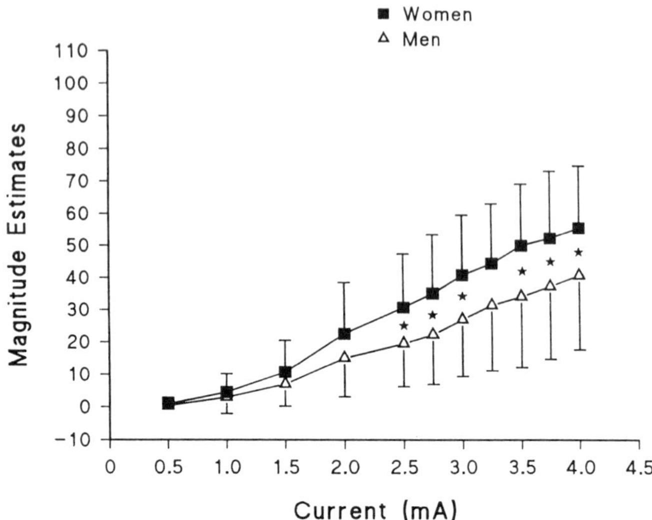

Fig 24–2.—Magnitude estimates of electrical stimuli applied to the hand ranging from .5 mA to 4 mA in women and men; mean and 1 SD are given; $n = 11$ for women and $n = 15$ for men. Significant sex differences at an intensity level are shown by *stars* (all $P < .05$). (Courtesy of Lautenbacher S, Rollman GB: *Pain* 53:255–264, 1993.)

ous and electrocutaneous responsiveness to both painful and nonpainful stimuli were studied.

Patients and Methods.—Forty participants, 20 men and 20 women, were included in the study. A Peltier thermode system was used to evaluate heat pain, warmth, and cold thresholds on the hand and foot. Participants, using magnitude estimation, also judged the sensation intensity elicited by temperatures ranging from 38°C to 48°C applied to the forearm. Detection, pain, and tolerance thresholds of electrocutaneous sensitivity were determined via electrical impulses applied to the hand. Magnitude estimates of sensation intensity were evaluated for stimuli of .5 mA to 4 mA (Figs 24–1 and 24–2).

Results.—No gender differences in heat pain, warmth, and cold sensations were noted. Significant gender differences were found in electrical detection and pain and tolerance thresholds, with lower thresholds observed in women. Magnitude estimates were comparable in both genders when using thermal stimuli. When electrical stimuli were used, women judged stimuli from 2.5 mA or more as more intense than did men. The measures for pain responsiveness from both methods were significantly correlated, in spite of these variances. Contrastingly, when the responsiveness to nonpainful stimuli was considered, no significant correlations between the 2 methods were observed.

Conclusion.—Gender differences in cutaneous responsiveness at nonpainful and painful levels depend on the stimulation method. Within a single physical dimension (e.g., electrical or thermal), stimulus parameters may have a strong effect on gender difference outcomes.

▶ The effects of differences in hormonal function on pain perception are of interest to many investigators. The high incidence of fibromyalgia in premenopausal women and the variation in pain with menses in some individuals attest to the importance of gender-associated differences in pain perception. This study illustrated some potential difficulties in investigating these differences.—S.E. Abram, M.D.

Role of Kinins in Pain and Hyperalgesia: Psychophysical Studies in a Patient With Kininogen Deficiency
Raja SN, Campbell JN, Meyer RA, Colman RW (Johns Hopkins Univ, Baltimore, Md; Temple Univ, Philadelphia)
Clin Sci 83:337–341, 1992   101-94-24-4

Introduction.—Bradykinin is considered to be an important mediator of pain and hyperalgesia associated with injury and inflammation. Psychophysical studies were conducted in a woman aged 79 years with complete kininogen deficiency to determine whether the absence of bradykinin affects pain sensibility. The patient had no apparent deficiencies in her capacity to detect or locate noxious stimuli.

Methods.—Sensitivity to heat stimuli was tested before and after localized burn to the thenar eminence. In addition, pain evoked by 3 intradermal injections of bradykinin, .1, 1, and 10 μg, into the forearm and the effects of bradykinin on pain induced by heat stimuli were studied. The intensity of pain evoked by all heat stimuli was rated relative to the pain induced by a 3-second 45°C stimulus.

Results.—The patient's heat pain threshold was 45°C for the glabrous skin, similar to that observed in 5 age-matched control subjects and to that previously observed in younger control subjects. As with normal subjects, burn injury resulted in a decrease in pain threshold and an increase in pain induced by suprathreshold stimuli. Intradermal injections of bradykinin produced pain and hyperalgesia to heat stimuli in control subjects, but in the patient, bradykinin injections induced minimal pain and no hyperalgesia to heat stimuli.

Conclusion.—Kinins are not essential for perception of noxious heat stimuli or for the development of hyperalgesia after heat injury. The absence of kininogens in the patient may be associated with a deficiency in bradykinin receptors.

▶ There seems to be some redundancy in our ability to experience hyperalgesia in response to tissue injury.—S.E. Abram, M.D.

Lack of Effect of Morphine-3-Glucuronide on the Spinal Antinociceptive Actions of Morphine in the Rat: An Electrophysiological Study

Hewett K, Dickenson AH, McQuay HJ (Univ College London; Univ of Oxford, England)
Pain 53:59–63, 1993
101-94-24-5

Background.—Morphine is metabolized by glucuronide conjugation to 2 major metabolites, morphine-3-glucuronide (M3G) and morphine-6-glucuronide (M6G). The latter has a relatively high affinity for the μ-opioid receptor and is substantially more potent than morphine. Although M3G has no affinity for the μ-opioid receptor and lacks analgesic activity in behavioral antinociceptive tests, intracerebroventricular and intraperitoneal M3G reportedly antagonize the antinociceptive effect of morphine in the rat tail flick test.

Objective and Methods.—The interaction of morphine with M3G was examined in halothane-anesthetized rats. The noxious C-fiber–evoked responses of convergent dorsal horn neurons and the innocuous A-beta-fiber responses were recorded extracellularly.

Results.—Intrathecally administered M3G by itself did not exhibit any antinociceptive effect. Pretreatment with M3G slightly reduced the antinociceptive effect of a 5-μg dose of morphine, but pretreatment with as much as 500 μg of M3G did not affect the action of a 50-μg dose of morphine.

Conclusion.—The metabolite M3G has, at most, a minor effect on the spinal antinociceptive action of morphine, and it is not likely to significantly antagonize the spinal antinociceptive effect of morphine in the clinical setting.

▶ This study suggests that under normal circumstances, M3G does not affect spinal analgesic effects of morphine. Perhaps when much higher morphine doses are administered, this metabolite may have significant effects, such as in the development of hyperalgesia after very-high–dose intrathecal morphine administration.—S.E. Abram, M.D.

T-Lymphocyte Subsets in Otherwise Healthy Patients With Herpes Zoster and Relationships to the Duration of Acute Herpetic Pain

Higa K, Noda B, Manabe H, Sato S, Dan K (Fukuoka Univ, Japan)
Pain 51:111–118, 1992
101-94-24-6

Background.—Subjects with impaired cell-mediated immunity have a higher incidence of herpes zoster (HZ). However, most HZ occurs in otherwise healthy patients. Serial changes in peripheral blood T-lymphocyte subsets were examined to determine whether these otherwise healthy patients have abnormalities in cell-mediated immunity.

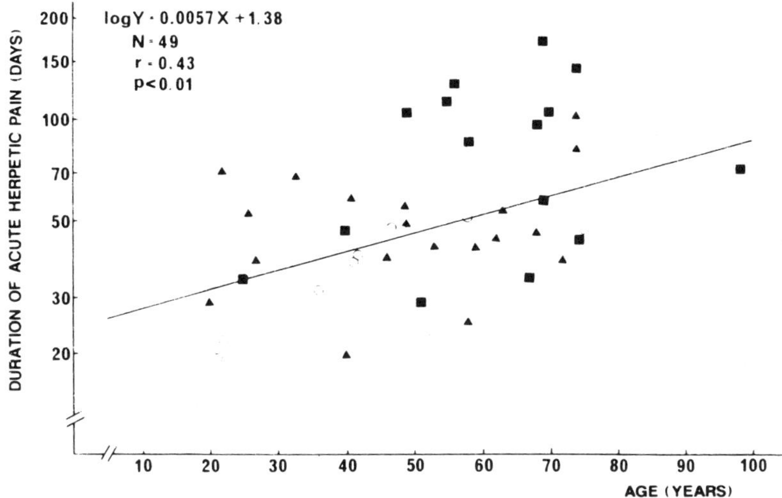

Fig 24–3.—Relationship between age and duration of AHP. All patients were treated with repeated SNBs. *Circles,* mild group; *triangles,* moderate group; *squares,* severe group, with all patients being represented. The mean ages of mild, moderate, and severe groups were 48.7, 49.3, and 61.5 years, respectively. These differences were not statistically significant. (Courtesy of Higa K, Noda B, Manabe H, et al: *Pain* 51:111–118, 1992.)

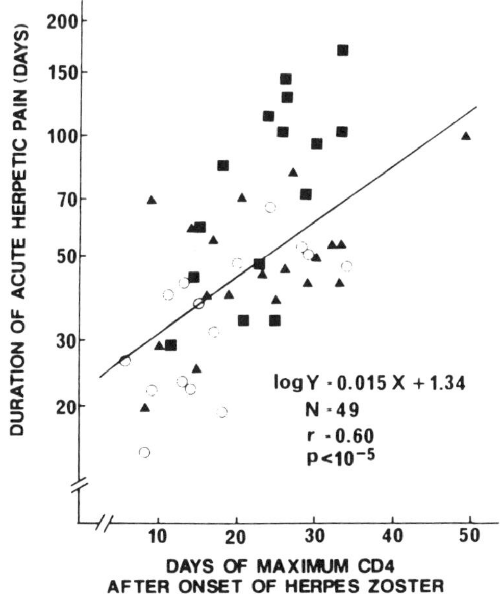

Fig 24–4.—Relationship between number of days on which percentage of CD4 lymphocytes showed maximum value after onset of HZ and duration of AHP. All patients were treated with repeated SNBs. *Circles,* mild group; *triangles,* moderate group; *squares,* severe group, with all patients being represented. (Courtesy of Higa K, Noda B, Manabe H, et al: *Pain* 51:111–118, 1992.)

Methods.—The subjects were 62 Japanese patients with a mean age of 52 years who had acute herpetic pain (AHP). In 22 the pain was mild, in 24 it was moderate, and in 16 it was severe. Treatment was with repeated sympathetic nerve blocks (SNBs) until pain was relieved. This was done in the hospital for those with severe AHP and on an outpatient basis for those with mild-to-moderate AHP. Thereafter, nerve blocks were performed 3 times a week. All patients underwent weekly measurement of T-lymphocyte subsets, beginning at their initial visit. Twenty normal controls were also studied.

Results.—There was no significant difference between patients and controls in the percentage of CD3 lymphocytes. The mild AHP group had significantly higher percentages of CD4 lymphocytes than controls in the first 3 weeks after the onset of HZ. These percentages were also higher than in the moderate and severe AHP groups, but not significantly so. The patient groups all had elevated percentages of CD8 lymphocytes, which decreased gradually with time. Patients had lower CD4/CD8 ratios than controls, with subsequent decreases resulting from increased percentages of CD8 lymphocytes rather than decreased percentages of CD4 lymphocytes. In 49 patients who had measurement of T lymphocytes on more than 2 occasions, a weak but significant positive linear correlation was found between age and duration of AHP (Fig 24–3). In addition, highly significant positive linear correlations were noted between number of days on which percentages of CD3 and CD4 lymphocytes and CD4/CD8 ratios reached minimum values after the onset of HZ and the duration of AHP (Fig 24–4).

Conclusion.—There are significant alterations in peripheral blood T-lymphocyte subsets after the onset of HZ, even in otherwise healthy patients. Cell-mediated immunity probably plays an important role in recovery from AHP.

► This study raises the issue of the possible role of immunotherapy in preventing herpes zoster in older patients with a history of varicella infection. With the probability that a vaccine will be available soon, perhaps immunization in exposed older individuals will raise numbers of T lymphocytes sufficiently to prevent the occurrence of shingles.—S.E. Abram, M.D.

Low Back Pain

Role of Psychosocial Risk Factors in Work-Related Low-Back Pain
Feyer A-M, Williamson A, Mandryk J, de Silva I, Healy S (Natl Inst of Occupational Health and Safety, Sydney, Australia)
Scand J Work Environ Health 18:368–375, 1992   101-94-24–7

Introduction.—Low back pain has been consistently associated with psychological factors. Both industrial and general population research has found a connection between job dissatisfaction and low back pain, although a cause-effect relationship has yet to be determined. The experience of low back pain and its psychosocial associates in blue-collar workers, white-collar workers, and a group of patients with chronic low back pain was examined.

Methods.—Both worker groups were considered to be at high risk for low back pain. The white-collar group included 257 members of the registered nursing staff at a large teaching hospital. Blue-collar workers were 256 mail sorters and postal carriers. Fifty-one patients attending a pain management clinic volunteered to participate. All participants were given a questionnaire dealing with the presence and degree of disability related to low back pain, psychological components of ill health, and perceptions of their work environment.

Findings.—Questionnaires were completed by 64% of the nurses, 45% of the postal workers, and 88% of the patients. The patients were a much older group than either of the 2 working populations. The lifetime prevalence of low back pain was 77% among nurses and 73% among postal workers. Twenty-eight percent of the nurses and 48% of the postal workers who reported low back pain had sought professional help. Similar pain sites were reported by both patients and those still at work. Disability, as expected, was more common in the patient group; low back pain was of more recent origin in the workers. Only among patients did the presence of psychological disturbance modify the relationship between severity of pain and disability. In working groups, disability from low back pain was positively linearly related to severity of pain; work dissatisfaction did not account for disability from low back pain.

Conclusion.—In a working population, low back pain patients did not differ from nonpatients on psychological indices. Psychological dysfunction among patients might be the result of the duration and persistence of their back pain.

▶ This article is important because it helps stratify the causes of pain and the causes of disability with pain. We clearly need more of this type of study, and we can hope that government agencies seek to fund more of this type of work, as the disability related to low back pain is an enormous expense for society. Fundamental and applied research into human pain behaviors may result in substantial reductions in disability and the financial consequences of disability.—M.F. Roizen, M.D.

Conventional and Acupuncture-Like Transcutaneous Electrical Nerve Stimulation Excite Similar Afferent Fibers
Levin MF, Hui-Chan CWY (McGill Univ, Montreal)
Arch Phys Med Rehabil 74:54–60, 1993   101-94-24–8

Background.—Two types of transcutaneous electric nerve stimulation (TENS) are commonly used for the therapeutic alleviation of pain in the clinic: conventional TENS and acupuncture-like TENS. The former consists of low-intensity (2–3 times sensory threshold [T]) and high-frequency (60–100 Hz) stimulation, whereas the latter is applied at high-intensity (more than $3 \times$ T) and low-frequency (2–4 Hz). Which type(s) of afferent fiber(s) is activated by either type of TENS was investigated.

Methods.—Seventeen healthy volunteers were studied. Electric stimulation was delivered to the median nerve at the wrist. For conventional TENS, single pulses were applied at an intensity of $3 \times$ T. Two kinds of acupuncture-like TENS were studied: single pulses at .1 Hz and trains of 100 Hz pulses at 4 Hz, both delivered at an intensity greater than $3 \times$ T. Thirty compound action potentials per type of stimulation were recorded over the median nerve in the cubital fossa and averaged.

Results.—The mean conduction velocities of the afferent fibers excited by conventional TENS ranged from 50.3 to 65.4 m/sec; by single-pulse acupuncture-like TENS, 50–63.5 m/sec; and by short-train acupuncture-like TENS, 41.3–54.8 m/sec. These conduction velocities did not differ significantly from each other.

Conclusion.—Both conventional and acupuncture-like TENS at intensities used clinically for relief of pain activate similar fiber types, predominantly large-diameter $A\alpha\beta$ fibers. The pain-alleviating effects of these 2 types of TENS may be mediated by the activation of similar peripheral afferent fibers.

▶ This study dispels the notion that low-frequency, high-intensity TENS, delivered at intensities high enough to cause discomfort, recruit $A\delta$ and possibly C fibers. The pain associated with stimulus intensities 3 times threshold appears to be related to changes in dorsal horn processing rather than to activation of nociceptors, which occurs at stimulus intensities 6 to 7 times sensory threshold. Such intensities are not easily tolerated.—S.E. Abram, M.D.

Dorsal Column Stimulation Induces Release of Serotonin and Substance P in the Cat Dorsal Horn
Linderoth B, Gazelius B, Franck J, Brodin E (Karolinska Hosp, Stockholm; Karolinska Inst, Stockholm)
Neurosurgery 31:289–297, 1992   101-94-24–9

Background.—Electric stimulation to the dorsal aspect of the spinal cord is the last resort for many patients with intractable pain. Dorsal column stimulation (DCS) may cause a segmental suppression of nociceptive transmission by inhibiting impulse propagation in second-order neurons of the spinothalamic tract. However, hypotheses centering on supraspinal loops have also been suggested. A series of experiments was done to determine whether serotonin and substance P (SP) are released in the dorsal horn by DCS.

Methods.—Twenty-one cats were used. In some experiments the cats were anesthetized, and in some they were decerebrated at the midcollicular level. Microdialysis probes were bilaterally implanted in the lumber dorsal horns and perfused. Dialysates were analyzed for serotonin. Dorsal column stimulation was then applied to the thoracolumbar junction, using a technique comparable to that used in humans.

Findings.—Dorsal column stimulation induced a significant release of serotonin in the dorsal horn of decerebrated animals. Metabolite 5-hydroxyindoleacetic acid levels were not significantly affected. By contrast, there was no release of SP in response to DCS in the decerebrated cats, although peripheral nociceptive stimulation and noxious electric dorsal root stimulation induced an increase in SP levels. In intact cats, DCS provoked a substantial SP release in the dorsal horn.

Conclusion.—Serotonin and SP may participate in the mediation of the pain-alleviating effect of DCS. Dorsal column stimulation and nociceptive stimulation may release SP from separate neuron populations, possibly with different functional properties.

▶ I wonder why this study was confined to the analysis of serotonin and SP. I suspect a great many substances are released during spinal stimulation, and the net effect is a reflection of relative changes in levels of a number of algogenic and analgesic substances.—S.E. Abram, M.D.

Autologous Nucleus Pulposus Induces Neurophysiologic and Histologic Changes in Porcine Cauda Equina Nerve Roots

Olmarker K, Rydevik B, Nordborg C (Univ of Gothenburg, Sweden)
Spine 18:1425–1432, 1993   101-94-24–10

Objective and Methods.—The neurophysiologic and pathologic results of applying autologous nucleus pulposus to the hog cauda equina were studied to determine whether disk herniation could produce nerve injury by means other than mechanical deformation. Electric stimulation studies and histologic examination were carried out 1, 3, and 7 days after the epidural application of nucleus pulposus or retroperitoneal fat, each in a semiliquid state, to the sacrococcygeal cauda equina.

Results.—Application of autologous nucleus pulposus without compression of the nerve root led to a marked reduction in nerve conduction velocity in the cauda equina nerve roots after 1 to 7 days. Nerve fiber injury was more marked in these animals than when retroperitoneal fat was applied.

Conclusion.—Autologous nucleus pulposus can injure nerve root tissues by means other than mechanical compression, possibly biochemically and via microvascular alterations, including inflammation. Also, nucleus pulposus might have a direct irritating effect or produce an autoimmune reaction.

▶ The idea that substances from the nucleus pulposus can produce a chemical neuropathy is old. The nucleus contains high levels of phospholipase A_2 and proteoglycans that have been shown to have tissue-irritating properties. This concept of a chemical radiculopathy helps explain the occurrence of radicular symptoms in patients who have no evidence of mechanical nerve root compression. Such patients are probably particularly amenable to treatment with epidural steroids.—S.E. Abram, M.D.

The Natural Course of Acute Sciatica With Nerve Root Symptoms in a Double-Blind Placebo-Controlled Trial Evaluating the Effect of Piroxicam

Weber H, Holme I, Amlie E (Ullevaal Hosp, Oslo, Norway; Norsk Hydro A/S Porsgrunn, Norway)
Spine 18:1433–1438, 1993   101-94-24-11

Background.—Although it is frequently seen, acute sciatica with nerve root involvement is incompletely understood. Most studies are retrospective, begun only when the patients are admitted to the hospital. A prospective study is necessary to obtain a true picture of the natural course of the disease. Such a study was reported.

Methods.—A total of 208 patients with obvious signs and symptoms of lumbar radiculopathy, L-5 or S-1 level, within 2 weeks of onset, were examined. All patients had radiating pain, with or without sensory or motor deficits, and all had a positive straight-leg–raising test with reduced mobility of the lumbar spine. The same physician repeated the examination after 2 and 4 weeks. Patients were confined to strict bed rest for 1 week, followed by gradual mobilization. They were randomized to receive either piroxicam, 40 mg/day for 2 days then 20 mg/day for 12 days, or placebo. If additional analgesia was needed, paracetamol with or without codeine or levomeprozine was given.

Results.—Back and leg pain decreased significantly, as recorded on a visual analogue scale, during the first 4 weeks (Fig 24–5). Functional ability improved to a similar extent. There were no significant differences between the 2 treatment groups in need for supplementary analgesics, although adverse effects were twice as common in the piroxicam group. Specialist referral was arranged for 12 patients in the placebo group vs. 3 in the piroxicam group. Almost 60% of patients went back to work in the first 4 weeks, which was the mean duration of sick leave. Back pain and activity restrictions persisted in 40% of patients after 3 months and more than 30% after 1 year (Fig 24–6). Twenty percent of the patients were still unable to work after 1 year. Previous sciatica was the only poor prognostic factor (table).

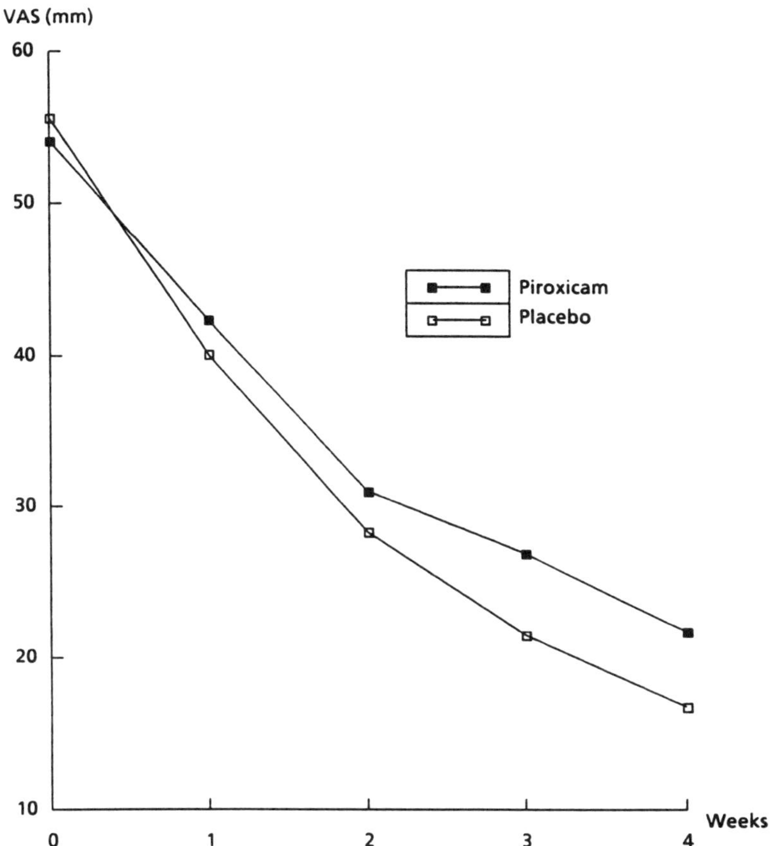

Fig 24–5.—Development of registered pain in back by visual analogue scale (1–100 mm) in randomized groups. (Courtesy of Weber H, Holme I, Amlie E: *Spine* 18:1433–1438, 1993.)

Conclusion.—This prospective study helps to clarify the natural history of acute sciatica with nerve-root symptoms. Encouraging results are noted with initial conservative treatment, although one third of patients may still have pain and activity restrictions after 1 year. When a patient with acute sciatica is seen by a general practitioner, neuroradiologic examinations are of theoretical interest only, as long as "acute back syndrome" is ruled out and the patient's condition improves.

▶ This study confirmed the high rate of resolution of lumbar radiculopathy during the first several weeks after onset and the 70% long-term success rate with conservative management reported in several other studies. These data must be kept in mind when assessing the success rates for treatment regimens for radiculopathy, including epidural steroid injections and surgery.—S.E. Abram, M.D.

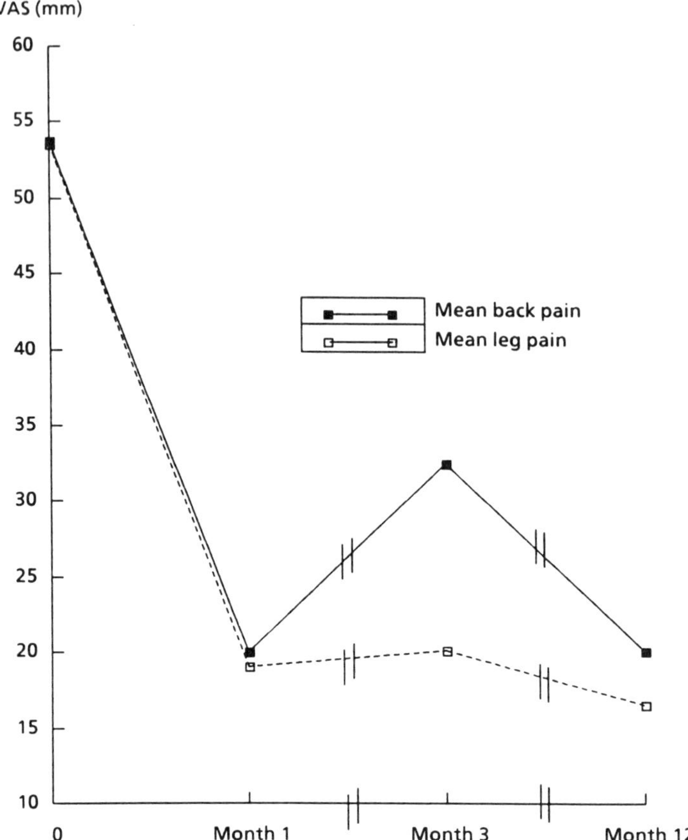

Fig 24–6.—Development of mean back and leg pain by time (visual analogue scale 1–100 mm at zero to 4 weeks, questionnaires from 1–12 months). (Courtesy of Weber H, Holme I, Amlie E: *Spine* 18:1433–1438, 1993.)

Relationship Between Freedom of Pain in Both Back and
Leg (Visual Analogue Scale < 10) and Previous Attacks
of Sciatica

	Painfree	
Previous Attacks	4 Weeks	1 Year
Yes	35.0%	44.3%
No	50.9%	63.2%
	(*P* = 0.023)	(*P* = 0.007)

(Courtesy of Weber H, Holme I, Amlie E: *Spine* 18:1433–1438, 1993.)

Spinal Cord Stimulation in Failed Back Surgery Syndrome

De La Porte C, Van de Kelft E (Universitair Ziekenhuis Antwerpen, Edegem, Belgium)
Pain 52:55–61, 1993   101-94-24–12

Introduction.—High failure rates have been reported with spinal cord stimulation for the control of pain, with the biggest problem being patient selection. No specific predictors of a good outcome have been identified to date. An experience with SCS in 78 consecutive patients with chronic intractable pain associated with the failed back surgery syndrome (FBSS) was reviewed.

Patients.—The patients, who had undergone an average of 3.6 previous lumbar operations, had epidural fibrosis and adhesive arachnoiditis or nerve root injury causing lumbar and radicular pain. Symptoms had been present for an average of 6.5 years. Selection criteria were proven FBSS with no surgically treatable lesion; no significant psychiatric complaint; treatment as needed for depression, anxiety, and insomnia; and an excellent response to temporary percutaneous stimulation. Most patients had monoradicular sciatica, and many had a radicular deficit as well. Patients were followed for a mean of 4 years, with evaluation in the stimulator clinic every 3 months.

Outcome.—The system was internalized after trial stimulation in 64 of 78 patients. Pain relief of at least 50% was reported by 97% of patients immediately after implantation, decreasing to 58% by 1 year. The device was removed because of poor results in 6 patients. By the end of follow-up, 55% of patients reported at least 50% relief, with 11 excellent, 24 good, 12 fair, and 14 poor results. The percentage of patients who needed no medications increased from 18% to 45%, and 90% of patients were able to switch from major to minor analgesics (table). Eighty-three percent of the patients were still using their device at the end of follow-up. Fifty-five percent of patients needed reinterventions. Compli-

Class	Medication	Patients (n = 60)		
		Admission	Implant	Latest follow-up
0	None	11	34	27
1	Minor analgesics	20	10	16
2	Tranquilizers and antidepressants	16	14	9
3	Major analgesics		5	2
4	Morphine or derivatives	8	0	6

(Courtesy of De La Porte C, Van de Kelft E: *Pain* 52:55–61, 1993.)

cations included spontaneous electrode migration, wire breakage, and superficial wound infection.

Conclusion.—A 54% long-term success rate of spinal cord stimulation was seen in patients with intractable pain resulting from FBSS. Well-defined selection criteria do not improve outcome, although they do reduce the number of failed trial stimulations. Important reductions in medication and improvements in life-style are possible, although technical problems still occur.

▶ A 54% long-term success rate seems rather low until one considers the extremely chronic (mean, 6.5 years) and intractable types of pain for which these devices are used. A cost-benefit analysis of this procedure would be useful. On the other hand, we must consider the benefits to the patient independently of the cost to society in determining the advisability of using epidural stimulation.—S.E. Abram, M.D.

Pain After Arthroscopy

Postarthroscopy Analgesia With Intraarticular Bupivacaine/Morphine: A Randomized Clinical Trial
Allen GC, St Amand MA, Lui ACP, Johnson DH, Lindsay MP (Pennsylvania State Univ, Hershey; Univ of Ottawa, Ont, Canada; Ottawa Civic Hosp, Ont, Canada)
Anesthesiology 79:475–480, 1993   101-94-24–13

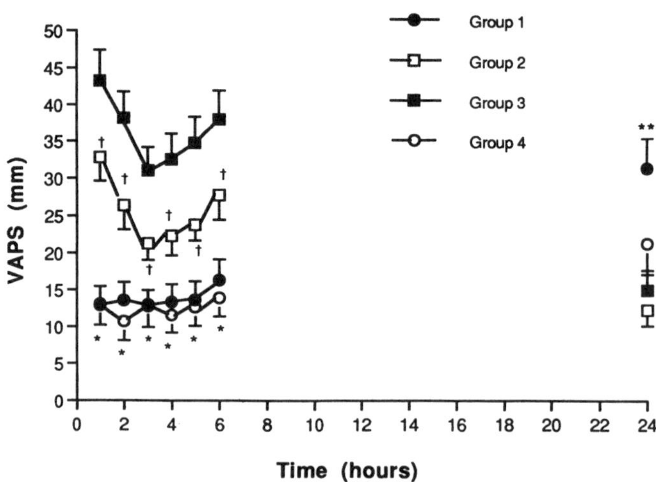

Fig 24–7.—Visual analogue pain scale scores (mean ± SEM) vs. time (hours). *P < .05 for groups 1 and 4 vs. 2 and 3 at 1–6 hours; †P < .05 for group 2 vs. 3 at 1–6 hours; **P < .05 for group 1 vs. 2, 3, and 4 at 24 hours. (Courtesy of Allen GC, St Amand MA, Lui ACP, et al: *Anesthesiology* 79:475–480, 1993.)

Background.—Satisfactory analgesia after arthroscopic knee surgery can be achieved with intra-articular bupivacaine but only for a few hours. In contrast, intra-articular morphine provides longer-lasting analgesia but at a delayed onset. Because the time of onset and duration of action of these agents appear to complement each other, the combination of intra-articular morphine and bupivacaine should provide ideal analgesia after knee arthroscopy.

Study Design.—A total of 120 American Society of Anesthesiologists physical status I–II outpatients underwent knee arthroscopy under general anesthesia with intravenously administered fentanyl, propofol, nitrous oxide, oxygen, and isoflurane. At the end of surgery, before tourniquet release, the patients received, in a random manner, intra-articular injections of .25% bupivacaine (group 1); 1 mg of morphine in saline (group 2); 2 mg of morphine in saline (group 3); or 1 mg of morphine in .25% bupivacaine (group 4). The volume injected was 30 mL and all solutions contained 1:200,000 epinephrine. For postoperative analgesia, the patients received intravenously administered fentanyl and/or orally administered acetaminophen.

Outcome.—At 1–6 hours after surgery, scores on the Visual Analogue Pain Scale (VAPS) and the McGill Pain Questionnaire were lowest in groups 1 and 4 (Fig 24–7). Despite receiving a larger dose, group 3 patients had significantly greater VAPS scores than group 2. At 24 hours, VAPS scores were lowest in groups 2, 3, and 4. Furthermore, patients in groups 1 and 4 required less supplemental analgesia for the first 12 hours, but no differences were observed between groups at 24 hours. There were no adverse effects to treatment.

Conclusion.—Intra-articular morphine (1 mg) in 30-mL .25% bupivacaine with 1:200,000 epinephrine provides superior analgesia for as many as 24 hours after knee arthroscopy, compared with bupivacaine or morphine alone.

▶ It is not clear why intra-articular morphine appears to have some benefit in this study but none in others.—S.E. Abram, M.D.

Comparison of Postoperative Analgesic Effects of Intraarticular Bupivacaine and Morphine Following Arthroscopic Knee Surgery

Raja SN, Dickstein RE, Johnson CA (Johns Hopkins Univ, Baltimore, Md)
Anesthesiology 77:1143–1147, 1992   101-94-24–14

Introduction.—Patients undergoing outpatient surgery require an analgesia that is site-specific, long-lasting, easily administered, and safe. Whether intra-articular administration of opiates provides analgesia after arthroscopic surgery, a common outpatient procedure, was investigated.

Methods.—Forty-nine patients were enrolled in the double-blind study; data from 47 patients were available for analysis. The patients were randomized to receive 1 of 3 intra-articular medications at the conclusion of the procedure. Sixteen received normal saline with 100 μg of epinephrine (group 1); 15 were given .25% bupivacaine with 100 μg of epinephrine (group 2); and 16 received 3 mg of morphine sulphate and 100 μg of epinephrine in normal saline (group 3). A visual analogue pain scale (VAS) was used by the patients to mark the intensity of their pain. The VAS scores were noted on arrival in the recovery unit, each hour until discharge, and at postdischarge follow-up at 48 or 72 hours.

Results.—The 3 groups had similar VAS scores before surgery and on arrival in the recovery room. Patients in the morphine group requested pain medication earlier than those in the bupivacaine group. During the first postoperative hour, supplemental analgesics were required by 9 patients in group 3; no patients in group 2, and 2 patients in group 1. The VAS scores during the first 2 postoperative hours were higher in the morphine group than in the bupivacaine group. Twenty capsules of Tylox had been given to each patient for use at home as needed, and the consumption per day did not differ by group.

Conclusion.—Patients who underwent arthroscopic knee surgery with regional anesthesia did not experience significant postoperative analgesia from intra-articular morphine. Patients in the group randomized to intra-articular bupivacaine had better pain relief. The findings failed to demonstrate functional opiate receptors in the knee joint, an idea suggested by several animal studies.

▶ The debate regarding the possible role of intra-articular opioid receptors continues. This well-controlled study suggests a very limited role for intra-articular opioids.—S.E. Abram, M.D.

Intraarticular Analgesia Following Knee Arthroscopy
Joshi GP, McCarroll SM, O'Brien TM, Lenane P (Cappagh Orthopaedic Hosp, Dublin; Mater Misericordiae Hosp, Dublin)
Anesth Analg 76:333–336, 1993   101-94-24–15

Purpose.—Patients undergoing knee arthroscopy receive intra-articular morphine, which yields effective and long-lasting pain relief. Intra-articularly administered bupivacaine is also effective, with a faster onset of action but a short duration of analgesia. Thus, the combination of the 2 agents might be complementary, providing a quick onset with a long duration.

Methods.—In a randomized, double-blind, controlled study, the analgesic effect of intra-articular morphine and bupivacaine, alone and in combination, was examined in 40 consecutive outpatients undergoing elective knee arthroscopy. Patients were assigned to 1 of 4 intra-articular injection groups. Group 1 patients received 5 mg of morphine in 25 mL of saline; group 2, 25 mL of .25% bupivacaine; group 3, 5 mg of morphine plus 62.5 mg of bupivacaine in 25 mL dilution; and group 4, 25 mL of saline. Pain was assessed according to a visual analogue scale up to 24 hours after injection and by the need for supplemental analgesia.

Results.—Group 1 and 3 patients showed no significant difference in either measure of pain. However, they had significantly lower pain scores and lower supplementary analgesic requirements than group 2 and 4 patients. All patients in groups 2 and 4 needed supplementary analgesia by 24 hours, compared with just 20% in groups 1 and 2.

Conclusion.—The effectiveness of intra-articular morphine in relieving pain after knee arthroscopy was confirmed; however, combining bupivacaine with morphine did not improve results. Intra-articular morphine analgesia is mediated locally and has a long duration of action and few or no side effects.

▶ If, indeed, intra-articular opioids exert an analgesic effect, it is not clear what the role of opioid receptors in the synovium might be.—S.E. Abram, M.D.

Beneficial Impact of Epidural Anesthesia on Recovery After Outpatient Arthroscopy
Parnass SM, McCarthy RJ, Bach BR Jr, Corey ER, Hasson S, Werling MA, Ivankovich AD (Rush-Presbyterian-St Luke's Med Ctr, Chicago)
Arthroscopy 9:91–95, 1993 101-94-24–16

Introduction.—Regional anesthesia is recommended rather than general anesthesia for ambulatory patients after surgery because it has fewer side effects likely to prolong hospital stay. Epidural anesthesia, combined with light levels of sedation, is well suited for lower extremity procedures. The effects of general and epidural anesthesia on discharge times, incidence of side effects, and overall patient satisfaction were studied in patients scheduled for knee arthroscopy.

Methods.—The study group consisted of 260 consecutive patients, 181 who received general anesthesia and 79 who received epidural anesthesia. The choice of anesthesia was decided by the anesthesia team and the patient. Patients were assessed before discharge and at 24-hour follow-up for side effects, pain, amount of time spent in the postanesthesia care unit (PACU), and satisfaction with the anesthetic method.

Results.—Demographic data on the 2 anesthesia groups were generally comparable. Those receiving epidural anesthesia were, on average, older than those receiving general anesthesia. Patients in the epidural group were discharged earlier from both the PACU and the outpatient recovery room. Compared with patients in the general anesthesia group, they had a lower incidence of pain and nausea/vomiting. Fewer patients in the epidural group needed analgesic treatment; those requiring analgesics used less medication. Backache during follow-up evaluation was the only problem reported more frequently in the epidural group. Patient satisfaction was similar for the 2 groups. Most patients in both general and epidural (81.3% and 87.3%, respectively) said they would request the same anesthesia for a further similar surgery.

Conclusion.—Epidural anesthesia offers a number of advantages in outpatient arthroscopy. The patient can view the procedure, reducing the potential for misunderstandings or dissatisfaction. The lower incidence of side effects with epidural anesthesia leads to earlier discharge and may save costs in medication and staffing.

▶ This study adds to the now overwhelming evidence that blockade of afferent impulses before the onset of the noxious stimulation of a surgical procedure reduces the level of postoperative pain and reduces analgesic requirements. The neurophysiology of the CNS changes that occur during intense painful stimulation and that lead to a hyperalgesic state postoperatively are now fairly well understood (1).—S.E. Abram, M.D.

Reference

1. Coderre TJ et al: *Pain* 52:259, 1993.

Post-Thoracotomy Pain

Effect of Interpleural Morphine on Postoperative Pain and Pulmonary Function After Thoracotomy
Welte M, Haimerl E, Groh J, Briegel J, Sunder-Plassmann L, Herz A, Peter K, Stein C (Ludwig-Maximilians-Universität München; Max-Planck-Institut für Psychiatrie, Martinsried, Germany)
Br J Anaesth 69:637–639, 1992   101-94-24-17

Background.—A previous study has shown that opioid agonists produce peripheral antinociceptive effects in inflamed tissue of rats through opioid receptors located on peripheral terminals of primary afferent neurons. Encouraged by the profound postoperative analgesia achieved with intra-articularly administered morphine, it is hypothesized that administration of interpleural (ip) morphine may occupy receptors in intercostal nerves and produce analgesia.

Methods.—The effects of ip morphine on postoperative pain and pulmonary function were studied in 17 patients after thoracotomy. At the end of surgery, an ip catheter was inserted percutaneously in the anterior axillary line. In a double-blind, randomized manner, the patients received either a bolus of ip morphine, 2.5 mg, and intravenous saline or intravenous morphine, 2.5 mg, and ip saline.

Outcome.—Neither postoperative pain scores—as assessed on the visual analogue scale, a numerical rating scale, and the McGill Pain Questionnaire—nor pulmonary function differed significantly in patients given morphine interpleurally or intravenously after thoracotomy. In addition, supplementary analgesic requirements were similar in the 2 groups.

Conclusion.—Interpleurally administered morphine does not provide superior analgesia or improve pulmonary function compared with the same dose given intravenously. This finding is in contrast with that observed after arthroscopic knee surgery. Postoperative bleeding and secretion after thoracotomy may dilute the morphine solution, whereas gravity-dependent pooling in dependent areas of the pleural space may preclude the action of morphine on nerve terminals. In addition, any drug injected into the interpleural space may be lost partially through the chest drains.

▶ Interpleural local anesthetics have been ineffective in some studies of post-thoracotomy pain because of pleural bleeding and loss of drug from chest drains. It is not clear why these authors chose to try this technique in light of the unlikelihood of its benefit.—S.E. Abram, M.D.

Continuous Intercostal Analgesia With 0.5% Bupivacaine After Thoracotomy: A Randomized Study
Deneuville M, Bisserier A, Regnard JF, Chevalier M, Levasseur P, Hervé P (Université Paris-Sud, Le Plessis Robinson, France)
Ann Thorac Surg 55:381–385, 1993   101-94-24–18

Introduction.—Methods of postoperative pain relief are needed that do not cause depressed pulmonary function. Intercostal nerve blockade using intermittent injections of bupivacaine hydrochloride can provide effective pain relief after abdominal and thoracic surgeries. Continuous intercostal analgesia using infusion of .5% bupivacaine hydrochloride via an extrapleurally placed indwelling catheter was studied to determine whether it provided prolonged analgesia after thoracotomy.

Methods.—This randomized study assessed the efficacy of continuous intercostal analgesia with .5% bupivacaine, 360 mg/day, in comparison to fixed-schedule or on-demand intramuscular narcotics. Studied were 86 patients undergoing lobectomy or wedge resection via posterolateral thoracotomy. Patients were randomized to receive intercostal bupivacaine (group 1); intercostal saline solution (group 2); or intramuscular buprenorphine (group 3). Groups 1 and 2 received supplementary buprenorphine as needed.

Technique.—A multiperforated epidural catheter was inserted percutaneously via the anterior part of the fifth intercostal space before thoracotomy closure. The catheter was advanced under direct vision to the neck of the second rib and positioned 3–4 cm from the spine. The pleura was stitched, the catheter secured to the skin, and saline solution injected through the catheter as a check against intrapleural leakage. The chest was closed with anterior and posterior chest tubes connected to water-sealed drainage with 20 cm of water suction. The chest tubes were removed on the fifth postoperative day. Patients received either .5% bupivacaine hydrochloride or .9% saline solution via catheter into the extrapleural space. Solution was continuously infused at a rate of 3 mL/hr for the first 5 days, after which the catheter was removed.

Results.—In the first 8 hours after surgery, patients in group 1 had lower pain scores than those in group 2. For the first 3 days, the mean pain scores of 5 or above were noted in 9% of group 1; 40% of group 2; and 13% of group 3. These differences were nonsignificant, however. The mean total buprenorphine dose was about 2 mg in groups 1 and 2, compared with 5 mg in group 3. Five patients in group 2 had respiratory complications compared with none in groups 1 and 3.

Conclusion.—For patients undergoing thoracotomy, continuous intercostal bupivacaine appears to provide early pain control similar to that of fixed-schedule narcotics but better than that of on-demand narcotics, with fewer complications. This form of analgesia is safe, effective, and easily administered. It is suitable for routine use but is especially beneficial for patients with impaired preoperative ventilatory function.

▶ Continuous intercostal analgesia with bupivacaine offers little benefit compared with scheduled buprenorphine, and patients in both of these groups fared better than the patients receiving placebo plus on-demand buprenorphine. Perhaps the limited benefit of intercostal bupivacaine is related to catheter migration. No mention was made of sensory testing after institution of bupivacaine infusion. The benefits of this technique remain to be determined.—S.E. Abram, M.D.

A Randomized Comparison of Intravenous Versus Lumbar and Thoracic Epidural Fentanyl for Analgesia After Thoracotomy

Guinard J-P, Mavrocordatos P, Chiolero R, Carpenter RL (Centre Hospitalier Universitaire Vaudois, Lausanne, Switzerland; Virginia Mason Med Ctr, Seattle)
Anesthesiology 77:1108–1115, 1992   101-94-24–19

Introduction.—There have been several reports that epidural administration of fentanyl provides better pain relief than intravenous administration of the drug to patients undergoing thoracic (T) surgery. Placement of the epidural catheter at the T level rather than at the lumbar (L) level may also enhance analgesia. The efficacy of fentanyl administered intravenously by the T epidural route was compared with administration by the L epidural route.

Methods.—Fifty consecutive patients scheduled for elective lung surgery were randomized to receive an 18-gauge epidural catheter placed under local anesthesia either at the T4–5 level (T group) or at the L4–5 level (L group), or to receive no epidural catheter (intravenous group). On the day before surgery, the patients were instructed in the use of a portable spirometer and a visual analogue scale (VAS) for pain. The fentanyl infusions were started after surgery and adjusted to maintain a score of 30 or less/100 at rest using the VAS. Data were collected before surgery, at fixed intervals during the 48 hours of fentanyl analgesia, and the day of discharge.

Results.—No differences were observed between the groups on most measures of efficacy: overall quality of analgesia at rest and after coughing, quantity of fentanyl delivered, incidence of pruritus needing treatment, and need to decrease fentanyl infusion rate because of side effects. Patients in the T group had a shorter hospital stay; patients in the intravenous group were more frequently nauseated.

Conclusion.—At the time of discharge after thoracotomy all investigated parameters were identical in the T, L, and intravenous groups. The T epidural administration of fentanyl has only a slight advantage over L epidural administration. Although the intravenous group patients had a slightly increased incidence of side effects, this method provides pain relief equivalent to that of the epidural routes.

▶ This is one of several recent studies that failed to show substantial benefit of epidural vs. intravenous fentanyl. The routine epidural use of lipid-soluble drugs, at least when used without concomitant local anesthetic, may not be justifiable.—S.E. Abram, M.D.

Preoperative Morphine Pre-Empts Postoperative Pain
Richmond CE, Bromley LM, Woolf CJ (Univ College London)
Lancet 342:73–75, 1993   101-94-24-20

Introduction.—The conventional approach to postoperative analgesia—administration of drugs in response to pain—is often inadequate. Studies of the mechanisms of acute pain have suggested that preinjury use of analgesia can prevent the sensitization of central neurons. The effects of morphine given before or after surgery were investigated.

Methods.—Seventy-six women scheduled for elective total abdominal hysterectomy were recruited for the double-blind study. The patients were randomized to receive 10 mg of morphine sulfate intramuscularly mixed with prochlorperazine 1 hour before operation, intravenously at induction of anesthesia, or intravenously at closure of the parietal peritoneum. Response was assessed by morphine consumption from patient-controlled analgesia (PCA) machines during the 24-hour postoperative period. Von Frey hairs were applied at 24 and 48 hours to assess pain sensitivity. Pain scores on visual analogue scale (VAS) were recorded at rest and on movement at 4, 24, and 48 hours after surgery.

Results.—Sixteen patients who did not remain on the PCA machine for 24 hours were excluded from analysis. Patients in the intravenous preoperative group used a significantly lower mean dose of morphine than patients in the intravenous postoperative group. The intramuscular preoperative group also used less morphine than the intravenous postoperative group, but the difference was not significant. The touch detection thresholds did not differ significantly between the groups. The relative pain thresholds, however, were significantly greater in the intravenous postoperative group. The VAS pain scores were similar at 4 and 24 hours, confirming the correct use of the PCA machine.

Conclusion.—Preemptive analgesia with a small dose of intravenous morphine reduced postoperative pain, analgesia requirements, and secondary hyperalgesia, compared with the same dose given after surgery. The reduction in dosage in the intravenous preoperative group relative to the intravenous postoperative group was 27%. The findings support central sensitization as the mechanism of postoperative pain.

▶ This study provides some justification for the preoperative administration of opioids, which is now almost routine. The lack of effect when the preoperative dose was given intramuscularly may reflect improper timing of the injection. It is not clear how important opioid premedication might be in patients receiving regional anesthesia.—S.E. Abram, M.D.

Preoperative Indomethacin for Pain Relief After Thoracotomy: Comparison With Postoperative Indomethacin
Murphy DF, Medley C (Sir Charles Gairdner Hosp, Nedlands, Australia)
Br J Anaesth 70:298–300, 1993   101-94-24–21

Background.—Various preemptive strategies for preventing postoperative pain reduce the quality of perceived pain and the need for analgesia after surgery. Nonsteroidal anti-inflammatory drugs inhibit prostaglandin synthesis, and when administered after thoracotomy, they significantly reduce pain and the cumulative need for opioid.

Study Design.—The value of preoperative administration of indomethacin in reducing postoperative pain and opioid needs was examined in a randomized, prospective trial of 50 patients having elective thoracotomy. Patients were assigned to receive 200-mg indomethacin suppositories beginning the night before surgery and 100-mg doses twice daily thereafter or to receive the same regimen starting on completion of surgery. Premedication and anesthesia were comparable in the 2 groups.

Results.—There were no significant differences in pain scores on the first and second postoperative days between the 22 patients who began indomethacin before surgery and the 28 who started treatment after surgery. Cumulative opioid requirements were also similar in the 2 groups. No adverse effects were ascribed to indomethacin.

Conclusion.—Indomethacin, given either before or after thoracotomy, lessens the need for opioid therapy.

▶ A great deal of attention has been given to the concept of preemptive analgesia. Although there is some evidence that regional anesthetic techniques administered before incision are more effective at diminishing postoperative pain than those begun postoperatively, it appears unlikely that the same phenomenon holds for nonsteroidal anti-inflammatory drugs (NSAIDs). Although spinally administered NSAIDs are capable of reducing hyperalgesia induced by subcutaneous formalin injection (1), such interventions appear to be effective, even if begun *after* the noxious stimulus.—S.E. Abram, M.D.

Reference

1. Malmberg AB, Yaksh TL: *J Pharmacol Exp Ther* 263:136, 1992.

A Randomized Double-Blind Comparison of Epidural Fentanyl Infusion Versus Patient-Controlled Analgesia With Morphine for Post-thoracotomy Pain

Benzon HT, Wong HY, Belavic AM Jr, Goodman I, Mitchell D, Lefheit T, Locicero J (Northwestern Mem Hosp, Chicago)
Anesth Analg 76:316–322, 1993   101-94-24–22

Background.—Although earlier studies suggested that epidural administration of opiate provided better postoperative analgesia than intravenous administration, more recent studies have shown no difference. Most of these studies examined the use of continuous intravenous infusion; however, patient-controlled analgesia (PCA) has come to be more commonly used.

Methods.—In a prospective, randomized, double-blind study, the use of epidural fentanyl infusion was compared with the use of PCA with morphine in 36 post-thoracotomy patients. Both groups received an epidural infusion and PCA, 1 placebo and the other active. The active treatment consisted of epidural fentanyl, 10 µg/mL, in the epidural group and morphine, 1 mg/mL, in the PCA group. If the patient perceived pain relief as inadequate, the infusion was escalated.

Results.—Analgesia appeared to be better in the epidural group, based on lower visual analogue scores and higher Total Pain Relief scores. The difference in pain was more pronounced during coughing. Forced vital capacity measurements were about the same in both groups after surgery. On the first day after surgery, greater degrees of sedation were more common in the PCA group, and pruritus was more often a problem in the epidural group. There was no difference in the incidence of nausea and vomiting.

Conclusion.—For patients who have undergone thoracotomy, epidural fentanyl infusion appears to give better analgesia than intravenous PCA morphine. If adequate personnel are available, epidural fentanyl infusion is the preferred method of treatment.

▶ This is a difficult study to interpret because it compared different drugs by different routes. It does, however, offer some clinical insight because it compared 2 commonly used alternative techniques.—S.E. Abram, M.D.

A Randomized, Double-Blind Comparison of Lumbar Epidural and Intravenous Fentanyl Infusions for Postthoracotomy Pain Relief: Analgesic, Pharmacokinetic, and Respiratory Effects

Sandler AN, Stringer D, Panos L, Badner N, Friedlander M, Koren G, Katz J, Klein J (Univ of Toronto; Toronto Hosp)
Anesthesiology 77:626–634, 1992   101-94-24–23

Background.—Lumbar epidural opioids provide very effective postthoracotomy pain relief and improve pulmonary function. Several investigators have reported that intravenous fentanyl infusions are as effective as epidural fentanyl for post-thoracotomy analgesia. A randomized, double-blind trial was designed to compare the analgesic, pharmacokinetic, and respiratory effects of lumbar epidural fentanyl and intravenous fentanyl infusions for post-thoracotomy pain relief.

Methods.—Twenty-nine patients undergoing elective thoracotomy were randomly assigned to epidural fentanyl plus intravenous normal saline or to epidural normal saline plus intravenous fentanyl. Additional fentanyl was given by the prescribed route as needed. Pain was assessed using a 10-point visual analogue scale. Patients were monitored for respiratory depression with continuous respiratory inductance plethysmography and sequential arterial blood gas analysis for the first 20 postoperative hours. Blood samples for plasma fentanyl assays were collected at regular intervals.

Results.—Both routes of fentanyl administration produced good postoperative analgesia. However, patients receiving epidural fentanyl required a significantly larger infusion dose than those in the intravenous infusion group. The time course for the plasma fentanyl concentrations was similar in the 2 groups, and plasma levels did not differ significantly at any sampling period. The prevalence of mild-to-moderate respiratory depression was also similar.

Conclusion.—Lumbar epidural fentanyl is equivalent to intravenous fentanyl for post-thoracotomy analgesia. Epidural fentanyl acts primarily by systemic reabsorption to provide postoperative analgesia and, thus, confers little advantage over intravenous fentanyl.

► The evidence that epidural infusions of fentanyl are no more effective than intravenous infusions continues to mount. Whether bolus epidural fentanyl injections have substantial spinal effects remains to be determined.—S.E. Abram, M.D.

Thoracic Epidural Bupivacaine Plus Sufentanil: High Concentration/ Low Volume Versus Low Concentration/High Volume
Laveaux MMD, Hasenbos MAWM, Harbers JBM, Liem T (Univ of Nijmegen, The Netherlands)
Reg Anesth 18:39–43, 1993   101-94-24–24

Introduction.—In previous studies, effective pain relief and decreased pulmonary complications after thoracotomy were demonstrated in patients given high thoracic epidural nicomorphine. Better pain relief can be achieved with the combination of an epidural local anesthetic and an opioid than with either agent alone. The analgesic and side effects of a continuous epidural infusion of bupivacaine with sufentanil in a high concentration /low volume (LV) were compared with the effects of an infusion with a low concentration/high volume (HV) of the same combination.

Methods.—A thoracic epidural catheter was placed at the T3–4 interspace in 30 patients undergoing lateral thoracotomy. All received postoperative analgesia via a 3-day continuous epidural infusion. Patients were randomized to receive either a LV with a high drug concentration of bupivacaine, .5%, 1.5–2 mL/hr, plus sufentanil, 4 μg/mL^{-1}; or a HV with a relatively low drug concentration of bupivacaine, .125% , 6–8 mL/hr, plus sufentanil, 1 μg/mL^{-1}. The 2 groups were compared for postoperative analgesia and side effects.

Results.—There was no apparent difference in pain on visual analogue scales, either at rest or with exercise. Half of both groups required supplementary analgesia. Hypercapnia, defined as a partial pressure of carbon dioxide in arterial blood ($PaCO_2$) of more than 7 kPa, occurred in the first postoperative hour in 24% of the LV group vs. 15% of the HV group. Both groups showed a significant increase over baseline in the mean $PaCO_2$, to about 6 kPa, on the first postoperative day, but not thereafter. There was never any significant between-group difference in $PaCO_2$ or in side effects.

Conclusion.—In post-thoracotomy patients receiving thoracic epidural bupivacaine and sufentanil, a high drug concentration in LV volume or a low concentration in HV gave equally good pain relief. Either way, there was no significant ventilatory depression and no difference in side effects. Total dose, not concentration or volume, is the more important factor in the efficacy of epidural block.

▶ There is growing evidence that epidural infusions of highly lipid-soluble opioids exert much, if not most, of their effect by systemic absorption. In light of such evidence, the results of this study are not surprising.—S.E. Abram, M.D.

Cancer Pain

Celiac Plexus Block Versus Analgesics in Pancreatic Cancer Pain
Mercadante S (SAMOT, Palermo, Italy)
Pain 52:187–192, 1993   101-94-24-25

Introduction.—Neurolytic celiac plexus block is claimed as the most satisfactory treatment for pancreatic cancer pain, but its effectiveness and duration of block remain controversial because of methodologic difficulties. A study was conducted to assess the course and effectiveness of celiac plexus block when compared with traditional treatment with analgesics by considering the previous and subsequent consumption of narcotics until death.

Study Design.—Twenty patients with pancreatic cancer and severe pain were treated. All patients were treated with oral analgesics using the nonsteroidal anti-inflammatory drug–narcotic sequence for the first week. Thereafter, the patients were randomly assigned to continue analgesic treatment, increasing opioid dosage to achieve a visual analogue score less than 4 cm until death, or to undergo celiac plexus block with subsequent use of analgesics as in the former group. The visual analogue score and opioid consumption were used to calculate the effective analgesic dose at weekly intervals until death.

Outcome.—During a mean survival time of 51 days, patients treated with celiac plexus block had significantly less opioid consumption than those treated with analgesics only, even on the day before death. Although both traditional analgesic treatment and celiac plexus block provided equally effective reduction in the visual analogue score, treatment with analgesics only was associated with more undesirable side effects. Complications caused by the block were limited and easily controlled and included prolonged diarrhea, orthostatic hypotension, and back pain at the site of injection.

Conclusion.—In controlling pancreatic cancer pain, celiac plexus block permits pain control with a reduction in opioid consumption, and this effect persists partially until the day before death in advanced patients.

▶ Although most physicians who employ neurolytic celiac plexus blocks for pancreatic cancer pain are convinced of the benefits, there have been little hard data to support those convictions. This randomized study shows that pain can indeed be controlled as well with analgesics, but at considerable cost in terms of side effects. The celiac block patients clearly used less medication and had fewer problems with side effects.—S.E. Abram, M.D.

Morphine Attenuates Surgery-Induced Enhancement of Metastatic Colonization in Rats

Page GG, Ben-Eliyahu S, Yirmiya R, Liebeskind JC (Univ of California, Los Angeles; Hebrew Univ of Jerusalem)
Pain 54:21–28, 1993   101-94-24–26

Background.—Several studies have indicated that surgery suppresses immune function and enhances tumor development. It is not clear whether the immune system mediates the tumor-enhancing effects of surgery or whether postoperative pain contributes to such effects.

Study Design.—The mammary adenocarcinoma MADB106 tumor cell line, which is syngeneic to the inbred Fischer 344 strain of rat used in this study and known to be sensitive to natural killer (NK) cell activity, was used in 2 experiments. In the first experiment, animals were assigned to anesthesia plus standard laparotomy, anesthesia only, or no treatment to investigate the effects of surgery on metastatic colonization. The MADB106 tumor cells were injected at 5 hours after surgery. In the second experiment, the animals were randomly assigned to surgery vs. anesthesia only and morphine vs. vehicle to assess the impact of an analgesic dose of morphine on surgery-induced enhancement of metastatic colonization.

Findings.—Animals that were injected with MADB106 and underwent surgery had twice the number of surface lung metastases than those found in the anesthesia-only and untreated controls. In the second study, this effect was significantly pronounced when MADB106 cells were injected at 5 or 24 hours after surgery, but not when injected 8 or 21 days after surgery. Compared with control levels, the number of large granular lymphocytes/NK cells per mL of blood increased significantly at 24 hours but not at 4 hours after surgery. The administration of an analgesic dose of morphine significantly attenuated surgery enhanced metastatic colonization without affecting metastasis in unoperated animals.

Implications.—Surgery enhances metastatic colonization only at a time when the MADB106 tumor is known to be sensitive to NK cell control, suggesting that suppression of NK cell activity mediates the surgery-induced enhancement of metastatic colonization. Morphine blocks the surgery-induced enhancement of metastatic colonization, suggesting that postoperative pain can enhance metastatic spread. Should a similar relationship between pain and metastasis be found in humans, pain control must be considered a vital component of postoperative care.

▶ This study has obvious implications. The changes in immune function associated with pain-induced stress responses may actually affect survival in some individuals.—S.E. Abram, M.D.

Morphine and Hydromorphone Epidural Analgesia: A Prospective, Randomized Comparison
Chaplan SR, Duncan SR, Brodsky JB, Brose WG (Stanford Univ, Calif; Univ of Pittsburgh, Pa)
Anesthesiology 77:1090–1094, 1992   101-94-24-27

Background.—Epidural opioid analgesia often causes troublesome side effects that restrict its usefulness in the clinical setting. Some anecdotal evidence points to epidural hydromorphone as having fewer side effects than epidural morphine. The side effects of equi-analgesic doses of epidural hydromorphone and morphine in the postoperative setting were compared.

Methods.—Of 54 patients undergoing major operations requiring postoperative analgesia, 27 were randomly allocated to epidural morphine infusion for the first 2 postoperative days. The other 27 received epidural hydromorphone. Epidural infusions were titrated to patient comfort. Pain, sedation, nausea, and pruritus were assessed twice daily. Prophylactic anti-emetics or antipruritics were not allowed.

Results.—Both drugs provided adequate and equal analgesia during the first 2 postoperative days. No significant difference was apparent between the 2 groups in the prevalence of sedation or nausea. However, moderate-to-severe pruritus was significantly less prevalent among hydromorphone-treated patients than among those treated with epidural morphine.

Conclusion.—The use of hydromorphone instead of morphine for postoperative epidural analgesia reduces the occurrence of moderate-to-severe pruritus.

▶ There seems to be no advantage to epidural hydromorphone over morphine with respect to nausea, sedation, or respiratory depression. There is an obvious benefit in terms of itching, which may represent a real advantage in obstetrics where pruritis is a major problem with epidural morphine. Because the total daily doses of each drug were not reported, it is difficult to assess whether the total daily doses of hydromorphone were substantially lower than what would be required by other parenteral routes. It is not clear, therefore, whether the case of respiratory depression from hydromorphone reported in this study was related to CSF migration or to systemic accumulation.—S.E. Abram, M.D.

A Comparison of Postoperative Epidural Analgesia Between Patients With Chronic Cancer Taking High Doses of Oral Opioids Versus Opioid-Naive Patients

de Leon-Casasola OA, Myers DP, Donaparthi S, Bacon DR, Peppriell J, Rempel J, Lema MJ (Roswell Park Cancer Inst, Buffalo, NY; State Univ of New York, Buffalo)
Anesth Analg 76:302–307, 1993   101-94-24–28

Background.—Patients with intractable cancer pain of moderate-to-severe intensity are usually treated with large doses of opioids. Increasing doses are required because of disease progression, tolerance, or both. Perioperative pain control can be a problem in patients taking high doses of oral opioids. A comparison was made between the postoperative epidural and intravenous opioid requirements of surgical patients with cancer who were taking opioids in doses larger than 50 mg of morphine (MS) daily, and others who were opioid naive.

Methods.—Ninety-nine patients were opioid naive (group 2), and 17 had been taking doses of MS greater than 50 mg/day for at least 3 months (group 1). For 5 days after epidural-light general anesthesia, these surgical patients received epidural analgesia with bupivacaine (BUP) (.1%) and MS (.01%). Postoperative infusions were started at 10 mL/hr $^{-1}$ for group 1 and 5 mL/hr $^{-1}$ for group 2. Patients were evaluated every 6 hours for pain, withdrawal, and overdosing. Dynamic pain scores were kept below 4 (on a scale in which 10 equals excrutiating pain) by titrating infusions or giving intravenous MS, 4 mg every hour as needed, or both.

Results.—The mean daily oral dose of MS in group 1 patients had been 183 mg. After surgery, these patients used 3 times more MS epidurally and 5 times more MS intravenously for breakthrough pain than did opioid-naive patients. When compared with group 2, group 1 patients had a longer requirement for analgesic therapy (9 days vs. 3 days). Daily

	Total Usage		
	Epidural morphine (mg)	Breakthrough IV morphine (mg)	Length of therapy (h)
Group I *n* = 17	137 ± 28	48 ± 4	218 ± 42
Group II *n* = 99	44 ± 15	10 ± 6	76 ± 35

Abbreviation: IV, intravenous.
Note: P < .0001 I vs. II for all comparisons. Values are mean ± standard deviation.
(Courtesy of deLeon-Casasola OA, Myers DP, Donaparthi S, et al: *Anesth Analg* 76:302–307, 1993.)

epidural and intravenous MS usage was always 2–3 times greater for group 1 patients (table). All patients experienced adequate analgesia and none experienced respiratory depression or opioid withdrawal during hospitalization.

Conclusion.—Chronic opioid users can achieve adequate postoperative analgesia with epidural BUP-MS, although 3 times the normal dosage and duration of therapy may be required. These larger doses of morphine did not result in respiratory depression, hyperesthesia, or other side effects. Nevertheless, such patients must be carefully monitored.

▶ This study provides documentation of the pharmacologic tolerance that develops to both neuraxial and systemic opioids after chronic use and provides some useful guidelines for predicting epidural MS doses for patients taking oral opioids chronically. It is particularly interesting that the patients treated with chronic opioids required a much longer period of epidural analgesia. Perhaps their preexisting cancer pain was responsible for the development of sensitization of sensory neurons in the CNS that did not develop in the opioid-naive patients because of the intraoperative epidural analgesia.—S.E. Abram, M.D.

Perineal Pain After Rectal Amputation: A 5-Year Follow-Up
Boas RA, Schug SA, Acland RH (Univ of Auckland, New Zealand; Auckland Hosp, New Zealand)
Pain 52:67–70, 1993   101-94-24–29

Introduction.—Patients undergoing rectal amputation commonly have perineal pain. Some aspects of the etiology and treatment of such pain are unclear. Previous retrospective studies may have addressed differing subsets of patients. A long-term follow-up study of 286 patients undergoing perineal resection for rectal cancer was reported.

Methods.—The initial study sample consisted of 286 cancer patients undergoing classic abdominoperineal resection of the rectum. One hundred and seventy-seven patients responded to a questionnaire concerning their postsurgical pain. Those who reported pain were reexamined at 2 and 5 years.

Findings.—Thirty-three patients (11.5%) reported persistent perineal pain. Twenty-three had early-onset pain, occurring within a few weeks of surgery. It was most often described as a shooting, bursting, or tight, aching pain of mild-to-moderate intensity. In three fourths of cases, it was intermittent or spontaneous in presentation and was usually felt around the inner level of the resected anorectal margin. Only 1 patient obtained good relief with conventional analgesics. Of 12 patients traced after 5 years, 9 still had undiminished pain.

In the other 10 patients, pain developed 3 months or more after surgery (Fig 24–8). This pain was sharp and aching in nature and severe in

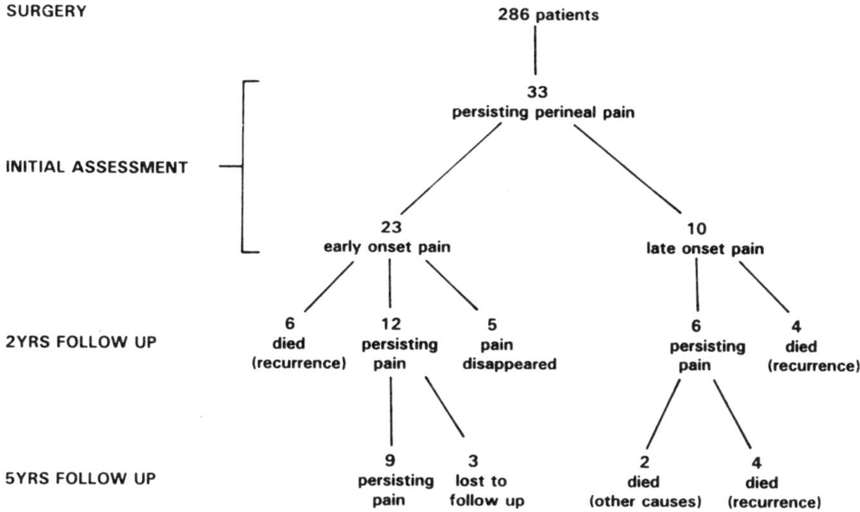

Fig 24–8.—Time course of patient outcome. (Courtesy of Boas RA, Schug SA, Acland RH: *Pain* 52:67–70, 1993.)

half of the cases. It was continuous and deep in most cases and was aggravated by pressure and sitting. About half of the patients responded well to nonsteroidal anti-inflammatory drugs. The tumor recurrence rate was 80%, compared with 26% in the patients with early-onset pain.

Conclusion.—Two distinct groups of patients with perineal pain after rectal resection were identified. Their difference may reflect different etiologic factors, either local tumor recurrence or neuronal deafferentation after excision of the pudendal nerve supply to the lower rectum and anus. Although early-onset phantom pain may account for most cases, late perineal pain is a highly significant predictor of tumor recurrence.

▶ This is a meaningful study that pointed out 2 important concepts: the prevalence of recurrent tumor associated with late-onset pain, and the extremely resistant nature of perineal pain after rectal amputation. Presumably, many of the mechanisms associated with pain after limb amputation are at work here.—S.E. Abram, M.D.

Enhancement of Morphine Analgesia by Fenfluramine in Subjects Receiving Tailored Opioid Infusions

Coda BA, Hill HF, Schaffer RL, Luger TJ, Jacobson RC, Chapman CR (Univ of Washington, Seattle; Fred Hutchinson Cancer Research Ctr, Seattle; Univ of Innsbruck, Austria)
Pain 52:85–91, 1993   101-94-24–30

Purpose.—Systemic morphine offers a relatively narrow therapeutic window, with concentrations of about 20 ng/mL producing initial pain reduction and 100 ng/mL causing respiratory depression. In theory, morphine analgesia could be enhanced, with no increase in side effects, by serotonin releasers such as fenfluramine. Whether fenfluramine itself had analgesic effects and whether it could increase the analgesic effect of morphine across a range of concentrations were investigated.

Methods.—The study sample comprised 10 healthy volunteers, all of whom had undergone previous study of individual morphine pharmacokinetics. Patients were evaluated for their response to repetitive, painful electrical stimuli to a central incisor at strong but tolerable intensities. Four treatments were tested on 4 different days: oral placebo followed by placebo infusion; fenfluramine, 60 mg by mouth, followed by placebo infusion; oral placebo followed by morphine infusion; and oral fenfluramine followed by morphine infusion. The fenfluramine dose was chosen because it was in the therapeutic range for weight control. Morphine infusion was given by a counter-pump system that, using the individual pharmacokinetic data, maintained consecutive, steady plasma concentrations at the target values of 16, 32, and 64 ng/mL. Each value was maintained for 45 minutes. Evaluation included pain reports and dental evoked potentials.

Results.—Fenfluramine had no effect on the pharmacokinetics of morphine. Given alone, the serotonin releaser appeared to have some borderline analgesic effects. It also appeared to significantly increase the analgesic effect of morphine, especially at the lower morphine concentrations. Fenfluramine was associated with slight but significant sedation but did not increase the side effects of morphine.

Conclusion.—The serotonin releaser fenfluramine might increase the analgesia of morphine without increasing its side effects. These effects do not result from inhibition of morphine clearance. Although fenfluramine would not be effective in long-term pain management, other drugs that increase synaptic serotonin without depleting the serotonergic neurons might be useful in persistent pain states.

▶ Relatively few systemic drugs have been shown to appreciably enhance the analgesic effect of systemic morphine. The approach used in this study was much more scientific than most pharmaceutical industry–sponsored studies done in the past. Perhaps some reasonable candidates will turn up.—S.E. Abram, M.D.

CSF Neuropeptides in Cancer Pain: Effects of Spinal Opioid Therapy
Samuelsson H, Ekman R, Hedner T (Central Hosp, Borås, Sweden; Univ of Lund, Sweden; Univ of Gothenburg, Sweden)
Acta Anaesthesiol Scand 37:502–508, 1993   101-94-24–31

Objective.—Levels of several opioid and nonopioid peptides in CSF were estimated in 10 patients with severe nociceptive pain caused by malignant disease, before and after initiation of spinal opioid treatment. Ten control patients without pain also were studied.

Methods.—The opioid peptides quantified in the CSF included met-enkephalin (ME), B-endorphin (BE), and dynorphin (DYN). In addition, several putative sensory neuropeptides were estimated, including substance P (SP), somatostatin, calcitonin gene-related peptide, and vasoactive intestinal polypeptide (VIP). Pain intensity was estimated using a 100-mm visual analogue scale. Eight of the patients with pain caused by cancer received chronic epidural opioid therapy, and 2 received a combination of morphine and bupivacaine intrathecally.

Results.—The patients with pain had significantly higher CSF levels of ME- and DYN-like immunoreactivity than control subjects and significantly lower levels of VIP- and BE-like immunoreactivity. Spinal opioid treatment did not significantly alter the CSF content of any of the peptides, although SP-like immunoreactivity tended to decline. Compared with somatic pain, visceral pain was associated with low levels of immunoreactive SP and ME. Levels of SP and ME were correlated to a highly significant degree.

Conclusion.—Nociceptive pain caused by cancer is associated with significantly altered levels of endogenous opioid peptides and VIP in the CSF. The decline in SP immunoreactivity noted after spinal opioid therapy may reflect decreased transmitter release from primary afferents.

▶ This study illustrates some of the complexities involved in determining the role of endogenous peptides in pain modulation. Relatively little can be learned by measuring the level of CSF peptides because the sample represents 1 point in time during a dynamic process. However, several findings in this study help to crystallize our understanding: (1) the high degree of correlation between SP and ME levels, (2) higher SP levels with somatic pain compared with visceral pain, and (3) a tendency toward lower SP levels after spinal opioid administration. These findings help to confirm the evidence that SP is released from C-fibers from somatic structures, that spinal opioids reduce the release of SP from C-fibers, and that ME is released in the dorsal horn in response to C-fiber stimulation. These observations also help explain the observation that spinal opioids are most effective for tonic, C-fiber–induced somatic pain and are less effective for phasic, or incident pain, which is associated with Aδ-fiber activation, or visceral pain.—S.E. Abram, M.D.

Clinical Efficacy of Methadone in Patients Refractory to Other μ-Opioid Receptor Agonist Analgesics for Management of Terminal Cancer Pain: Case Presentations and Discussion of Incomplete Cross-Tolerance Among Opioid Agonist Analgesics

Crews JC, Sweeney NJ, Denson DD (Univ of Cincinnati, Ohio)
Cancer 72:2266–2272, 1993　　　　　　　　　　　　　　　101-94-24-32

Background.—In patients with pain related to advanced cancer, tolerance to opioid analgesics frequently occurs. In such patients, cross-tolerance among opioid analgesics represents a significant management problem. Incomplete cross-tolerance among opioid analgesics has been reported in both animals and humans and is frequently attributed to opioids with different opioid-receptor subtype affinities. Clinical evidence of the incomplete cross-tolerance of methadone with a number of μ-opioid agonist analgesics was reported.

Patients and Findings.—Six patients had cancer-related pain unresponsive to other μ-opioid receptor agonist analgesics, as indicated by their inability to obtain analgesia in spite of increased opioid doses. However, when opioid doses were converted to methadone doses, all patients achieved adequate analgesia. Compared with their previous dose requirements, the methadone dose needed to establish and sustain analgesia in these patients was modest. When conversion to other opioids was tried, no patient exhibited variability in the analgesic response, other than to methadone.

Conclusion.—Methadone is a powerful opioid analgesic that shows incomplete cross-tolerance with other μ-opioid receptor agonist analgesics. In the opioid-tolerant patient with cancer-related pain, conversion to methadone may provide an effective therapeutic alternative.

▶ The reason for methadone's efficacy in the face of tolerance to other agents is unclear. Occasionally, the converse is true: Methadone is less effective than other opioids. Perhaps there are effects on non–μ-opioid receptors or on nonopioid analgesic receptors.—S.E. Abram, M.D.

Blood Pressure and Heart Rate During Orthostatic Stress and Walking With Continuous Postoperative Thoracic Epidural Bupivacaine/Morphine

Møiniche S, Hjortsø N-C, Blemmer T, Dahl JB, Kehlet H (Hvidovre Univ Hosp, Denmark)
Acta Anaesthesiol Scand 37:65–69, 1993　　　　　　　　　　101-94-24-33

Background.—Thoracic epidural anesthesia combined with light general anesthesia followed by postoperative balanced analgesia has been proposed for patients undergoing upper abdominal surgery to provide stable intraoperative hemodynamics and effective alleviation of postop-

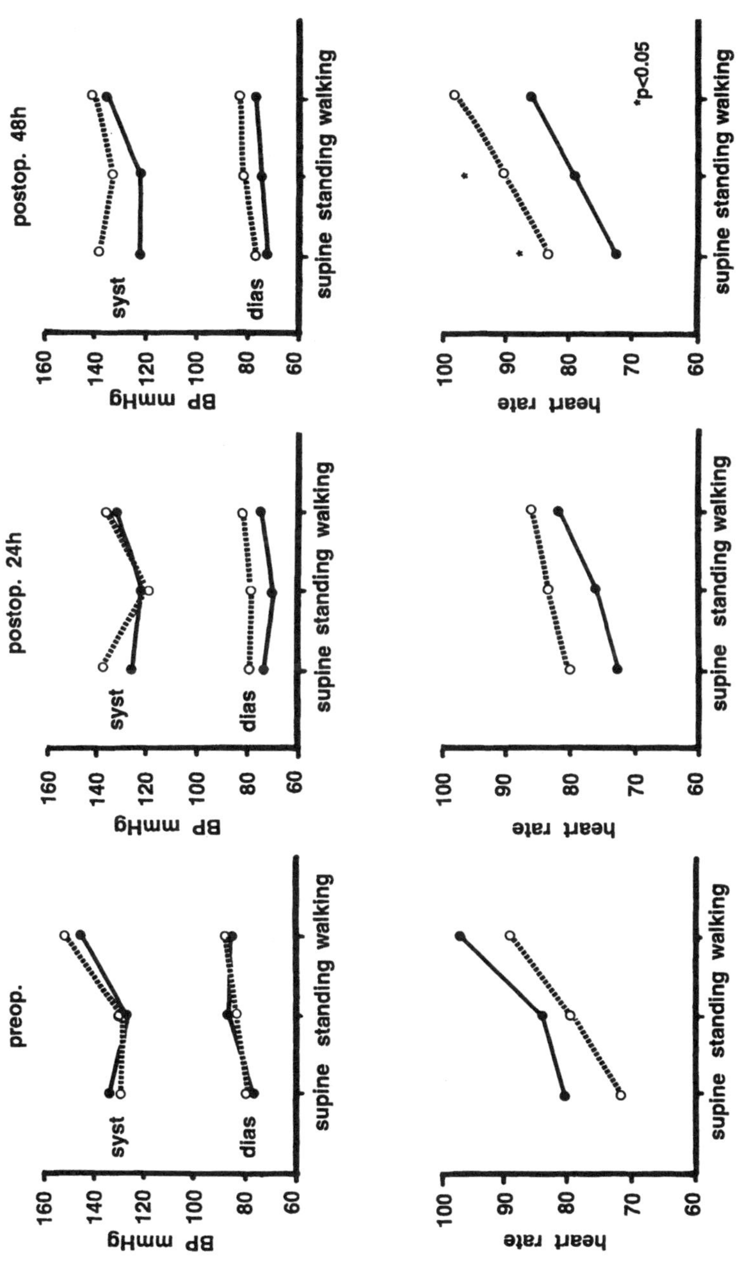

Fig 24–9.—Systolic and diastolic blood pressure *(BP)* and heart rate at rest, during orthostatic stress, and after 40 minutes of walking. *Filled circles,* epidural group; *open circles,* control group. Measurements at 24 hours were performed during continuous epidural analgesia, and measurements at 48 hours were performed 10 hours after cessation of epidural analgesia. * Significant ($P < .05$) difference between epidural and control group. (Courtesy of Møiniche S, Hjortsø N-C, Blemmer T, et al: *Acta Anaesthesiol Scand* 37:65–69, 1993.)

erative pain. The effects of postoperative balanced analgesia with low-dose epidural bupivacaine and morphine plus systemic nonsteroidal anti-inflammatory drugs (NSAIDs) vs. systemic morphine and NSAIDs on heart rate and blood pressure during rest, orthostatic stress, and walking were studied.

Methods.—The subjects were 31 patients undergoing elective cholecystectomy through a minilaparotomy. By random assignment, 15 patients received combined thoracic epidural anesthesia with light general anesthesia and postoperative balanced analgesia with continuous epidural bupivacaine and morphine for 38 hours after surgery, plus systemic ibuprofen. The remaining 16 patients received general anesthesia and postoperative analgesia with systemic morphine and ibuprofen.

Findings.—During postoperative epidural infusion, the sensory blockade to pinprick was T4 to L1. Analgesia at rest and during mobilization was better than with systemic morphine and NSAIDs. Hemodynamic responses (blood pressure and heart rate) during rest, orthostatic stress, and after walking did not differ significantly between groups (Fig 24–9). There was also no significant between-group difference in the number of patients with a reduction of more than 20 mm Hg in systolic blood pressure during orthostatic stress. The number of episodes of dizziness, nausea, and vomiting during rest or mobilization was also similar in the 2 groups.

Conclusion.—No significant differences were found in hemodynamic responses to orthostatic stress and walking in the 2 groups studied. These findings do not support the belief that low-dose continuous thoracic epidural analgesia with local anesthetic and opioid may prevent ambulation in patients after surgery because of sympathetic blockade or impaired cardiovascular adaptation to the upright position.

▶ Our concepts regarding the sympathetic vs. the somatic blocking effects of epidural anesthesia have been changing. Perhaps widespread sympathetic blockade is not a necessary consequence of epidural analgesia with local anesthetics. Once again, a "barrier" to the use of regional anesthesia appears to be a small one, indeed.—S.E. Abram, M.D.

Effects and Side Effects of a Percutaneous Thermal Lesion of the Dorsal Root Ganglion in Patients With Cervical Pain Syndrome
van Kleef M, Spaans F, Dingemans W, Barendse GAM, Floor E, Sluijter ME (Univ Hosp, Maastricht, The Netherlands)
Pain 52:49–53, 1993   101-94-24–34

Background.—Patients who fail initial conservative therapy for cervical pain may go on to more aggressive forms of treatment. Percutaneous partial rhizotomy (PPR) to create a radiofrequency lesion of the dorsal root ganglion may now be done by using a small-diameter, temperature-

		Pain Score After 3, 6, and 9 Months			
Follow-up	No.	Pain free	Good	Moderate	No effect
3 months	20	2 (10%)	8 (40%)	5 (25%)	5 (25%)
6 months	20	4 (20%)	2 (10%)	4 (20%)	10 (50%)
9 months	17	2 (11%)	2 (11%)	3 (17%)	10 (58%)

Note: Pain free indicates 100% relief; *good,* 50% to 100% relief; *moderate,* 30% to 50% relief; and *no effect,* less than 30% relief.

(Courtesy of van Kleef M, Spaans F, Dingemans W, et al: *Pain* 52:49–53, 1993.)

monitoring electrode system. The safety and efficacy of this modification were investigated.

Methods.—Percutaneous partial rhizotomy was performed on 20 consecutive patients with intractable, chronic cervical pain. Lesions were created at the level of C4, C5, or C6. Patients were studied before and 3 weeks after treatment by electromyography (EMG) and sensory evoked potentials (SEPs); pain was assessed at 6 weeks on numeric rating scales. Follow-up interviews were conducted at 3, 6, and 9 months after PPR.

Results.—Twelve patients reported a vague-to-troublesome burning pain in the dermatome of the affected nerve root after 3 weeks, and 7 had hyposensibility in the area after 3 weeks. The side effects resolved by 6 weeks in all patients but 1. There was no evidence of denervation on EMG, and only 1 patient had a persistently abnormal SEP recording. Seventy-five percent of patients reported pain relief after 3 months and 50% reported relief after 6 months (table).

Conclusion.—There was no evidence of motor denervation and no long-term signs of deafferentation after PPR for chronic, intractable cervical pain. Although initial pain relief was good, there was a tendency for pain to recur in 3 to 9 months, suggesting the possibility of nerve root recovery.

▶ Analysis of long-term benefits of neurodestructive lesions for nonmalignant pain invariably demonstrates sharp declines in benefit over a period of months. Unless we find better ways of predicting which small subset is likely to have persistent benefits, we should probably think twice about utilizing such techniques. However, this might be a very helpful technique for patients with severe cancer pain in a radicular distribution.—S.E. Abram, M.D.

How Frequent Is Anesthesia Dolorosa Following Spinal Posterior Rhizotomy? A Retrospective Analysis of Fifteen Patients

Pagni CA, Lanotte M, Canavero S (Univ of Turin, Italy; CTO Hosp, Turin, Italy)
Pain 54:323–327, 1993   101-94-24–35

Background.—Anesthesia dolorosa (AD) is characterized by constant unpleasant sensations localized to areas of skin and mucous membrane with pronounced loss of sensibility. It has been suggested that this condition is an infrequent complication after spinal posterior rhizotomy. Data on all patients who underwent rhizotomy at one institution between 1962 and 1972 were reviewed to determine the incidence of AD.

Patients and Findings.—Fifteen patients aged 20–76 years, had undergone multiple rhizotomy for chronic, unrelenting nondeafferentative neoplastic and nonneoplastic pain. Thirteen patients had cancer and 2 had non-neoplastic conditions. Eight patients, 53% of the study sample, had a typical deafferentation pain (AD) 1.5 to 8 months after rhizotomy. One of the 6 remaining patients died after 6 days; 3 with brain metastasis remained pain free; and 2 with rectal cancer did not have AD during follow-up of 2–15 months.

Conclusion.—Although rhizotomy is still advocated by some, this center no longer performs this operation because of the high incidence of AD. Because AD may trigger worse pain than that experienced before rhizotomy, this procedure should be considered high-risk surgery.

▶ Our present level of understanding of dorsal horn neurophysiology provides an explanation of the high failure rates for rhizotomy. Fortunately, most centers have given up this technique except in the most unusual circumstances.—S.E. Abram, M.D.

Grand Mal Seizures Associated With High-Dose Intravenous Morphine Infusions: Incidence and Possible Etiology

Gregory RE, Grossman S, Sheidler VR (Johns Hopkins Univ, Baltimore, Md)
Pain 51:255–258, 1992   101-94-24–36

Background.—High doses of continuous infusion (CI) intravenous opiates are important in treating severe pain in patients with cancer. Generalized seizures recently occurring in 2 patients receiving high-dose intravenous morphine by CI prompted a retrospective review of toxicities related to this treatment.

Methods and Findings.—Seven years of pharmacy records at 1 oncology center were reviewed retrospectively. In that time, 6 patients received more than 4 g of morphine sulfate per day by CI. Three patients were given high-dose infusions for longer than 24 hours, 2 of whom had grand mal seizures. The third patient was receiving a neuromuscular blocking agent that made detection of seizures difficult. The development of seizures may be attributable to prolonged administration of high concentrations of the sodium bisulfite preservative in the morphine solution.

Conclusion.—Prolonged intravenous infusions of high-dose morphine may place patients at risk for seizures. In this series, 2 of 3 patients given more than 4 g/day of intravenous morphine sulfate for more than 24 hours had grand mal seizures after 46 and 62 hours of therapy, respectively. Caution should be used when high-dose, preservative-containing morphine is given in a continuous infusion.

▶ The concept of limitless escalation of systemic opioid dose in cancer patients is bringing us to the threshold of some new complications (see Abstract 101-94-24–65). The concept of beneficial drug interactions is an important one to explore in our efforts to reduce the incidence of such problems.—S.E. Abram, M.D.

Neuropathic Pain/Chronic Pain

Successful Treatment for Phantom Pain

Davis RW (Pain Review, Inc, Colorado Springs, Colo)
Orthopedics 16:691–695, 1993   101-94-24–37

Introduction.—Phantom pain usually refers to pain perceived in a missing body part, whereas deafferentation pain occurs despite total anesthesia of the affected area. Treatment of these pain syndromes is often difficult and incomplete. Data on a series of patients with phantom pain were reviewed.

Methods.—Thirty-one of 47 consecutive patients seen at an amputee clinic reported having phantom pain. Most of these patients also had phantom sensation (91%) and nearly half had stump pain (43%). In an open-label study, each patient received mexiletine orally, 150 mg per day, initially. The dose was gradually increased every 3 or 4 days until side effects appeared, a plateau of pain relief was reached, or there was no change after reaching a maximum dose of 900 mg/day. Thirteen patients who did not benefit from mexiletine alone also used a clonidine TTS-1 patch. Pain relief was evaluated by a visual analogue scale (VAS) and a verbal pain report at 2, 4, 6, and 12 months.

Results.—The patient group had an average age of 62.1 years and a male-female ratio of 2.1:1. The ratio of above-knee to below-knee amputation was 7.7:1. Twelve patients had excellent results, with a mean decrease in their VAS score of 7.8 points. Six patients with a mean decline in their VAS score of 4.75 points were judged to have a good result. The decline in VAS scores for these groups was significant. The remaining 13 patients had a mean decrease of only 1.82 points, which was not statistically significant. Eleven of these patients subsequently achieved excellent results with the addition of a clonidine TTS-1 patch to mexiletine. Responders had retained their low VAS scores at 1-year follow-up. Three patients discontinued mexiletine after 1 year because of nausea.

Conclusion.—Mexiletine may be safe and effective in treating phantom pain, deafferentation pain, spinal cord injury pain, and nerve root avulsion. The drug, a congener of lidocaine, works primarily by blocking fast sodium channels. After amputation, activation of the wide dynamic range neurons found in the dorsal horn results in excessive calcium leakage. Clonidine, an alpha-2 agonist, relieves phantom pain only in combination with mexiletine.

▶ The dramatic benefits associated with mexiletine treatment in this series must be accepted with caution. There were no controls, and there was no mention of the duration of pain in these patients. If many of the patients were recent amputees, spontaneous resolution of pain would be a likely possibility.—S.E. Abram, M.D.

Reduced Pain-Related Behavior by Adrenal Medullary Transplants in Rats With Experimental Painful Peripheral Neuropathy

Hama AT, Sagen J (Univ of Illinois, Chicago)
Pain 52:223–231, 1993   101-94-24-38

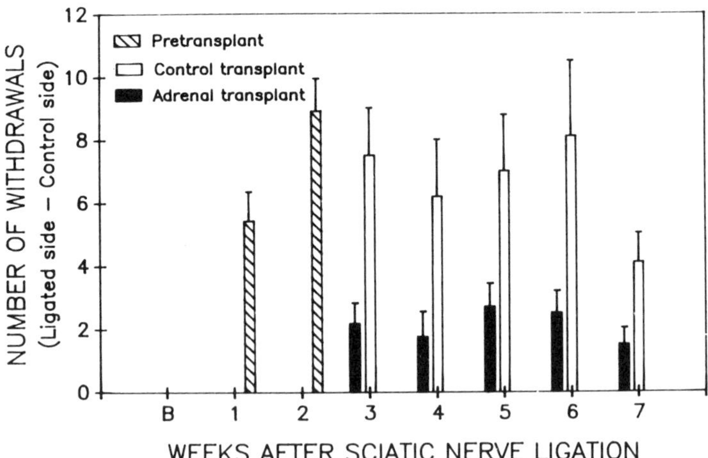

Fig 24–10.—Changes in degree of thermal allodynia with time after peripheral nerve injury as assessed by the number of hind paw withdrawals on a cold copper plate (5°C). The abscissa is time (weeks) after unilateral sciatic nerve ligation. *B* represents pre–nerve injury baseline scores, which were 0, indicating no difference between right and left paw withdrawals before ligation. Control striated muscle or adrenal medullary transplants were given 2 weeks after nerve ligation. Difference scores were calculated by subtracting left hind paw (control side) scores from right hind paw (nerve-injured side) scores. Each determination represents the mean ± SEM; $n = 8$–9 animals per transplant group. (Courtesy of Hama AT, Sagen J: *Pain* 52:223–231, 1993.)

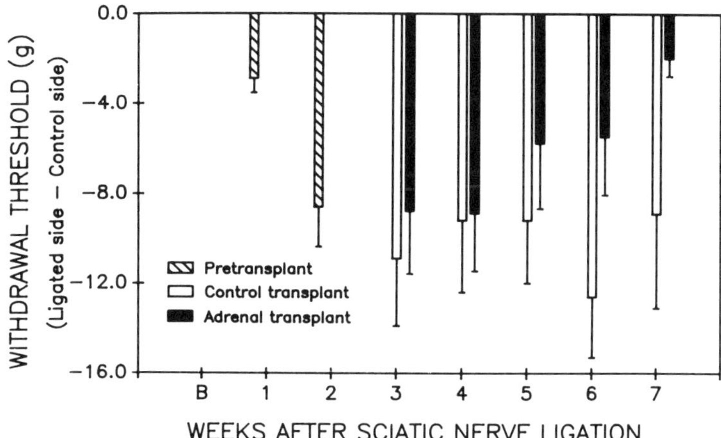

Fig 24–11.—Changes in degree of tactile allodynia with time after peripheral nerve injury as assessed by calibrated von Frey hairs directed at the rat's hind paw midplantar skin. The weight at which the rat's paw lifted was recorded at threshold (g). Withdrawal difference scores (mean ± SEM) were calculated by subtracting left hind paw (control side) thresholds from right hind paw (nerve-injured side) thresholds. Control striated or adrenal medullary tissue transplants were given 2 weeks after unilateral sciatic nerve ligation. *B*, baseline difference scores before nerve ligation. Each determination represents the mean ± SEM; *n* = 8-9 animals per transplant group. (Courtesy of Hama AT, Sagen J: *Pain* 52:223–231, 1993.)

Background.—Previous animal studies have shown that transplanting adrenal medullary tissue into the spinal subarachnoid space can reduce nociception to several types of noxious stimuli. These transplants, which work by providing a continual source of opioid peptides and catecholamines, could play an important adjunctive role in the management of chronic pain. However, their efficacy must first be demonstrated in long-term and abnormal pain syndromes.

Methods.—A new model of peripheral neuropathy in rats was used to evaluate the effects of transplanting adrenal medullary chromaffin cells into the subarachnoid space. Anesthetized adult Sprague-Dawley rats underwent unilateral chronic constriction injury of the right common sciatic nerve at the mid-thigh. Injury was followed 2 weeks later by adrenal medullary or control striated muscle transplants to the subarachnoid space at the level of the lumbar enlargement. Before and 7 weeks after nerve injury, the animals were subjected to behavioral testing, including cold and tactile allodynia and thermal hyperalgesia.

Results.—The peripheral nerve procedure was followed by eversion of the injured hind paw with ventroflexion and adduction of the toes. The rats appeared to guard the paw while stationary or asleep and walked with a limp. Guarding appeared reduced and mobility better in animals receiving adrenal transplants. Response to cold allodynia increased significantly after nerve injury but decreased significantly in animals receiving adrenal medullary transplants (Fig 24–10). In the tactile allodynia test, between-group scores were only slightly lower in animals receiving

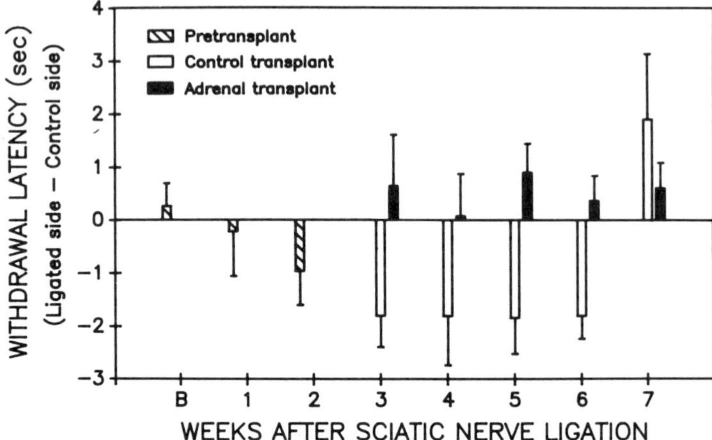

Fig 24–12.—Changes in degree of thermal hyperalgesia with time after peripheral nerve injury as assessed by measurement of the animal's response to a radiant heat source aimed at the hind paw planter skin. Hind paw withdrawal latency difference scores (mean ± SEM) were calculated by subtracting left hind paw (control side) latencies from right hind paw (nerve-injured side) latencies. Baseline differences scores before nerve ligation are shown at *B*. Control striated muscle or adrenal medullary transplants were given 2 weeks after ligation. Each determination represents the mean ± SEM; n = 8–9 animals per transplant group. (Courtesy of Hama AT, Sagen J: *Pain* 52:223-231, 1993.)

adrenal medullary tissue (Fig 24–11). Hyperalgesia completely resolved in the active treatment group, with withdrawal latencies returning to baseline by 1 week after adrenal medullary transplantation (Fig 24–12).

Conclusion.—Adrenal medullary transplants into the subarachnoid space can effectively reduce neuropathic pain in rats. Significant reductions are noted in allodynia and hyperalgesia, as well as in spontaneous pain-related behavior. If it could be applied clinically, this novel treatment would avoid the need for frequent drug injections in patients with neuropathic pain.

▶ This study provided some of the animal data that set the stage for a limited human study that appeared in the fall of 1993 (1). This novel approach raises many more questions than it answers, such as, How long will the implanted cells function? Will tolerance develop to the neurotransmitters they produce? What is the appropriate "dose" of implanted cells? The approach to determining whether this procedure is effective in humans is far from simple (2).—S.E. Abram, M.D.

References

1. Winnie AP, et al: *Anesthesiology* 79:644, 1993.
2. Yaksh TL, Foley KM: *Anesthesiology* 79:637, 1993.

Morphine Injected Around the Stellate Ganglion Does Not Modulate the Sympathetic Nervous System Nor Does it Provide Pain Relief

Glynn C, Casale R (Churchill Hosp, Oxford, England; Clinicia del Lavoro, Pavia, Italy)
Pain 53:33–37, 1993

101-94-24-39

Background.—For several decades, the stellate ganglion block (SGB) with local anesthetics has been used in the diagnosis and treatment of pain mediated by the sympathetic nervous system. It has been suggested that SGB using morphine would provide longer-lasting relief of pain than local anesthetics, but there has been no neurophysiologic evidence to support this idea.

Methods.—In a pilot study, the effects of SGB using morphine and bupivacaine were compared in 7 patients with pain believed to involve the sympathetic nervous system. All patients received stellate ganglion injection with both drugs, first 10 mL of .5% bupivacaine and, at least 1 week later, 5 mg of morphine in 10 mL of saline. Sympathetic activity was assessed by the sympathetic skin response (SSR) (based on a change in the electric potential of the skin), the inspiratory gasping response (IGR) (electric response to a deep inspiration), finger plethysmography, and clinical assessment. All measures were recorded bilaterally, thus providing a control response in the untreated extremity.

Results.—With bupivacaine injection the IGR and SSR were abolished in all patients in the treated extremity but not in the untreated extremity. The amplitude of finger plethysmography increased in the treated extremity, and all patients had Horner's syndrome on the side of the injection. Complete pain relief was obtained for as long as 24 hours in 4 patients. With morphine injection, however, there was no evidence of sympathetic modulation in either extremity in any patient. No analgesic effect was shown in any of the patients.

Conclusion.—Morphine is not an appropriate drug for SGB in patients with pain mediated by the sympathetic nervous system. It neither modulates sympathetic activity nor provides pain relief. Designing a confirmatory placebo-controlled study would be problematic, especially from an ethical standpoint.

▶ Much work remains to be done in defining the role of opioid receptors located outside the neuraxis in modulation pain perception.—S.E. Abram, M.D.

Painful Neuropathy: Altered Central Processing Maintained Dynamically by Peripheral Input

Gracely RH, Lynch SA, Bennett GJ (Natl Inst of Dental Research, Bethesda, Md)
Pain 51:175–194, 1992

101-94-24–40

Introduction.—In many patients with painful peripheral neuropathies, lightly touching or brushing the skin will evoke intense pain; this situation is known as mechano-allodynia. Increasing evidence suggests that allodynia is mediated by input from large-diameter, rapidly conducting $A\beta$ low-threshold mechanoreceptor ($A\beta$ LTM) primary afferents, implicating a central process in which the subject perceives input from these afferents as pain.

Methods and Results.—The results of sensory assessments before and during diagnostic tourniquet-cuff and local anesthetic block in 4 patients with reflex sympathetic dystrophy and mechano-allodynia were reported. All 4 patients perceived electric stimuli as painful at detection levels, suggesting $A\beta$ LTM mediation of mechano-allodynia. Reaction time latencies to painful electrical stimuli at the threshold for A-fiber activation supported this conclusion. In 1 case, differential cuff blocks abolished $A\beta$ function and allodynia with no effect on thermal sensation. When local anesthetic blocks were administered to painful foci associated with previous trauma, mechano-allodynia, cold allodynia, and spontaneous pain were abolished in all patients. In 1 case, local anesthetic block relieved tonic contractures of the toes. All symptoms returned as the local anesthetic block declined.

Discussion.—A new model of neuropathic pain is proposed: Nociceptive afferent input from a peripheral focus maintains the altered central processing that accounts for allodynia and other sensory and motor abnormalities. The central processing returns to normal when the peripheral input—which can be independent of sympathetic activity or determined completely or partly by sympathetic efferent activity or circulating catecholamines—is blocked. Thus, the model also accounts for sympathetically maintained and sympathetically independent pain, which may share a common final pathway.

▶ This study deserves reading in detail, as does an earlier hypothesis of the role of large afferents in the pathophysiology of neuropathic pain (1).—S.E. Abram, M.D.

Reference

1. Roberts WJ: *Pain* 24:297, 1986.

The Role of Peripheral Sudomotor Blockade in the Treatment of Patients With Sympathetically Maintained Pain

Glynn CJ, Stannard C, Collins PA, Casale R (Churchill Hosp, Headington, England; Rehabilitation Ctr of Montescano, Italy)
Pain 53:39–42, 1993　　　　　　　　　　　　　　　　　　　101-94-24-41

Purpose.—Bier's block with guanethidine has long been used as a treatment for patients with sympathetically maintained pain (SMP). Although this treatment acts mainly on the vasomotor components of the sympathetic nervous system, the sudomotor component may also play a role in the initiation and maintenance of SMP. Acetylcholine governs sudomotor function, and increased cholinergic activity may be related to the pain of SMP. The role of the peripheral cholinergic blockade using Bier's block with atropine in the treatment of SMP was studied.

Methods.—The subjects were 33 patients with a confirmed clinical diagnosis of SMP. They were randomized to receive Bier's block with either .6 mg of atropine in 10 mL of saline or 10 mL of saline only in double-blind fashion. Patients received the other injection 7 days later if pain relief was inadequate or when pain returned. Pain intensity, pain relief, and mood were evaluated by a visual analogue scale, and pain intensity was also measured by a categorical scale.

Results.—The 2 treatments were no different in their initial effects on any of the 3 parameters. During the week after injection, the atropine group consistently reported less pain and more pain relief, but the difference was nonsignificant. No patient preference could be confirmed for either treatment.

Conclusion.—There was no significant difference in pain relief for patients with SMP who received Bier's block with atropine vs. those receiving placebo. Thus, the cholinergic component of the peripheral sympathetic nervous system does not appear to play an important role in the initiation or maintenance of SMP.

▶ The role of sympathetic cholinergics in the pathophysiology of SMP seemed unlikely, but this study was needed to assure their lack of importance.—S.E. Abram, M.D.

Local Anesthetic-Induced Conduction Block and Nerve Fiber Injury in Streptozotocin-Diabetic Rats

Kalichman MW, Calcutt NA (Univ of California, San Diego)
Anesthesiology 77:941–947, 1992　　　　　　　　　　　　　　　101-94-24-42

Background.—The presence of peripheral neuropathy in diabetic patients may have clinical implications regarding the use of regional nerve block. Local anesthetic–induced conduction block and nerve fiber injury were studied in streptozotocin-diabetic rats.

Methods.—The effects of local anesthetics on nerve conduction and nerve fiber injury were assessed in control rats and experimental rats 4 weeks after the onset of diabetes induced by streptozotocin injection. Evoked electrical activity in hindpaw muscles was recorded after ipsilateral electrical stimulation of the sciatic nerve near the hip to assess nerve conduction. Motor nerve conduction block was quantified by recording the amplitude of the evoked response at 1-minute intervals for as long as 15 minutes after lidocaine or procaine injection in the midthigh next to the sciatic nerve.

Findings.—Procaine was much less effective than lidocaine in producing conduction block in control rats. The rate and magnitude of lidocaine-induced conduction block did not differ significantly between control and diabetic animals. However, procaine-induced conduction block was sufficiently enhanced in diabetic animals to become comparable to that of lidocaine-treated control nerves. In both control and diabetic nerves, lidocaine induced edema. However, 4% lidocaine induced significantly more edema in diabetic nerves than in control nerves. Nerve fiber injury did not occur in saline-treated nerves. Injury, evident in all lidocaine groups, was significantly increased in lidocaine-treated diabetic nerves compared with lidocaine-treated control nerves.

Conclusion.—The local anesthetic requirement is reduced in diabetes. A dose reduction may be necessary in diabetic patients to prevent nerve injury caused by standard doses.

▶ Diabetic patients are particularly susceptible to mechanical nerve injury. This study suggests that they may be more susceptible to local anesthetic–induced nerve dysfunction. Perhaps high concentrations of local anesthetics for spinal analgesia, e.g., 5% lidocaine, should be used with particular caution in such patients.—S.E. Abram, M.D.

The Safety of Intravenous Phentolamine Administration in Patients With Neuropathic Pain
Shir Y, Cameron LB, Raja SN, Bourke DL (Johns Hopkins Hosp, Baltimore, Md)
Anesth Analg 76:1008–1011, 1993   101-94-24–43

Background.—Sympathetically maintained pain (SMP) syndromes are chronic pain states dependent on sympathetic efferent function. Conventionally, SMP is diagnosed by local anesthetic block of the appropriate sympathetic ganglia. Regional intravenous block also has been used to diagnose and treat SMP syndrome, but, like local block, it has disadvantages including false-negative results and problems in identifying placebo responders. Peripheral α-adrenergic receptors may have a role in SMP.

Methods.—In this institution, patients suspected of having SMP have received 25–75 mg of phentolamine intravenously over 20 minutes. Patients are pretreated with intravenous fluids, and usually with 1–2 mg of propranolol as well, 10 minutes before the start of phentolamine infusion. In this retrospective study of 100 consecutive patients with chronic pain, given a dose of phentolamine usually at 35 mg, the safety of the test was evaluated.

Results.—No major complications occurred during or after the test. Changes in arterial pressure and heart rate were limited. Mild nasal stuffiness was a consistent observation, but oxygen saturation did not decline. Five patients had minor effects such as sinus tachycardia, premature ventricular beats, dizziness, or wheezing that resolved spontaneously.

Conclusion.—Intravenous phentolamine administration is a safe procedure for patients with neuropathic pain.

▶ Although the safety of this technique has been confirmed, its utility has not. If one makes a diagnosis of SMP on the basis of this diagnostic procedure, what are the therapeutic implications? Will oral sympatholytic agents be helpful? What about local anesthetic sympathetic blocks, sympathectomy, or prolonged epidural analgesia? Outcome studies are still needed to answer these questions. It would also be interesting to study the relationship between the results of this test and those of a 3-phase bone scan and thermography.—S.E. Abram, M.D.

Dose-Response for Analgesic Effect of Amitriptyline in Chronic Pain
McQuay HJ, Carroll D, Glynn CJ (Churchill Hosp, Oxford)
Anaesthesia 48:281–285, 1993   101-94-24-44

Introduction.—Antidepressants are effective in treating a variety of chronic pain syndromes, although the mechanism by which these drugs exert an analgesic action is unclear. The dose-response curve for analgesia in chronic pain is reportedly shifted to the left of the dose-response curve for depression. Whether a dose-response for amitriptyline occurred when given for chronic pain was determined.

Methods.—Three oral doses (25, 50, and 75 mg) of amitriptyline were compared in a double-blind, randomized, crossover study. There were 3 treatment periods of 3 weeks each and no washout period. Eligible patients were adults with chronic nonmalignant pain of more than 2 months' duration who had already taken antidepressants or for whom antidepressants were to be prescribed. The patients measured their daily pain intensity on a 4-point scale and were interviewed at the clinic after each of the 3 treatment periods.

Results.—Twenty-nine patients entered the study. One was withdrawn before analysis, 2 withdrew during the first week of treatment, and 8 other patients did not complete the full 9 weeks because of adverse effects or inadequate relief. Global scores did not differ significantly for the 3 doses for any week of treatment. The mean daily pain relief as recorded by patients was significantly higher with 75 mg of amitriptyline compared with 25 mg for the first and third weeks of treatment. Overall, amitriptyline at 75 mg provided significantly greater efficacy than did the lower doses of the drug. The 75-mg dose also produced a significantly higher incidence of adverse effects, primarily dry mouth and drowsiness.

Conclusion.—Even with a limited dose range, the analgesic effect of amitriptyline in chronic pain had a dose-response relationship, which was shown clearly when daily pain relief scores were compared within-patient. Although there was a dose-response relationship for the incidence of adverse effects, the dose response was unrelated to mood elevation.

▶ As with other pharmacologic interventions, the dose of tricyclic antidepressants should be titrated to optimize analgesic effect within the range of tolerable side effects. Unfortunately, many physicians give up on these agents because inadequate time is alotted for trials, which may require 2 to 3 weeks at a given dose.—S.E. Abram, M.D.

The Effect of Low-Level Laser Therapy on Musculoskeletal Pain: A Meta-Analysis
Gam AN, Thorsen H, Lønnberg F (Bispebjerg Hosp, Copenhagen; Univ of Copenhagen; Danish Inst of Clinical Epidemiology, Copenhagen)
Pain 52:63–66, 1993								101-94-24–45

Background.—Low-level laser therapy (LLLT) has been used to treat many musculoskeletal pain syndromes in clinical studies since the early 1970s. However, there has been no scientific evidence to show that laser light at the applied intensity and wave length can penetrate deeper structures, and the quality of many of the published clinical trials evaluating the effect of LLLT has been criticized.

Study Design.—A meta-analysis was conducted of published studies on the effect of LLLT on musculoskeletal pain. A Medline search was used to identify pertinent articles published before November 1, 1991.

Results.—A total of 23 LLLT trials were identified, 17 of which were controlled studies. Ten were double-blind and 7 were insufficiently blinded. Pain was evaluated by using a visual analogue scale or another pain index. In 9 of the double-blind trials and 4 of the controlled studies, the results were reported in a manner which allowed pooling of data. The mean difference in pain between LLLT and placebo was .3% in the double-blind studies. In the insufficiently blinded studies, the mean difference in pain was 9.5%.

Conclusion.—The primary indication for LLLT was pain reduction. Accordingly, 95% of the reviewed studies included a pain index completed by the patient. Results from this meta-analysis indicate that LLLT does not reduce musculoskeletal pain, yet it is a widely used treatment. Before accepting a new form of equipment for therapy, the physician and therapist should have the manufacturer demonstrate its effect, as is the case before introducing new pharmaceutical preparations.

▶ Here is an example of a new technology looking for a new application. The authors suggested that we seek substantiation of effect from the manufacturer before acceptance of new devices. I disagree. Manufacturers provide us with a great deal of substantiating material, much of it flawed. It is up to us to do the appropriate studies, such as this one, *without manufacturers' support,* and to make those data available to our colleagues.—S.E. Abram, M.D.

Relationship of Sexual and Physical Abuse to Pain and Psychological Assessment Variables in Chronic Pelvic Pain Patients
Toomey TC, Hernandez JT, Gittelman DF, Hulka JF (Univ of North Carolina, Chapel Hill)
Pain 53:105–109, 1993   101-94-24-46

Objective.—Mounting evidence suggests that chronic pain syndromes may be related to a history of physical or sexual abuse, or both. The association is particularly strong for patients with pelvic or abdominal pain, or both. However, there are few data on the effects of abuse on pain or psychosocial variables. The incidence of physical and sexual abuse was studied in patients at a chronic pelvic pain clinic, and the effects of sexual abuse on a series of pain and psychological variables were explored.

Methods.—The study sample comprised 36 women referred with chronic pelvic pain. Their average age was 30 years and the average duration of pain was 5 years. The patients were assessed for a history of abuse by using a reliable 6-item scale. Those considered to be sexually abused were then compared with the nonabused patients on 4 classes of variables potentially related to abuse: description of, functional impact of, others' response to, and psychosocial impact of pain.

Results.—Nineteen patients reported some form of physical or sexual abuse, with sexual abuse being more common. There were no differences between abused and nonabused patients in terms of demographics, pain description, or functional impact of pain. However, the abused patients had less perceived control over their lives, a higher punishing response to their pain, and more somatization and global distress.

Conclusion.—A high frequency of physical and sexual abuse among patients with chronic pelvic pain was suggested by this study. Psychosocial and psychological disturbance were more common among the abused patients, although they did not differ from nonabused patients in their descriptions of pain or reported interference with function. The physician and other health-care providers should be alert for opportunities to intervene in current or recent episodes of abuse.

▶ There has been a great deal of attention paid to issues of abuse history among chronic pain patients with facial or pelvic pain. A high incidence has been reported for both groups. However, a fairly high incidence of sexual and physical abuse is found in patients with other types of chronic pain as well, and the psychological issues associated with such a history often need to be addressed.—S.E. Abram, M.D.

Other Postoperative Pain

Intranasal Meperidine Titration for Postoperative Pain Relief
Striebel WH, Malewicz J, Hermanns K, Castello R (Free Univ of Berlin)
Anesth Analg 76:1047–1051, 1993   101-94-24–47

Introduction.—The intramuscular administration of opioids to relieve pain entails several pharmacokinetic problems. The slow onset of opioid action precludes individualized demand-adapted titration to minimize the risk of respiratory depression. Intranasal meperidine administration was evaluated in a prospective double-blind trial in 60 American Society

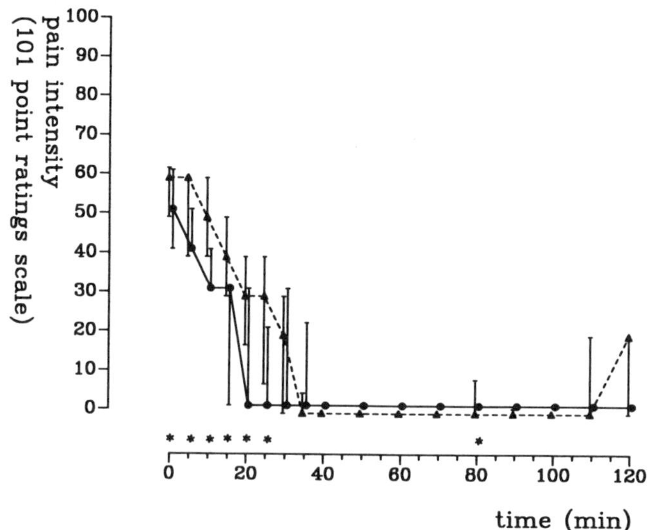

Fig 24–13.—Postoperative course of pain intensity evaluated by a 101-point numerical rating scale in the intravenous (*circles*) and nasal (*triangles*) group. *Significant intergroup difference, $P < .05$. (Courtesy of Striebel WH, Malewicz J, Hermanns K, et al: *Anesth Analg* 76:1047–1051, 1993.)

of Anesthesiologists physical status I and II women having vaginal or abdominal hysterectomy.

Methods.—After premedication with meperidine, promethazine, and atropine, general anesthesia was induced with fentanyl and thiopental and maintained with oxygen/nitrous oxide and isoflurane. Patients received meperidine by either intranasal spray or intravenous infusion, with physiologic saline used as a placebo for both routes of administration. The intranasal solution contained 4.5 mg of meperidine per .09 mL; the intravenous preparation contained 4.5 mg/mL.

Results.—Patients treated intravenously received a mean of 76.5 mg of meperidine, and those treated intranasally received 104.4 mg. Pain intensity was significantly lessened in both groups, but, at most intervals, pain scores were lower in the intravenously treated patients (Fig 24–13). Side effects did not differ significantly in the 2 groups.

Conclusion.—Demand-adapted titration of intranasal meperidine provides adequate and safe pain relief for women having hysterectomy in the early postoperative period.

▶ This technique has the advantage of rapid onset compared with transdermal systems and may be a reasonable alternative to intramuscular (IM) administration, particularly in children who undergo frequent painful interventions and have a phobia for needles. The study lasted only 2 hours, so it is difficult to assess the actual analgesic duration, but it is unlikely that it would last much beyond the 2-hour duration of IM meperidine. Because of the potential for toxic metabolite accumulation, the technique probably has limited application for cancer pain, except as a supplement for breakthrough or incident pain.—S.E. Abram, M.D.

Sucralfate in Alleviating Post-Tonsillectomy Pain

Freeman SB, Markwell JK (Naval Hosp, Portsmouth, Va)
Laryngoscope 102:1242–1246, 1992   101-94-24–48

Background.—Pain after tonsillectomy is caused by inflammation, nerve irritation, and spasm of the exposed pharyngeal muscles. Severe throat pain, ear pain, and trismus do not subside until the exposed and inflamed muscles are covered with regenerated mucosa. Sucralfate binds with the fibrinous exudate of duodenal ulcers, forming a protective barrier that promotes healing. Whether sucralfate would form a similar barrier in the tonsillar bed and reduce painful irritation and muscle spasm and promote healing was investigated.

Study Design.—In a double-blind, randomized study, 34 adult volunteers received, after tonsillectomy, either sucralfate or lactose solution to swish and swallow 4 times daily for 10 days. The average age of patients in both groups was 25 years.

Outcome.—Throat pain, otalgia, and trismus were significantly alleviated after surgery in patients using sucralfate, compared with those using placebo. The sucralfate group required significantly less pain medication immediately after surgery but subsequently showed only a trend toward using less narcotic. In addition, 62% of patients using sucralfate recovered half their strength the day after surgery and ate half their diet by the sixth day.

Conclusion.—Sucralfate substantially reduces the pain after tonsillectomy, hastens recovery, and may actually promote healing. It is well tolerated with minimal side effects.

▶ This is an innovative treatment that may have other applications, such as for painful oropharyngeal ulcers in patients with AIDS or cancer.—S.E. Abram, M.D.

Ventilatory Effects of Epidural Clonidine During the First 3 Hours After Caesarean Section

Narchi P, Benhamou D, Hamza J, Bouaziz H (Université Paris-Sud, Clamart, France)

Acta Anaesthesiol Scand 36:791–795, 1992   101-94-24-49

Background.—The use of epidural clonidine as an analgesic after cesarean section has recently been studied with higher doses at 400–800 µg. Prompted by concerns of the possibility of respiratory depression with as much as 300 µg of epidural or orally administered clonidine which could not be supported by other studies, the analgesic and ventilatory effects of 2 smaller doses of epidural clonidine after cesarean section were evaluated and compared with the effects of parenteral morphine.

Study Design.—In a randomized, double-blind study, 20 women who had elective cesarean section were assigned to 1 of 3 postoperative analgesic regimens. Seven patients received subcutaneous morphine, 10 mg, with epidural saline; 7 received epidural clonidine, 150 µg (EC150), and subcutaneous saline; and 6 received epidural clonidine, 300 µg (EC300), and subcutaneous saline. Arterial oxygen saturation, breathing pattern, and pain scored on the Visual Analogue Scale were monitored during the first 3 hours after cesarean section.

Outcome.—The duration of analgesia was significantly longer after EC150 (252 minutes), when compared with morphine (171 minutes), but it was not different from EC300 (233 minutes). The arterial blood pressure decreased significantly 30 minutes after injection in both epidural clonidine groups. Patients in the EC300 group were more sedated than those in the EC150 group. Furthermore, 6 episodes of severe oxygen desaturation occurred in 3 patients in the EC300 group, and these episodes were associated with a deep-sleep state, snoring, and episodes of obstructive sleep apnea.

Conclusion.—Epidural clonidine provides better and longer analgesia after cesarean section when compared with subcutaneous morphine. A dose of 150 μg of epidural clonidine is preferable to higher doses (300 μg), which are associated with unacceptable respiratory obstructive disturbances.

▶ Respiratory depression is not generally reported as a complication of epidural clonidine. This study reported the occurrence of respiratory depression with 300 μg but not 150 μg of epidural clonidine. The authors attributed this response to a central depressant effect. Another possibility is a decreased perfusion of respiratory centers because of hypotension. The latter explanation is difficult to document, as few data regarding blood pressure effect were reported.—S.E. Abram, M.D.

Neostigmine Counteracts Spinal Clonidine-Induced Hypotension in Sheep

Williams JS, Tong C, Eisenach JC (Wake Forest Univ, Winston-Salem, NC)
Anesthesiology 78:301–307, 1993   101-94-24-50

Background.—Intraspinal administration of clonidine produces analgesia without respiratory depression, but it also lowers the blood pressure and has a sedative effect. Spinal injection of neostigmine alone increases blood pressure in animals, and it enhances clonidine-induced analgesia. Reports of α_2-adrenergic–cholinergic interactions in spinal sensory processing indicate that combinations of these agents may produce better analgesia than α_2-adrenergic–opioid combinations while minimizing the risk of side effects. Unlike opioids, cholinergic agonists increase activity in the spinal preganglionic sympathetic nervous system, thereby increasing the blood pressure and heart rate.

Objective.—The effect of neostigmine on clonidine-induced hypotension was examined in chronically prepared sheep. They received intrathecal injections of neostigmine in doses of 150, 300, and 1,000 μg or saline, followed in 15 minutes by a 200-μg dose of clonidine.

Results.—Intrathecal clonidine lowered the mean arterial pressure and also produced minor reductions in heart rate and cardiac output. Hypotension was less evident after the higher doses of neostigmine. Neostigmine alone led to a prolonged increase in the mean arterial pressure (Fig 24–14). The protective effect of neostigmine was reduced by the coadministration of methylatropine.

Discussion.—This and other studies indicate that both clonidine and neostigmine, given intrathecally, influence blood pressure and heart rate by actions within the spinal cord. The effect of local cholinesterase inhi-

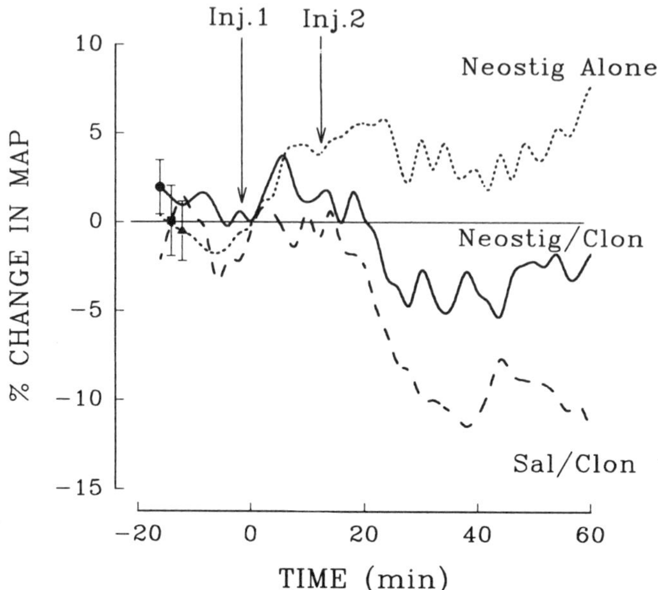

Fig 24–14.—Percentage change in mean arterial pressure after injection of 1,000 μg of neostigmine at time 0 (*dotted line*); saline at time 0 and clonidine at time 15 minutes (*dashed line*); and 1,000 μg of neostigmine at time 0 and clonidine at time 15 minutes (*solid line*). Time of injections is indicated by *arrows*. Pressure change is 0 at time of first injection. Each *line* represents the mean of 5–7 animals. Examples of individual data point's standard error of mean are shown for neostigmine-clonidine (*circles*), saline-clonidine (*squares*), and neostigmine alone (*triangle*). All 3 curves differ by 2-way analysis of variance ($P < .05$). Courtesy of Williams JS, Tong C, Eisenach JC: *Anesthesiology* 78:301–307, 1993.)

bition in increasing blood pressure and heart rate suggests that cholinergic systems must be tonically active.

▶ Although intrathecal neostigmine appears to complement the analgesic effect and offset the hypotensive effect of intrathecal clonidine, some disturbing side effects in rats, such as irritability and abnormal posturing (1), may be related to spinal nicotinic effects. No mention of behavioral abnormalities was made in this study. The mechanism by which cholinergic agonists produce analgesia is still unclear.—S.E. Abram, M.D.

Reference

1. Abram SE, Winne RP: Unpublished data.

Comparison of the Antinociceptive Effects of Pre- and Posttreatment With Intrathecal Morphine and MK801, an NMDA Antagonist, on the

Formalin Test in the Rat

Yamamoto T, Yaksh TL (Univ of California, San Diego)
Anesthesiology 77:757–763, 1992   101-94-24-51

Background.—Subcutaneous injection of small amounts of an irritant, such as formalin, produces an immediate, marked increase in the spontaneous activity of afferent C fibers. A prolonged small afferent input might evoke mechanisms that significantly potentiate spinal nociceptive processing.

Objective.—The behavioral correlates this form of spinal facilitation were investigated by studying the effects of intrathecal morphine, a μ-

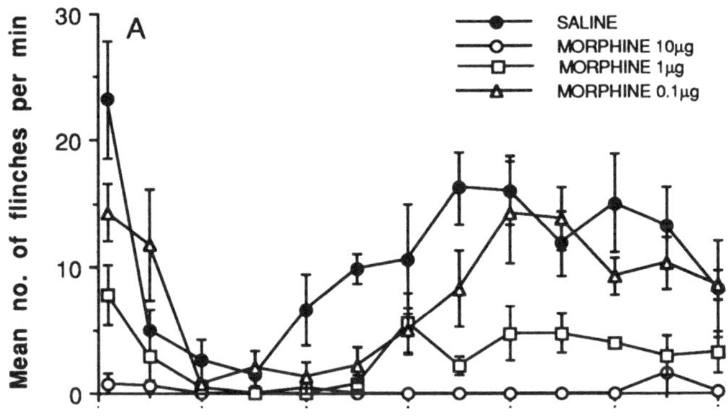

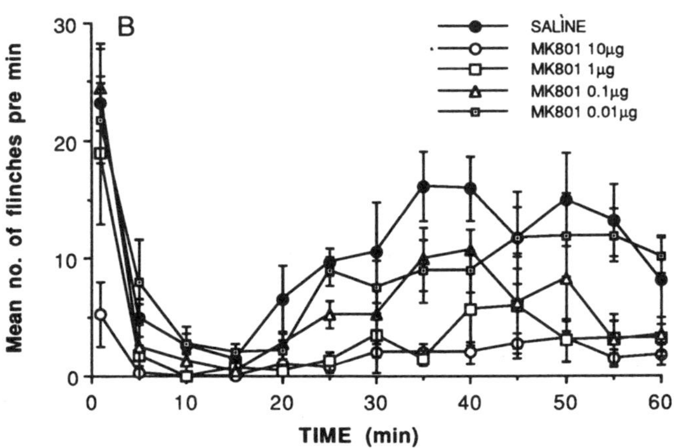

Fig 24–15.—Time-effect curve of morphine (**A**) and MK801 (**B**) before injections of formalin into right hind paw for number of flinches per minute observed after formalin. Each *line* represents the group mean and standard error of mean of 4-6 animals. Saline group is presented for comparison in both graphs. (Courtesy of Yamamoto T, Yaksh TL: *Anesthesiology* 77:757–763, 1992.)

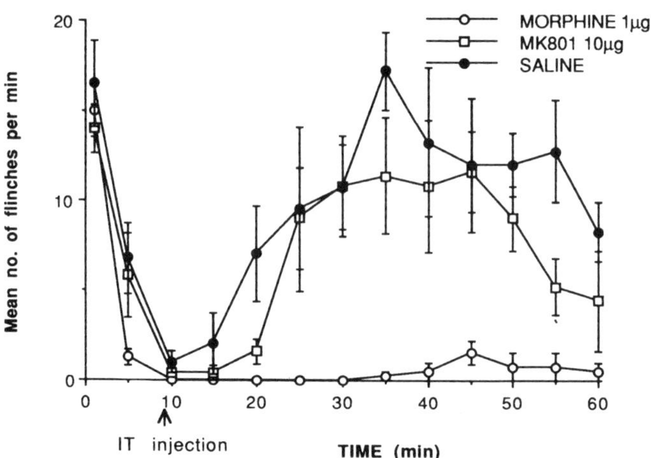

Fig 24–16.—Time-effect curve for number of flinches per minute observed after subcutaneous injection of formalin in right hind paw. As indicated, each *line* represents group mean and standard error of mean of 4–6 animals. Groups received MK801 or morphine 9 minutes after intrathecal injection of formalin. Mean phase 2 flinch per minute response: saline = MK801 > morphine; 1-way analysis of variance, $P < .05$. (Courtesy of Yamamoto T, Yaksh TL: *Anesthesiology* 77:757–763, 1992.)

opioid agonist, and MK-801, an N-methyl-D-aspartate (NMDA) antagonist, on the formalin test in male Sprague-Dawley rats.

Results.—Intraplantar injection of formalin led to biphasic flinching behavior in the first 5 minutes and again from 10 to 60 minutes after injection. Pretreatment with intrathecal morphine suppressed both phases of flinching behavior in a dose-dependent manner (Fig 24–15), and posttreatment with morphine suppressed the later response. Pretreatment with MK801 primarily inhibited the second-phase response, but posttreatment had no such effect at the highest intrathecal doses (Fig 24–16).

Interpretation.—A local irritant appears to exert a direct excitatory effect and evoke pain behavior that is independent of spinal NMDA sites but is subject to modulation by opioid. In a second-phase response, the acute afferent barrage upregulates the response to a stimulus that is already noxious. The NMDA sites are needed to initiate this facilitatory component but not to sustain it.

▶ The concept of providing a selective reduction in the sensitization of dorsal horn neurons without exerting a true analgesic effect is new and exciting. Unfortunately, many of the NMDA receptor antagonists, such as MK801, are phencyclidine derivatives and have undesirable psychic effects. This study did not show any difference between intrathecal morphine given before the noxious stimulus and that given afterward, suggesting a lack of preemptive effect on sensitization. A subsequent study from the same laboratory showed that intrathecal morphine administered before formalin, in anesthetized animals, blocked spinal sensitization despite naloxone reversal of analgesia shortly after the formalin injection (1).—S.E. Abram, M.D.

Reference

1. Abram SE, Yaksh TL: *Anesthesiology* 78:713, 1993.

Oral Transmucosal Fentanyl Citrate (OTFC) for the Treatment of Postoperative Pain

Ashburn MA, Lind GH, Gillie MH, de Boer AJF, Pace NL, Stanley TH (Univ of Utah, Salt Lake City)
Anesth Analg 76:377–381, 1993   101-94-24-52

Objective.—Oral transmucosal fentanyl citrate (OTFC) is useful in a variety of clinical situations, such as for preoperative medication in children and for analgesia in cancer patients. In a prospective study, its analgesic efficacy in patients with acute pain after major orthopedic surgery was examined.

Methods.—The subjects were 38 patients, American Society of Anesthesiologists (ASA) physical status I–III, undergoing total hip replacement or total knee arthroplasty. They were randomly assigned to receive either OTFC, 7–10 µg/kg, or placebo. All patients received general anesthesia for surgery and patient-controlled analgesia with morphine. The study drugs were given at 0, 4, and 8 hours during a 12-hour study.

Results.—Twenty-eight patients completed the study, with no significant differences between groups as to age, sex, ASA classification, or surgical procedure. No significant differences were noted in the number of patient-controlled analgesia attempts or delivered morphine dose before or after the study period. However, during the study period, the OTFC group had a significant decrease in morphine dose delivered compared with the control group (mean, 6 mg vs. 15 mg). There were no differences in side effects.

Conclusion.—Oral transmucosal fentanyl citrate can reduce the need for other analgesics in patients undergoing major orthopedic surgery; 1 mg of OTFC is as potent as 5 mg of intravenous morphine sulfate. The specific role of OTFC in the management of acute pain remains to be determined.

▶ Although OTFC appears to be a reasonable preoperative sedative/analgesic when administered to patients who can be monitored closely, it would not seem to be ideal for postoperative pain management because of its short duration, imprecise dosing, and potential for overdose. On the other hand, it might be a useful technique for supplementing transdermal fentanyl for cancer pain. However, the potential for disaster if children find these administration systems gives one pause when considering outpatient applications.—S.E. Abram, M.D.

A Randomized, Double-Blind Evaluation of Ketorolac Tromethamine for Postoperative Analgesia in Ambulatory Surgery Patients

Wong HY, Carpenter RL, Kopacz DJ, Fragen RJ, Thompson G, Maneatis TJ, Bynum LJ (Northwestern Univ, Chicago; Virginia Mason Clinic, Seattle; Syntex Labs Inc, Palo Alto, Calif)

Anesthesiology 78:6–14, 1993   101-94-24–53

Purpose.—More and more operations are being done on an ambulatory basis, raising new concerns about the provision of effective and safe analgesia. Despite their side effects, the opioid drugs are still the main form of postoperative analgesia. The new nonsteroidal anti-inflammatory drug ketorolac tromethamine, given intravenously then orally, was compared with fentanyl and oral codeine in ambulatory patients up to 1 week postoperatively.

Methods.—The randomized, double-blind, multidose-design study included 221 patients with moderate-to-severe pain after surgery. Patients in 1 group, designated K30, received 2 intravenous doses of 30 mg of ketorolac, followed by as many as 6 intravenous doses of 10 mg every 30 minutes as needed, then 10 mg orally every 4–6 hours. Another group, designated F50, received 50 μg of fentanyl intravenously at the same time intervals, followed by 60 mg of codeine and 600 mg of acetaminophen orally every 4–6 hours. The third group, designated F10, received the same combination of drugs as group F50 but only 10 μg of fentanyl per dose.

Results.—The analgesic effects of the intravenous portion of the K30 regimen were delayed but otherwise equivalent to those of the F50 regimen. Side effects were also similar. The side effects of nausea, somnolence, and delayed return of bowel function were less common with oral ketorolac than with codeine and acetaminophen. The 2 oral treatments were no different in pain relief, tolerability, quality of life, or psychological well-being.

Conclusion.—The K30 regimen appears to give safe and effective analgesia for patients undergoing ambulatory surgery. The onset of pain relief is slower than with fentanyl, but side effects are less common than with codeine plus acetaminophen. Further studies of intraoperative ketorolac are needed to address the issues of delayed onset of action, reduction of adverse effects during recovery, and the use of a more costly medication.

▶ Once again, ketorolac measures up well when compared with opioids for postoperative pain. It is not clear whether this drug is exceptional when compared with other nonsteroid anti-inflammatory drugs (NSAIDs), a difficult proposition since other NSAIDs are not available as injectables in the United States. Ketorolac's pharmacologic profile is one of relatively good analgesia and relatively weak anti-inflammatory effect, which may, indeed, make it an ideal drug for postoperative use.—S.E. Abram, M.D.

Quantitative Sensory Examination During Epidural Anaesthesia and Analgesia in Man: Effects of Morphine

Brennum J, Arendt-Nielsen L, Horn A, Secher NH, Jensen TS (Gentofte Hosp, Hellerup, Denmark; Aalborg Univ, Denmark; Rigshospitalet, København, Denmark; et al)

Pain 52:75–83, 1993   101-94-24-54

Background.—Morphine and other opiates have been shown to inhibit nociception in the spinal dorsal horn. Development of new, rationally based treatments for pain—including an understanding of why different types of pain can and cannot be treated with opiates—requires improved knowledge of the neurophysiologic mechanisms of opiate analgesia. Recently, improved psychophysical methods for quantification of somatosensory functions were used to examine the effects of epidural morphine in humans.

Methods.—The double-blind, placebo-controlled, crossover study included 10 healthy volunteers who received epidural morphine, 4 mg, or saline. Naloxone was given intravenously 180 minutes after epidural administration. Before and for 10 hours after administration, sensory detection, pain detection, and pain tolerance thresholds to thermal, mechanical, and electric stimuli were measured. Magnitude ratings of short-lasting stimuli of the same modalities were also carried out.

Results.—With morphine administration came a naloxone-reversible increase in the pain detection threshold to heat and mechanical stimuli. The pain tolerance threshold to heat and mechanical and electric stimuli increased as well. There was a more marked increase in pain tolerance than in pain detection threshold. Epidural morphine decreased the magnitude rating of a short-duration argon laser stimulus but had no significant effect on the magnitude rating of short-lasting mechanical and electric stimuli. Morphine also induced a naloxone-reversible increase in the warm-detection threshold. Most subjects reported a segmental pruritus after epidural morphine, which changed to a short-lasting burning sensation after naloxone. There was no change in somatosensory functions when a .1-mg dose of naloxone per kg was given before placebo.

Conclusion.—Epidural morphine causes differential increases in pain detection and tolerance thresholds, depending on the type and duration of the stimuli. The somatosensory effect of epidural morphine appears to be mediated by unmyelinated C afferents. Morphine may also decrease temporal facilitation of spinal cord neurons.

▶ This is an elegant example of how detailed clinical testing can provide insights into the mechanism of action of spinally administered opioids. More of this type of study is needed.—S.E. Abram, M.D.

The NMDA-Receptor Antagonist CPP Abolishes Neurogenic 'Wind-Up Pain' After Intrathecal Administration in Humans

Kristensen JD, Svensson B, Gordh T Jr (Univ Hosp, Uppsala, Sweden; Uppsala Univ, Sweden)
Pain 51:249–253, 1992　　　　　　　　　　　　　　　　　101-94-24-55

Introduction.—When neurogenic pain resulting from peripheral nerve injury becomes chronic in nature, conventional treatment is often ineffective. The pathophysiologic background of such pain conditions may involve central sensitization and a wind-up phenomenon at the spinal or supraspinal level. There is currently an interest in drugs affecting the N-methyl-D-aspartate (NMDA)–receptor system. A patient with a severe and intractable pain condition was benefited by administration of the NMDA-receptor antagonist 3-(2-carboxypiperazin-4-yl)propyl-1-phosphonic acid (CPP). A previous study showed that CPP can prevent establishment of central sensitization.

Case Report.—Woman, 51, had undergone several operations for varicose veins in her left leg. She subsequently had a severe and intractable neuralgia in the left thigh, probably attributable to injury of the anterior cutaneous branches of the femoral nerve. The pain syndrome consisted of a continuous deep pain, an allodynia, and a wind-up–like component. The deep pain component and allodynia were unchanged after intrathecal administration of 200 nmol of CPP, but the wind-up phenomenon was abolished. Pain relief was not improved by another 500 nmol of CPP administered over 2 hours. The patient's blood pressure, heart rate, sensitivity, and reflexes were not affected by CPP, but she did experience marked anxiety for a short period after the treatment.

Conclusion.—Use of the NMDA-receptor antagonist CPP in a patient with neuropathic pain blocked the spread of pain outside the area of the injured nerve. The following wind-up phenomenon with afterdischarge and radiation to the left side of her body were completely abolished. Outcome in this case supports the theory that the NMDA-receptor antagonists influence only pathologic pain transmission. The psychotomimetic ketamine-like side effects of CPP were probably the result of the rostral spread of the agent.

▶ Other than a few studies done with ketamine, a relatively nonspecific NMDA antagonist, this is the first such study done in humans. The possibilities are exciting, but we will need to find agents without appreciable psychotomimetic effects.—S.E. Abram, M.D.

Redistribution of Sufentanil to Cerebrospinal Fluid and Systemic Circulation After Epidural Administration in Dogs

Stevens RA, Petty RH, Hill HF, Kao T-C, Schaffer R, Hahn MB, Harris P (Med College of Wisconsin, Milwaukee; Uniformed Services Univ of the Health

Sciences, Bethesda, Md; Fred Hutchinson Cancer Research Ctr, Seattle)
Anesth Analg 76:323–327, 1993   101-94-24–56

Introduction.—Sufentanil, a highly lipophilic opioid, is thought to be less likely than morphine to migrate rostally in the CSF, a cause of respiratory depression after epidural administration. However, early respiratory depression, attributed to systemic drug uptake, has been reported after large doses of epidural sufentanil. The pharmacokinetics of sufentanil in the lumbar and cisternal CSF and in plasma were studied.

Methods.—Experiments were performed in 6 female mongrel dogs. Sampling catheters were placed in the lumbar subarachnoid space, cisterna magna, and femoral arteries. Each animal received 50 μg of sufentanil via epidural catheter. Samples of cisternal CSF, lumbar CSF, and blood were drawn at 0, 1, 5, 15, 30, 60, 90, 120, and 180 minutes after sufentanil injection. Drug concentrations were measured by gas chromatography–mass spectrometry.

Results.—At each sampling time, sufentanil concentrations in lumbar CSF were significantly greater than in plasma or cisternal CSF. Mean cisternal CSF concentrations were significantly greater than mean plasma concentrations at 30 and 60 minutes after epidural administration. Sufentanil appeared rapidly in lumbar CSF; a maximum concentration of 57 ng/mL was reached at 6.5 minutes. Corresponding findings for cisternal CSF and plasma were 1.2 ng/mL at 21 minutes and .35 ng/mL at 6 minutes, respectively. The area under the concentration-time curve of sufentanil in cisternal CSF was approximately 6 times higher than the corresponding value for plasma. The amount of sufentanil reaching the lumbar CSF was about 140 times that reaching plasma, whereas the sufentanil reaching cisternal CSF was only 5% of that reaching lumbar CSF. All of these differences were significant.

Conclusion.—The absence of a rostral spread of lipophilic opioids in the CSF after lumbar epidural injection was not confirmed. Thus, sufentanil may not be safer than morphine for epidural analgesia. Small patient-controlled doses of epidural sufentanil may be the preferred way to administer this drug.

▶ One should be cautious in extrapolating these dog data to humans, because CSF volumes and circulation may not be comparable, and there is considerable difference in the physical properties of canine and human dura (1). The authors' suggestion of limiting epidural sufentanil administration to small patient-controlled doses may reduce the likelihood of delayed respiratory depression, but there is growing evidence that such administration may not be appreciably more effective than intravenous patient-controlled analgesia administration.—S.E. Abram, M.D.

Reference

1.   Patin DJ, et al: *Anesth Analg* 76:535, 1993.

Comparison of Intrathecal Fentanyl Infusion With Intrathecal Morphine Infusion or Bolus for Postoperative Pain Relief After Hip Arthroplasty

Niemi L, Pitkänen MT, Tuominen MK, Rosenberg PH (Helsinki Univ, Central Hosp)

Anesth Analg 77:126–130, 1993   101-94-24-57

Objective.—Good postoperative analgesia can be achieved through intrathecal administration of opioid. Morphine achieves good relief of pain, but complications such as pruritus, vomiting, somnolence, and even late respiratory depression occur. Fentanyl plus bupivacaine is also effective but relatively short lasting. Continuous infusion may avoid side effects in many patients. In a double-blind, randomized study, intrathecal infusion of fentanyl was compared with intrathecal administration of morphine, given as a continuous infusion or bolus, for postoperative analgesia in 60 patients undergoing hip joint replacement.

Methods.—In 11 patients, a 28- or 22-gauge spinal catheter was introduced through the L3-4 interspace and 3-4 cm into the subarachnoid space. After induction of spinal anesthesia with 2mL of plain .5% bupivacaine, with additional bupivacaine in .5-mL increments as needed, the patients were randomized into 3 groups of 20. Group I patients received .5 mL of saline followed by infusion of fentanyl, 120 μg over 24 hours. Group II patients received .5 mL of saline followed by infusion of morphine, 200 μg over 24 hours. Group III subjects received morphine, 200 μg as a single bolus, followed by a 3-mL infusion of saline over 24 hours. Oxycodone was given for postoperative pain at the operation site and ketoprofen was used for pain elsewhere in the body.

Results.—Group II and III patients obtained good postoperative analgesia, but nearly all patients in group I required additional opioid anesthesia during the first 24 hours. Group I patients requested additional opioids an average of 480 minutes after the study infusion, significantly earlier than group III patients (Table 1). Group I patients required a total of 46 doses of oxycodone, compared with 18 doses in group II. Patients in group III received more oxycodone at the end of the observation period than did those in group II. Group III patients were the most likely to have urinary retention, but there were no significant differences in the number of patients with nausea or pruritus (Table 2).

Conclusion.—Intrathecal infusion of fentanyl, 120 μg over 24 hours, was inadequate for analgesia in patients who had undergone hip replacement surgery. Better analgesia was achieved with intrathecal morphine, given either as a continuous infusion or as a single 200-μg bolus. The latter group required more supplemental analgesics after 18 hours. Side effects continued to present problems with intrathecal morphine therapy.

TABLE 1.—Need for Supplementary Intramuscular (IM) Oxycodone and Time to First Oxycodone Administration

	Group I (fentanyl infusion)	Group II (morphine infusion)	Group III (morphine bolus)	Statistical significance
Need for additional IM opioids				
Total number of doses/24 h	46	18	24	$P < 0.01$, Group I vs II
0–6 h	8	4	2	
6–12 h	13	7	4	$P < 0.01$, Group I vs III
12–18 h	12	4	6	$P < 0.05$, Group I vs II
18–24 h	13	3	12	$P < 0.01$, Group I vs II and II vs III
Number of patients	18	8	13	$P < 0.01$, Group I vs II
Analgesic time (mean, min)	480	490	786	$P < 0.01$, Group I vs III
SD	267	328	411	

Note: Time to first oxycodone administration from initial intrathecal drug injection in 24-hour postoperative period.
(Courtesy of Niemi L, Pitkänen MT, Tuominen MK, et al: *Anesth Analg* 77:126–130, 1993.)

TABLE 2.—Side Effects During 24-Hour Postoperative Observation Period

	Group I (fentanyl infusion) $n = 20$	Group II (morphine infusion) $n = 20$	Group III (morphine bolus) $n = 20$
Urinary catheter (no. of patients)	6^a	11	13^a
Pruritus (no. of patients)	4	3	5
Nausea (no. of patients)	6	7	9

[a]$P < .05$.
(Courtesy of Niemi L, Pitkänen MT, Tuominen MK, et al: *Anesth Analg* 77:126–130, 1993.)

▶ Here is more evidence that epidural morphine exerts more spinally mediated analgesic effect than epidural infusions of lipid-soluble opioids.—S.E. Abram, M.D.

Tonsillectomy and Adenoidectomy Pain Reduction by Local Bupivacaine Infiltration in Children

Jebeles JA, Reilly JS, Gutierrez JF, Bradley EL Jr, Kissin I (Univ of Alabama, Birmingham)
Int J Pediatr Otorhinolaryngol 25:149–154, 1993   101-94-24–58

Rationale.—Controlling pain from tonsillectomy and tonsillectomy with adenoidectomy (T/A) is important because both children and parents are affected by the days lost from school and work. Recent studies have suggested that even with general anesthesia, pain impulses from the periphery alter the properties of dorsal horn neurons and lead to a hyperexcitable neural state, prolonging postoperative pain. Blocking peripheral pain impulses to the CNS during surgery should reduce postoperative pain.

Study Design.—Twenty-two consecutive children aged 8–18 years who were scheduled for tonsillectomy or T/A were enrolled in a double-blind study in which general anesthesia was accompanied by local administration of either bupivacaine or saline. After general anesthesia was induced, the peritonsillar region was infiltrated with either .25% bupivacaine or .9% saline, both with epinephrine (1:200,000).

Results.—Pain scores were significantly lower in the bupivacaine-treated patients on the day of surgery and for 5 days afterward. Less marked differences persisted through postoperative day 10. Pain on swallowing also was significantly less marked in patients given local anesthesia, and deglutition times were shorter in this group. No adverse effects were noted.

Conclusion.—Postoperative throat pain may be significantly lessened in patients having tonsillectomy or T/A if the tonsillar fossa is infiltrated preincisionally with bupivacaine during general anesthesia.

▶ It is particularly interesting that the local infiltration group had some demonstrable benefit to as many as 10 days postoperatively. It is not clear whether the reduced postoperative pain is related to blockade of intraoperative afferent traffic. A comparison with a group receiving postoperative infiltration is needed to answer that question.—S.E. Abram, M.D.

Analgesic Action of Metoclopramide in Prosthetic Hip Surgery

Kandler D, Lisander B (Sahlgrenska Hosp, Göteborg, Sweden; Univ Hosp, Linköping, Sweden)
Acta Anaesthesiol Scand 37:49–53, 1993   101-94-24–59

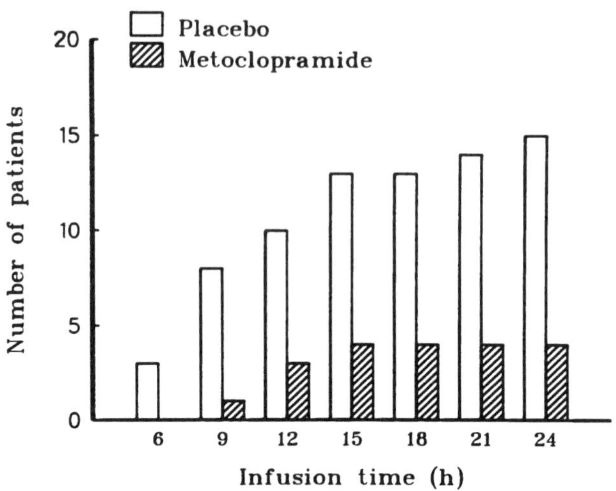

Fig 24–17.—Cumulative number of patients receiving analgesics during the 24 hours after start of intravenous infusion containing placebo (23) or metoclopramide (17). (Courtesy of Kandler D, Lisander B: *Acta Anaesthesiol Scand* 37:49–53, 1993.)

Background.—Previous clinical reports have attributed the pain-relieving effects of metoclopramide to an action on smooth muscle activity. Another study has suggested that this agent has a true analgesic effect. In a double-blind study of patients undergoing prosthetic hip surgery under spinal anesthesia with bupivacaine and morphine, metoclopramide was given as an intravenous infusion.

Methods.—Forty-seven patients were included in the study. Prosthetic hip surgery was done with the patients under subarachnoidal anesthesia with bupivacaine, 16–20 mg, and morphine, .2 mg. Before surgery, 17 patients received metoclopramide, 1 mg/kg, intravenously followed by an infusion of 1.5 mg/kg^{-1} over 9 hours. The 23 patients in the control group received corresponding amounts of solvent.

Findings.—The characteristics of the spinal block (level of analgesia to pinprick and muscular block) and postoperative visual analogue pain scores were comparable in the 2 groups. During the 24 hours after the infusion was begun, 4 patients in the metoclopramide group and 15 in the control group needed intravenous opioids (Fig 24–17). The metoclopramide patients had a longer pain-free period. Arterial levels of carbon dioxide pressure were increased, peaking within 6 hours of infusion, with no significant differences between groups.

Conclusion.—The current findings may be explained by a metoclopramide action on the 5-HT$_3$ receptor. In a previous study of postoperative emesis, however, the specific 5-HT$_3$ blocker ondancetron did not reduce the need for analgesics after surgery.

▶ Proposals for a mechanism of analgesic action include a serotoninergic and a dopaminergic mechanism. The role of metoclopramide as an analgesic remains to be determined.—S.E. Abram, M.D.

Can Pre-Emptive Lumbar Epidural Blockade Reduce Postoperative Pain Following Lower Abdominal Surgery?

Pryle BJ, Vanner RG, Enriquez N, Reynolds F (Univ of Buenos Aires, Argentina; St Thomas' Hosp, London)
Anaesthesia 48:120–123, 1993   101-94-24-60

Background.—According to the concept of neuroplasticity, pain impulses are not conducted along a fixed pathway but a pathway that adapts to its input. If these experimental findings on neuroplasticity were applied to clinical practice, it might be expected that a preoperative local anesthetic block would decrease postoperative pain more effectively than a block administered after surgery. This hypothesis was tested in a double-blind trial.

Methods.—Thirty-six women receiving a standard general anesthetic for elective abdominal hysterectomy or myomectomy were enrolled in the study. All received 15 mL of .5% bupivacaine with epinephrine by lumbar epidural injection, either 15 minutes before surgery (group A) or the same dose after surgery before waking (group B). Pain was assessed for 24 hours by cumulative self-administered morphine dose and visual analogue scale and verbal rating scores.

Findings.—No significant between-group differences were found in morphine dose or by visual analogue scale scores (table) or verbal rating scores at 6 or 24 hours after waking. However, as expected, there was a significant difference in the mean time of first use of patient-controlled analgesia (4.3 hours in group A and 5.1 hours in group B). However, when 23-hour pain scores in group A were compared with 24-hour pain scores in group B, no significant differences emerged.

Mean (Range) Values for Postoperative Analgesic Requirements and Pain Scores

Group	A	B
1st use PCA; h	4.26 (2.3–5.2)	5.06 (2.5–7.0)
6 h morphine dose; mg	9.87 (4–26)	9.57 (0–28)
24 h morphine dose; mg	49.3 (24–88)	50.7 (16–86)
6 h VAS; cm	2.71 (0.5–5)	2.97 (0–7.5)
24 h VAS; cm	2.63 (0–7)	2.9 (0–9)

Abbreviations: PCA, patient-controlled analgesia; VAS, visual analogue pain score.
(Courtesy of Pryle BJ, Vanner RG, Enriquez N, et al: *Anaesthesia* 48:120–123, 1993.)

Conclusion.—This study did not demonstrate that epidural blockade administered before surgery had a significantly better effect than blockade administered after surgery in relieving postoperative pain. Although experimental evidence for the efficacy of preemptive analgesia is clear, comparable clinical evidence is still lacking.

▶ This study failed to support the evidence that regional anesthesia begun before incision provides better analgesia. Perhaps the difference between this and other studies is the liberal intraoperative opioids used here.—S.E. Abram, M.D.

Interaction of Intrathecal Morphine With Bupivacaine and Lidocaine in the Rat

Penning JP, Yaksh TL (Ottawa Civic Hosp, Ont, Canada; Univ of California, San Diego)
Anesthesiology 77:1186–1200, 1992   101-94-24-61

Background.—There is extensive evidence that the addition of opioid significantly increases the analgesic efficacy of epidurally administered local anesthetics. Few studies, however, have attempted to define systematically the effects of jointly administering local anesthesia and an opioid by the spinal route, and few animal data are available.

Objective and Methods.—The interaction between intrathecal morphine and local anesthetics (bupivacaine and lidocaine) on motor and autonomic functions and on nociceptive responses was examined. Nociception involved use of a hot plate at 52.5°C and the application of paw pressure.

Results.—Both the local anesthetics produced a rapid, dose-dependent but transient reduction in hindlimb motor function. Adding 1 μg or 10 μg of intrathecal morphine did not influence the degree or duration of motor dysfunction. Low doses of either local anesthetic led to a significant leftward shift in dose-response curves for intrathecal morphine for both hot plate and paw pressure (Fig 24–18). Intrathecal morphine did not influence the dose-dependent effects of intrathecal bupivacaine or lidocaine on motor function or autonomic blockade.

Clinical Implications.—It seems possible that concentrations of local anesthetic that may not obviously affect behavior can lead to changes in spinal sensory processing when spinal opioid receptors are occupied. Neuraxial administration of low doses of bupivacaine along with morphine may limit the occurrence of side effects, such as respiratory depression, and may lessen the risk that opiate tolerance will develop. In addition, low levels of local anesthesia may alter afferent input into the dorsal horn and thereby enhance the postsynaptic action of opioid.

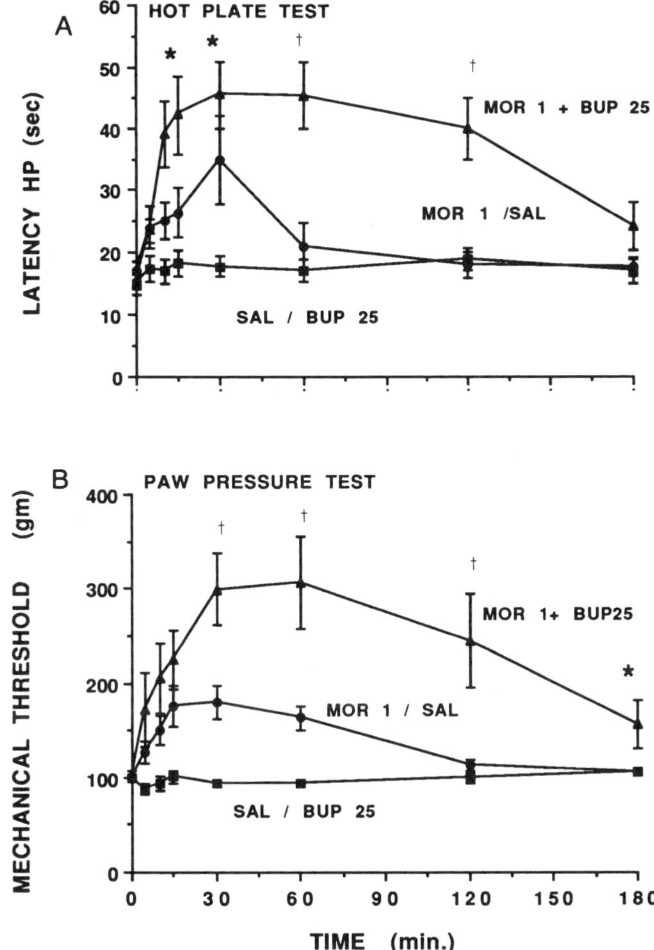

Fig 24–18.—Time course of changes in hot plate (**A**) response latencies and paw pressure (**B**) withdrawal pressures after intrathecal administration of morphine (MOR), 1 μg, together with bupivicaine (BUP), 25 μg, as a mixture, compared with agents administered alone; for all groups, $n = 7$. Data are presented as mean ± standard error of mean. MOR 1 + BUP 25 significantly greater than MOR 1 at individual time points: *$P < .05$; †$P < .01$. (Courtesy of Penning JP, Yaksh TL: *Anesthesiology* 77:1186–1200, 1992.)

▶ Low doses of local anesthetics that have no appreciable analgesic effect significantly increase the analgesic effect of intrathecal morphine in models of both thermal and mechanical antinociception. The clinical evidence for such synergy remains to be definitively shown.—S.E. Abram, M.D.

Anaphylactoid Reaction Following Local Anaesthesia for Epidural Block

Thomas AD, Caunt JA (Gloucestershire Royal Hosp, England; Northern Gen Hosp, Sheffield, England)
Anaesthesia 48:50–52, 1993　　　　　　　　　　　　　101-94-24-62

Background.—Epidural anesthesia is commonly used in women undergoing elective cesarean section. Most complications associated with this anesthesia have been related to placement, inadvertent intrathecal block, convulsions after high blood concentrations, and hypotension from the sympathetic block. One woman had a probable immunologic reaction to epidural anesthesia that was potentially serious.

Case Report.—Woman, 27, was scheduled for a repeat cesarean section with epidural anesthesia. She had had a cesarean section with epidural bupivacaine anesthesia 2.5 years earlier. Three days after this procedure, an allergic rash had developed over her face, body, and arms. It was subsequently considered an Elastoplast allergy and not further investigated. For the new procedure, bupivacaine, .5% plain, was injected, for a total dose of 18 mL. Twenty-five minutes later, the patient complained of a tingling of her tongue, faintness, and nausea. Her systolic arterial pressure dropped, and she became bright red and itchy. Her lips, eyelids, fingers, and toes were obviously swelling. She was treated with 100% oxygen through a face mask, additional intravenous fluids, and ephedrine, followed by chlorpheniramine and hydrocortisone. The patient responded well but was still in obvious distress. She agreed to continue with the now urgent cesarean section with the existing epidural block. After delivery, the patient was given intravenous oxytocin, metoclopramide, alfentanil, and methylprednisolone. At birth, the male infant was limp, cyanosed, and edematous peripherally. Copious pulmonary edema fluid was noted after tracheal intubation. In the special care baby unit, his trachea was extubated 30 minutes later, and he and his mother improved during the next 3 hours. Six weeks after delivery, skin testing on the mother produced an intradermal wheal positive to lidocaine 2%, but not to bupivacaine.

Conclusion.—This patient reacted with erythema, itching, and generalized and pulmonary edema after epidural bupivacaine was used for cesarean section. Subsequently, the baby had pulmonary edema. The cause of the mother's reaction was probably an immunologic hypersensitivity to bupivacaine or lidocaine.

▶ Given the extreme rarity of true allergy to local anesthetics, other sources of allergens should be considered in this case. Latex is a likely candidate.—S.E. Abram, M.D.

Pain Relief for Infants Undergoing Abdominal Surgery: Comparison of Infusions of I.V. Morphine and Extradural Bupivacaine

Wolf AR, Hughes D (Univ of Bristol, England)
Br J Anaesth 70:10–16, 1993   101-94-24–63

Background.—Variable-rate intravenous opioid infusions are used even in young infants for postoperative analgesia, but they may have serious adverse effects, such as impaired consciousness or ventilatory depression. Opioids can be avoided by the use of extradural infusions of bupivacaine, but this alternative may produce hypotension and complications from extensive local block or systemic absorption of local anesthetic. The effects of intravenous morphine infusions were compared with those of extradural infusions of bupivacaine in infants and young children after abdominal surgery.

Methods.—Thirty-two children younger than age 4 years were enrolled in the prospective, randomized, double-blind trial. Sham extradural or intravenous catheters were used to maintain the blinded nature of the study.

Findings.—Both techniques produced adequate analgesia for most of the 36-hour postoperative period. There were no differences in the pat-

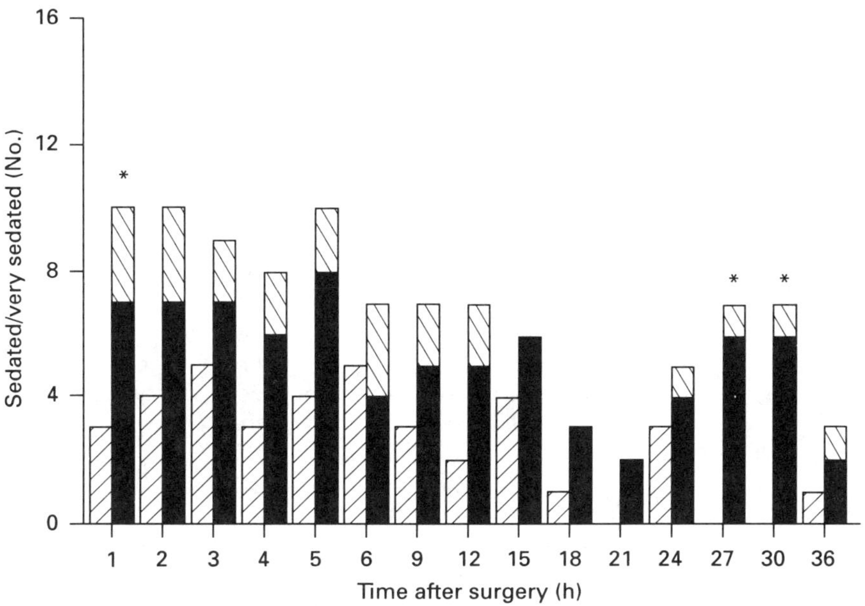

Fig 24–19.—Numbers of patients in extradural and morphine groups observed as sedated (sedation score 2) or very sedated (sedation score 3) during the first 36 hours after surgery. *Leftward-slanting-striped bars,* bupivacaine group with sedation score 2; *filled bars,* morphine group with sedation score 2; *right-slanting–striped bars,* morphine group with sedation score 3. **P < .05.* (Courtesy of Wolf AR, Hughes D: *Br J Anaesth* 70:10–16, 1993.)

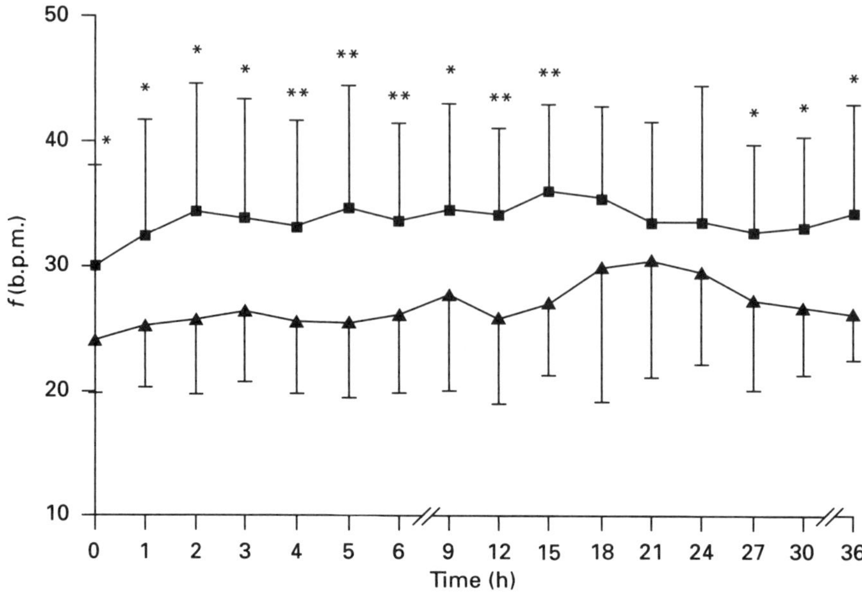

Fig 24–20.—Ventilatory frequencies (*f*) for patients receiving extradural bupivacaine (*squares*) or morphine (*triangles*) analgesia (mean, standard deviation). *$P < .05$; **$P < .01$. (Courtesy of Wolf AR, Hughes D: *Br J Anaesth* 70:10–16, 1993.)

tern or quality of analgesia. Children given intravenous morphine were significantly more sedated and had slower ventilatory frequencies than the extradural group (Figs 24–19 and 24–20). Oxygen saturation was also significantly lower in children given morphine (Fig 24–21). The 2 groups had similar mean systolic arterial pressures. No life-threatening complications occurred. Three children in the extradural group had a troublesome lack of sedation.

Conclusion.—Extradural analgesia with bupivacaine administered through a caudal catheter gave excellent postoperative analgesia in young children after abdominal surgery. This technique may be preferable to morphine infusion in neonates and younger infants sensitive to ventilatory depression and in whom sedation is not necessary or desirable. Older children may need more sedation or analgesia to prevent restlessness after surgery.

▶ The lack of problems with hypotension and improved oxygen saturations for the bupivacaine group is encouraging. Safe limits for bupivacaine infusion rates in small children have not been established.—S.E. Abram, M.D.

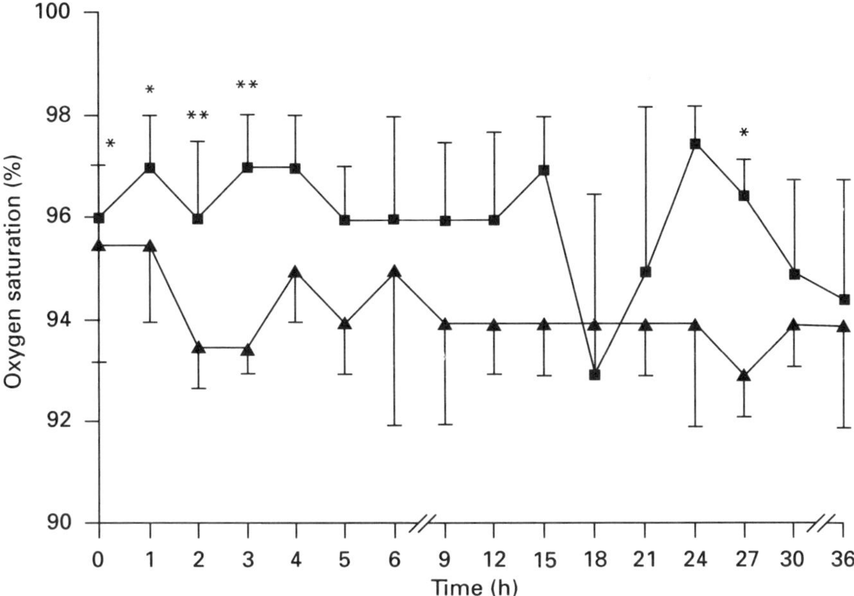

Fig 24–21.—Oxygen saturation for patients receiving extradural bupivacaine (*squares*) or morphine (*triangles*) analgesia (median, quartiles). **P < .05; **P < .01.* (Courtesy of Wolf AR, Hughes D: *Br J Anaesth* 70:10–16, 1993.)

Intravenous or Epidural Clonidine for Intra- and Postoperative Analgesia

De Kock M, Crochet B, Morimont C, Scholtes J-L (Univ of Louvain, Brussels, Belgium)
Anesthesiology 79:525–531, 1993   101-94-24–64

Introduction.—The α_2-adrenoreceptor agonist clonidine may be given either intravenously or epidurally for postoperative analgesia. Research suggests that the analgesic effects of clonidine have a spinal site of action. In a randomized, prospective study, the analgesic effects of epidural vs. intravenous administration of clonidine were examined.

Methods.—The subjects were 40 patients undergoing intestinal surgery with general propofol/nitrous oxide anesthesia. At the time of induction, clonidine was given either epidurally or intravenously. The dose was the same in both groups: 4 μg/kg in 10 mL over 20 minutes, then 2^{-1} μg/kg/hr^{-1} at a rate of 5 mL/hr over 12 hours. Alfentanil was given intraoperatively for increased blood pressure and heart rate not responding to additional propofol. Morphine was given postoperatively as needed.

Results.—The intraoperative alfentanil requirement was .93 mg in the epidural group, compared with 2.4 mg in the intravenous group. Mor-

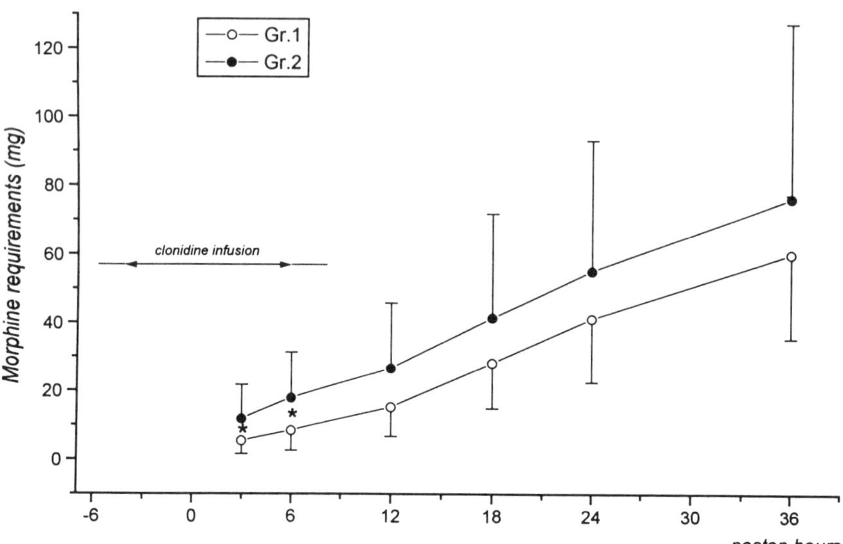

Fig 24–22.—Postoperative morphine requirements (mg) in patients having received epidural (group 1; $n = 20$) or intravenous (group 2; $n = 20$) clonidine at different postoperative times. Results are means ± 1 SD. *$P < .001$ (comparison between group 1 and group 2). (Courtesy of De Kock M, Crochet B, Morimont C, et al: *Anesthesiology* 79:525–531, 1993.)

phine requirements in the first 6 hours postoperatively were also lower in the epidural group (Fig 24–22). Pain scores on a visual analogue scale were similar in the 2 groups, although the epidural group had a better patient's analgesia score during the first 12 hours. There were no differences in sedation score or heart rate and blood pressure response. The epidural group had lower plasma clonidine concentrations only after their loading doses.

Conclusion.—Giving clonidine by the epidural rather than the intravenous route reduces intraoperative and early postoperative analgesic requirements. Although this study noted no significant differences in side effects, the possible complications of epidural catheter placement must be considered.

▶ The analgesic effect of epidural clonidine compared with intravenous clonidine is quite modest. Perhaps combinations of epidural clonidine plus epidural morphine will provide more dramatic results.—S.E. Abram, M.D.

Opioid Hyperexcitability: The Application of Alternate Opioid Therapy

MacDonald N, Der L, Allan S, Champion P (Univ of Alberta, Edmonton, Canada; British Columbia Cancer Agency, Victoria, Canada; Queen Elizabeth

Hosp, Charlottetown, PEI, Canada)
Pain 53:353–355, 1993   101-94-24–65

Introduction.—Experience with 3 cases suggests that the extent of cross-tolerance may change as the dose of opioid increases. This implies that caution is needed when using equivalency conversion tables for patients receiving very high doses.

Case 1.—Man, 69, was given hydromorphone to control pain from a malignant fibrous histiocytoma arising from the right buttock. His opioid needs escalated during the ensuing months, from 2 mg/hr by continuous subcutaneous infusion to 200 mg/hr by continuous intravenous infusion. Marked generalized myoclonus and delirium occurred. The myoclonus resolved when hydromorphone was replaced by morphine infusion at a rate of 200 mg/hr, 20% of the usual equianalgesic dose. The patient was also given methotrimeprazine, indomethacin suppositories, methadone, and clonazepam. The delirium cleared when the morphine dose was reduced to 130 mg/hr. Pain was well controlled until the patient died 6 weeks later of pneumonia.

Case 2.—Woman, 41, had pain in the thoracic spine 16 months after primary treatment for adenocarcinoma of the breast. Progressive metastatic bone disease developed, producing uncontrolled pain. Liver and pituitary metastases also were present. The patient had myoclonus when receiving 200 mg/hr of hydromorphone; she was changed to morphine at the same rate by continuous subcutaneous infusion. Myoclonus resolved, and pain control was maintained with morphine, 160 mg/hr.

Case 3.—Woman, 32, had recurrent ovarian cancer with widespread abdominal metastases and pain in the left back and hip secondary to lumbar nerve root involvement. Increasing intermittent doses of hydromorphone had been required to control pain, and control remained poor with 65 mg/hr. The patient became agitated and confused and had paranoid ideation and myoclonus. She was given morphine by continuous intravenous infusion at a rate of 75 mg/hr, 23% of the equivalent dose of hydromorphone. Myoclonus and agitation promptly resolved. Pain was controlled by 50 mg/hr of morphine.

Discussion.—In these patients, tolerance to hydromorphone and myoclonus developed rapidly. Two of them were also delirious. Hyperexcitability, confusion, and myoclonus are recognized side effects of high-dose opioid treatment. The specific metabolites responsible have not been identified. Hydromorphone and morphine can produce similar symptoms.

▶ It would be interesting to know whether simply decreasing the dose of hydromorphone might have resulted in alleviation of symptoms and preservation of analgesia.—S.E. Abram, M.D.

25 Psychological Aspects of Anesthesiology and Pain

Awareness, Recall, Learning

Midazolam Enhances Anterograde but Not Retrograde Amnesia in Pediatric Patients

Twersky RS, Hartung J, Berger BJ, McClain J, Beaton C (Long Island College Hosp, Brooklyn, NY)

Anesthesiology 78:51–55, 1993   101-94-25-1

Introduction.—In children undergoing surgery, premedication with an amnestic drug can inhibit recall of stressful postoperative experiences. Ideally, this drug will inhibit recall of events occurring after the drug was given but not before. Although the benzodiazepines have been shown to inhibit recall, the extent of this amnesia is unknown.

Patients and Methods.—A randomized, double-blind study sought to determine the effect of midazolam sedation on recall before and after drug administration in children. The subjects were 40 patients, aged 4 to 10 years, undergoing elective operations. The children were assigned to receive premedication with either intranasal midazolam, .2 mg/kg, or distilled water via an atomizer. Recall and recognition were tested by using series of picture cards that were shown to the children before administration of midazolam/placebo and after administration of midazolam/ placebo but before induction of general anesthesia.

Results.—Children receiving midazolam showed significant reductions in the ability to recall and recognize cards shown to them after the drug was administered. Patients in the placebo group both recalled and recognized twice as many cards, on average, as did the midazolam patients. On the other hand, the 2 groups were no different in their ability to recall or recognize cards shown to them before midazolam/placebo administration.

Conclusion.—Given to children as a preanesthetic amnestic, midazolam inhibits recall and recognition of events occurring after administra-

tion of the drug. It does not, however, affect memory of events occurring before the child received the drug.

▶ Midazolam seems to be emerging as the preferred drug for pharmacologic premedication in children. The ability to administer this drug by oral or nasal routes further adds to its acceptance.—R.K. Stoelting, M.D.

The P3a Wave of the Auditory Event-Related Potential Reveals Registration of Pitch Change During Sufentanil Anesthesia for Cardiac Surgery

Plourde G, Joffe D, Villemure C, Trahan M (McGill Univ, Montreal; Royal Victoria Hosp, Montreal)
Anesthesiology 78:498–509, 1993

101-94-25-2

Background.—It has proven difficult to detect unintentional awareness during cardiac surgery. The N1 and P3 waves of the auditory event-related potential (ERP) vary with the level of consciousness. The N1 wave is lowered during states of low vigilance, whereas P3 is seen only with stimuli that capture the subject's attention. The P3a component predominates in the frontal region and likely occurs when the subject notices a stimulus. The P3b component occurs parietally and connotes conscious awareness of the stimulus.

Study Design.—Auditory event-related potentials were recorded in 12 adult patients scheduled for coronary artery bypass surgery or cardiac valve replacement. The patients were premedicated with diazepam, morphine, and scopolamine and received sufentanil for induction and maintenance of anesthesia. No other anesthetics were used. Auditory event-related potentials were recorded at intervals before, during, and after induction and before the institution of cardiopulmonary bypass, using 1,000-Hz tone bursts at 85 dB as frequent stimuli and 2,000-Hz tone bursts as rare stimuli.

Observations.—The N1 component was significantly attenuated but not abolished by sufentanil. The P3b was recorded only before induction of anesthesia. A P3a component was recorded after intubation and before the start of cardiopulmonary bypass.

Interpretation.—Cortical discrimination of pitch is often observed during sufentanil anesthesia even if the electroencephalogram is maximally slowed. It is not associated with clinically inadequate anesthesia. Attenuation of N1 from the time of induction suggests reduced arousal caused by sufentanil. Whether the P3a reflects the return of consciousness remains uncertain.

▶ Although the title of this paper does not even remotely give away its importance, this, I predict, will be a very important paper. Dr. Plourde and his colleagues at McGill have made some real progress on a problem that has plagued us since the invention of muscle relaxants, namely, awareness under anesthesia. It is entirely possible that the auditory evoked potentials these investigators are studying might eventually be incorporated into a legitimate "awareness monitor." I have been interested in this issue for many years. I do not think that anyone is closer to understanding how to do this than is this group at Montreal. I hope they persist in these potentially enormously important efforts.—J.H. Tinker, M.D.

Awareness and Recall During General Anesthesia: Facts and Feelings

Moerman N, Bonke B, Oosting J (Univ of Amsterdam; Erasmus Univ, Rotterdam, The Netherlands)
Anesthesiology 79:454–464, 1993   101-94-25–3

Introduction.—A number of case reports in the literature of awareness and recall result from insufficient general anesthesia during surgery. Many types of anesthetic techniques have been involved. Because such an experience can be distressing and have lasting consequences, systematic information on patients who reported awareness and recall during general anesthesia was obtained.

Methods.—Patients were referred by anesthesiologists at a large university hospital. After talking freely about their experiences, the patients were interviewed in a semistructured way. An attempt was also made to trace the anesthetic records. For each awareness case, 2 similar cases in which no awareness had been reported were chosen for comparison. Three experienced anesthesiologists, without knowledge of the occurrence of awareness, then rated the case and control records for the likelihood that awareness and recall might have taken place.

Results.—Twenty-six patients were available for in-depth interviews. They had undergone anesthesia for clinical elective surgery in 10 cases,

Recollections of 26 Patients		
	N	%
Sounds	23	89
Paralysis	22	85
Pain	10	39
Visual perception	7	27
Intubation or tube	6	23
Feeling the operation without pain	5	19
Anxiety, panic	24	92
Helplessness, powerlessness	12	46
Aftereffects	18	69

(Courtesy of Moerman N, Bonke B, Oosting J: *Anesthesiology* 79:454–464, 1993.)

acute trauma surgery in 7, day-case surgery in 5, and cesarean section in 4. The mean age at the time of awareness was 35 years. Almost all patients experienced some auditory perception. A sensation of paralysis and pain at the site of the operation were commonly reported. Most recalled feelings of anxiety, panic, and helplessness (table). Twenty patients had tried unsuccessfully to alert someone to their condition. Long-term effects, such as sleep disturbances and flashbacks, were reported by 18 patients. Most said they had become more afraid of anesthesia. The anesthesiologists who reviewed the records of cases and controls were unable to distinguish those who might have experienced awareness and recall.

Conclusion.—The main aspects of awareness reported here—the ability to hear and sensations of weakness or paralysis followed by pain—are similar to the findings of previous studies. The anesthetic record does not explain why certain patients have insufficient anesthesia. Anesthesiologists should ask about their patients' previous anesthetic experiences and visit them after surgery to determine whether reassurance or psychological help is needed.

▶ This is a startling compilation of case studies of awareness and recall during general anesthesia. Anybody who thinks this does not occur should read this article. If you think it cannot happen to you, you should also read this article. If you think that one or another of your favorite "anesthetic depth" monitoring methods will guarantee freedom from this problem, please read this article. We need an awareness monitor.—J.H. Tinker, M.D.

Recall of Music: A Comparison Between Anaesthesia With Propofol and Isoflurane

Oddby-Muhrbeck E, Jakobsson J (Karolinska Inst, at Danderyd's Hosp, Sweden)
Acta Anaesthesiol Scand 37:33–37, 1993   101-94-25-4

Introduction.—The advent of new intravenous anesthetics and the practice of combining regional anesthesia with light general anesthesia have renewed concern about patients being aware during anesthesia. What really makes patients sleep while anesthetized remains unknown, and it is not clear how to determine whether patients unconsciously register anything during anesthesia.

Objective and Methods.—Auditive recall was sought in 60 American Society of Anesthesiologists status I women who underwent laparoscopy under either total intravenous anesthesia with propofol or inhalational anesthesia with isoflurane. All patients received midazolam as premedication and fentanyl before intubation. All were ventilated with nitrous oxide in oxygen. Some patients in each anesthesia group were randomly assigned to hear a piece of soft music at a speaking voice level (50–60 dB) or to hear a piece of hard rock music at 70–80 dB. The music was played through earphones at least once during anesthesia. Control patients were exposed to a blank tape. Patients were asked about their experience 24 hours postoperatively.

Findings.—Ten patients anesthetized with propofol and 2 in the isoflurane group reported having heard music. Eleven of the 12 had, in fact, been exposed to music. Thirteen other patients claimed to have heard music after listening to a tape containing a number of musical pieces, but only 2 patients specified the correct piece. Patients who were exposed to music or a blank tape while inhaling 66% nitrous oxide in oxygen were able to recall accurately whether music had been played, and to identify the correct piece.

▶ This paper tells us that recall and learning do occur with both intravenous and inhalation anesthesia. There is a hint that the total intravenous anesthesia group may have had somewhat more awareness as they were inclined more often to state that they had been exposed to music. I selected this paper so that readers can be aware of the kinds of studies that are going on in this important and currently "hot" area of study in anesthesiology.—J.H. Tinker, M.D.

Effects of Isoflurane and Nitrous Oxide in Subanesthetic Concentrations on Memory and Responsiveness in Volunteers
Dwyer R, Bennett HL, Eger E III, Heilbron D (Beaumont Hosp, Dublin; Univ of California, Sacramento; Univ of California, San Francisco)
Anesthesiology 77:888–898, 1992   101-94-25–5

Purpose.—Since the introduction of neuromuscular relaxants, conscious memory of events occurring during anesthesia has been a recur-

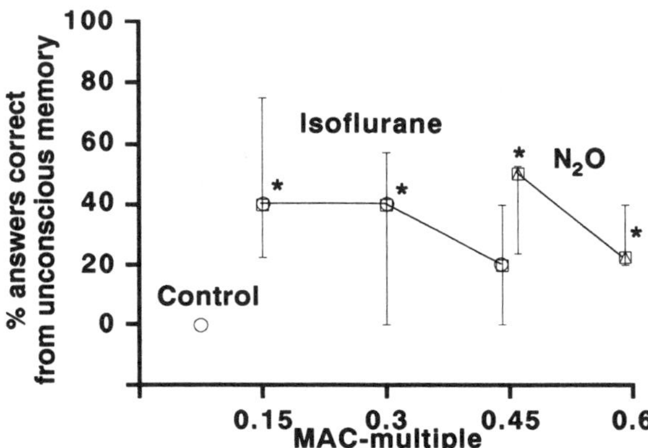

Fig 25–1.—Percentage of correct answers from unconscious memory (without conscious recognition), for each anesthetic concentration. * *P* < .05 compared with control questions (medians, quartiles). (Courtesy of Dwyer R, Bennett HL, Eger II, et al: *Anesthesiology* 77:888–898, 1992.)

rent problem. Questions remain concerning the ability of volatile anesthetics and nitrous oxide to prevent conscious memory. The effects of isoflurane and nitrous oxide on memory were examined in 17 healthy young men.

Methods.—The volunteers were assigned to receive both agents in random order, at least 1 week apart. At each test, they were studied at the following end-tidal concentrations: .15, .3, .45, and .15 times the minimum alveolar concentration (MAC) for isoflurane and .3, .45, .6, and .3 times MAC for nitrous oxide. At each concentration, the subjects were tested for voluntary response to command and given verbal information to remember after anesthesia. The next day, they were assessed for conscious and unconscious memory of the information presented.

Results.—Isoflurane was more potent than nitrous oxide in preventing voluntary response; the mean end-tidal concentration necessary to prevent voluntary response in half the subjects was .38 times MAC for isoflurane vs. .64 times MAC for nitrous oxide. With both agents, memory decreased as anesthetic concentration increased. Isoflurane prevented conscious recall at .45 MAC, but nitrous oxide could not completely prevent it even at .6 MAC. The same was true for unconscious recall (Fig 25–1). Memory was more potently suppressed by isoflurane than by MAC-equivalent concentrations of nitrous oxide. The dose necessary to suppress memory by 50% was estimated to be .2 MAC for isoflurane and .5 MAC for nitrous oxide.

Conclusion.—Dose-dependent reductions in memory by both isoflurane and nitrous oxide were documented. At MAC-equivalent concentrations, however, isoflurane is better than nitrous oxide at preventing memory and voluntary response to command. It is unknown whether these are the concentrations needed to prevent memory during surgery.

▶ Eger and others have contended for quite some time now that volatile agents were somehow "better" at suppressing memory and awareness than "nitrous-narcotic"–type anesthetics. The authors had no choice in this study but to utilize so-called equipotent concentrations in the sense of so-called MAC-equivalent concentrations. It is possible to conclude from their study, as they did, that the volatile agent isoflurane is more effective at memory suppression, but it is also possible to conclude that "equi-MAC" means movement, not memory. I have had this discussion with Dr. Eger, who takes umbrage at my contention that studying cardiovascular phenomena, or other nonmovement-related phenomena, using equi-MAC concentrations may not be valid. I do believe that this is a viable alternative explanation for their findings. On the other hand, many experienced anesthetists would agree that when a volatile agent is present, in some concentration or other, during the anesthetic, awareness and memory seem, at least anecdotally, to be unlikely.—J.H. Tinker, M.D.

Preoperative Preparation

Effect of Preoperative Suggestion on Postoperative Gastrointestinal Motility

Disbrow EA, Bennett HL, Owings JT (Univ of California, Davis, Sacramento)
West J Med 158:488–492, 1993   101-94-25-6

Background.—There is evidence of visceral learning in humans. Because autonomic behavior is subject to direct suggestion, the return of intestinal function after major elective intra-abdominal operations was compared.

Study Design.—In a prospective study, 40 patients undergoing major elective intraperitoneal surgical procedures were randomly assigned to hear, preoperatively, 5 minutes of specific instructions for the early return of gastrointestinal motility or an equal-length interview offering reassurance and nonspecific instructions (control). Resolution of postoperative ileus was compared while accounting for such covariates as duration of operation, amount of intraoperative bowel manipulation, and amount of postoperative narcotics.

Outcome.—The suggestion group had a significantly shorter time to first passage of flatus (mean, 2.6 days), compared with the control group (mean, 4.2 days). The average time to taking clear liquids and the duration of nasogastric tube placement tended to be shorter in the suggestion group. Duration of hospital stay was shortened by an average of 1.5 days in the suggestion group. There was no correlation between the experimental condition and hypnotic ability scores, indicating that giving suggestions can be effective regardless of a patient's susceptibility to suggestion.

Conclusion.—Patients undergoing major operations can benefit from verbal suggestions given preoperatively in a believable manner. Patients who receive instructions for early return of bowel motility can reduce the duration of ileus with shorter hospital stay, resulting in an average savings of $1,200 per patient.

▶ Information provided in preoperative clinics can be beneficial, not only in helping patients get out of the hospital faster because they know more about pain therapy and pain treatments and about their operation, but also because their gastrointestinal tract starts functioning quicker—another rationale for why your hospital outpatient clinic should set up a preoperative clinic and why you should willingly staff it.—M.F. Roizen, M.D.

Preparation for Undergoing an Invasive Medical Procedure: Interacting Effects of Information and Coping Style

Ludwick-Rosenthal R, Neufeld RWJ (Univ of Western Ontario, London, Canada)

J Consult Clin Psychol 61:156–164, 1993   101-94-25-7

Background.—It is becoming increasingly common for hospitals to provide patients with stress management training so that they will be able to cope with their medical care. Various cognitive and combined cognitive-behavioral techniques have been used with the goal of changing the way the patient evaluates environmental stimuli. A common feature is to provide information about the stressful event to come.

Objective.—An information-based preparative program was evaluated in 72 patients having cardiac catheterization for the first time. It was hypothesized that coping efforts during the procedure would be enhanced or impeded according to the fit between the level of information supplied and the patient's dispositional preference for information.

Patients.—Thirty-six patients of each sex, aged from 38 to 75 years, participated. Their mean educational level was grade 12, and their mean intelligence quotient was 103. Nineteen patients had had myocardial infarction in the past year.

Methods.—The high-information program included an audiotape with written text that gave a reason for the procedure, described the operating environment, and outlined the steps of the procedure. In addition, patients were told of the sensations they could expect. The low-information condition consisted of a shorter tape giving a general description of the procedure. The dispositional desire for information was assessed using the Miller Behavioral Styles Scale, which estimates the tendency to seek out or avoid threat-relevant information in the context of hypothetical stress scenarios. In addition, the Krantz Health Opinion Survey was administered. The Information subscale of this measure estimates the desire to ask questions and to be informed about medical decisions. Another instrument determined the desire to control events in one's environment.

Findings.—A desire for information was independent of a desire for control. When the desire for information was matched with the level of preparatory information delivered, patients had less behavioral anxiety during catheterization. In addition, their coping activities were focused more on problems and less on emotions. The coping disposition itself did not influence the patient's adjustment during catheterization. Providing a large amount of preparatory information led to more positive self-statements and was associated with shorter procedural times.

Conclusion.—Those who seek information are best able to cope when it is made available, but information avoiders cope less well with problems when a high level of information is provided.

▶ This wonderful article has very great value and importance to us. We should be able to segregate by easy questions which patients want information about their procedure and which do not. From that, this article implies, we can better match the information we give with the patient's coping behavior and thus provide the right amount of information preparatory to anesthesia, surgery, and pain relief to patients. I believe this article and its implications should be taken seriously by anyone involved in preoperative preparation of patients.—M.F. Roizen, M.D.

Forum: The Effectiveness of Pre-Operative Advice to Stop Smoking: A Prospective Controlled Trial
Munday IT, Desai PM, Marshall CA, Jones RM, Phillips M-L, Rosen M (St Mary's Hosp Medical School, London; Univ of Alabama, Birmingham; Royal Free Hosp, London; et al)
Anaesthesia 48:816–818, 1993   101-94-25-8

Background.—Cigarette smoking is a major but avoidable cause of postoperative morbidity. Postsurgical respiratory status is likely to be improved in patients who stop smoking more than 6 weeks before their operation. The surgical outpatient clinic appears to be a good place to discuss this risk with patients and allow them time to improve their fitness for surgery.

Methods.—A prospective, controlled study was done to determine whether written preoperative advice given at outpatient consultation could induce patients to quit smoking before elective surgery. All patients received a leaflet titled "Smoking and Your Operation" that advised them to quit smoking at least 6 weeks before surgery. This advice was given to 136 regular smokers; no advice was given to 97 control patients who smoked.

Results.—Just 1 patient in each group stopped smoking before the operation. Similar percentages in the 2 groups reported abstinence for more than 3 days. There was a tendency for the study group patients to decrease their consumption and for the control group patients to increase their consumption. There was no difference between the groups in the time of the last cigarette before surgery, with 15% of patients smoking within 1 hour before their operation.

Conclusion.—Advising elective surgical patients to stop smoking before their operation does not appear to improve their ability to quit. However, it may reduce the amount of tobacco consumed. Stopping cigarette consumption on admission to the hospital would be beneficial, as many patients continue to smoke until just before their operation.

▶ This is one of the first descriptions other than our own work as reported in the Miller textbook (1) and other textbooks of using the preoperative clinic as an area in which to render preventive care. I worry that the American system of medical care will soon approach the British in the long delays, etc., for surgery, but it looked clear from this article that there was more than a 6-week queue before surgery, as each patient could be given the stop-smoking leaflet 6 weeks before his or her operation. Nevertheless, the authors found, as would be expected, that if all you give a patient is a leaflet, only 1 of 136 will stop smoking.

I think this article—plus several others that are reviewed in the YEAR BOOK OF ANESTHESIOLOGY AND PAIN MANAGEMENT this year—is an important step in highlighting the role of the anesthesiologist as the primary care physician in perioperative care, and the role of the anesthesiologist in instituting routine preventive care measures that not only affect perioperative outcome but may also affect long-term well-being.—M.F. Roizen, M.D.

Reference

1. Roizen MF: Preoperative evaluation, in Miller RD (ed): *Anesthesia,* 4th ed. New York, Churchill-Livingstone, 1994.

Patient Attitudes/Knowledge

Patient Knowledge of Operative Care

Williams OA (Chesterfield and North Derbyshire Royal Hosp, England)
J R Soc Med 86:328–331, 1993   101-94-25-9

Introduction.—Inadequate knowledge regarding perioperative events may be related to anxiety. A survey was conducted among patients undergoing elective surgery to evaluate knowledge of perioperative events.

Methods.—Preoperatively, 111 patients completed a questionnaire addressing 6 topics, namely, the operation, the anesthetic, time spent in the operating theater, amount of postoperative pain, duration of hospital admission, and time required to return to normal fitness. The source of information for each topic was identified and the degree of knowledge and satisfaction with the information was correlated with the level of anxiety, measured on a visual analogue scale.

Results.—More than 30% of the patients received no information about the anesthesia, time in the operating theater, return to fitness, and pain; only 17% had sufficient knowledge regarding the anesthesia and 24.5% had information on return to fitness. For each of the 6 topics in the survey, more than 40% of the patients desired further information, but only 19.8% made inquiries. The nursing staff were the main providers of information, although more than 60% of the patients reported that "nobody" had provided explanations about the anesthesia, time spent in theater, return to fitness, and pain. There was no correlation between the level of information per se and anxiety, but there was a significant correlation between satisfaction with the information provided and anxiety. There was a positive correlation between lack of information and desire for more information.

Conclusion.—There is a considerable need for information regarding perioperative events, particularly for patients in whom anxiety is associated with a desire for further explanation of operative care. Less dissatisfaction with the level of information given should prove beneficial in terms of reducing anxiety.

▶ It is not clear whether the patients' knowledge of operative care was deficient because the physicians did not give it or because of memory deficits after the anesthetic, but the phenomenon of greater patient satisfaction because they have more knowledge found in this study is an important rationale, in addition to better medical care, for initiating funding and running preoperative clinics. Perhaps the questionnaire should have been sent to the physicians as well to see how much knowledge they thought they imparted to patients.—M.F. Roizen, M.D.

The Effect of the Anaesthetist's Attire on Patient Attitudes: The Influence of Dress on Patient Perception of the Anaesthetist's Prestige
Hennessy N, Harrison DA, Aitkenhead AR (Univ Hosp, Nottingham, England)
Anaesthesia 48:219–222, 1993   101-94-25–10

Introduction.—Many patients view the anesthetist as a technician rather than as a medically qualified staff member. The anesthetist may not wear the "regulation" white coat or name tag of a doctor and has less contact with the conscious patient than do other professionals. A study was designed to relate the appearance of the anesthetist at the preoperative visit to the patient's perception of the anesthetist's prestige relative to other medical personnel.

Methods.—Adult patients scheduled for surgery were randomly selected and allocated to 1 of 2 groups. The same male anesthetist visited all patients before the operation. When visiting group A patients, he wore a suit and tie. For group B patients, the anesthetist wore jeans, athletic shoes, and an open-necked shirt. Half an hour later, a second individual interviewed the patients regarding their impressions of the anesthetist. The patients were also asked to grade 15 items of doctors' ward attire as desirable, neutral, or undesirable.

Results.—Each patient group comprised 27 men and 28 women. No statistical differences were noted in the adjectives chosen to describe the anesthetist in jeans or in a suit. Both groups used words related to professionalism and approachability when describing the anesthetist. When ranked in order of prestige, anesthetists were most often second, third, or fourth in a list of 10 health professionals. That ranking was not affected by the anesthetist's attire. Most (81.8%) patients knew that the anesthetist had a medical degree, but few (35.4%) thought that anesthetists were involved in the intensive care unit. Patients older than age 60 years were more likely to place a value on formal attire. Use of a name tag was thought desirable by 90% of patients and a white coat by 65.5%.

Conclusion.—Patients do not judge a physician's abilities by his appearance, although traditional dress and a name tag are favored. Patients appear to have an increasing awareness of the duties and qualifications of the anesthetist.

▶ Dr. Aitkenhead, one of the co-authors of this article, must live an interesting life. He has done fascinating studies, and this appears to be another one of them. Patients respond to a white coat, respond to a name tag, and respond to appropriate professional appearance. I only wish all the residents (and staff?) in America could read this article.—M.F. Roizen, M.D.

Attitudes of Anesthesiology Residents Toward Critical Care Medicine Training
Durbin CG Jr, McLafferty CL Jr (Univ of Virginia, Charlottesville)
Anesth Analg 77:418–426, 1993   101-94-25–11

Introduction.—In recent years, fewer anesthesiology residents have pursued fellowship training in critical care medicine (CCM). Consequently, a significant number of training positions now go unfilled each year.

Study Plan.—The causes of this situation were sought by surveying residents in 38 anesthesiology programs having accredited CCM fellowships with respect to their views toward CCM practice and training. The survey was developed by analyzing data from respondents in 4 of these programs and from 1 without CCM fellowships. A total of 640 responses were received, accounting for more than 30% of all residents.

Findings.—Fewer than 9% of residents intended to pursue a CCM fellowship. The respondents' interest in CCM training declined as they passed through their residencies. Those who had little responsibility for patient care during rotations on the intensive care unit expressed the least interest in CCM training. How large an administrative role was played by the anesthesiology department in the intensive care unit was also a factor in how much interest the residents had in CCM training. Frequently expressed concerns included the stress of chronic care, the cost of an added year of training, the load of intensive care unit care, and the ambiguity of the role in intensive care. Most respondents knew a CCM anesthesiologist whom they admired, and most knew that unfilled fellowship positions were available.

Suggestions.—Possible ways of getting anesthesiology residents more interested in CCM practice are to better define the job market, improve the curriculum and teaching, agree to defer student loans, and introduce medical students and residents to the intensive care unit at an earlier stage.

▶ It is truly amazing how many medical students profess to be interested in CCM as a reason for choosing an anesthesiology residency, and just how few remain committed to this field by the time they complete their training. This article provides those anesthesiologists involved in critical care education with insight into ways to maintain and stimulate enthusiasm in this field for those residents considering careers as intensivists.—D.M. Rothenberg, M.D.

26 Anesthesia Training and Continuing Education

Selecting Anaesthetists: The Use of Psychological Tests and Structured Interviews
Reeve PE, Vickers MD, Horton JN (People Dynamics, Cardiff, Wales; Univ of Wales, Cardiff; Univ Hosp of Wales, Cardiff)
J R Soc Med 86:400–403, 1993
101-94-26-1

Purpose.—Problems in the selection methods used in the appointment of physicians in the British National Health Service have been noticed. The use of psychological testing as a supplement to interviews for the selection of senior house officers and registrars in anesthesiology was examined.

Methods.—The study sample comprised 140 physicians short-listed from a group of 635 applicants. All underwent a semistructured interview conducted by specially trained consultant anesthetists, as well as a personality questionnaire, the Cattell 16PFQ-form C. The 62 physicians selected in this process were subsequently followed up for 3 to 8 years. Actual outcomes—as determined by academic, clinical, behavioral, and overall performance—were compared with predictions of future performance by the psychological test and the interviewers.

Findings.—On the personality questionnaire, selected applicants tended to be more practical and realistic, more self-disciplined, more dependable, and less subjective. Highly significant correlations were noted between prediction and outcome measures. Multiple regression analysis allowed creation of equations, based on 5 of the Cattell personality factors, to predict performance. They were detached/warmhearted, dull/bright, unstable/stable, timid/socially bold, and casual/controlled. Both personality measures and interview predictions were able to discriminate between the best and worst performers. Of those selected, 16% eventually left the specialty.

Conclusion.—The personality questionnaire used in this study is a valid tool for predicting which applicants will be successful in the specialty of anesthesia. A semistructured interview conducted by trained members represents an improvement over the ad hoc National Health Service selection system. Together, the 2 methods are highly predictive.

▶ I guess the ideal anesthesiologist is someone who is warm, intelligent, stable, bold, and in control. Eight of the 10 people who eventually left the National Health Service would not have been selected had these criteria been used. I wonder whether there is a role for this method in selecting residents, or even faculty, in an era when an over-supply of applicants and an undersupply of positions will be present.—M.F. Roizen, M.D.

Work Hours of Residents in Seven Anesthesiology Training Programs
Berry AJ, Hall JR (Emory Univ, Atlanta, Ga)
Anesth Analg 76:96–101, 1993   101-94-26–2

Introduction.—Problems resulting from the long hours of work required of residents in some medical specialties have led to calls for reform. The Accreditation Council for Graduate Medical Education now requires residency programs to establish policies on schedules and hours based on educational and patient needs. Trainees at 7 university-affiliated programs were surveyed to evaluate the work hours of anesthesiology residents.

Methods.—The survey form was distributed for use during the week of March 18–24, 1990. Residents in clinical anesthesia who volunteered to participate were asked to record their activities each day and the times to the nearest quarter hour for each activity.

Results.—A total of 158 surveys were returned for an overall response rate of 64.6%. The responses from 10 residents who were on vacation during the survey week were excluded. Residents in clinical anesthesia years 1, 2, and 3 spent an average of 66, 65, and 64 hours per week, respectively, in the hospital. Most of this time was devoted to patient care activities in the operating room. In-hospital work time did not differ by year of training, but 2 of the 7 programs differed significantly in the average number of hours per week (72 vs. 58). Some work-related activities were performed outside the hospital and some residents had moonlighting activities.

Conclusion.—The average total in-hospital time reported by these residents in clinical anesthesia was well within all published recommendations. However, this survey did not consider the specific hours of the day that the residents were in the operating room. The type of schedule and the time for sleep between shifts can affect wake-sleep cycles and produce fatigue. All training programs should be aware of the effect of resident work hours on vigilance tasks and management of critical incidents.

▶ My guess from discussions with chairs from around the country is that attendings are now spending more hours working in their professional activities than are residents. What have we come to? Maybe we should reduce the number of residents by 50% as the federal government wants, and just make each of them work twice as hard (only kidding). But in all seriousness, maybe the residents are not working hard enough to learn to make the necessary judgements and to deal with all the problems in a 2½-year training program. Do we have evidence for such inadequacies in learning processes?

Will we go the way of Great Britain with registrars working longer before they come on the faculty, and, thus, having faculty spending less time than trainees in anesthesia-related work? I do not know, but perhaps the current trend—which sees faculty working longer and longer and residents working shorter and shorter—cannot continue forever, or can it? Do Berry and Hall need to enlarge the study to look at the work hours of faculty as well as residents?—M.F. Roizen, M.D.

Continuing Medical Education: Perioperative Blood and Blood Component Therapy

Irving GA (Univ of Cape Town, Republic of South Africa)
Can J Anaesth 39:1105–1115, 1992   101-94-26-3

Introduction.—Anesthetists are probably responsible for the administration of as much as half of all red cell products, but more than half of the anesthetists at teaching hospitals may lack basic knowledge of the indications for blood and component treatment and of the problems involved. The critical aspect of all transfusions is that the microcirculation be maintained by an adequate intravascular volume.

Procedural Review.—An acceptable hemoglobin level for each patient should be calculated preoperatively, and a history should be obtained to identify potential bleeding problems. In most cases, perioperative anemia does not increase the risk of morbidity or mortality. The bleeding time does not predict the degree of perioperative blood loss, but it is a useful test when there is a known bleeding problem or if even minor bleeding will make surgery more difficult or lead to patient morbidity. If blood is necessary, packed red cells in a volume of 4 mL/kg will increase the hemoglobin by 1 g/dL. If bleeding results from thrombocytopenia, there will usually be time to check the number and function of platelets before ordering a transfusion. Fresh plasma is used much too often; it is indicated chiefly for replacing coagulation factors. Warming of blood is not important when 1–3 units are given during several hours. Drugs are never added to transfused blood.

Autotransfusion.—A healthy patient whose hematocrit exceeds 34% is able to donate a unit of blood every 4–7 days. As many as 4 units of blood may be collected preoperatively in this way, with the last unit taken 3 days before surgery. Shed blood may be salvaged if there is bleeding into the pleural or peritoneal cavity without bowel soiling, and if there is no risk of contamination by bacteria or tumor cells.

▶ This article is a useful overview of the indications, complications, and benefits of perioperative blood and blood component therapy.—M.F. Roizen, M.D.

27 Ethical Issues in Anesthesiology/Critical Care

Suspending Do-Not-Resuscitate Orders During Anesthesia and Surgery
Bernat JL, Grabowski EW (Dartmouth Med School, Hanover, NH; Univ of Vermont, Burlington)
Surg Neurol 40:7–9, 1993   101-94-27–1

Background.—Physicians writing do-not-resuscitate (DNR) orders for patients who either have refused or would not benefit from cardiopulmonary resuscitation, generally assume that cardiopulmonary arrest will be a spontaneous complication of the process of death. However, the issue is confused when a nonmoribund patient with a DNR order undergoes anesthesia and surgery. Most hospitals lack a written policy on temporary suspension of DNR orders during the perioperative period.

Suggested Policy.—A model hospital policy for the temporary suspension of DNR orders was described. A 24- to 72-hour moratorium encourages the optimal use of medical technology to alleviate the patient's suffering while maintaining his or her autonomy. The policy gives surgeons and anesthesiologists the right to attempt to reverse the complications of their procedures, given that such reversals can be achieved in a reasonable time. Informed consent, including a discussion of the benefits with the patient, is required. The surgeon decides on the exact duration of the moratorium, after which the previous DNR order goes back into effect. At this time, the patient or proxy is notified.

Discussion.—A suggested hospital policy for temporary suspension of DNR orders regarding surgical patients is outlined. This policy is believed to be justified because it contributes to the betterment of care by accommodating the needs of the surgeon and anesthesiologist as well as the patient. The most compelling argument for such a policy is that it differentiates between "natural" and iatrogenic cardiopulmonary arrest.

▶ This discussion of DNR and end-of-life decisions is an important one. I do not know whether most people believe they should follow the prescription stated or should follow a policy of mandatory reevaluation of DNR orders before surgery based on informed discussions with the patient. We personally do not follow the suspension policy but do follow mandatory rediscussion with the patients so that they understand what is going to happen and exactly what they will accept.

No matter what your hospital policy, I think it is important for you as a person in your department and as a department to come to grips with this issue and to voice your opinions to both the surgeons and the hospital administration as well as primary care physicians. This article can be a stimulant to such discussions.—M.F. Roizen, M.D.

Withholding and Withdrawal of Life Support From Surgical Neonates With Life-Threatening Congenital Anomalies

Hazebroek FWJ, Tibboel D, Mourik M, Bos AP, Molenaar JC (Erasmus Univ, Rotterdam, The Netherlands)
J Pediatr Surg 28:1093–1097, 1993   101-94-27–2

The Stages of the Decision-Making Process on Forgoing
Life-Support Treatment

Before death discussions between
  Responsible Senior Intensive Care Specialist (SICS) and
    other involved medical and surgical staff members
  SICS and nurses
  SICS and nurses and parents—"bad news talk"
  Feedback to other involved staff members
  (Repetition of "bad news talk" with parents)
  SICS with nurses and parents— discussion circum-
    stances of death such as presence of parents, child
    in arms of parents
  SICS with nurses—discussion about actual dying
    process
After death discussions between
  SICS and nursing team—evaluation of dying process,
    feedback and evaluation
  Treatment team—discussion, of complete medical
    history 1 week after death of the child
  On the initiative of the parents contact between SICS
    and parents—review medical history (including au-
    topsy results), questions about future risk of recur-
    rence, prenatal diagnosis, etc

(Courtesy of Hazebroek FWJ, Tibboel D, Mourik M, et al: *J Pediatr Surg* 28:1093–1097, 1993.)

Introduction.—Although many infants who previously would have died of life-threatening conditions can now be kept alive, not all survivors will lead normal lives. The expected quality of life of these children influences the decision to provide or continue life support. A protocol instituted at the Sophia Children's Hospital in Rotterdam for neonates with major congenital anomalies was described.

Methods.—The Rotterdam institution is a tertiary referral center admitting 120–140 neonates with major congenital anomalies each year. The records of all neonates admitted within 1 month after birth between January of 1988 and January of 1992 for whom life support was subsequently withheld (group A) or withdrawn (group B) were reviewed.

Results.—During the review period, 529 neonates were admitted to the pediatric surgical intensive care unit. Of the 52 deaths, 28 were from underlying disease and 24 were from the withholding (15 infants) or withdrawing (9 infants) of treatment. In group A, life support was withheld because of the severity of the anomalies, the presence of associated chromosomal anomalies, or conditions incompatible with life. Treatment was withdrawn from all group B infants because of serious postoperative complications. The parents of all 24 infants agreed with the decision to forego life support. All infants died in the lap of a parent or nurse and had received sedatives and analgesics as comfort care. The decision-making process involved lengthy discussions before and after death between medical and surgical staff members, nurses, and parents (table).

Conclusion.—Because medical technology can now keep many neonates with increasingly complex congenital anomalies alive, the need to withhold or withdraw life support has increased. Rapid confirmation of serious chromosomal anomalies allows the parents to know that the infant has a hopeless outlook and should not be subjected to invasive procedures. In other cases, the futility of treatment is only apparent after some procedures have been performed. The diagnosis must be reviewed and a consensus reached between parents and physicians. Including all members of the treatment team helps in dealing with grief and preventing burnout. Discussions about decision making must be part of the continuing education of physicians and nurses who treat seriously ill newborns.

▶ This thoughtful article emphasized 2 major points: (1) that end-of-life issues, such as withdrawal and withholding of life support, need to be carefully managed with a team approach, and (2) that medical-ethical committees may be a "valuable resource" for educating health-care professionals, but the ultimate decisions regarding infant care are the responsibility of the parent and physicians.—D.M. Rothenberg, M.D.

Biases in How Physicians Choose to Withdraw Life Support
Christakis NA, Asch DA (Univ of Pennsylvania, Philadelphia)
Lancet 342:642–646, 1993   101-94-27–3

Introduction.—The decision to withdraw life support is best made by patients themselves, but the manner in which this decision should be accomplished is usually entrusted to the physician. There is very limited data on the factors that influence physicians' decisions on which forms of life support to withdraw.

Methods.—A survey was specially designed to solicit physicians' preferences for the withdrawal of 8 life-sustaining medical therapies in critically ill patients in whom the decision to withdraw had already been made. In addition, the physicians' responses to 7 clinical vignettes were assessed. The survey was mailed to 862 American internists, with a response rate of 56%.

Findings.—Physicians had preferences on what form of life support to withdraw from critically ill patients. The most likely to be withdrawn was blood products, followed by hemodialysis, intravenous vasopressors, total parenteral nutrition, antibiotics, mechanical ventilation, tube feedings, and intravenously administered fluids. Physicians were more likely to withdraw therapy supporting organs that failed from natural causes rather than iatrogenic reasons, recently instituted rather than long-standing interventions, therapy that resulted in immediate death rather than delayed death, and therapy that resulted in delayed death when the diagnosis was uncertain.

Implications.—Physicians do have preferences regarding what forms of life support to withdraw from critically ill patients in whom the decision to withdraw therapy has already been made. Furthermore, these preferences are influenced by iatrogenic complications, duration of therapy with each form of life support, expected timing of death, and diagnostic uncertainty. These biases may have clinical, social, and ethical consequences that are not relevant to the patients' goals and may even represent impediments to rational and compassionate decision making in critical care.

▶ This small and predominantly in-house survey confirms what I have continually witnessed: that those with limited experience in direct patient care in the intensive care unit are less prepared to make complex medical and ethical decisions.—D.M. Rothenberg, M.D.

Subject Index

A

Abdomen
    compression, interposed, with
        cardiopulmonary resuscitation,
        outcome during asystole and
        electromechanical dissociation,
        94: 188
    interventions, screening laboratory tests
        before, 93: 66
    lower, surgery, pain after
        continuous epidural methadone for,
            93: 386
        pre-emptive lumbar epidural block
            for, 94: 461
    surgery
        bupivacaine 0.1% not improving
            epidural fentanyl after, 93: 388
        effects on liver blood flow, 93: 50
        oxygen desaturation risk during sleep,
            93: 265
        pain relief for infant undergoing,
            morphine vs. bupivacaine, 94: 465
Abortion
    prostaglandin-induced, metoclopramide
        enhancing analgesia for, 94: 106
Abuse
    cocaine, nonmedical, detracting from
        availability in hospital, 93: 7
    sexual and physical, and chronic pelvic
        pain, 94: 443
Acetaminophen
    perioperative effects in children
        undergoing myringotomy, 93: 231
Acetazolamide
    in acute mountain sickness, and gas
        exchange, 93: 304
Acetylcholine
    receptors, tolerance and upregulation
        after d-tubocurarine, 93: 39
Acid
    aspiration of gastric contents at
        emergency cesarean section, IV
        ranitidine reducing risk of, 94: 304
    gastroesophageal reflux, and ranitidine,
        94: 107
Acid-base
    management with carbon dioxide in
        phosphate concentration in
        hypothermic cardiopulmonary
        bypass, 94: 224
    status of newborn after spinal and
        extradural anesthesia for cesarean
        section, 93: 198
    variables, maternal and fetal, with
        propofol and thiopental (in
        pregnant ewe), 94: 286
Acidity

gastric, preoperative anxiety influencing,
    93: 69
Acidosis
    lactic
        bicarbonate effects on hemodynamics
            and tissue oxygenation in, 93: 329
        hypoxic, Carbicarb, sodium
            bicarbonate and sodium chloride in
            (in dog), 94: 341
    metabolic, contractile dysfunction
        during, and energy metabolism
        impairment, 93: 300
Acquired immunodeficiency syndrome (*see*
    AIDS)
Acupuncture
    discriminative sensation and, 93: 238
    like transcutaneous electrical nerve
        stimulation, 94: 401
    somatosensory evoked potentials by,
        and tactile skin stimulation, 93: 238
Adductor
    muscle
        of larynx and adductor pollicis
            rocuronium at, 93: 46
        pollicis, as monitor of atracurium
            block of laryngeal muscles, 94: 144
        pollicis, function and aging, 93: 253
Adenoidectomy
    bupivacaine after, in children, 94: 459
Adenosine
    low-dose, in myocardial performance
        after coronary artery bypass,
        94: 203
    for vasodilation after coronary artery
        bypass, 94: 206
Adenylate kinase
    CSF levels after heart surgery and CNS
        damage, 93: 137
Adjuvants
    pharmacology of, 94: 65
Adrenal
    cortex adaptation after etomidate, in
        newborn, 94: 90
    medulla transplant
        for painful peripheral neuropathy (in
            rat), 94: 434
        tissue, for chronic pain (in rat),
            93: 442
Aeromedical
    airway management, neuromuscular
        blockade in, 93: 327
Age
    in mechanical ventilation in ICU
        outcome, 93: 303
    in sevoflurane and isoflurane awakening
        concentrations, 94: 95
Aged, 93: 253
    carotid endarterectomy results, 93: 165

H

Author Index

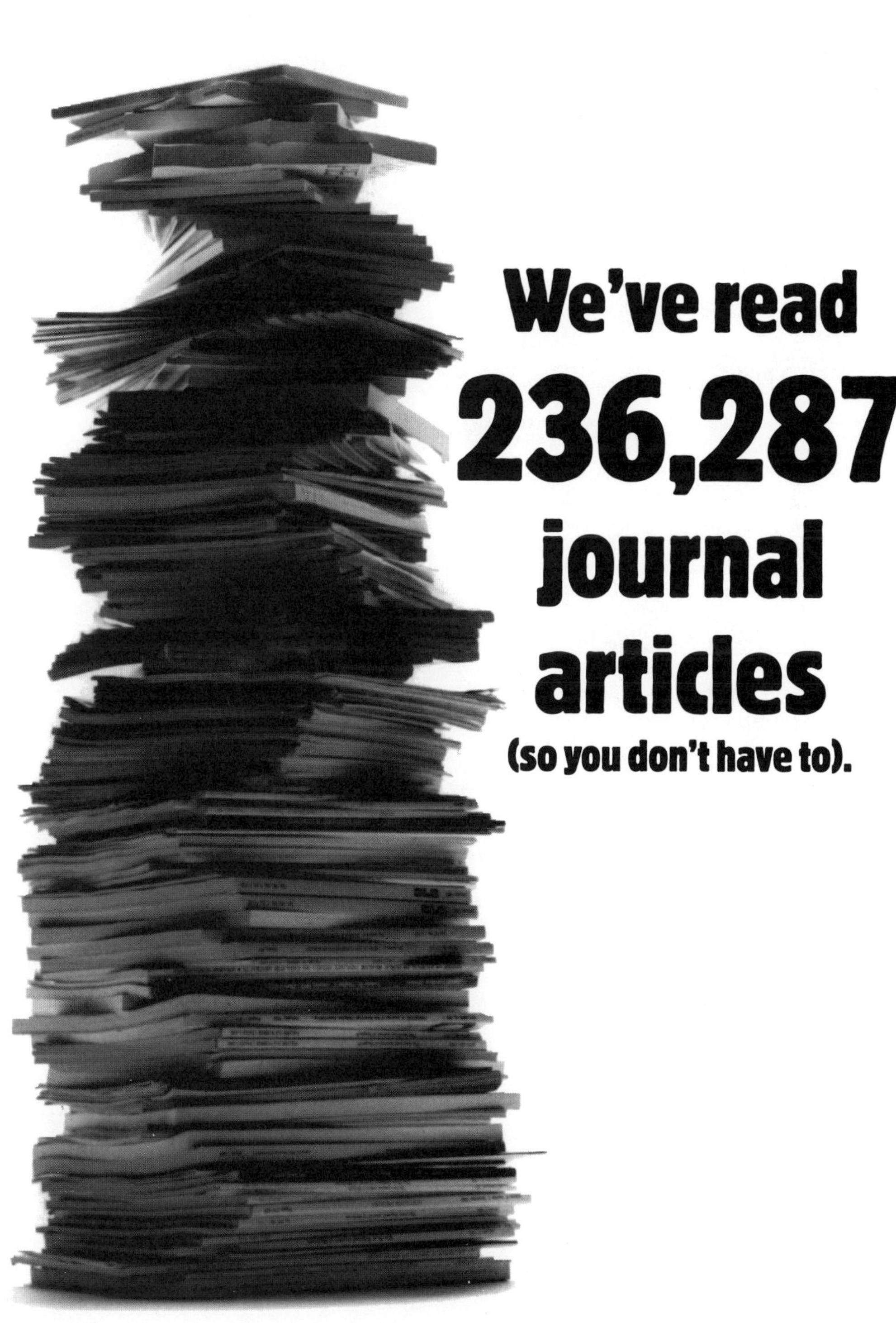

We've read
236,287
journal
articles
(so you don't have to).

The Year Books—
The best from 236,287 journal articles.

At Mosby, we subscribe to more than 950 medical and allied health journals from every corner of the globe. We read them all, tirelessly scanning for anything that relates to your field.

We send everything we find related to a given specialty to the distinguished editors of the **Year Book** in that area, and they pick out *the best*, the articles they feel *every practitioner in that specialty should be aware of.*

For the **1994 Year Books** we surveyed a total of 236,287 articles and found hundreds of articles related to your field. Our expert editors reviewed these and chose the developments you don't want to miss.

The best articles—condensed, organized, and with personal commentary.

Not only do you get the past year's most important articles in your field, you get them in a format that makes them easy to use.

Every article that the editors pick is condensed into a concise, outlined abstract, a summary of the article's most important points highlighted with bold paragraph headings. So you can quickly scan for exactly what you need.

In addition to identifying the year's best articles, the editors write concise commentaries following each article, telling whether or not the study in question is a reliable one, whether a new technique is effective, or whether a particular trend you've head about merits your immediate attention.

No other abstracting service offers this expert advice to help you decide how the year's advances will affect the way you practice.

With a special added benefit for Year Book subscribers.

In 1994, your **Year Book** subscription includes a new added benefit. Access to **MOSBY Document Express**, a rapid-response information retrieval service that puts copies of original source documents in your hands, in a little as a few hours.

With **MOSBY Document Express**, you have convenient, *around-the-clock-access to literally every article* upon which **Year Book** summaries are based. What's more, you can also order journal articles cited in references—or for that matter, virtually any medical or scientific article that can be located. Plus, at your direction, we will deliver the article(s) by FAX, overnight delivery service, or regular mail.

This new added benefit is just one of the enhanced services that makes your **Year Book** subscription an even better value—it's your key to the full breadth of health sciences information. For more details, see **MOSBY Document Express** instructions at the beginning of this book.